Surgery in and around the Brain Stem and the Third Ventricle

Anatomy · Pathology · Neurophysiology
Diagnosis · Treatment

Edited by M. Samii

With 370 Figures

Springer-Verlag Berlin Heidelberg New York
London Paris Tokyo

Dr. med. M. Samii
Professor and Chairman
Neurosurgical Clinic
City of Hanover
Nordstadt Hospital
Haltenhoffstraße 41
3000 Hannover 1, FRG

ISBN-13:978-3-642-71242-5 e-ISBN-13:978-3-642-71240-1
DOI: 10.1007/978-3-642-71240-1

Library of Congress Cataloging in Publication Data. Surgery in and around the brain stem and the third ventricle. Includes bibliographies and index. 1. Brain stem–Surgery. 2. Cerebral ventricles–Surgery. 3. Brain stem–Tumors–Surgery. 4. Cerebral ventricles–Tumors–Surgery. I. Samii, Madjid. [DNLM: 1. Brain Neoplasms–surgery. 2. Brain Stem–surgery. 3. Cerebral Ventricles–surgery. WL 310 S961] RD594.S9 1986 617′.481 86-15583 ISBN-13:978-3-642-71242-5 (U.S.)

Softcover reprint of the hardcover 1st edition 1986

2122/3130-543210

Foreword

It is, of course, a real challenge to summon together an International Symposium in and around the Brain Stem and Third Ventricle. Up to this moment the various experiences and papers on this subject were distributed throughout the world literature, making it very difficult for someone interested in the matter to have access to the actual state of knowledge. Therefore I believe such a meeting was long overdue and is a considerable attempt to open closed doors for present and future ambitious neurosurgical activities.

After succeeding in previous symposiums of similar interest in Hannover, it was obvious that Prof. Madjid Samii and his coworkers took the initiative of organizing such a meeting, bringing together – in the pure sense of the word – Neurosurgeons with Anatomists, Neurologists, Neurophysiologists, Neuroradiologists, ENT-, Maxillofacial-, Stereotactic-, and Radiosurgeons as well as other colleagues. One contribution after the other followed, from the basic sciences up to the operative management considering very new and actual concepts. Through the application of new microsurgical techniques and the incorporation of new understanding for the many problems afflicting the midline of the CNS, and based on a growing closer cooperation between the various disciplines, a wide field has opened up which concerns us all.

There were a number of facets covered by the Symposium: the recognition of the importance of microanatomy, arterial supply and venous drainage, contributions to understanding normal and abnormal functions, new techniques, useful in preserving anatomical and functional integrity, and an outline of new routes and new standards of quality for surgical management.

To pick up some facts of common interest it has been shown by anatomists that the brain stem is surrounded by arterial vessels like a circle, fed by larger vessels from the base, from Willis' circle. The veins do not follow the arteries and vice versa, not running hand in hand. The arteries provide landmarks outside the brain and the veins provide clear anatomical landmarks within the ventricles. These are important aspects for approaching the brain stem and ventricles for the neurosurgeon.

The studies on Evoked Potentials of the brain stem are indeed preliminary, but very interesting and encouraging for follow up of function. It is the desire of all to find out which signal would indicate reversible defects and which one permanent defects.

Concerning the neuroradiological achievements no method can fully replace the other. Each method has its own indication, and the neurosurgeon has to decide in every case what he needs to know. In general one can say that the Magnetic Resonance Imaging (MRI) information is superior in soft tissue lesions (intramedullary gliomas, hydromyelia etc.) to CAT-scan neuroimages. However, in osseous lesions of the skull base the high resolution cranial CT shows its superiority in comparison to the MRI information. But also the native X-ray examination retains its lasting value today.

With regard to the angiographic examinations it is to stress that the study of the venous system is as important as the examination of the arterial system in lesions of the brain stem and the third ventricle, particularly in connection with AVMs as well as space-occupying lesions. We learned that the neuroradiologist is a useful partner for the neurosurgeon and other colleagues. Especially with the selective and supraselective embolization technique he can help us treat AVMs as well as highly vascularized tumors at the skull base (meningiomas, chemodectomas, etc.).

The surgical management of AVMs of the brain stem presents specific difficulties. The size of the AVM is just one factor, location is another. There are great difficulties in approaching deep-seated angiomas, but if one maintains oneself in the sulci and anatomically bounded structures using stereoscopic magnification, then one does not need more space and minimizes additional damage. This concept should be followed in the future. Furthermore, we heard that indications for Prof. Jannetta's vascular decompression operations have enlarged and proved their effectiveness. They will have their place in the future. On the other hand, a new discussion about the bypass-revascularisation procedures for vertebro-basilar ischemia in respect to the Toronto Bypass Study has originated. Bypass operations seem, under certain circumstances, not to be as effective as one assumed them to be. In any case this chapter has not yet been closed to controversy.

New concepts on strategies for approaching clival and petroclival tumors as well as for the total removal of large chemodectomas of the jugular foramen were contributed by the Mainz group of neurosurgeons and otorhinolaryngologists. By subtotal removal of the pyramid with isolation and displacement of the facial nerve, they facilitated and widened the approach to these deep-seated tumors diminishing brain retraction with a subsequent decrease of the operative risk. From a surgical standpoint one can presumably underline once more, what the signer is expressing since years: the shortest and safest route to the lesion is usually the best one.

In general and above all this, the Symposium showed that processes in certain deep-seated regions, such as the pineal area, skull base and other deep regions, can be tackled by various surgical approaches as well as by other therapeutical modalities. This is demonstrated by contributions made by stereotaxy, radiosurgery, interstitial radiotherapy and chemotherapy which all have their particular indications.

This marvellous Symposium was an extraordinary event for all participants. It offered an intensive coverage by a distinguished faculty who has contributed to our understanding of new information in a very interesting but not easy to handle field of surgery in and around the brain stem and the third ventricle. Such a survey has not been available till now. However, with modesty and humility, it must be said that only the tip of the iceberg has been discovered and a long road is yet before us. This Symposium will have served its purpose if we follow the marked way.

Once more, we must thank the initiator, Prof. Madjid Samii, for his idea and for the excellent organization of this meeting.

Also our gratitude to the authors for their contributions and Springer-Verlag for their cooperation and efforts enabling this volume to reach you all modern day pioneers!

Mainz KURT SCHÜRMANN

Preface

After the pioneer work by such neurosurgeons as Foerster, Krause, Horsley, Cushing, Dandy, Olivecrona, Tönnis, Krayenbühl, and others, the surgery on cerebrum and cerebellum experimented a transformation, establishing neurosurgical techniques as standard surgical procedures as well as obtaining favorable results.

Whilst this was so, before the era of microsurgical operations, the surgery in and around the brain stem and third ventricle remained plagued with a high percentage of mortality and morbidity and therefore the indication for surgical treatment of pathological entities of this area was cautiously made and remained very limited.

With the introduction of the surgical microscope in the late 1960's the key was found for the beginning of a new era for surgical activities, at first around but now even in deep-seated brain structures.

My personal experience in this field started in 1967, supported by my honored teacher, Prof. K. Schürmann, in the Neurosurgical Department of the University of Mainz. With the growing knowledge of the microanatomy of structures surrounding the brain stem, some of us could extend the limited indications step by step and deeper each time during the past eighteen years. This progressive unmasking was stimulated by the major breakthroughs in diagnostic measures: CT scans, super selective angiography, and MRI. The new possibilities for neurophysiological recordings provide us with valuable information of the changes in brain stem parameters which appear often before manifestations capture the clinical eye. Continuous monitoring of brain stem evoked potentials has achieved a definite place in modern neurosurgery in this area.

On these different fronts and thanks to engaged neuroscientists, advances were made in the separate fields. It was a dream come true to have had the possibility of bringing together for discussion the leading specialists throughout the world at the International Symposium on Surgery in and around the Brain Stem and the Third Ventricle at Hannover, in February, 1985, to deal with the subject at hand and to share or exchange knowledge for the present and future.

All this was compiled as manuscript, and after hard efforts together with joy is presented to the public and interested circle of scientists, eager for the information gathered in what was a marathon and historical week of Symposium.

Full of gratitude to the man who has encouraged my work, allowing me to carry on in this field, seeing the course of things to come, I dedicated the first day of the Symposium to Prof. K. Schürmann to honor his 65th birthday.

To the colleagues and friends, who through their knowledge made it all possible, my everlasting acknowledgements for the great service rendered to our patients and to coming generations of colleagues, for we can now say that the surgery in and around the brain stem and the third ventricle, with good results, is a new chapter in our exciting field.

Last but not least, I would like to thank Mr. W. Bergstedt of Springer-Verlag and his team for their efforts in organizing the publication of this book, as well as Dr. F. Weber for his work on the subject index.

Special thanks must be given to Mrs. R. Nitsche and Dr. H. Khalil for their revision of the papers as far as translation and context. They were irreplaceable and a great help to me in every stage of the preparation of the manuscript for this book.

Hannover MADJID SAMII

Contents

Neuroradiology

Surgical Management of Specific Lesions: Vascular Lesions, Trauma

Surgical Management of Lesions in Specific Locations: Pineal Region, Anterior Third Ventricle

Posterior Fossa: IV Ventricle, Clivus, Foramen Magnum

Stereotactic Intervention, Radiotherapy, Chemotherapy

List of Contributors

Afshar, F.: Department of Neurosurgery, The London Hospital Medical College, University of London, Whitechapel, London E1 1BB, England

Appuzo, M. L. J.: Department of Neurological Surgery, University of Southern California, School of Medicine, 1200 N. State Street, Suite 5046, Los Angeles, CA, USA

Arita, N.: Department of Neurosurgery, Osaka University Medical School, 1-1-50Fukushima, Fukushima-ku, Osaka, Japan 553

Artero, J. C.: Department of Neurological Surgery, Henry Ford Hospital, 2799 West Grand Boulevard, Detroit, MI 48202, USA

Artigas, J.: Institute of Neuropathology, Free University Berlin, Hindenburgdamm 30, 1000 Berlin 45, FRG

Aruffo, C.: Institute of Neuropathology, Free University Berlin, Hindenburgdamm 30, 1000 Berlin 45, FRG

Ascher, P. W.: Universitätsklinik für Neurochirurgie Graz, Landeskrankenhaus, 8036 Graz, Austria

Ausman, J. I.: Department of Neurological Surgery, Henry Ford Hospital, 2799 West Grand Boulevard, Detroit, MI 48202, USA

Baethmann, A.: Institute for Surgical Research, Ludwig-Maximilians-University, Klinikum Großhadern, 8000 München 70, FRG

Balasubramaniam, V.: Madras Medical College, Madras-600 003, India

Basauri, L.: Neurosurgical Institute, Clinica Las Condes, Lo Fontecilla 441, Las Condes, Santiago, Chile

Basevska, R.: Clinic for Surgical Diseases, Department of Neurosurgery, Medical Faculty, University of "Cyril and Methody", Ivan Cankar 28 Vlae, 91000 Skopje, Yugoslavia

Basso, A.: Chief Department of Neurosurgery, Hospital Santa Lucia, Ayacucho 1342, Buenos Aires 1111, Argentina

Beil, C.: Max-Planck-Institut für neurologische Forschung, Ostmerheimer Str. 200, 5000 Köln 91, FRG

Berman, S. K.: Department of Neurological Surgery, Henry Ford Hospital, 2799 West Grand Boulevard, Detroit, MI 48202, USA

Bhagwati, S. N.: Medical Research Centre, Bombay Hospital, 19 Marine Lines, Bombay 400 020, India

Birk, P.: Neurological Department of the Technical University Munich, Möhlstraße 28, 8000 Munich, FRG

Bitoh, S.: Department of Neurosurgery, Osaka Kosei Nenkin Hospital, Osaka, Japan 553

Bock, W. J.: Neurochirurgische Universitätsklinik der Universität Düsseldorf, Moorenstraße 5, 4000 Düsseldorf, FRG

Boulos, R.: Departments of Neurosurgery and Neuroradiology, Henry Ford Hospital, 2799 West Grand Boulevard, Detroit, MI 48202, USA

Brock, M.: Institute of Neuropathology, Free University Berlin, Hindenburgdamm 30, 1000 Berlin 45, FRG

Bronec, P.: Department of Surgery, Division of Neurosurgery, Duke University Medical Center, Durham, North Carolina, USA

Brown, W. J.: Division of Neurological Surgery, UCLA School of Medicine, 760 Westwood Plaza, Los Angeles, CA 90024, USA
Buchfelder, M.: Neurochirurg. Klinik der Universität Erlangen, Schwabachanlage 6, 8520 Erlangen, FRG
Caputi, A.: Chief Endocrinological Unit, Hospital Alvarez, Buenos Aires, Argentina
Cedzich, C.: Neurochirurg. Klinik der Universität Erlangen, Schwabachanlage 6, 8520 Erlangen, FRG
Cervós-Navarro, J.: Institute of Neuropathology, Free University Berlin, Hindenburgdamm 30, 1000 Berlin 45, FRG
Chervin, A.: Chief Endocrinological Unit, Hospital Alvarez, Buenos Aires, Argentina
Chiu, M.: Service de Radiologie, Hôpital Bicêtre, Université XI-Orsay, 78, rue du Général Leclerc, 94270 Kremlin Bicêtre, France
Chodakiewitz, J.: Department of Surgery, Division of Neurosurgery, Duke University Medical Center, Durham, North Carolina, USA
Deck, J.: Department of Pathology, Toronto General Hospital and University of Toronto, Toronto, Canada
De Los Reyes, R. A.: Departments of Neurosurgery and Neuroradiology, Henry Ford Hospital, 2799 West Grand Boulevard, Detroit, MI 48202, USA
Diaz, F. G.: Departments of Neurosurgery and Neuroradiology, Henry Ford Hospital, 2799 West Grand Boulevard, Detroit, MI 48202, USA
Dujovny, M.: Departments of Neurosurgery and Neuroradiology, Henry Ford Hospital, 2799 West Grand Boulevard, Detroit, MI 48202, USA
Dzonov, I.: Clinic for Surgical Diseases, Department of Neurosurgery, Medical Faculty, University of "Cyril and Methody", Ivan Cankar 28 Vlae, Skopje, Yugoslavia
Ebeling, U.: Department of Neurosurgery, University Bern, Inselspital, Bern, Switzerland
Fahlbusch, R.: Neurochirurg. Klinik der Universität Erlangen, Schwabachanlage 6, 8520 Erlangen, FRG
Fasano, V. A.: Institute of Neurosurgery, University of Turin, Via Cherasco 15, 10126 Turin, Italy
Frowein, R. A.: Neurochirurg. Universitätsklinik Köln, Joseph-Stelzmann-Str. 9, 5000 Köln 41, FRG
Fuse, T.: Department of Neurosurgery, Tokyo Jikei University, School of Medicine, 3 25 8, Nishi Shimbashi, Minato ku, Tokyo, Japan
Gádor, I.: National Institute of Neurosurgery, Amerikai út 57, 1145 Budapest, Hungary
Geiger, T.: Division of Neurological Surgery, UCLA School of Medicine, 760 Westwood Plaza, Los Angeles, CA 90024, USA
Grote, E.: Neurochirurg. Universitätsklinik, Calwerstraße 7, 7400 Tübingen, FRG
Gürtner, P.: Neurosurgical Clinic City of Hanover, Nordstadt Hospital, Haltenhoffstraße 41, 3000 Hannover 1, FRG
Guitelman, A.: Chief Endocrinological Unit, Hospital Alvarez, Buenos Aires, Argentina
Hadley M. N.: Division of Neurological Surgery, Barrow Neurological Institute, 350 West Thomas Road, Phoenix, Arizona 85013, USA
Haferkamp, G.: Neurologische Klinik der Henriettenstiftung, Schwemannstraße 19, 3000 Hannover 71, FRG
Hakuba, A.: Department of Neurosurgery, Osaka City University Medical School, 1-5-7, Asahi-machi Abeno-ku, Osaka, Japan
Hamer, J.: Neurochirurg. Abteilung des Chirurgischen Zentrums der Universität Heidelberg, Im Neuenheimer Feld 110, 6900 Heidelberg 1, FRG
Hartmann, A.: Neurological Hospital of the University of Bonn, Sigmund-Freud-Straße 25, 5300 Bonn 1, FRG
Hasegawa, H.: Department of Neurosurgery, Osaka Kosei Nenkin Hospital, Osaka, Japan 553

Hayakawa, T.: Department of Neurosurgery, Osaka University Medical School, 1-1-50 Fukushima, Fukushima-ku, Osaka, Japan 553
Heiss, W.-D.: Max-Planck-Institut für neurologische Forschung, Ostmerheimer Straße 200, 5000 Köln 91, FRG
Helms, J.: ENT Department, University Hospital Mainz, Langenbeckstraße 1, 6500 Mainz, FRG
Heppner, F.: Universitätsklinik für Neurochirurgie Graz, Landes-Krankenhaus, Auenbruggerplatz, 8036 Graz, Austria
Herholz, K.: Max-Planck-Institut für neurologische Forschung, Ostmerheimer Straße 200, 5000 Köln 91, FRG
Herrmann, H.-D.: Neurosurgical Department, University Hospital Hamburg (UKE), Martinistraße 52, 2000 Hamburg 20, FRG
Hochstetter, H.: Neurochirurg. Klinik der Universität Erlangen, Schwabachanlage 6, 8520 Erlangen, FRG
Holl, K.: Neurosurgical Clinic City of Hanover, Nordstadt Hospital Haltenhoffstraße 41, 3000 Hannover 1, FRG
Holly, E.: Department of Radiation Oncology, UCLA School of Medicine, 760 Westwood Plaza, Los Angeles, CA 90024, USA
Huber, P.: Department of Neuroradiology, University Bern, Inselspital, Bern, Switzerland
Ikeda, T.: Department of Neurosurgery, Osaka University Medical School, 1-1-50 Fukushima, Fukushima-ku, Osaka, Japan 553
Jelicic, I.: Central Institute for Tumors and Allied Diseases, Ilica 197, 41000 Zagreb, Yugoslavia
Kamiyama, H.: Department of Neurosurgery, Hokkaido University of Medicine, Sapporo, Japan
Kamm, C.: Neurosurgical Department, University Hospital Hamburg (UKE), Martinistraße 52, 2000 Hamburg 20, FRG
Kano, M.: Department of Neurosurgery, Osaka Rosai Hospital, Osaka, Japan 553
Katakura, R.: Division of Neurosurgery, Institute of Brain Diseases, Tohoku University School of Medicine, Seiryo-Cho 1-1, Sendai, Japan 980
Kayama, T.: Division of Neurosurgery, Institute of Brain Diseases, Tohoku University School of Medicine, 1-1, Seiryo-cho, Sendai, Japan 980
Khonsary, A.: Division of Neurological Surgery, UCLA School of Medicine, 760 Westwood Plaza, Los Angeles, CA 90024, USA
Klein, H. J.: Department of Neurosurgery, University of Ulm, District Hospital Günzburg, FRG
Klug, N.: Department of Neurosurgery, University of Giessen, Klinikstr. 29, 6300 Giessen, FRG
Knipprath, R.: Neurochirurgische Universitätsklinik Köln, Joseph-Stelzmann-Straße 9, 5000 Köln, FRG
Kohmura, E.: Neurosurgical Clinic City of Hanover, Nordstadt Hospital, Haltenhoffstraße 41, 3000 Hannover 1, FRG
Krämer, M.: Neurochirurgische Universitätsklinik Düsseldorf, Moorenstraße 5, 4000 Düsseldorf 1, FRG
Krauseneck, P.: Neurologische Universitätsklinik, Josef-Schneider-Straße 11, 8700 Würzburg, FRG
Kreutel, H.: Chief Endocrinological Unit, Hospital Alvarez, Buenos Aires, Argentina
Laitinen, L. V.: Department of Neurosurgery, University Hospital, Umea, Sweden
Lang, J.: Anatomical Institute of the University of Würzburg, Koellikerstraße 6, 8700 Würzburg, FRG
Lasjaunias, P.: Service de Radiologie, Hôpital Bicêtre, Université XI-Orsay, 78, rue du Général Leclerc, 94270 Kremlin Bicêtre, France
Lavyne, M. H.: Division of Neurosurgery, The New York Hospital, 525 East 68th Street, New York, N.Y. 10021, USA

Lerch, K.-D.: Neurosurgical Clinic City of Hanover, Nordstadt Hospital, Haltenhoffstraße 41, 3000 Hannover 1, FRG
Lopes, H.: Department of Surgery, Division of Neurosurgery, Duke University Medical Center, Durham, North Carolina, USA
Lopez Ibor, L.: Service de Radiologie, Hôpital Bicêtre, Université XI-Orsay, 78, rue du Général Leclerc, 94270 Kremlin Bicêtre, France
Lorenz, R.: Department of General Neurosurgery, Center of Neurology and Neurosurgery, Clinics of the Johann Wolfgang Goethe-University Frankfurt/ Main, Schleusenweg 2–10, 6000 Frankfurt 71, FRG
Lorenz, R.: Neurological Clinic City of Hanover, Nordstadt Hospital, Haltenhoffstraße 41, 3000 Hannover 1, FRG
Ludwig, B.: Department of Neuroradiology, University Hospital Mainz, Langenbeckstraße 1, 6500 Mainz, FRG
Lumenta, C. B.: Neurochirurgische Universitätsklinik der Universität Düsseldorf, Moorenstraße 5, 4000 Düsseldorf 1
Lupret, V.: Central Institute for Tumors and Allied Diseases, Ilica 197, 41000 Zagreb, Yugoslavia
Lye, R. H.: University Department of Neurosurgery, Manchester Royal Infirmary, Oxford Road, Manchester M13 9PL, England
Macpherson, P.: Department of Neuroradiology, Institute of Neurological Sciences, Southern General Hospital, Glasgow G51, England
Maeda, Y.: Department of Neurosurgery, Osaka Rosai Hospital, Osaka, Japan 553
Malik, G. M.: Department of Neurosurgery, Henry Ford Hospital, 2799 West Grand Boulevard, Detroit, MI 48202, USA
Manelfe, C.: Service de Radiologie, Hôpital Bicêtre, Université XI-Orsay, 78, rue du Général Leclerc, 94270 Kremlin Bicêtre, France
Mehta, B.: Departments of Neurosurgery and Neuroradiology, Henry Ford Hospital, 2799 West Grand Boulevard, Detroit, MI 48202, USA
Meinig, G.: Department of Neurosurgery, University Hospital Mainz, Langenbeckstraße 1, 6500 Mainz, FRG
Mircevski, M.: Clinic for Surgical Diseases, Department of Neurosurgery, Medical Faculty, University of "Cyril and Methody", Ivan Cankar 28 Vlae, 91000 Skopje, Yugoslavia
Mirchandani, H. G.: Department of Neurological Surgery, Henry Ford Hospital, 2799 West Grand Boulevard, Detroit, MI 48202, USA
Mogami, H.: Department of Neurosurgery, Osaka University Medical School, 1-1-50 Fukushima, Fukushima-ku, Osaka, Japan 553
Mokrusch, T.: Neurochirurg. Klinik der Universität Erlangen, Schwabachanlage 6, 8520 Erlangen, FRG
Mori, S.: Department of Neurosurgery, The Center for Adult Diseases, Osaka, Japan 553
Mundinger, F.: Neurochirurg. Universitätsklinik, Abt. Stereotaxie und Neuronuklearmedizin, Hugstetter Straße 55, 7800 Freiburg i. Br., FRG
Nadjmi, M.: Department of Neuroradiology of the University of Würzburg, Josef-Schneider- Straße 11, 8700 Würzburg, FRG
Nagamine, Y.: Division of Neurosurgery, Institute of Brain Diseases, Tohoku University School of Medicine, 1-1, Seiryo-cho, Sendai, Japan
Nakamura, N.: Department of Neurosurgery, Tokyo Jikei University, School of Medicine, 3-25-8, Nishi-Shimbashi, Minato-ku, Tokyo, Japan
Nashold, B. S.: Department of Surgery, Division of Neurosurgery, Duke University Medical Center, Durham, North Carolina, USA
Neidhardt, M. K.: 1. Kinderklinik des Krankenhauszweckverbands, Postfach 10 19 20, 8900 Augsburg, FRG
Nemati, N.: Neurosurgical Clinic City of Hanover, Nordstadt Hospital, Haltenhoffstraße 41, 3000 Hannover 1, FRG
Niizuma, H.: Division of Neurosurgery, Institute of Brain Diseases, Tohoku University School of Medicine, Seiryo-Cho 1-1, Sendai, Japan 980

Oberbauer, R. W.: Universitätsklinik für Neurochirurgie Graz, Landeskrankenhaus, 8036 Graz, Austria
Ohta, H.: Department of Surgical Neurology, Research Institute for Brain and Blood Vessels–Akita, 6–10, Senshu-kubota-machi, Akita 010, Japan
Oku, Y.: Department of Neurosurgery, Kansai Rosai Hospital, Osaka, Japan 553
Oppel, F.: Neurosurgical Department, Free University Berlin, Hindenburgdamm 30, 1000 Berlin 45, FRG
Otsuki, T.: Division of Neurosurgery, Institute of Brain Diseases, Tohoku University School of Medicine, Seiryo-Cho 1-1, Sendai, Japan 980
Pannek, H. W.: Neurosurgical Department, Free University Berlin, Hindenburgdamm 30, 1000 Berlin 45, FRG
Pásztor, E.: National Institute of Neurosurgery, Amerikai út 57, 1145 Budapest, Hungary
Patel, S.: Departments of Neurosurgery and Neuroradiology, Henry Ford Hospital, 2799 West Grand Boulevard, Detroit, MI 48202, USA
Patterson, R. H., Jr.: Division of Neurosurgery, The New York Hospital, 525 East 68th Street, New York, N.Y. 10021, USA
Pawlik, G.: Max-Planck-Institut für neurologische Forschung, Ostmerheimer Straße 200, 5000 Köln 91, FRG
Pearce, J.: Departments of Neurosurgery and Neuroradiology, Henry Ford Hospital, 2799 West Grand Boulevard, Detroit, MI 48202, USA
Pedroza, A.: Department of Neurological Surgery, Henry Ford Hospital, 2799 West Grand Boulevard, Detroit, MI 48202, USA
Pendl, G.: Department of Neurosurgery, University of Vienna Medical School, Währinger Gürtel 18–20, 1090 Vienna, Austria
Perneczky, A.: Neurosurgical Clinic, University of Vienna, Währinger Gürtel 18–20, 1090 Vienna, Austria
Piffkó, P.: National Institute of Neurosurgery, Amerikai út 57, 1145 Budapest, Hungary
Ponzio, R. M.: Institute of Neurosurgery, University of Turin, Via Cherasco 15, 10126 Turin, Italy
Popovski, A.: Clinic for Surgical Diseases, Department of Neurosurgery, Medical Faculty, University of "Cyril and Methody", Ivan Cankar 28 Vlae, 91000 Skopje, Yugoslavia
Potthoff, P. C.: Neurochirurgie, Knappschafts-Krankenhaus, „Bergmannsheil", Schernerweg 4, 4650 Gelsenkirchen-Buer, FRG
Ramamurthi, B.: Department of Neurosurgery, Voluntary Health Services Medical Centre, Madras 600 113, India
Ramina, R.: Neurosurgical Clinic City of Hanover, Nordstadt Hospital, Haltenhoffstraße 41, 3000 Hannover 1, FRG
Rand, R. W.: Division of Neurological Surgery, UCLA School of Medicine, 760 Westwood Plaza, Los Angeles, CA 90024, USA
Reulen, H. J.: Department of Neurosurgery, University Bern, Inselspital, Bern, Switzerland
Richard, K.-E.: Neurochirurgische Universitätsklinik Köln, Joseph-Stelzmann-Straße 9, 5000 Köln 41, FRG
Richter, H.-P.: Neurosurgical Clinic, City Hospital Fulda, Pacelliallee 4, 6400 Fulda, FRG
Rogers, J. S.: Department of Neurosurgery, Henry Ford Hospital, 2799 West Grand Boulevard, Detroit, MI 48202, USA
Ruškov, P.: Clinic for Surgical Disease, Department of Neurosurgery, Medical Faculty, University of "Cyril and Methody", Ivan Cankar 28 Vlae, 91000 Skopje, Yugoslavia
Samii, M.: Neurosurgical Clinic City of Hanover, Nordstadt Hospital, Haltenhoffstraße 41, 3000 Hannover 1, FRG
Sanker, P.: Neurochirurgische Universitätsklinik Köln, Joseph-Stelzmann-Straße 9, 5000 Köln 41, FRG

Sano, K.: Department of Neurosurgery, Teikyo University, 2-11-1 Kaga, Itabishi-ku, Tokyo 173, Japan
Schirmer, M.: Neurochirurgische Universitätsklinik, Moorenstraße 5, 4000 Düsseldorf 1, FRG
Schramm, J.: Neurochirurg. Klinik der Universität Erlangen, Schwabachanlage 6, 8520 Erlangen, FRG
Schrell, U.: Neurochirurg. Klinik der Universität Erlangen, Schwabachanlage 6, 8520 Erlangen, FRG
Schürmann, K.: Department of Neurosurgery, University Hospital Mainz, Langenbeckstraße 1, 6500 Mainz, FRG
Sekino, H.: Department of Neurosurgery, Tokyo Jikei University, School of Medicine, 3-25-8, Nishi-Shimbashi, Minato-ku, Tokyo, Japan
Shindo, K.: Department of Neurosurgery, Yuri General Hospital, Akita 010, Japan
Shrontz, C.: Departments of Neurosurgery and Neuroradiology, Henry Ford Hospital, 2799 West Grand Boulevard, Detroit, MI 48202, USA
Siegfried, J.: Neurosurgical Department, University of Zürich, Rämistrasse 100, 8091 Zürich, Switzerland
Sima, A. A. F.: Department of Pathology, University of Manitoba, Winnipeg, Canada
Sindou, M.: Department of Neurosurgery, Hôpital Neurologique, 59 Bd. Pinel, 69003 Lyon, France
Snow, H. D.: Department of Diagnostic Radiology, UCLA School of Medicine, 760 Westwood Plaza, Los Angeles, CA 90024, USA
Spetzler, R. F.: Division of Neurological Surgery, Barrow Neurological Institute, 350 West Thomas Road, Phoenix, Arizona 85013, USA
Sprick, C.: Neurochirurgische Universitätsklinik der Universität Düsseldorf, Moorenstraße 5, 4000 Düsseldorf, FRG
Struppler, A.: Neurological Department of the Technical University Munich, Möhlstraße 28, 8000 Munich, FRG
Suzuki, A.: Department of Surgical Neurology, Research Institute for Brain and Blood Vessels–Akita, 6–10, Senshu-kubota-machi, Akita 010, Japan
Suzuki, J.: Division of Neurosurgery, Institute of Brain Diseases, Tohoku University School of Medicine, 1-1, Seiryo-cho, Sendai, Japan
Szapiro, J.: Department of Neurosurgery, Hôpital Neurologique, 59, Bd. Pinel, 69003 Lyon, France
Szelies, B.: Max Planck Institut für neurologische Forschung, Ostmerheimer Straße 200, 5000 Köln 91, FRG
Taguchi, Y.: Department of Neurosurgery, Tokyo Jikei University School of Medicine, 3-25-8, Nishi-Shimbashi, Minato-ku, Tokyo, Japan
Takahashi, A.: Division of Neurosurgery, Institute of Brain Diseases, Tohoku University School of Medicine, 1-1, Seiryo-cho, Sendai, Japan
Tasker, R. R.: Division of Neurosurgery, Toronto General Hospital, University of Toronto, Room 7-221E Eaton Wing, 101 College Street, Toronto, M5G 1L7, Canada
Teasdale, E.: Department of Neuroradiology, Institute of Neurological Sciences, Southern General Hospital, Glasgow G51, England
Teasdale, G.: Department of Neurosurgery, Institute of Neurological Sciences, Southern General Hospital, Glasgow G51, England
Ter Brugge, K.: Service de Radiologie, Hôpital Bicêtre, Université XI-Orsay, 78, rue du Général Leclerc, 94270 Kremlin Bicêtre, France
Urciuoli, R.: Institute of Neurosurgery, University of Turin, Via Cherasco 15, 10126 Turin, Italy
Ushio, Y.: Department of Neurosurgery, Osaka University Medical School, 1-1-50 Fukushima, Fukushima-ku, Osaka, Japan 553
Vajda, J.: National Institute of Neurosurgery, Amerikai út 57, Budapest, Hungary
Van den Bergh, P.: Department of Neurology, Tufts New England Medical Center, Boston, MA 02111, USA

Van den Bergh, R.: Department of Neurology and Neurosurgery, Catholic University of Leuven, Academic Hospital St. Rafaël, Kapucijnenvoer 33, Leuven, Belgium
Van Loveren, H.: Neurosurgical Department, University of Zürich, Rämistrasse 100, 8091 Zürich, Switzerland
Vitale, M.: Chief Endocrinological Unit, Hospital Alvarez, Buenos Aires, Argentina
Voges, J.: Neurosurgical Department, Free University Berlin, Hindenburgdamm 30, 1000 Berlin 45, FRG
Wackenheim, A.: Service de Radiologie I, Pavillon Clovis Vincent, CHR de Strasbourg – B.P. No. 426, 67091 Strasbourg Cedex, France
Wagner, R.: Max-Planck-Institut für neurologische Forschung, Ostmerheimer Str. 200, 5000 Köln 91, FRG
Wappenschmidt, J.: Neurosurgical Hospital of the University of Bonn, Sigmund-Freud-Straße 25, 5300 Bonn 1, FRG
Watanabe, K.: Department of Neurosurgery, Southern Tohoku Research Institute for Neuroscience, Koriyama, Japan
Wienhard, K.: Max-Planck-Institut für neurologische Forschung, Ostmerheimer Straße 200, 5000 Köln 91, FRG
Wilson, G. H.: Division of Neurological Surgery, UCLA School of Medicine, 760 Westwood Plaza, Los Angeles, CA 90024, USA
Winter, J.: Department of Diagnostic Radiology, UCLA School of Medicine, 760 Westwood Plaza, Los Angeles, CA 90024, USA
Yampolsky, C.: Chief Endocrinological Unit, Hospital Alvarez, Buenos Aires, Argentina
Yasui, N.: Department of Surgical Neurology, Research Institute for Brain and Blood Vessels–Akita, 6–10, Senshu-kubota-machi, Akita 010, Japan
Yoshida, M.: Department of Neurosurgery, Kurume University, School of Medicine, Kurume, Japan
Yoshimoto, T.: Division of Neurosurgery, Institute of Brain Diseases, Tohoku University School of Medicine, 1-1, Seiryo-cho, Sendai, Japan 980
Zülch, K. J.: Max-Planck-Institut für neurologische Forschung, Ostmerheimer Straße 200, 5000 Köln 91, FRG

Problems of Surgery in and around the Brain Stem and the Third Ventricle. A General Perspective

M. Samii, Hannover/FRG

The process affecting the human brain stem and diencephalon has been the source of great challenge to all scientists engaged in their diagnosis and treatment. In recent times there has been intense activity to that effect, resulting in new technical discoveries. This naturally produces great hope for future possibilities.

The understanding of problems of surgery in this region starts with its complicated anatomic relationship. We are dealing with hundreds of nuclei and millions of connecting pathways. The knowledge of some of them is available and has been helpful, amongst other illnesses, in the treatment of painful conditions and abnormal movement disorders. However, much pertaining to functional neuroanatomy still remains enigmatic. With the existing knowledge serving as a base and with the support of newer technologic aids we have to build up storeys of their different function.

Technologic advances have made it recently possible to study metabolic disturbances and blood flow measurements in this area. We are aware of the anatomy, but are still speculating on the exact role of the brain stem perforating vessels. With PET and CBF measurements one hopes to get some more information. The study of neurotransmitter substances is another great field which holds promise towards diagnosis and treatment of disorders of the brain stem and the deep-seated nuclei.

A major breakthrough in diagnostic measurement of neurologic function is the development of brain stem evoked potential studies. They can signal disorders not only when symptoms are early but even before they have appeared; they have not only a preoperative diagnostic value but are useful in monitoring the operative procedure and postoperative follow-up.

With the advent of CT and MRI and superselective angiography neurodiagnosis has been revolutionized. The CT and MRI of today can pick up very small lesions, and equally important, demonstrate the pathologic disturbances of its surrounding area (Figs. 1, 2).

Superselective angiography with development of various balloon techniques and selective occlusions of certain vessels provide us with the opportunity of hemodynamic studies of individual vessels supplying different parts of the brain stem. Embolization procedure done by this method may preclude or even eliminate the need for surgery.

Based on an accurate preoperative assessment with modern diagnostic aids, the fundamentals of surgery of processes in the brain stem are the selection of the proper surgical approach to the disorder and the use of microsurgical technique.

As the brain stem is located in the center of the head a pathologic process can be reached from a variety of directions. The diversity of the choice of approaches, both

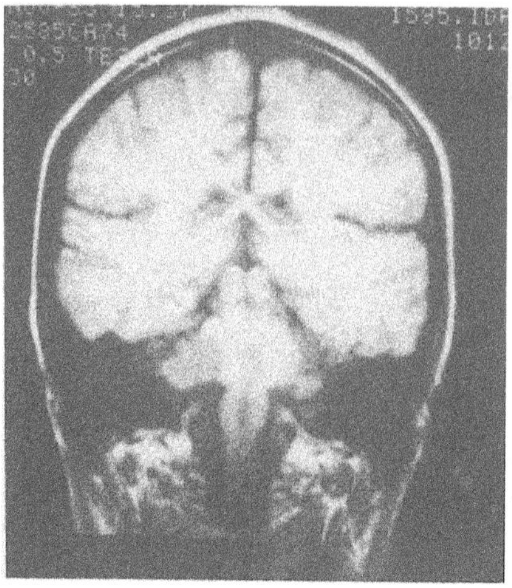

Fig. 1

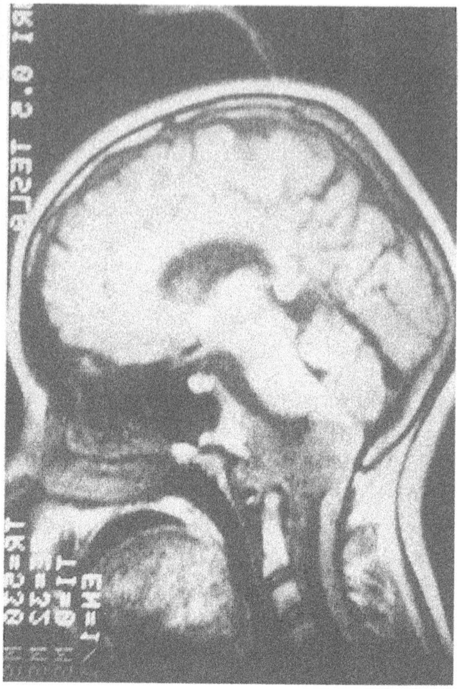

Fig. 2

Fig. 1. MRI (coronal section) showing a right acoustic neurinoma in the cerebellopontine angle indenting the pons

Fig. 2. MRI (sagittal section) demonstrating a large clivus chordoma compressing the medulla oblongata and extending downwards through the foramen magnum till the level of C_3

old and new, will be presented in this book, and are bound to raise controversies. However, the fundamental requirement of any approach is that it should reach the lesion with the least possible trauma and the best possible exposure.

For example, what approach would you take for the removal of a large craniopharyngioma (Figs. 3, 4) – transcranial or transsphenoidal? And if transcranial, subfrontal or subtemporal; transcortical or transcallosal? And what about the stereotactic procedure? Such questions are bound to come up during the planning of surgery.

For a second example see this pineal region tumor (Fig. 5). To operate, or not to operate – *that is the question!* If to operate, to biopsy it, or remove it totally – and again, how to approach it – supratentorially or infratentorially?

Another example is a large tentorial notch tumor (Fig. 6). Which approach should one take, and what will be the outcome?

The problem of intrinsic lesions is to know if the deficits are due to tumor compression or infiltration. The question again is whether to operate or not. Is stereotaxic surgery with interstitial radiotherapy safer and more effective than an open operation? The answers may be different and may be colored by personal bias. The papers presented in this book discuss the merits and demerits of various approaches and therapeutic modalities to the same problem.

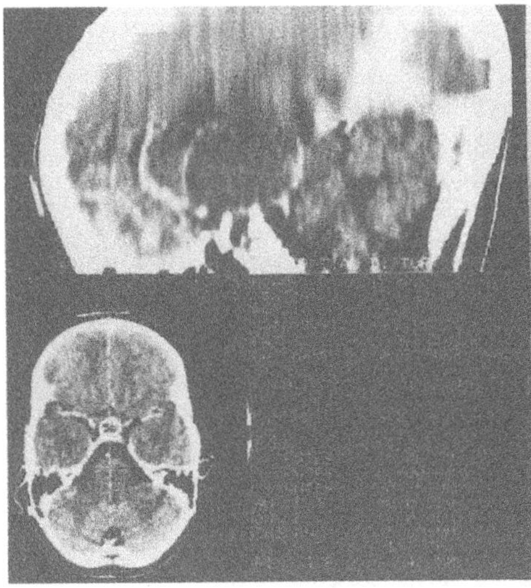

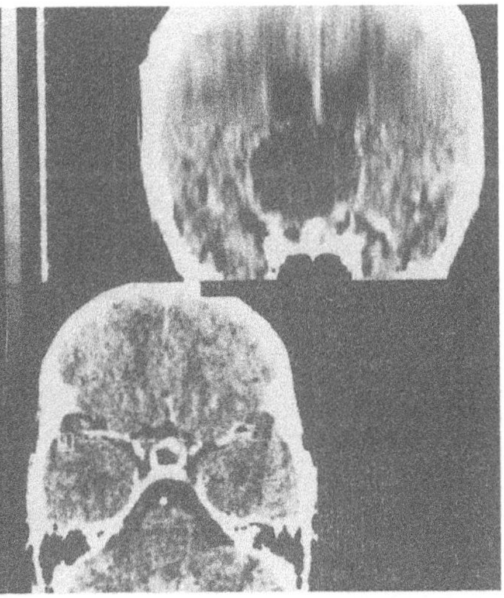

Fig. 3 **Fig. 4**

Fig. 3. CT scan with sagittal reconstruction showing a large craniopharyngioma. Note the posterior extension to the interpenduncular region

Fig. 4. CT scan with coronal reconstruction of the same case. Note the upward extension of the tumor indenting the third ventricle and reaching up to the lateral ventricles

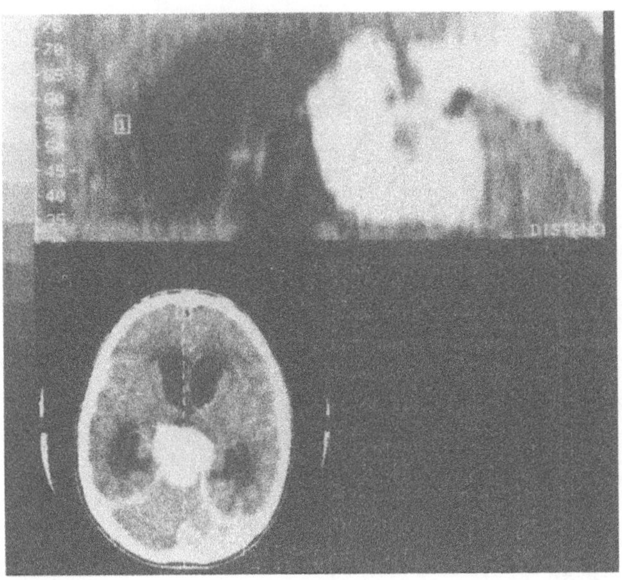

Fig. 5. CT scan with sagittal reconstruction showing a large pineal tumor with secondary (obstructive) hydrocephalus

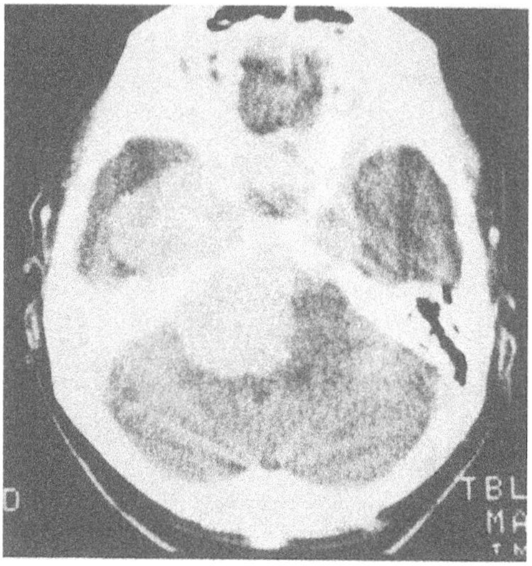

Fig. 6. CT scan showing a large tentorial notch tumor extending from the middle to the posterior fossa

With the introduction of operative microscope there was a tremendous improvement in results of vascular neurosurgery. However, the problem of AVMs in and around the brain stem and the basal ganglia continues to challenge the neurosurgeon. The first question is, are they treatable? The second question is, what options do we have in their successful management? There has been a surge of activity in

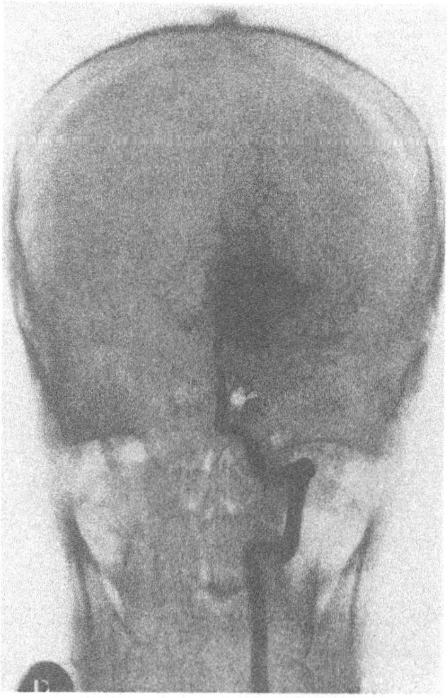

Fig. 7

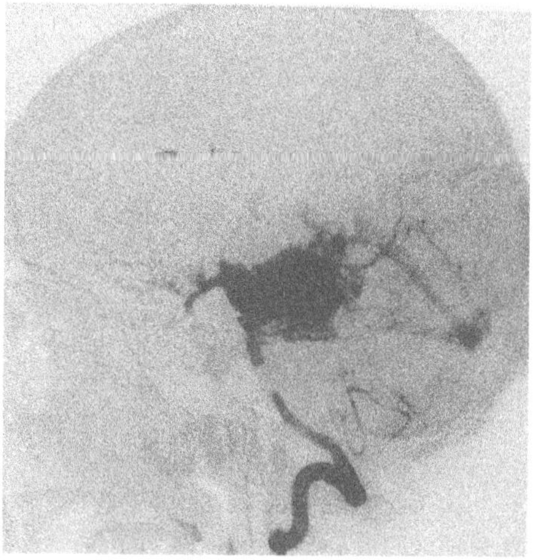

Fig. 8

Figs. 7, 8. Left vertebral angiography showing a large angioma in and around the brain stem

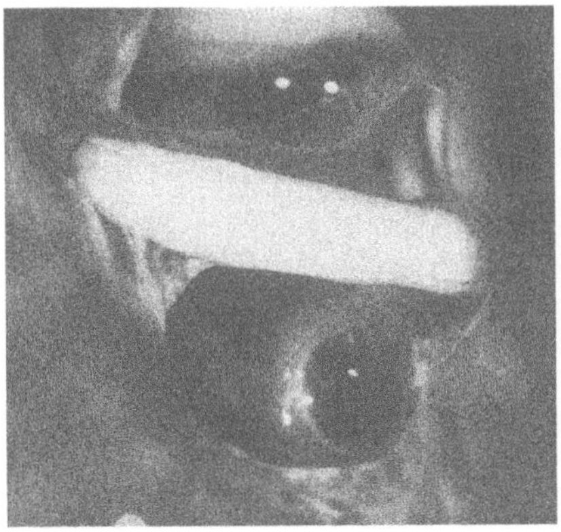

Fig. 9

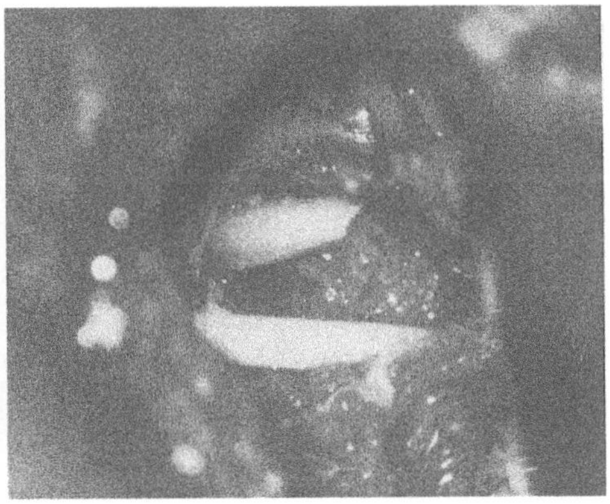

Fig. 10

Figs. 9, 10. A case of hemifacial spasm. Note in Fig. 9 the vascular loop compressing the 7th nerve from below at the brain stem. Fig. 10 shows decompression of the nerve using a muscle piece

the treatment of angiomas, aneurysms, and vascular fistulae by embolization techniques. Can they be successfully employed for brain stem angiomas? What is the role of radiotherapy? The third option is microsurgery. What should be the strategy? To get to the angioma or first to its feeders? The surgical exposure may vary considerably; the approach for the angioma and for the feeders may be one and the same, but can be quite different (Figs. 7, 8).

Surgery of neurovascular compression syndromes at the brain stem is now an established procedure at many centers. Nevertheless it still generates controversy and therefore forms a theme for discussion (Figs. 9, 10).

Revascularization of the brain stem using different bypass techniques has added a new dimension to the treatment of brain stem ischemia and we are eager to know about their efficacy.

With some examples I could only superficially touch the vast magnitude of the problems that we as neuroscientists encounter in and around the brain stem and the third ventricle.

In this book experienced and knowledgeable scientists share and discuss their views, trying to give us some answers to the different questions that face neurosurgeons when dealing with lesions in this very difficult and dangerous part of the brain.

Anatomy

Microanatomy of and around the Brain Stem and the Third Ventricle

J. Lang, Würzburg/FRG

Introduction

The brain stem consists (in the anatomical sense) of the myelencephalon (medulla oblongata), metencephalon (pons) and mesencephalon (midbrain). The third ventricle is bordered mainly from the diencephalon structures, hypothalamic and thalamic areas. Only the most anterior part of the hypothalamus and the lamina terminalis, according to their development, belong to the telencephalon. Of course it is impossible to demonstrate all important structures of these brain parts, their nerves and vessels in a short time. Therefore, I will begin with some remarks to the important anatomical structures, which are situated along the neurosurgical approaches.

Third Ventricle

The third ventricle and its surrounding structures can be reached (besides the transsphenoidal approach) by frontal, frontolateral, pterional, transcortical-transventricular, transcallosal and posterior supra- and infratentorial approaches. Another approach to the third ventricle is the transcortical-transventricular approach through the trigone of the lateral ventricle.

Frontal Approaches to the Third Ventricle (Fig. 1)

To avoid the danger of damaging the orbital surface of the frontal lobe, the approaches have to be performed as deep as possible at the bottom of the anterior cranial fossa. The bottom of the anterior fossa is situated deeper in medial parts (fovea endofrontalis medialis) and in lateral parts (fovea endofrontalis lateralis). Between both of these areas we described an eminentia endofrontalis (Lang et al. 1976). If the approach is chosen in the medial deep area, it should be remembered, that the frontal sinus has a height in the frontal squama of 24.3 (5–66) mm. Also the thickness of the frontal bone in this area is in men 4.1, in women 4.2 mm (mean values), Roche (1953). The frontal sinus was not included.

In the mediansagittal plane is situated: the falx cerebri and the crista galli (which is pneumatisized in about 10%). The length of the crista galli in our material is 21.5 (15–31) mm, its height 12.1 (7–18) mm.

In the superior sagittal sinus the first prefrontal vein drains from the facies superolateralis. The first prefrontal vein in anteroposterior level is between 0 and 10 mm from the frontal pole (but in different heights). The largest diameter of this vein measured in our material at the left side 1.59 (0.7–3.9) mm and at the right 1.51

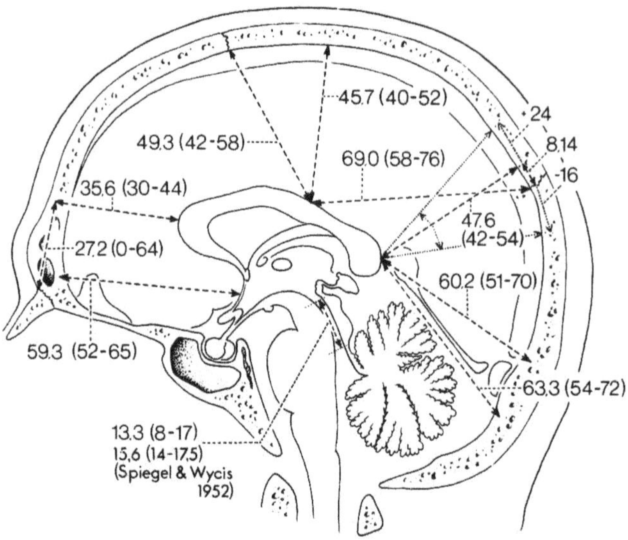

Fig. 1. Distances between the dura mater of calvaria and different areas and brain parts. From left to right distance between the frontal pole and lamina terminalis, between the genu corporis callosi and the squama frontalis (here are also given the shortest distances to the nasion), distance from the coronal suture to the corpus callosum, shortest distance of corpus callosum to the parietal bone, distance to the lambda, shortest distance of the splenium corporis callosi to the skull (situated 8.14, +24—26) mm frontal and occipital of the lambda, distances at supratentorial and infratentorial approaches to this area. Given are also our measurements about the length of the lamina tecti and results from Spiegel and Wycis about the length of the aqueduct. All measurements are given in mm

(0.8–3.0) mm. We found between one and six prefrontal veins on the facies superolateralis. From the medial surface of the forebrain in our material two prefrontal veins were counted on the left side in 60% and on the right side in 40%. The number varies between one (6% on the left and 14% on the right) and five. The sagittal distance of the lower and anterior one of these veins from the frontal pole (but upwards of this) is 2.9 (0–12) mm. The width of the most anterior vein (veins) is 1.06 (0.6–2.2) mm.

Between the frontal pole area and the lamina terminalis we found a length of 59.3 (52–65) mm in our material (Fig. 1). It should be mentioned that the bottom of the anterior fossa between the anterior rounded transition in the calvaria and the entrance in the optic canal measures 44.75 (36–54) mm. This value includes a 3.1 (1–8.5) mm long dural fold above the intracranial pore of the optic canal. The distance between the medial borders of the optic canals amounts to 14.0 (9–24) mm, the distance between the tuberculum sellae and the midpoint of the chiasma measures 5.5 (2–10) mm, and the medial length of the optic nerve 10.5 (7–15) mm (Fig. 2). Of course for the neurosurgeons it is important to know the length between the dural opening of the optic nerve to the lower border of the lamina terminalis: this distance varies in our material between 13 and 19 mm (mean value 15.1 mm). The distance to the lateral lower part of the lamina terminalis to the upper border of the optic canal measures 19.2 (16–25) mm. It is well known, that the anterior cere-

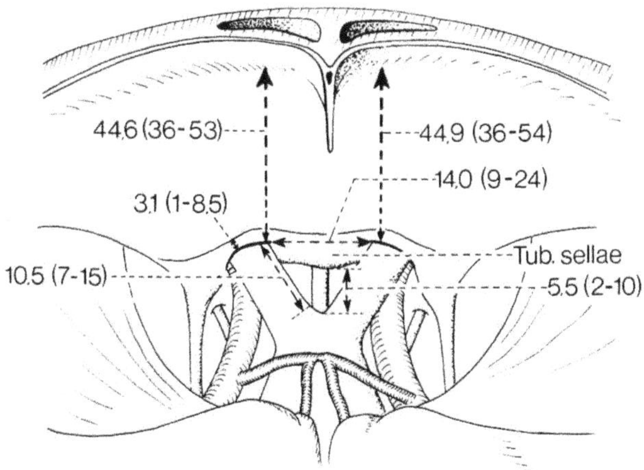

Fig. 2. Distances between the rounded transition of the anterior cranial fossa in the squamous part of the frontal bone to the dural membrane over the internal opening of the optic canal, the length of this membrane, the length of the medial border of the optic nerve and the distance between the tuberculum sellae and the chiasm. Given is also the distance between the two medial borders of the optic nerves. Measurements in mm (extremals)

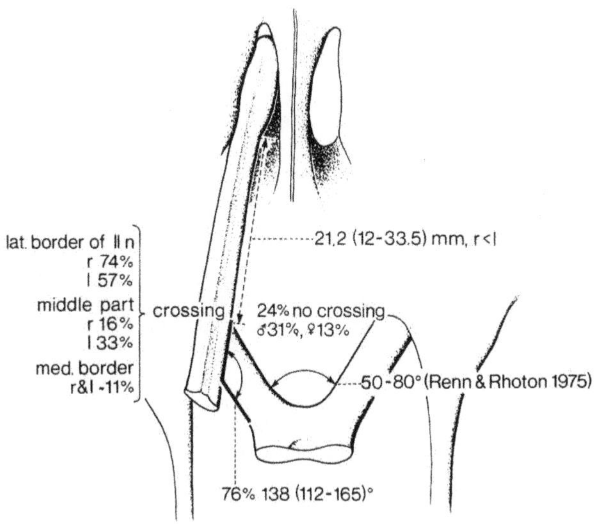

Fig. 3. Length of the olfactory tract and its crossing area with the optic nerve. No crossing olfactory tracts are found in our material in 24%. The angle between the optic nerves is measured by Renn and Rhoton (1975). Measurements in degrees and mm. The olfactory bulb has a length of 12.2 (7–24) mm in our material

bral artery curves (in different loops or nearly rectilineal) above the optic nerve or the optic chiasm to the midline.

The length of the olfactory bulb and olfactory tract and its crossing with the optic nerve are shown in Figs. 3 and 4. It should be noted, that in rare conditions small branches of the frontopolar branch or of the medial orbitofrontal branch supply the olfactory bulb and pierce the cribriform plate to the nasal cavity. Also some small veins of the anterior part of the forebrain rarely take this way.

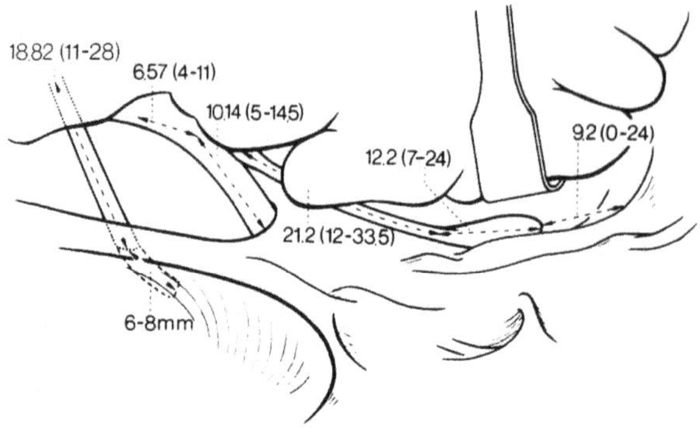

Fig. 4. Shown are our measurements about the distance of the anterior border of the olfactory bulb to the most anterior part of the anterior cranial fossa, the length of the bulb, the length of the olfactory tract, the lateral length of the optic nerve, the length of the chiasm and the length of the third cranial nerve in the hypophyseal area and inside its dural and arachnoideal sheaths in the sidewall of the cavernous sinus. Measurements in mm

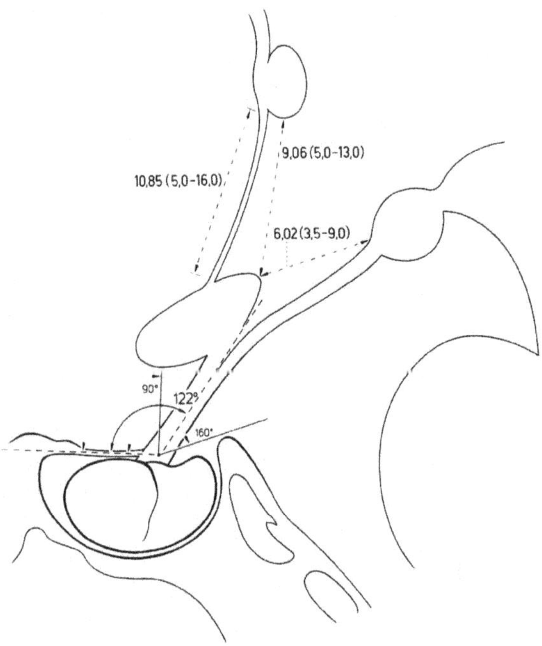

Fig. 5. Anterior and lower part of the third ventricle and the infundibulum. Given are the length of the lamina terminalis, the distance between the chiasm and the anterior commissure and the anterior border of the corpus mamillare and the angle between the hypophyseal stalk and the planum sphenoidale. Measurements in mm and degrees

About the intracisternal length of the nerves in the hypophyseal region and the infundibulum see Fig. 4. It should be noted, that the intracranial part of the optic nerve in our material (255 nerves) is 3.16 (1.5–5.0) mm in height and 5.03 (2.5–7.0) mm in width. The optic chiasma has a thickness (on median-sagittal section) of 3.41 (2.0–7.0) mm and an antero-posterior length of 6.57 (4.0–11.0) mm (Lang et al. 1983). The width of the optic chiasm is in our material 11.57 (8.5–15.0) mm. It should be noted, that the optic tract from the midpoint of the chiasm to the lateral geniculate body has a length of 40.37 (22.5–52.0) mm. Most values have been estimated between 42 and 47 mm.

The measured distance between the anterior communicating artery and the lamina terminalis was 4.9 (0–10) mm and above this level the distance between the posterior border of the A_2 segment and the lamina terminalis amounted to 6.2 (2–11) mm. The length of the lamina terminalis varies between 5.0 and 16 mm. On Fig. 5 are also given other measurements of structures of the third ventricle including the angle between the hypophyseal stalk and the planum sphenoidale (mean 122°). Very important are the small branches of the distal part of the A_1 segment and the anterior communicating artery to the anterior inferior diencephalon: Rami diencephalici inferiores anteriores. In our material we found in the mean 4.3 branches from the anterior communicating artery and 5.3 branches from the distal part of the A_1 segment. The recurrent artery of Heubner arises in about 60% from the A_2 segment and in 30% from the A_1 segment of the anterior cerebral artery. From the anterior communicating artery there also arises sometimes a thicker branch which reaches the rostrum and the genu of the corpus callosum (according to definition in about 12%). A few small branches of this segment also supply the upper surface of the chiasm and the intracranial (intracanalicular) part of the optic nerve. It should be mentioned, that the medial frontobasal branch arises 3.55 (0–15) mm distal from the anterior communicating artery and in 8.5% from the frontopolar ramus, which has its origin in about 60% 9.18 (2–25) mm distal of the anterior communicating artery. The frontobasal branch has a diameter of 0.64, the frontopolar branch is about 0.97 mm in diameter. The latter one arises in 30.4% from the frontal anteromedial branch. Both branches supply the different areas of the frontal pole and the medial and basal surface of the forebrain. It should be mentioned, that also the artery of Heubner has in most cases branches to the posteromedial part of the lower surface of the forebrain. If the branches of the forebrain are disturbed (if the pial anastomoses are not sufficient), disturbances of the frontal lobe are bound to follow. This refers also to cutting off medial and lateral prefrontal veins (Figs. 6a and 6b).

The anterior inferior diencephalic branches supply the anterior hypothalamic area with the nuclei preoptici medialis and lateralis, the septal nuclei, the anterior hypothalamic nucleus a.o. Vascular alterations with resulting destruction of these nuclear areas can lead to functional disturbances of the pituitary gland and thus influence the hormonal water and electrolyte balance as well as the centers for temperature sensation and regulation. It should be mentioned that the fibers of the paraventricular nuclei also pass to the spinal nuclei of the sympathetic nervous system. Therefore this nucleus participates in the regulation of vasodilatation and sweet glands. According to Yaşargil (1984) the occlusion of these arteries is partially responsible for mental changes and electrolyte disturbances.

The long central artery (anterior recurrent artery, Heubner's artery) was in our material duplicated in approximately 30%, a tribble artery exists in approx. 1%. In roughly ⅔ of cases the artery has branches which contribute to the supply of the olfactory bulb, olfactory tract and the orbital part of the frontal lobe. Sometimes the vessel is thick and supplies also brain parts, which belong in most cases to the middle cerebral artery (MCA). According to Yaşargil (1984) the recurrent artery runs anterior to the A_1 segment in 60% and posterior superior to it in 40%, back-

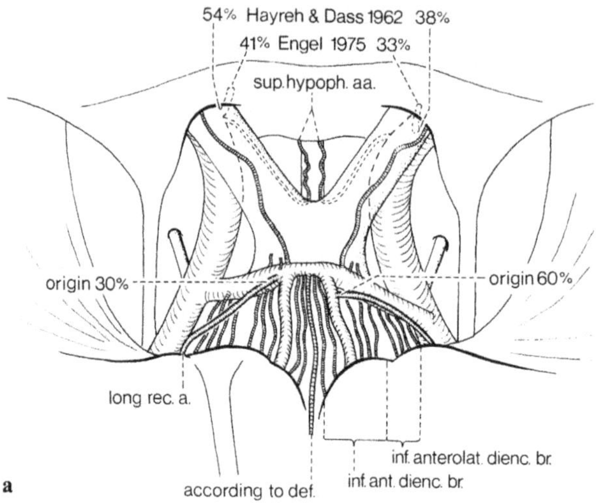

a

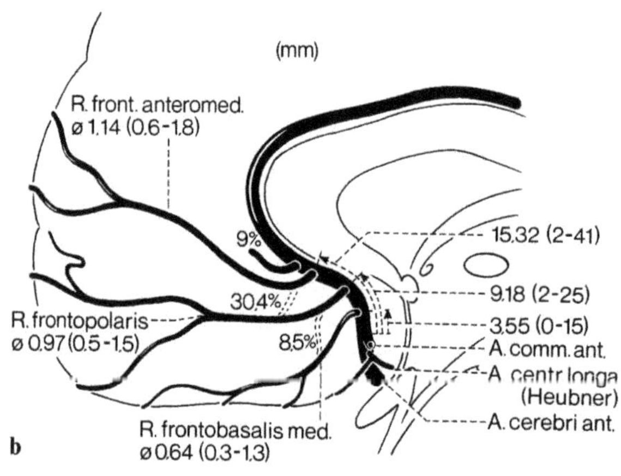

b

Fig. 6. a Most important brain vessels in the anterior hypophyseal region, given are also the most common origin zones (Hayreh and Dass 1962) and course of the ophthalmic artery in the optic canal (Engel 1975). **b** Origin zones of the most important arteries to the lower part of the frontal lobe and their diameters. Measurements in mm

wards to the medial part of the anterior perforate substance. Superficial twigs are found in this area. The main artery perforates the substance and supplies the anterior parts of the nucleus caudatus and the putamen, a part of globus pallidus and the anterior limb and middle part of the internal capsule. Occlusion of this vessel can result in aphasia, hemiparesis and paralysis of the face and tongue on the dominant hemisphere (Yaşargil 1984). From the MCA normally arises the lateral frontobasal branch for the lateral part of the orbital gyri of the forebrain. Therefore I think that thick vessels, which arise from the anterior cerebral artery, should not be termed as accessory middle cerebral arteries.

By frontal approach also the configuration of the arteries distal the anterior communicating artery is important. The median artery of corpus callosum arises from the anterior communicating artery and exists in 12% (3.6), Kleiss (1941/42), to 20%, McCormick (1969). The artery sometimes runs around the genu and divides above the trunk of the corpus callosum in 2 or more terminal branches. A middle anterior cerebral artery is an arterial trunk, which arises from the fusion area of both anterior cerebral arteries (behind the anterior communicating artery). This trunk has a variable length – Decker, 1960 – who had seen such vessels in 3%. For details see Lang (1981) and Yaşargil (1984).

Cingulomarginal Artery

If a larger twig of the pericallosal artery branches off and has twigs to at least two or more different areas of the brain, crosses the cingulate gyrus and runs into the cingulate sulcus for a short distance, we called this vessel cingulomarginal artery. Such vessels we found in about 60% (Lang and Häckel 1980). In 10% the main stem of the A_2 segment runs in the cingulate sulcus. In these cases a small pericallosal artery exists. In about 4% this vessel arises proximal to the anterior communicating artery and has 3 to 5 anastomoses with this vessel. In 29% this vessel branches off in the anterior quarter of the corpus callosum, in 26% a little bit more behind and in 35% over the middle part of the trunk of corpus callosum.

Frontolateral Approach

By the frontolateral approach also tumors (chiasma, hypothalamic a.o.) and aneurysms of the anterior communicating artery and A_1 segment can be reached. Dorsal located structures can be approached between the optic nerve and the internal carotid artery and also between the internal carotid artery and the 3rd nerve. The starting point of the approach is the frontozygomatic point, which is the narrowest zone of the superior temporal line. In German it is called the "Stirnenge". This zone is situated 17.8 (11–26) mm above the frontozygomatic suture. Inside the skull in this area is the lateral area of the bottom of the anterior cranial fossa: Fovea endofrontalis lateralis which deepens more posteriorly. The lower surface of the forebrain (Gyrus frontalis inferior) in this part is normally supplied by the lateral frontobasal branch of the middle cerebral artery.

In our anatomical specimens we found a thick arachnoid membrane between the so-called vallecula between the frontal and temporal lobe which sometimes has to be cut. Then the middle cerebral artery and its branches and also the middle superficial cerebral vein are visible. In our specimen the middle cerebral artery has a length of 16.2 (5–24) mm (Lang and Brunner 1978). Its external diameter is 2.7 (1.5–3.5) mm. In most cases we found a trifurcation, a quadrifurcation, bifurcation and quintafurcation of this vessel (Lang and Dehling 1980). Bifurcations we only found in 20% (according to our definition). From this vessel the central branches arise to the anterior perforate substance. Figure 7 shows that a medial group of branches exists in 71% and intermediate in 86% and a lateral one in 100%. Also the diameters (mean) are visible. Some authors gave different numbers of the central rami (perforators) of the middle cerebral artery. We discussed this problem and

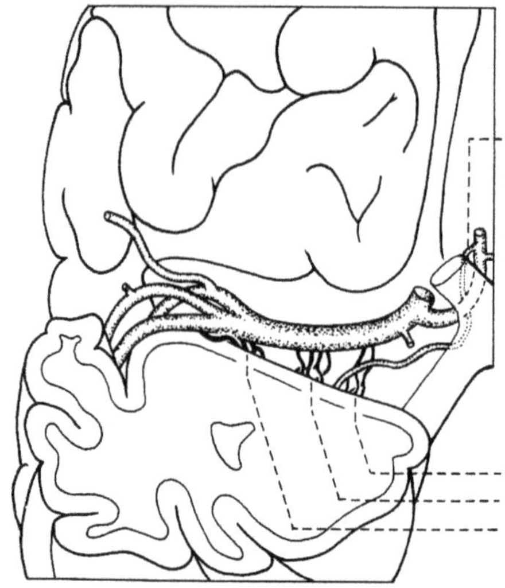

Fig. 7. Most important arteries to the anterior perforate substance (central rami of the middle cerebral artery and anterior recurrent artery), origin zones and diameters in mm

pointed out that these rami may extracerebrally bifurcate in smaller branches before they enter the brain substance (Lang and Brunner 1978). The fact that the rami centrales of the distal portion or the twigs of the middle cerebral artery are usually larger than the proximal arising branches was seen from other researches (f.e. Grand 1980).

Pterional Approach

The pterional area is defined in most cases as a H-shaped area between the frontal bone, parietal bone, temporal squama and ala major ossis sphenoidalis.

There are also some other combinations of this sutural zone (see Lang 1983). In the new-born the anterolateral fontanelle is situated in this area. One to one and a half cm behind the frontozygomatic suture an impression (fossa alaris) is situated in over 80%. Inside the skull in this area the crista alaris is build up, a prolongation of the lesser wing of the sphenoid bone. This crista alaris is a crest in most of its medial parts and flattens laterally and posteriorly. It divides the areas of the temporal lobe below and the frontal lobe above and is bordered by the arachnoid membrane of the lateral cerebral sulcus. In about 33% in our material we found a canal in this bone-part for the frontal ramus of the middle meningeal artery and its concomitant veins. In about 20% we found a vessel canal to the orbit in this area, especially a connection between the middle meningeal artery and the lacrimal artery. During the approach the anterior part of the temporal muscle has to be displaced posteriorly. In the upper part this displacement may be without disturbances to lower areas (fossa temporalis) medial of the zygomatic arch. The deep anterior temporal nerve and vessel branches reach the temporal muscle. These branches can be fixed below the skull in about 5%, in canals of a pterygospinose lamina. It should be noted that the temporal muscle area is drained by superficial and deep lymph vessels.

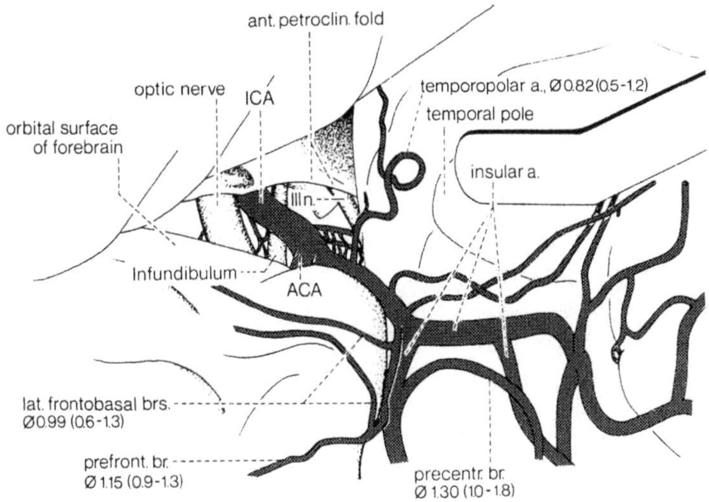

Fig. 8. Pterional approach, main arteries, diameters of some branches of the middle cerebral artery are given in mm

At the pterional approach (Fig. 8) to the third ventricle and adjacent structures the optic nerve area can be reached without division of the arachnoid membrane between the frontal and temporal lobe. Posterior areas are visible after cutting this membrane. In most cases anteriorly the superficial middle cerebral vein is situated, which drains into the sphenoparietal sinus or into the cavernous sinus sidewall. Sometimes this vein runs on the lower surface of the temporal lobe to the upper knee of the sigmoid sinus or into the superior petrosal sinus. In other preparations we saw a thick bridging vein, inwoven in the dura mater of the middle cranial fossa, which we called paracavernous sinus. Sometimes in this sinus the ophthalmic vein also runs. In rare conditions this paracavernous sinus was running through the roof of the middle ear cavity. By this approach it is possible to see the bifurcation area of the middle cerebral artery which is situated 20 mm medial the Sylvian part and the central rami of this vessel and its branches. After opening the lateral fissure the insula with the insular arteries are visible. In our material the distance between the pterional area (lateral endofrontal fovea) to the sideborder of the optic nerve on the optic canal is about 38.5 (33–43) mm (Lang 1984). Important is also the height of the temporal lobe in this area. We measured in the anterior part this height on the right side with 29.2 (20–36) mm, on the left 28.4 (15–35) mm in men and 28.4 (20–33) mm on the right and 30.0 (22–35) mm in women. The subarachnoid part of the internal carotid artery (ICA) has a length between 8.0 and 18.0 mm. Of course a greater length of this vessel normally allows an easier approach to the hypophyseal area and adjacent structures. The first branches of the internal carotid artery are the ophthalmic and the superior hypophyseal artery, which is doubled sometimes. Its origin is situated in the transition zone between the cavernous part and the subarachnoid part of the ICA. Distally from this area the internal carotid artery gives off some branches to the infundibulum and to the lower surface of the optic chiasm. The first larger branch is the posterior communicating artery. Its inferior dien-

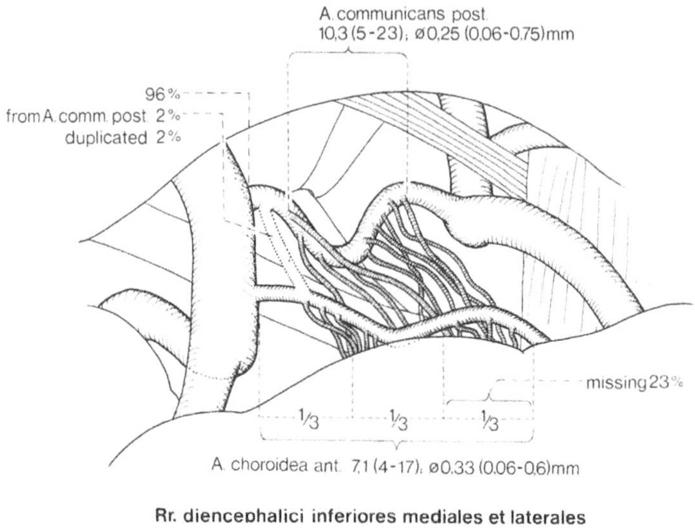

Fig. 9. Central branches of the posterior communicating artery and the anterior choroideal artery. The origin of the anterior choroideal artery in our material was found in 96% from the internal carotid artery and in 2% from the posterior communicating artery, in 2% this vessel was duplicated. Given are the numbers of the inferior diencephalic branches, its origin areas and diameters in mm

cephalic branches, 10.3 (5–23) in number, with a width of 0.25 (0.06–0.75) mm supply the inferior medial diencephalic area (Fig. 9). It should be noted, that we found the origin zone of the posterior communicating artery on the medial side of the internal carotid artery in 28.5%, on its lower surface in 58.6% and on its lower lateral surface in 11.5%.

The distance between the origin zone of the posterior communicating artery and the anterior choroideal artery measures in our material 3.47 (1.5–7.0) mm (Lang 1982). In 96% of our material this vessel is a branch of the internal carotid artery, in 2% we found this branch arising from the posterior communicating artery and a duplicated origin of this vessel was seen in 2%. To the lower surface of the diencephalon we found 7.1 (4–17) branches with a width of 0.33 (0.06–0.6) mm. These branches pierce the lower surface of the diencephalic area medial, through and lateral of the optic tract. For further details see Lang (1983).

The veins in the area of these arteries we studied in 1981 (Lang et al. 1981). We stated, that we found the course of the basal vein (and its efflux), which is given in textbooks, only in 41% (more frequently on the right than on the left). In 34% the basal vein is formed by the confluence of the peduncular vein and the inferior ventricular vein, while the vessels, which normally form the basal vein in the region of the rostral perforate substance, run directly to the cavernous sinus, to the sphenoparietal sinus or even into a paracavernous sinus. In 14% the vein arises in the neighborhood of the rostral perforate substance in the normal way, its main affluent being the deep middle cerebral vein. At the lateral border of the crus cerebri the vein curves sharply in a caudal direction and runs as a lateral peduncular vein to the petrosal vein or directly to the superior petrosal sinus. In 12% we found a draining

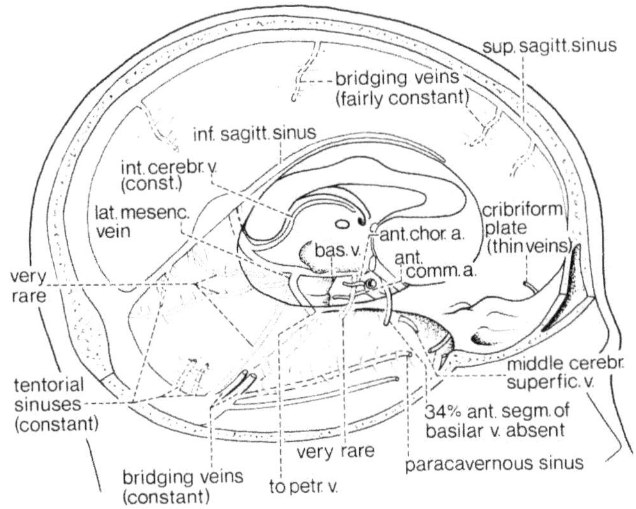

Fig. 10. Shown are constant and rare cerebral veins, which should be known by pterional and other approaches

from the deep (and superficial) middle cerebral veins, the anterior cerebral vein, the inferior thalamostriate veins, the vein of the olfactory gyrus and the orbital veins to the cavernous sinus or to the sphenoparietal sinus or paracavernous sinus. In this type the basal vein arises from the peduncular vein and the inferior ventricular vein and it discharges its blood (completely in about 50% and partially in the remainder) into the petrosal vein. In rare conditions we found a vein from the anterior tributaries to the side-wall of the cavernous sinus, the peduncular vein and its affluents to

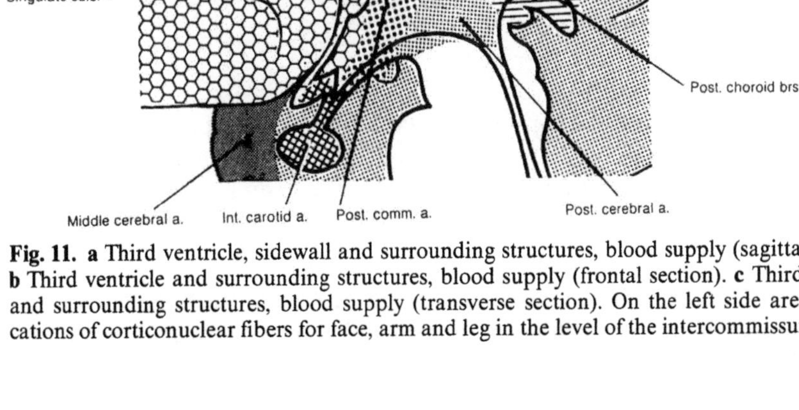

Fig. 11. a Third ventricle, sidewall and surrounding structures, blood supply (sagittal section). **b** Third ventricle and surrounding structures, blood supply (frontal section). **c** Third ventricle and surrounding structures, blood supply (transverse section). On the left side are given locations of corticonuclear fibers for face, arm and leg in the level of the intercommissural line

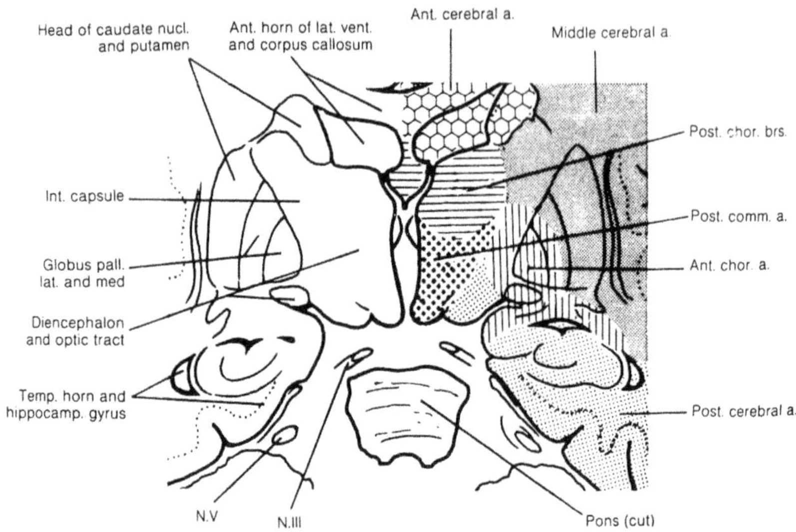

Fig. 11b

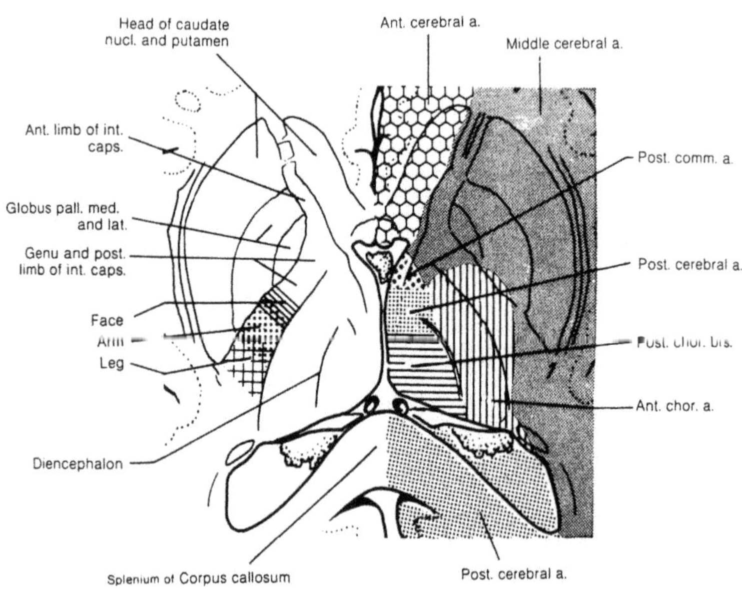

Fig. 11c

the superior petrosal sinus (see Fig. 10), or to the superior knee of the sigmoid sinus. The areas of arterial distribution in the walls of the 3rd ventricle and surrounding structures are given in Figs. 11a, b, c.

Transcortical – Transventricular Approach to the Third Ventricle

According to Koos et al. (1985) this approach can be used to reach the lateral ventricle in the area of the interventricular foramen and also the upper part of the third

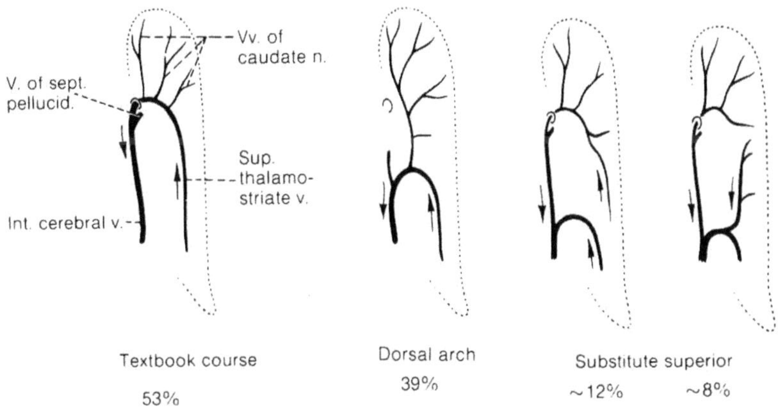

Fig. 12. Superior thalamostriate vein and veins of the caudate nucleus. Given are also some variations of the courses and bloodflow (Lang et al. 1981)

ventricle. The central sulcus of the brain is situated (according to Passet 1883 and others) on the left side 5.58 (3.5–7.4) cm behind the coronal suture in men and 5.29 (3.4–6.6) cm in women in the paramedian area. According to our resul'ts the superior frontal gyrus has a width of 21 mm and the prefrontal gyrus is about 23 mm broad (Lang and Belz 1981). Therefore, if the approach should go to the middle frontal gyrus. The posterior border of the incision in this gyrus has to be at least 21 mm paramedian and about 15 mm behind the coronal suture. According to Torkildsen (1933/34) and our observations the anterior horn of the lateral ventricle is situated about 40 mm below the cerebral surface projected (in the midline) and the distance to the interventricular foramen in this direction is 19.4 mm (mean value). Koos et al. (1985) mentioned that the anterior vein of the septum pellucidum and the choroid plexus of the lateral ventricle is a guide structure to find the interventricular foramen. In most cases the venous angle is situated at the level of the interventricular foramen. The superior thalamostriate vein as a rule curves around the anterior tubercle of the thalamus and then turns dorsally and medially. In most cases the superior choroid vein joins this venous curve, less commonly it runs dorsal to the curve into the internal cerebral vein or very uncommonly into the vein of the septum pellucidum. The confluence of the veins of the septum pellucidum and the superior thalamostriate vein in our material is situated on an average of 6.05 (0–27) mm dorsal to the posterior margin of the column of the fornix (in the region of the interventricular foramen). In about 87% the vein of the septum pellucidum passes lateral to the fornix to reach its termination, in 12.5% it transverses the fornix and in 0.8% it runs medial to it. An important fact at this approach to the third ventricle is the fornix. Its vessels and the structure itself should not be damaged. Therefore it is important to know that we found only in 53% the course of the superior thalamostriate vein and the vein of the septum pellucidum, as given in the text book. The so-called dorsal arch of the thalamostriate vein (and the venous angle) existed in 39% and a double arch (affluence in the area of the foramen interventriculare and a dorsal one) together in 8%. In these cases the superior thalamostriate vein has a blood flow dorsally (8%) or a double affluent medially (12%) (Fig. 12).

Transcallosal Approach to the Third Ventricle (see Fig. 1)

At the transcallosal approach in my opinion it is important to know the situation of the postcentral gyrus and the location of the posterior border of the paracentral lobule. In this area the representation zones of the foot, genitalia, micturition centers a.o. are situated. The central sulcus of the brain is located in the median plane between 3.4 and 7.4 cm behind the coronal suture and 4.0–10.0 cm anterior to the lambda. The postcentral gyrus in our material has a width of 12.3 mm (mean). The approach should be behind this area. In this way we found beside small vessels of the pericallosal or cingulomarginal artery anastomoses between dural and brain arteries and bridging veins to the superior sagittal sinus on the superolateral surface, to the falx cerebri and to the inferior sagittal sinus. The distance between the inner surface of the skull and the truncus corporis callosi measures in our material 45.7 (40–52) mm, Fig. 1. After dividing the corpus callosum, the corpus fornicis and the cisterna fissurae transversae the roof of the third ventricle is reached. In the cistern of the transverse fissure the internal cerebral veins and their affluence and the medial posterior choroid branches are situated. These branches supply a part of the fornix and the corpus callosum and also the upper parts of the thalamus. We found small end-twigs of these branches also to the upper surface of the caudate nucleus.

At subtemporal approach the mesencephalon and its surrounding structures are seen.

Mesencephalon

The mesencephalon is the smallest brain part and connects those parts of the brain in the hypophyseal region (diencephalon) with those of the posterior cranial fossa. Its weight is according to Jenkins and Truex (1963) 8.9 g. Its parts are the pedunculi cerebri with the pars ventralis and the pars dorsalis, the fossa interpeduncularis and the substantia perforata interpeduncularis. The basis pedunculi is the crus cerebri and the area above the mesencephalic aqueduct is called tectum mesencephali. On our material we measured the width of the mesencephalon, its caudal and cranial parts, the height and the length of the crus cerebri, the length and width of the trigonum lemnisci superius, the size of the cranial and caudal collicle and the length and width of the brachia colliculi cranialis et caudalis (see Figs. 13, 14). The colliculus cranialis on the right side is larger than its counter part and the caudal colliculus also has on its right side a greater width than on its left. Figure 15 shows the height of the lamina tecti, the length of the lamina tecti and the length and inferior height of the tegmentum mesencephali. Also measurements are given about the interpeduncular fossa (Lang and Deymann-Bühler 1984). The exit-zone of the third nerve in the interpeduncular fossa (and partly through the crus cerebri) is situated 4.15 (1.5–7.5) mm behind the anterior recess of the interpeduncular fossa and 4.77 (2.0–9.5) mm rostral to the posterior recess of the interpeduncular fossa (Lang et al. 1983). The length of the exit-zone of the third nerve we estimated with 3.26 (2.0–5.5) mm. Like other brain nerves the third nerve has also a central = glial segment, which has a length of 1.88 (1.0–4.0) mm (Lang 1982). Concerning the nuclei of the mesencephalon and the course of the most important fiber system see Figs. 16, 17. On the dorsal side and a little bit behind the caudal colliculus there is the exit-zone

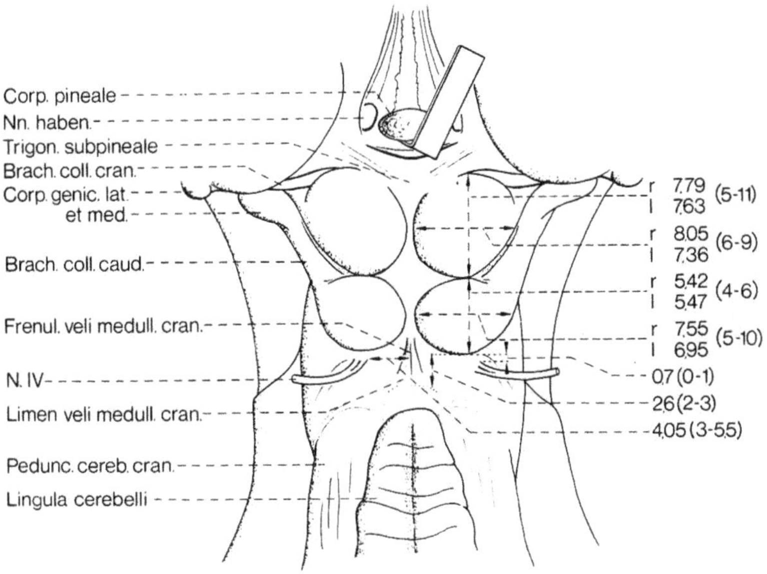

Fig. 13. Mesencephalon and surrounding structures, dorsal view. Measurements of the colliculi and the exit zone of the trochlear nerve in mm (Lang and Deymann-Bühler 1984)

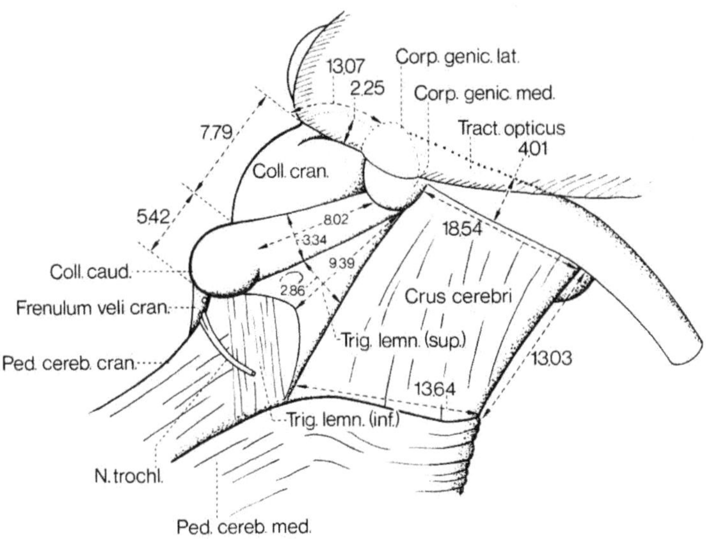

Fig. 14. Measurements of the mesencephalon from the lateral side in mm (main values)

of the trochlear nerve. In our material the exit-zone of this nerve is 0.7 (0–1) mm caudal to the lower border of the colliculus caudalis and 4.05 (3–5.5) mm lateral to the median plane. The intracerebral decussation of the nerve fibers is called limen veli medullaris cranialis, it has a thickness up to 1.5 mm. This limen is situated 2.6 (2–3) mm posterior and inferior to the caudal colliculus. Further caudally in our preparations the thin velum medullare craniale is located, which has a length of 2.6

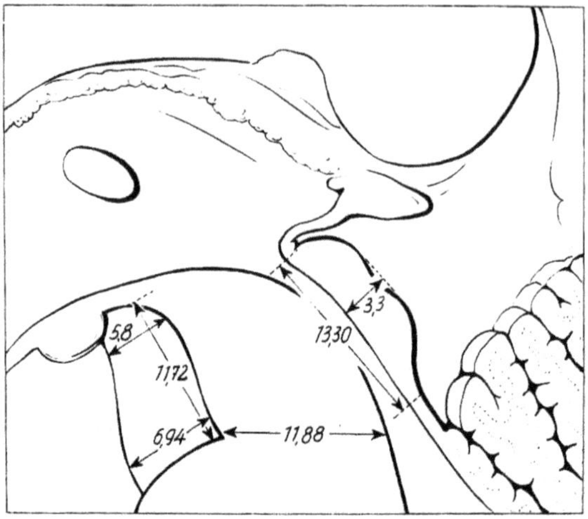

Fig. 15. Mesencephalon from medial on sagittal section, measurements of different parts (main values in mm)

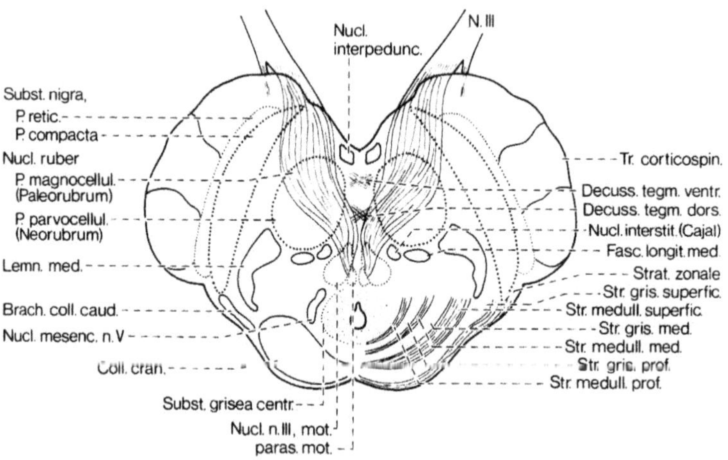

Fig. 16. Transverse section of mesencephalon in the level of the cranial colliculus, main important fiber systems and nuclei

(1–3.5) mm to the anterior border of the lingula cerebelli. In most cases the fourth nerve leaves the cerebrum with more than one fiber bundle and runs in the cistern of the lamina tecti and in the cisterna in the peripeduncular part of the cisterna ambiens. The dorsal part of the nerve in most cases is situated between the rami vermis superioris of the superior cerebellar artery, the caudal intercisternal inwoven in the arachnoid membrane. Its intracisternal length between the exit-zone and the entrance in the dura mater has a length of 32.65 (20–42) mm. Then the nerve pierces the dura mater together with prolongation of the arachnoid membrane in the sidewall of the cavernous sinus. In about 80% the entry-zone in the dura mater is situated between the anterior and posterior petroclinoideal folds, in 20% on the lower

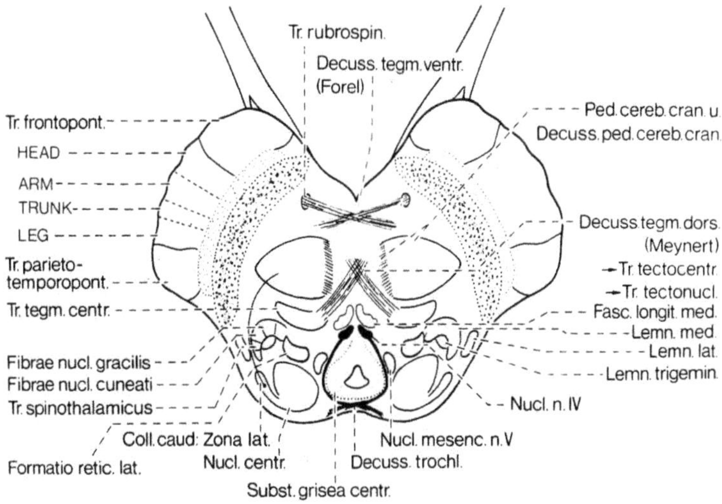

Fig. 17. Transverse section through the mesencephalon in the level of the colliculus caudalis, fiber systems and nuclei

surface of the tentorium cerebelli (see Fig. 18, in which is also given the length of the 3rd nerve).

Mesencephalon, Arteries

The mesencephalon is surrounded by many arteries all giving twigs into this brain part. From the basal side the rami mesencephalici inferiores (et diencephalici inferiores posteriores) pierce the interpeduncular substance and supply middle parts of the mesencephalon up to the aqueductus mesencephali. These interpeduncular arteries have their origin from the posterior cerebral artery, the superior cerebellar artery and the basilar artery. The pedunculus cerebri, crural and tegmental parts, are also supplied from twigs of the anterior choroideal artery, the posterior cerebral artery, the superior cerebellar artery, the artery of the tectal part of the mesencephalon and the posterior choroideal branches (Figs. 19, 20). It should be noted, that the mesencephalon in the level of the inferior colliculi is also supplied by an artery, which we call pontomesencephalic artery (PMA) and is found in 60%. These vessels also supply parts of the cerebellum and its cranial peduncle. In 13.7% of our material the tectal artery and in 4% the posterior medial choroid branches pierce the third nerve (Lang and Fischer, in press). Once we found one medial branch of the superior cerebellar artery (which had an isolated origin from the basilar artery) perforating the third nerve. A doubled origin of the superior cerebellar artery was found in 14–22%, an origin of this vessel from the posterior cerebral artery in 4%.

It should be noted, that the oculomotor nerve exit-zone is not only situated in the medial crural sulcus of the mesencephalon. Some fibers after piercing the red nucleus and the substantia nigra, forming a series of curves with a lateral convexity, pierce the lower and medial parts of the crus cerebri.

The central part of the 3rd nerve has a length of 1.88 (1.0–4.0) mm (Lang 1982). This part is covered by a prolongation of the pia mater, in which in most cases pig-

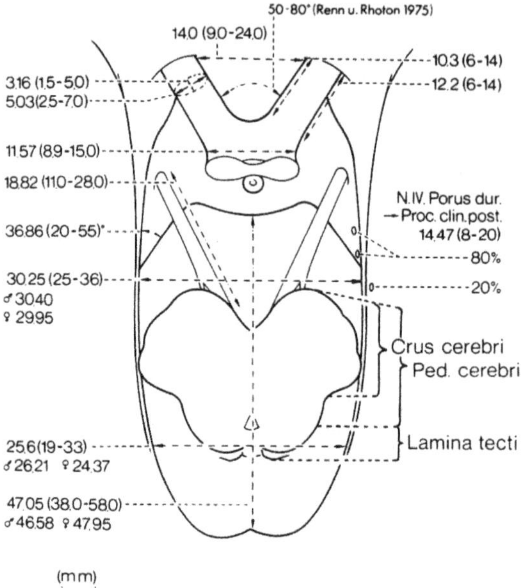

Fig. 18. Mesencephalon and incisura tentorii, measurements in mm and degrees (extremals). Given are also measurements of the optic nerve and chiasm, the angle between the two optic nerves was estimated by Renn and Rhoton (1975). Included are the entrance zones of the trochlear nerve

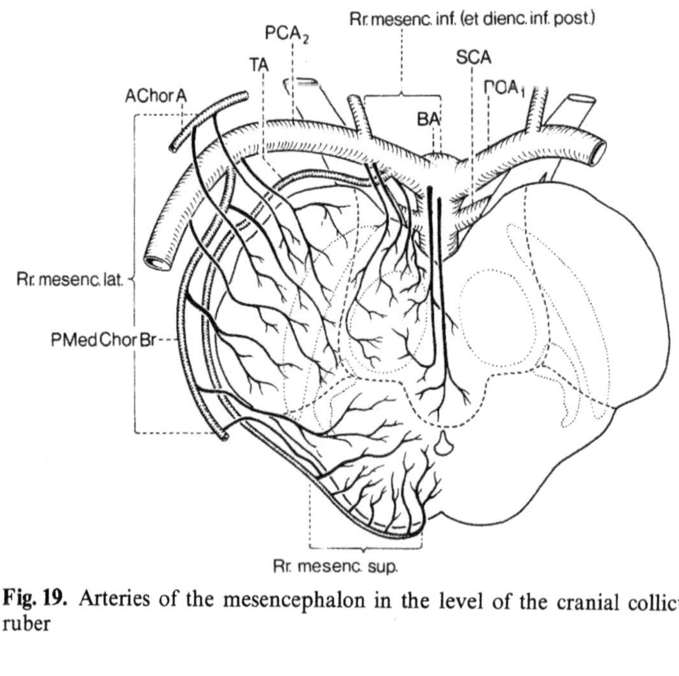

Fig. 19. Arteries of the mesencephalon in the level of the cranial colliculus and the nucleus ruber

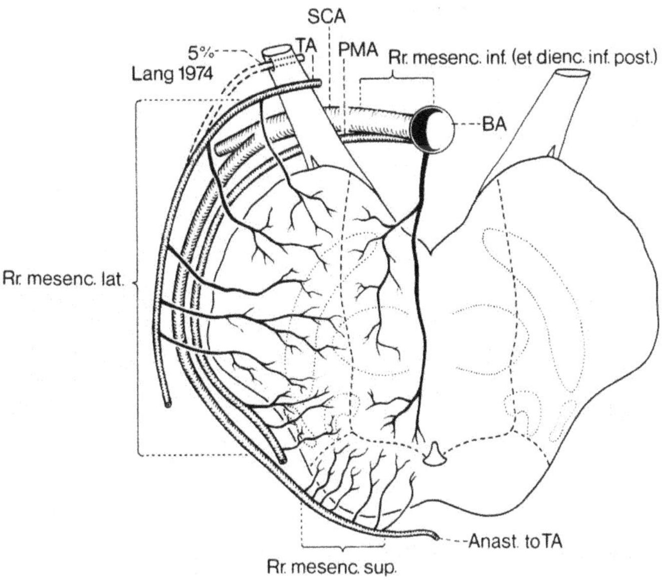

Fig. 20. Arteries of the mesencephalon in the level of the caudal colliculus

ment cells are visible (at larger magnification of the operating microscope). After a short distance from this zone the nerve fibers are bundled in one stem, which is round or ovale and has diameters between 2 and 3 mm on transverse section and a cross-section between 2.77 and 4.55 mm². The third nerve in its cisternal segment contains in our material 15000 (11360–21351) fibers with a diameter of 5 μm and more. Björkman and Wohlfart (1936) using silver staining counted between 25000 and 35000 fibers. Surprisingly we found in the cavernous sinus wall up to 50% more, but thinner fibers than in the proximal segment (Thorsteinsdottir 1982). According to Sunderland (1957/58) the fibers for the sphincter muscle of the pupil are situated on the anterior and upper surface of the nerve and can be compressed by pressure on the posterior petroclinoideal fold (herniations and space occupying processes of the brain). This fiber situation leads first to a constriction of the pupils (= irritation) and later to a widening and loss of pupilar reflexes (= paralysis). Later on, disturbances of the external eye muscles, which are supplied from the third nerve, are found to occur. The nerve sometimes is stretched and displaced by the P_1 or P_2 segment of the posterior cerebral artery or the posterior communicating artery. It should be noted, that as early as 1884 Nothnagel described lesions of the third nerve like Boeri and Passerini (1964) following a megalodolichobasilare anomaly. In one case (Ricker and Mertens 1970) there was a spasm of the eye muscles, which was possibly caused by a compression of the central segment of the third nerve (Lang 1982).

The autonomic and motor nuclei of the third nerve are situated below the mesencephalic aqueduct in the level of the cranial colliculus. On each side of the midline the large cell oculomotor mass is topographically divided into dorsolateral, intermediate and ventromedial nuclei (Warwick 1953). In monkeys the motor pools of the rectus inferior, obliquus inferior and rectus medialis are situated in a dorsoventral order. The caudal central nucleus is the motor pool of the two levators of

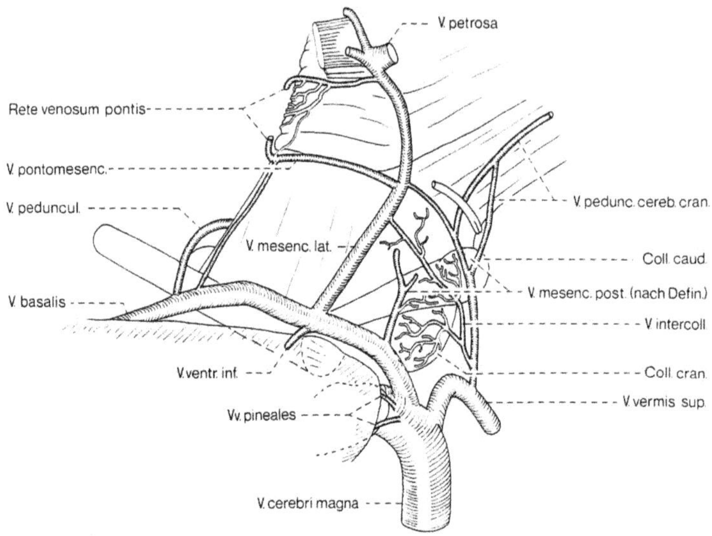

Fig. 21. The most important veins on the outer surface of the mesencephalon

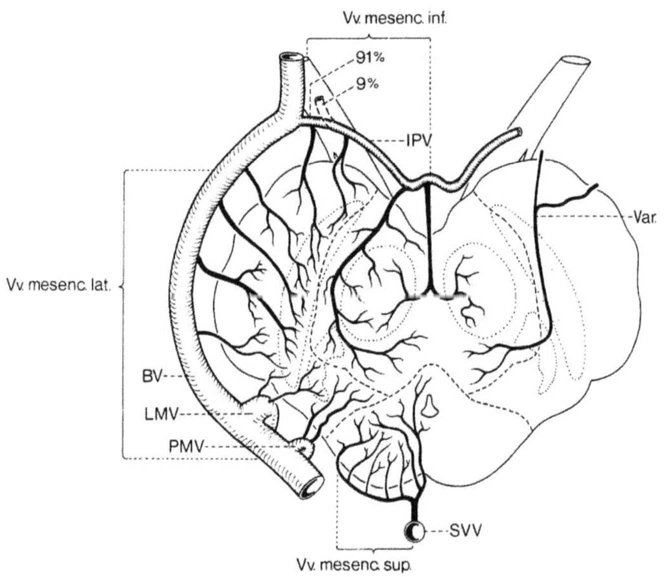

Fig. 22. Veinous drainage of the mesencephalon

the upper eyelids. Porter et al. (1983) stated like Warwick (1953) that each extraocular muscle receives solely unilateral innervation, with contralateral representation of only the superior rectus and the superior oblique muscles. The superior rectus motor neurons were distributed along the medial aspect of the contralateral nucleus with the predominant representation at caudal to midnuclear levels. Inferior oblique motor neurons filled the gap lateral to those of the superior rectus and ventral to the

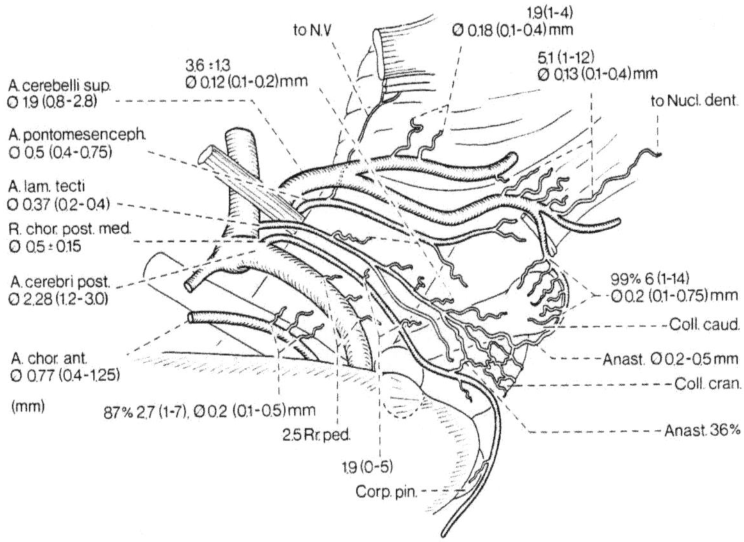

Fig. 23. Arteries on the outer surface of the mesencephalon and its twigs to the mesencephalon and anastomoses, numbers and diameters in mm (extremals)

medial rectus muscle (dorsal subgroup) and inferior rectus representation. The autonomic nuclei (Edinger and Westphal) are composed of smaller multipolar nerve cells and developed at cranial oculomotor levels, where they fuse together and argue ventrally over the cranial end of the main oculomotor nuclei. In more caudal levels nuclei frequently show a tendency to splitting in paired parts. The central nucleus of Perlia consists, according to Warwick (1955), as a few scattered large motor cells in the midline raphe between the right and left oculomotor masses, but they never constitute clear nuclear mass in mankind. In any case such nerve cells appear to innervate the superior rectus and not the medial rectus muscle. The connection of the oculomotor nuclei includes corticonuclear fibers from both sides, which reach the cells directly or via interneurons. The medial longitudinal fasciculus connects the nuclei of the fourth, sixth and eighth nerves (especially the medial and superior vestibular nuclei) according to Tarlov (1972) and also the anterior horn cells of the spinal cord, the tectobulbar tract, the pretectal nuclei of both sides for the light reflexes, a.o. About the main nuclei and fiber tracts in the mesencephalon see Figs. 16, 17. In Figs. 21, 22 the veins on and in the mesencephalon and in Fig. 23 the arteries of the mesencephalon are visible.

Trochlear Nerve

The nucleus of the trochlear nerve is situated below the floor of the mesencephalic aqueduct in the level of the caudal colliculus. The medial longitudinal fasciculus ventral to this nucleus is visible (like other nuclei and fibers) in the level of the caudal colliculus in Fig. 17. Its fiber connections in the brain stem are similar to those of the oculomotor nuclei. But the corticonuclear fibers run chiefly homolaterally. After leaving the nucleus the fibers of the trochlear nerve first run downwards and laterally through the tegmentum and then turn backwards around the central grey matter to the upper part of the anterior medullary velum. Here they decussate with the contralateral fibers in the limen veli medullaris cranialis. This is a thicker zone of the velum medullare craniale (up to 1.5 mm) and is situated 2.6 (2–3) mm behind the caudal colliculus (Lang and Deymann-Bühler 1984). In most cases more than 1 fiber bundle is seen in the exit-zone of the fourth nerve (Lang 1979; Lang 1981; Lang 1983). Their central glial segments are 0.3 (0.0–1.0) mm long (Lang 1982). In most cases of the first part of the peripheral segment of the nerve, in which the fibers are bundled to one stem, the nerve is surrounded by one branch of the vermal branches of the superior cerebral artery. In this area anastomoses are also situated between the superior cerebellar artery and the tectal artery. These twigs have a width of 0.2 mm or less. The trochlear nerve then curves around the mesencephalon to its dural pore in the cavernous sinus region. Its length between the exit- zone and its dural pore we estimated to be 32.65 (20.0–42.0) mm (Lang and Reiter, in press). We found a mean length of 33.6, in females of 30.94 mm (T=2.28). Its cross-section area was 0.41 (0.247–0.671) mm^2 (Thorsteinsdottir 1982). In our material we found in the cisternal segment of the fourth nerve 1800 (823–2589) fibers of 5 μm and more in diameter. Björkman and Wohlfahrt (1936) counted 34000 fibers. Then the nerve pierces the dura mater in 80% between the posterior and anterior petroclinoideal fold, in about 20% the lower surface of the tentorium cerebelli (Lang 1974). In the sidewall of the cavernous sinus it is concomitated by arachnoideal sheath of different lengths (up to 2 mm dorsal the dural pore for the oculomotor nerve). Inside the sidewall of the cavernous sinus the nerve has different courses, which are important for approaches to the posterior knee of the internal carotid artery (Parkinson's triangle). The length of the 4th nerve in the sidewall of the cavernous sinus forward to the vertical level of the lower border of the orbital opening of the optic canal measures in our material 31.16 (23–39) mm (Lang and Reiter 1984). Similar to our results from the oculomotor nerve we found in distal parts of the trochlear nerve more fibers than the proximal (cisternal) segment. In the sidewall of the cavernous sinus we found about 24% more fibers than in the proximal one and especially more fibers of A-Gamma-type with a thickness between 4.9 and 8 μm (including myelin sheaths). With silver staining of course the nerve contains more fibers (3000–3500).

At retrosigmoideal posterolateral or pterional approaches the lower cranial nerves and the pons are available.

Pons

The pons is the anterior part of the rhombencephalon and can be divided into a pars ventralis and pars dorsalis pontis. The pars ventralis contains the corticospinal, corticonuclear, corticoreticular, corticopontine, more longitudinal running fibers and in fibrae pontis transversae, which build the middle cerebellar peduncle. Between these fiber tracts the scattered nuclei pontis are situated.

The pars dorsalis pontis (tegmentum pontis) contains sidewards of the raphe the medial and dorsal longitudinal fascicles, the lemnisci medialis, spinalis, trigeminalis and lateralis. Also in the pars dorsalis pontis the tractus tectospinalis, spinalis n. V., mesencephalicus n. V are running and the nuclei of the 5th, 6th, 7th, 8th nerves and their intracerebral fiber connections and afferent and efferent fiber bundles are situated.

In our material the lower surface of the pons has a length of 28.6 (22–33) mm (Schubert 1976). Kazda and Putz (1981) measured the entry-zone of the medial border of the trigeminal nerve. According to their measurements the trigeminal nerve entry- and exit-zone is on the right 18.6 and on the left 19.7 mm paramedian and on the right has angles with the median plane of 39.5 (10–70)°, on the left of 41.5 (10–65)°. In our material the width of the radix sensoria is 3.74 (2.3–5.4) mm, according to Gudmundsson et al. (1971) 3–4.5 mm. These authors estimated the thickness of the sensory root with 1.5 to 3.0 mm. The central segment of the radix sensoria has a length of 3.57 (2–6) mm (Lang 1982) (Fig. 24). In most cases there are developed 2 or 3 radices motoriae, which have an exchange of fiber bundles with the radix sensoria in different levels. Vidic and Stefanatos (1969) estimated in the upper one of the motor roots fibers of 8 (3.5–13.2) μm and in the lower one fibers of 5.5 (2.0–13.0) μm. Young and Stevens (1979) counted in the motor roots between 3140 and 7462 fibers and noted, that 12–20% are unmyelinated (equal percentage in the ventral roots of the spinal cord). In our material the central segment of the motor roots have a length of 0.67 (0.0–1.5) mm. 1984 we estimated the length of the medial and lateral borders of the trigeminal nerve between its exit(entry-)zones and the trigeminal pore of Meckel's cave in the posterior fossa. This was on the medial border 13.38 (8–20) and on the lateral 12.01 (7.5–17) mm.

Sjöquist (1938) counted in the radix sensoria 140000 (76842–150079) fibers. According to Young 50% of them are nonmyelinated. The central or glial segment is vulnerable against pressures from neighboring arterial loops, veins, arachnoid adhesions and tumors. Especially the superior cerebellar artery or one of its twigs is sometimes situated near the central segment of the 5th nerve. Also the anterior inferior cerebellar artery, the posterior inferior cerebellar artery and the petrosal vein or the pontomesencephalic artery (developed in 60%) can run to this zone. These nerve-vessel-relations can cause hyperactive reactions of the trigeminal nerve and in my opinion this is the most common reason for the trigeminal neuralgy.

Abducent Nerve (see Fig. 24)

The nucleus of the 6th nerve is situated immediately below the facial colliculus in the anterior medial part of the rhomboid fossa. According to Olszewski and Baxter (1954) the nucleus has a length of 3 mm and contains 3970–7270 cells (Blinkov 1963). According to Konigsmark et al. (1969) the nucleus contains 22000 cells! The nucleus is connected with the corticonuclear fibers of the contralateral hemisphere, the medial longitudinal fasciculus, the tectobulbar tract and the formatio reticularis.

Its axons descend ventrally through the pons and emerge in the sulcus between the caudal border of the pons and the cranial end of the pyramid, sometimes also the lower transverse fibers of the pons. The exit-zone of the medial border of the 6th nerve is situated 3.93 (2.0–6.5) mm paramedian. In most cases in this area there are visible two or more fiber bundles, which, after a short distance – build up to one nerve, which contains 6600 (Björkman and Wohlfahrt 1936) and 5124 (4058–6039) myeliniated nerve fibers according to Abdullaev (1965). In our material we found 3700 (1946–8136) myelinated fibers with diameters from 4.9 μm and more (Thorsteinsdottir 1982). The central segment of this nerve measures in our material 0.3 (0.1–1.0) mm (Lang 1982). In 7.5% Nathan et al. (1974) found two nerve bundles in the posterior fossa of the 6th nerve. In the posterior fossa the nerve runs to its dural pore and is situated dorsally to the inferior anterior artery in 79%, basal to this vessel in 16%. In 5% the vessel was found between a doubled abducent nerve (Brunner 1978). The course of the 6th nerve in the posterior fossa has a length of 15.9 (11.0–22.0) mm. It should be noted, that doubled nerves can pierce the dura mater in a distance up to 4.5 mm. In our material the dural pore for the 6th nerve is situated 6.14 (4.0–9.5) below the lower border of the trigeminal pore and 13.9 (10.5–17.0) mm medial of the medial lip of the internal acoustic pore. Then the nerve runs, imbedded in an arachnoid sheath and a prolongation of the dura mater inside of the inferior petrosal sinus to Dorello's canal in the area of the apex of the petrous bone and then curves around the lateral wall of the internal carotid artery.

In about 80% (more often on the right side) the nerve is situated below the upper pole of the trigeminal ganglion. In the other cases the nerve runs above the ganglion pole and then medially to the ophthalmic nerve (Strobel 1980). Inside the posterior part of the cavernous sinus we found doubled nerves in 18.2% (on the right side in 14%, on the left in 22%). In 2.2% the nerve in this area was fan-shaped and flattened (Lang and Reiter 1985). A short distance in front of the posterior ascending part of the internal carotid artery in most cases there is an autonomic ganglion and its connection with sympathetic nerves of the internal carotid plexus (see Lang 1979, Fig. 29).

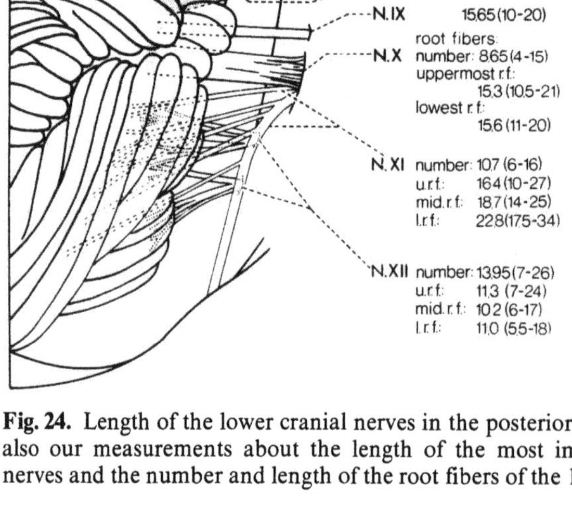

Fig. 24. Length of the lower cranial nerves in the posterior fossa in mm (extremals). Given are also our measurements about the length of the most important central segments of these nerves and the number and length of the root fibers of the 10th, 11th and 12th nerves

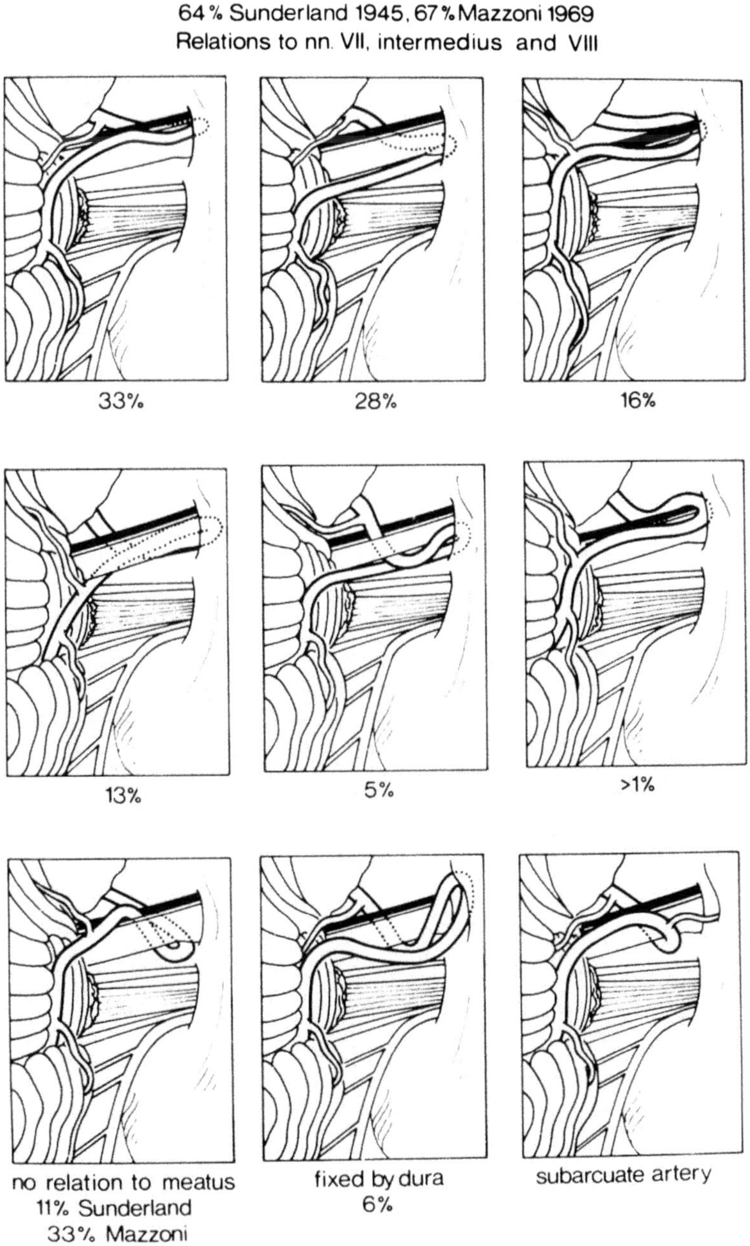

Fig. 25. Inferior anterior cerebellar artery on or in meatus

Facial Nerve

The nucleus of the facial nerve is situated 4–5 mm below the rhomboid fossa and below the spinal nucleus of the 5th nerve and the medial vestibular nucleus. Szentagothai described an inferior, a median, dorsal, superior and ventral nuclei area. According to Vraa-Jensen (1942) the nucleus has a length between 3.0 and 3.5 mm, a width of 2.5–3 mm and a height of about 1 mm. It is situated in the formatio reticularis lateralis and with its largest part inside of the pons and a smaller one in the medulla oblongata. According to Shindo (1959) the length of the nucleus is between 2.0 and 5.6 mm. It contains 5196–6270 cells (Maleci 1934). Blinkov (1963) found between 6040 and 13640 cells. Concerning the somatotopic organisation of this nucleus see Lang (1981).

The axons of the facial nucleus are first orientated dorsally and upwards to the medial surface of the abducent nucleus, then curve around this nucleus (inner knee of the facial nerve) and downwards and laterally to its exit-zone. The intracerebral course of the nerve has a length of about 16 mm. The medial border of the facial nerve exit-zone is situated 11.81 (9.5–14.5) mm paramedian. The nerve has an ovale cross area with a largest diameter of 1.82 mm on the right and 1.72 mm on the left side. According to van Buskirk (1945) it contains 11600 fibers (76% myelinated and 24% nonmyelinated). The central segment of the facial nerve in our material measures 2.05 (0.5–4.0) mm (Fig. 24). This vulnerable segment can be touched by the anterior inferior cerebellar artery, by the vertebral artery or the posterior inferior cerebellar artery. These nerve-vessel-relations are important to hemifacial spasm. The length of the facial nerve in the posterior fossa in our material (Lang and Reiter, in press) is 15.8 (9–26) mm, the nerve is situated medially to the 8th nerve. In about 65% a loop of the anterior inferior cerebellar artery or the posterior inferior cerebellar artery is found in different relations to the 7th, intermediate and 8th nerves in the area of the internal pore of the internal acoustic meatus (Sun-

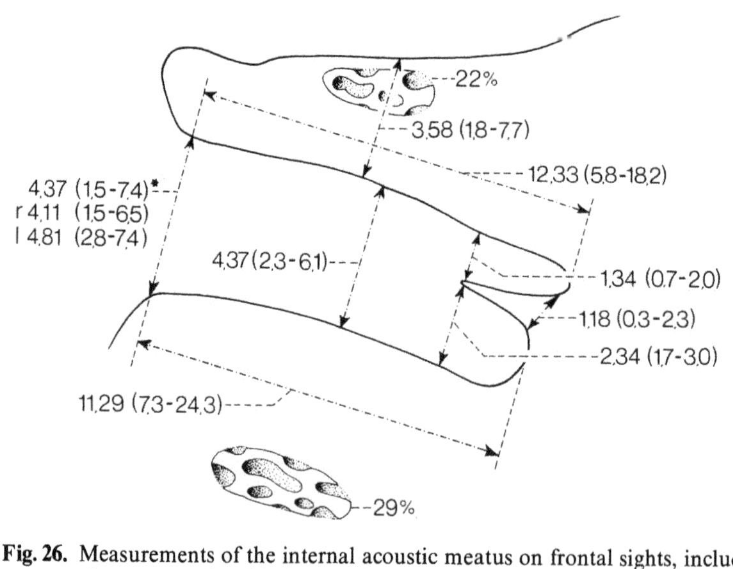

Fig. 26. Measurements of the internal acoustic meatus on frontal sights, included is the development of suprameatal and inframeatal mastoid cells. Measurements in mm (extremals)

derland 1945; Mazzoni 1969 and in our own material, see Fig. 25). The internal meatus of adults is about 12 (7.3–24.3) mm long (measured distally to the pores of the facial and eighth nerve canals) Fig. 26. The height on the pore we found in our sections was 4.37 (1.5–7.4) mm. In the middle part we measured a height of 4.37 (2.3–6.1) mm. Above the meatus we found suprameatal cells in 22% and below the meatus inframeatic cells in 29%. Distal to the foramen meatale the Fallopian canal begins with its labyrinthine, geniculate, tympanic, pyramidal and mastoid segments. For further details see Lang (1974).

Vestibulocochlear Nerve

Vestibular Part

The superior vestibular part has fibers from the anterior and lateral ampullary nerves (about 6000) from the utricular nerve (about 6000) and from the superior saccular nerve. The ganglion is situated inside the meatus acusticus internus near the fundus. It contains bipolar ganglion cells (together with the inferior ganglion: 18440) according to Naufal and Schuknecht (1972). The superior part is running first above and then medially to the inferior vestibular part and the cochlear part of the 8th nerve to the brain stem. Bergström (1973) counted in the superior vestibular part 11800 fibers. The inferior vestibular part has fibers from the posterior ampulla (about 2500), from the cochlear saccular nerve, from the vestibulocochlear nerve and the sacculus (4000). This nerve part posterior to the ganglion is situated in the porus area laterally and downwards and on the brain stem laterally to the superior vestibular part. Bergström (1973) counted about 6500 fibers in the inferior vestibular part. Between the internal acoustic pore to the brain stem we measured a length of 15.1 (9.0–22.0) mm (Lang and Reiter, in press). On the brain stem its medial border is situated 15.04 (13.0–17.5) mm paramedian and 1.36 (0.5–2.0) mm laterally to the facial nerve. It should be noted that about 200 efferent fibers are counted in the vestibular part. According to Henschen (1961) the central segment of the 8th nerve has a length between 10 and 13 mm in men and 7 and 10 mm in women. In our material we measured a length of 10 (6–15) mm (Lang 1982), see Fig. 24. The transition dome (glial dome) is situated in the area of the internal acoustic pore, in the internal acoustic meatus or in the posterior fossa. Tarlov (1937) found the glial segment of the cochlear part of the 8th nerve longer than the glial segment of the vestibular part in 13 out of 18 nerves. The glial dome between the apex and the lateral border has a length of about 1.1 mm. A hyperactive reaction after compression of the 8th nerve is followed by tinnitus, hyperacusis, diplacusis, vertigo and hearing loss. According to Jannetta the anterior inferior cerebellar artery, the posterior inferior cerebellar artery and the labyrinthine arteries may be responsible for such disturbances. If the vestibular part is touched, then the patients have vertigo, nerve-vessel-relations at the cochlear part cause tinnitus. Jannetta saw such compression zones in most of his cases near the brain stem. It should be mentioned that more distal vessel loops between the 7th and 8th nerves in our material were seen in about 40% (for further details see Lang 1979; Lang 1981; Lang 1982). According to Lazorthes et al. (1961) the diameter of the nerve fibers in the vestibular part of the vestibulocochlear nerve is between 2 and 6 μm in 89% and in 10% between 8 and 10 μm. The central fibers of the vestibular nerve reach the vestibular nuclei. According to Ponomarev (1958) the superior vestibular nucleus has a length of 4.4 (3.4–5.4) mm, the medial vestibular nucleus of 6.6 (5.0–8.3) mm, the lateral vestibular nucleus is 4.0 (2.9–5.8) mm long and the caudal vestibular nucleus 2.8 (2.0–3.8) mm. According to Blinkov and Glezer (1968) 120000 cells were found in the medial nucleus, in the lateral 50000, in the cranial nucleus 35000 and in the caudal nucleus about 50000. About the fiber connections of these nuclei with the cerebellum, the longitudinal medial fascicle and the spinal cord see Lang (1985).

Cochlear Part

In our material the distance between the hair cells in the organ of Corti of the cochlea and in the ventral cochlear nucleus measures about 26 mm, the distance to the dorsal cochlear nucleus is about 4 mm longer. In the internal meatus and near the fundus the cochlear part is placed medially from the inferior vestibular part in the posterior fossa on the lower surface of the vestibulocochlear nerve and on the entry-zone in the brain stem, this part is placed laterally to the superior vestibular part below the inferior vestibular part of the 8th nerve, Figs. 27, 28. According to Bergström (1973) and others the cochlear part contains about 30000 fibers with a diameter between 1 and 9 μm (Larsell 1951). 75% of the fibers have diameters between 2 and 5 μm, 14% between 5 and 9 μm (Engström and Rexed 1940). According to Olszewski and Baxter (1954) the ventral cochlear nucleus has a length of about 3 mm and the dorsal one of 2–3 mm. The ventral nucleus therefore is larger and has a volume of 1.3 mm^3, the dorsal one of 1.2 mm^3 (Zvorykin 1959, cited by Blinkov and Glezer 1968). The average distance between the cochlear nuclei and the opposite trapezoid and upper olivary nuclei measures about 16 mm and between these nuclei and the caudal colliculus 30 mm. The distance from these nuclei areas (central and lateral) to the medial geniculate body we estimated to be 15 mm and from this nucleus area to the Heschl's gyri (area 41) about 50 mm, see Fig. 29. It should be

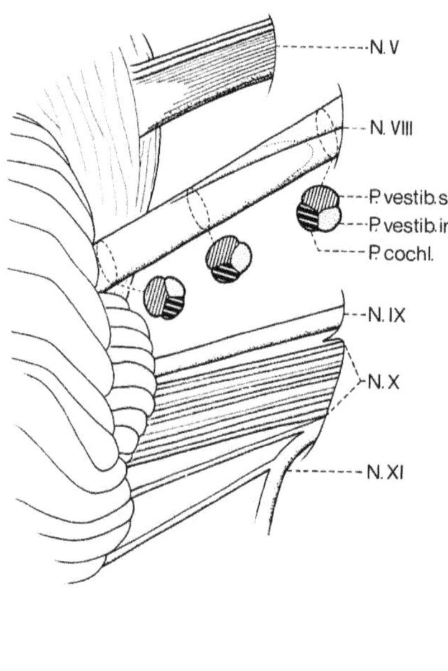

Fig. 27. Course of the parts of the vestibulocochlear nerve in the posterior fossa and near the brain stem (after gentle dividing the nerve parts between the fundus of the meatus and the brain stem)

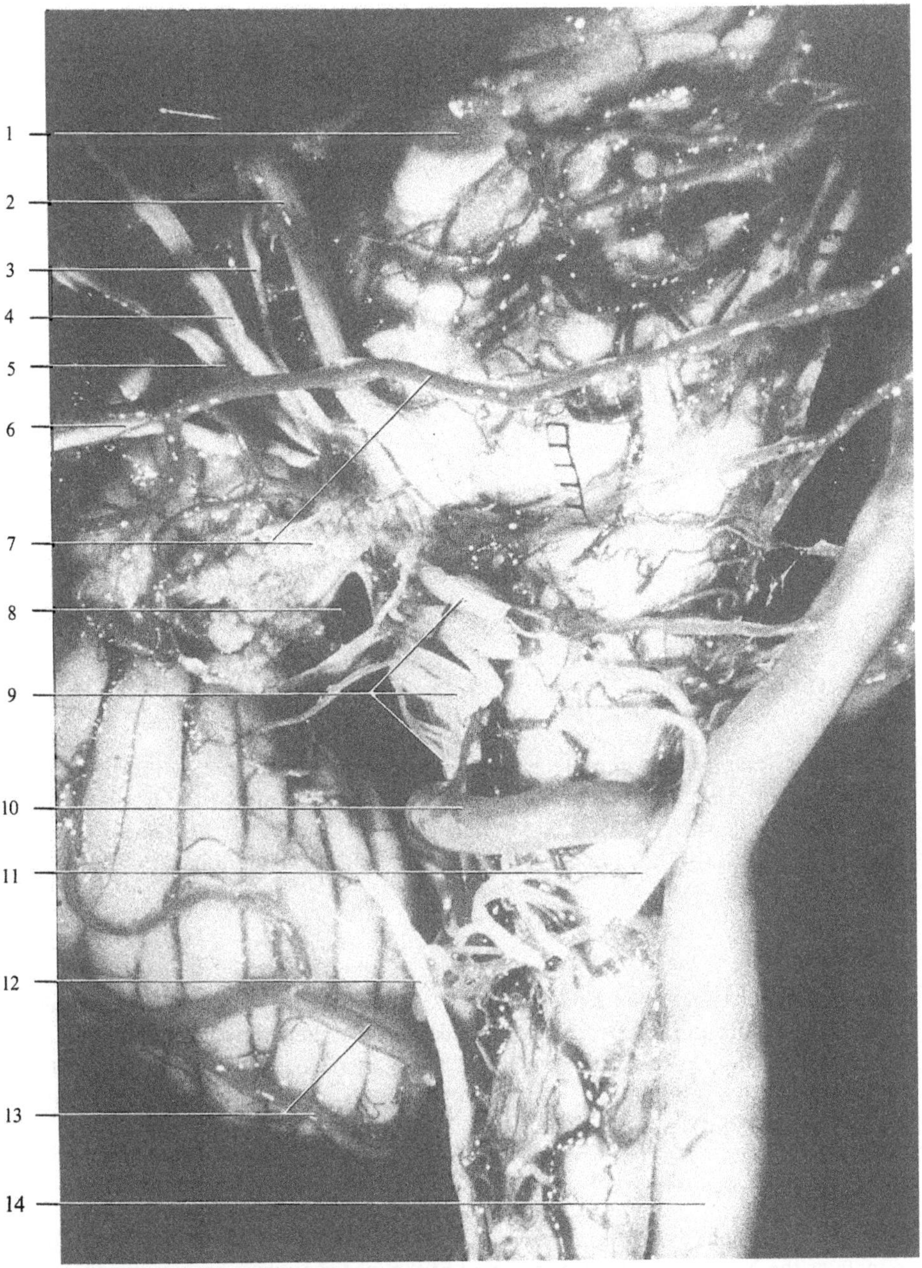

Fig. 28. Vestibulocochlear nerve parts divided (brain stem from ventrally).
1 = Trigeminal nerve, *2* = Facial nerve, *3* = Intermediate nerve, *4* = Sup. vestib. part, *5* = Inf. vestib. part, *6* = Cochlear part, *7* = AICA and plexus of lateral aperture of 4th ventricle, *8* = Lateral aperture of 4th ventricle, *9* = Nn. IX, X and cranial roots of the XIth nerve, displaced medially, *10* = AICA, *11* = Root fibers of XIIth nerve (displaced medially), *12* = Spinal root of XIth nerve, *13* = Branches of PICA, *14* = Vertebral artery

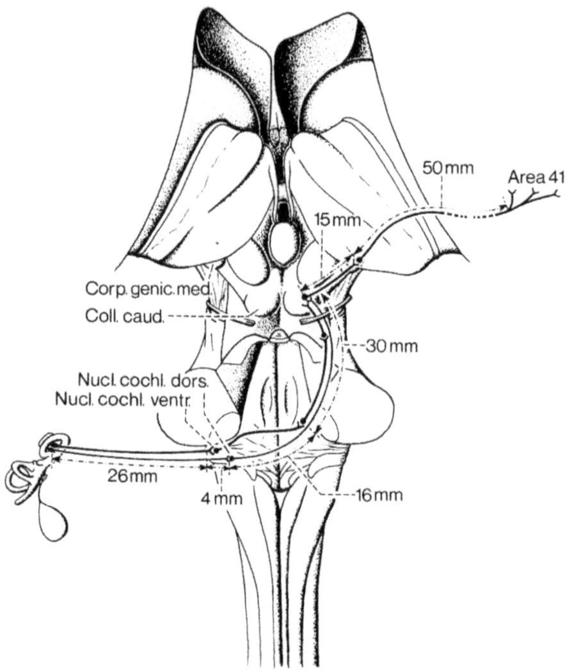

Fig. 29. Overview of the main important cochlea, pathways in mm

noted, that Rasmussen's bundle from the trapezoid nuclei to Corti's organ has 200–400 fibers. The thickness of the vestibulocochlear nerve near the brain stem in our material measured 3.05 (2.0–5.0) mm: 1.3 (1.0–2.5) mm. The entry-zone is situated 15.04 (13.0–17.5) mm paramedian and 1.36 (0.5–2.0) mm laterally to the facial nerve.

N. intermedius

The intermediate nerve has a diameter of 0.09 mm^2, leaves the brain in most cases near the vestibular part of the vestibulocochlear nerve, then between the 7th and 8th nerves. Often this nerve is incorporated in the 8th nerve near the brain stem. Most of the fibers of the intermediate nerve have diameters between 1.5 and 10 μm with a peak between 2 and 4 μm.

N. glossopharyngeus

The 9th cranial nerve has the same nuclei areas in the pons and the medulla oblongata as the Xth nerve. The anterior part of the motor nucleus ambiguus, which is 10–20 mm in length and 3 mm in width, is situated about 7 mm below the bottom of the rhomboid fossa in the level of the striae medullaris. Dorsal to this nucleus are placed the nuclei vestibularis medialis et caudalis, the nucleus of the solitary tract and the formatio reticularis lateralis. In more caudal levels dorsal of this nucleus the spinal nucleus and tract of the 5th nerve and the nucleus cuneatus are placed. The nucleus (according to different authors) contains 1100–2700 cells. In rostral levels the cells for the muscles of the pharynx and the velum palatinum are situated. Intracerebral the fibers like the facial nerve fibers build an inner knee and then run basolaterally to the exit-zone of the 9th nerve. The secretory fibers are axons of the inferior salivatory nucleus, which is situated in the reticular formation.

It should be noted, that lateral to this nucleus band according to most authorities a nucleus for afferent fibers of the viscera is placed, which is supplied from both nerves. Lateral to this nucleus area and deep to it the nucleus of the tractus solitarius is found (taste fiber system). The sensitive impulses are transmitted to the spinal nucleus of the fifth nerve. The glossopharyngeal nerve has its exit-zone in the retro- olivary area 3.19 (1.5–5.0) mm sidewards to the lateral border of the inferior oliva and 1.79 (1.0–3.0) mm caudal to the bulbopontine sulcus. Like Tarlov (1937) we found in our material medial roots with a short central segment and lateral roots, a little bit longer, in the 9th (and 10th) cranial nerve. The motor roots are placed a little bit more medially and have a central segment from 0.1 mm and less, the lateral one have a central segment of 1.1 mm. The extracerebral fiber length in the posterior fossa is measured in our material with a mean length of 15.65 (10.0–20.0) mm. On the right side the nerve was a little bit shorter than on the left. In men we estimated a mean length of 16.03, in women of 14.86 mm.

Neuralgy of the 9th Nerve

According to Garretson and Elvidge (1963) Harris (1926) described for the first time the neuralgy of the 9th nerve. Jannetta operated up to 1977 two patients with glossopharyngeus neuralgy and found in each case a compression of the 9th nerve near the brain stem, which was caused from the vertebral artery. It should be noted, that in our material in 22% the cranial loop of the posterior inferior cerebellar artery reaches the 9th nerve and in further 13.1% the 7th nerve before the artery runs dorsally. In my opinion also this vessel can touch the 9th nerve. Extremely long styloid processes can also compress the nerve and cause a neuralgy of the 9th nerve area (tonsillar area and surrounding structures, pharynx and middle ear cavity). About the relations of the 9th, 10th, 11th and 12th nerves in the foramen jugulare see Fig. 30. It should be noted, that the superior ganglion of the 9th nerve is placed immediately below the cochlear aqueduct and cochlear vein and its upper surface is reached by the cerebrospinal fluid. The lower one is imbedded into the dura mater and connective tissue. The inferior ganglion of the 9th nerve is placed near the fossula petrosa. Distal of the ganglion the nerve (and its perineurium) has a diameter of 1.0 (0.4–1.9) to 0.6 (0.2–1.0) mm. In the area of the inferior ganglion or a little bit distal or proximal to it the tympanic nerve branches off from the 9th nerve (which anastomoses with the ramus auricularis n. X) and distal to it the rr. sinus carotici leave the 9th nerve to the pressoreceptor area of the sinus and the glomus caroticum. Between 3 and 4 rami pharyngei reach the pharynx and together with similar branches of the 10th nerve, build up the pharyngeal plexus, in which a number of ganglion cells were found. The nerve also supplies the stylopharyngeal muscle and with the plexus tonsillaris the tonsillary bed on the outer surface of the palatine tonsil and the mucosal membrane of the tonsil and neighboring parts of the soft palate. The end twigs of the nerves are the rr. linguales in which a number of small ganglion cells are imbedded. For further details see Lang (1985).

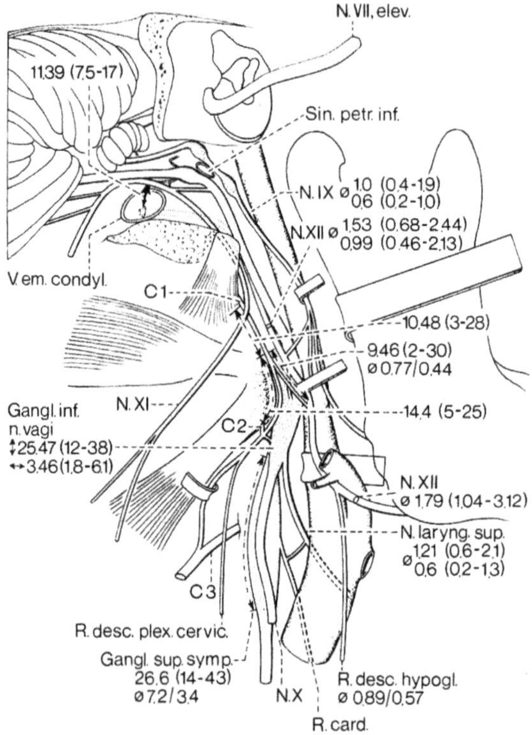

Fig. 30. Course of the nerves IX, X, XI and XII through the foramen jugulare (after resection of the internal jugular vein). Given are also measurements of the diameters and length values of different structures in mm (extremals)

N. vagus

The nucleus dorsalis n. vagi has a length of about 10 mm and contains about 9500 cells (general visceral efferent and general visceral afferent columns) (Etemadi 1961). The cranial end of this nucleus is placed below the trigonum n. vagi, the caudal one below the nucleus gracilis. The nucleus ambiguus is connected with the corticonuclear fibers of both hemispheres (about the fibers to the tractus and nucleus solitarius and the spinal trigeminal nucleus see n. glossopharyngeus). The fibers for the voluntary muscles build inside the brain also an inner knee (the other one have a straight course to their nuclei). In our material (Lang and Reiter 1985) we counted 8.65 (4.0–15) root fibers of the 10th nerve in the retro-olivary fossa. The uppermost fiber bundle of the 10th nerve has a length of 15.33 (10.5–21.0) mm, the lowermost one a length of 15.6 (11.0–20.0) mm between the brain stem and the superior ganglion of the 10th nerve. The exit-(and entry-)zone of the upper fiber bundles of the 10th nerve is placed 2.70 (1.5–4.0) mm lateral to the lateral border of the oliva. Like the fibers of the 9th nerve Tarlov studied the fibers of the 10th nerve. According to this authority the medial bundles are thinner and contain motor fibers. The lateral ones are thicker and composed of sensible and sensory fibers. The medial ones have a short central segment (up to 0.1 mm), the lateral ones a longer (up

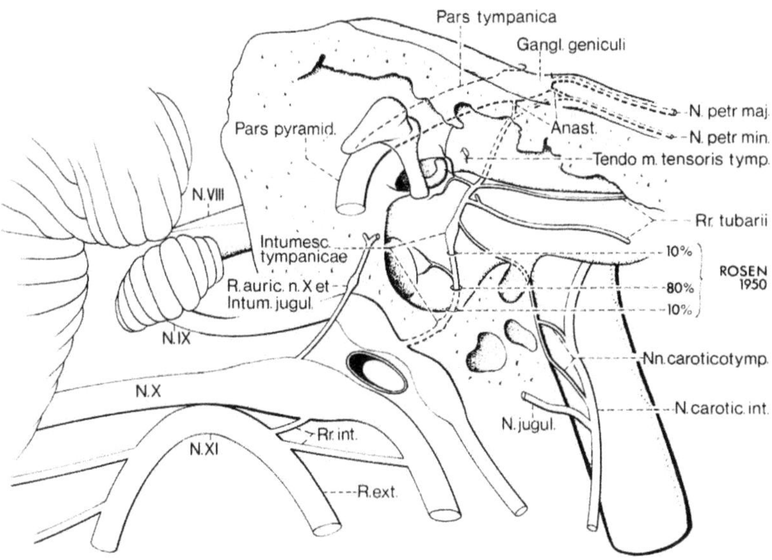

Fig. 31. Intumescenses (from which can develop chemodectomas) of the 9th and 10th nerve branches and surrounding structures. The entrance portals of the tympanic nerve werė estimated by Rosen (1950)

to 2.0 in length) in our material (Lang 1982). Jannetta et al. (1981) mentioned that a vascular compression of the left vagus nerve or the medulla oblongata cause an essential hypertension. A small, but important, branch is the r. auricularis n. X, because in this nerve are imbedded (like in the tympanic nerve) intumescences from which can arise chemodectomas (Fig. 31).

N. accessorius (see Fig. 24)

The nucleus of accessory nerve is placed in the medulla spinalis and reaches from the first cervical segment downwards to the 4th (3.–5.) cervical segment. Its cranial fibers have efferent neurons of the nucleus ambiguus and have the exit-zone in the same area, but further caudal than the vagus nerve fibers. In our material we found 10.66 (6–16) fiber bundles inside of the posterior fossa. The length of the uppermost fiber bundles we estimated to be 16.42 (10.0–27.0) mm, the length of the lowest fiber bundles of the pars cranialis 22.81 (17.5–34.0) mm. The axons of this pars cranialis (ramus internus of the 11th nerve) reach the vagus nerve in different levels below the superior ganglion of the 10th nerve. One or two filaments of the cranial fibers are connected with the superior ganglion of the n. vagus. According to Gray's Anatomy it is probable that this is the source of the motor fibers, which run with the vagus nerve supplying the muscles of the soft palate (with exception of the tensor veli palatini) and the superior and recurrent laryngeal nerves, possibly also the cardiac nerves of the 10th nerve. About the spinal roots, which build up the spinal part of the accessory nerve, see Lang (1981). These nerve parts supply the sternocleidomastoid and the trapezius muscles (together with fibers of the 2nd and 3rd cervical segment). In our material extracranially the accessory nerve was found running anterior to the internal jugulare vein in about 83%, posterior to this vein in 15% and through a hole of the vein (or between the inferior petrosal sinus and the vein) in 2%.

N. hypoglossus (see Figs. 24 and 30)

The nucleus n. hypoglossi has a length between 6.7 and 12 mm and contains about 5800 cells (Larina 1965). Its uppermost part is placed below the trigonum n. hypoglossi, the lower one lies in the ventral part of the central grey matter, close to the median plane. The efferent fibers of this nucleus pass ventrally through the medulla oblongata and leave the medulla between the pyramid and the oliva. We counted 13.95 (7–26) root fibers which are collected in most cases in two bundles: The uppermost root fiber has a length of 11.3 (7–24) mm, the lower one of 11.0 (5.5–18.0) mm to the dural pore course. In 65% (more on the left than on the right) we found two pori durales for the 12th nerve, their distance from one another being 4.16 (0.5–9) mm. The distance of the lower pore to the vertebral artery in our measurements was 8.71 (7–15) mm. The distance of the upper pore to the lower border of the pore for 11th nerve in our material amounted to 11.39 (7.5–17.0) mm. The central segment of the 12th nerve fibers has a length less than 1 mm (like other motor nerve fibers). Inside the hypoglossal canal the fiber bundles unite with each other before the nerve leaves this canal. The nerve fibers are surrounded by an arachnoid sheath and a prolongation of the dura mater and surrounded by the plexus venosus hypoglossi. In most cases one of the meningeal arteries of the posterior fossa runs through the canalis hypoglossalis. Outside the skull the measured diameter of the nerve was 1.53 (0.68–2.44) : 0.99 (0.46–2.13) mm. As a rule, the nerve has anastomoses with the 9th nerve, with the ventral bundle between the 1st and 2nd cervical nerve, with the inferior ganglion of the vagus nerve and in most cases also with the superior ganglion of the sympathetic nerve. In our material we found in rare cases nerve fiber bundles of the 12th nerve anterior to the vertebral artery in the posterior fossa (see Fig. 35, Lang 1981), or fibers which pierce a hole in the vertebral artery, see Lang (1979), and fiber bundles of the 12th nerve which were stretched from a loop of the vertebral or of the posterior inferior cerebellar artery (see Fig. 36, Lang 1981). In all of our cases the nerve extracranially surrounds the occipital artery, especially its proximal branch to the sternocleidomastoid muscle. For further details see Lang (1979), Lang (1981), Lang (1983) and Lang (1985).

References

Abdullaev MS (1965) Connections between the nerve of the oculomotor apparatus. Arkh Anat Gistol Embriol 486:70–77

Bergström B (1973) Morphology of the vestibular nerve. Acta Otolaryngol (Stockh) 76:162–172

Björkmann A, Wohlfahrt G (1936) Faseranalyse der Nn. oculomotorius, trochlearis und abducens des Menschen und des N. abducens verschiedener Tiere. Z Mikrosk Anat Forsch 39:631–647

Blinkov SM (1963) cited at Blinkov SM, Glezer II (1968)

Blinkov SM, Glezer II (1968) Das Zentralnervensystem in Zahlen und Tabellen. Fischer, Jena

Boeri R, Passerini A (1964) The megadolichobasilare anomaly. J Neurol Sci 1:475–484

Brunner FX (1978) Über die Arterien des Hirnstammes. Vorkommen, Zahl, Durchmesser und Variationen. Inaug. Diss., Würzburg

Buskirk C van (1945) The seventh nerve complex. J Comp Neurol 82:303–333

Decker K (1960) Klinische Neuroradiologie. Thieme, Stuttgart

Engel A (1975) Ursprungs- und Verlaufsvariationen der ersten Ophthalmica-Strecke. Med. Diss., Würzburg

Engström H, Rexed B (1940) Über die Kaliberverhältnisse der Nervenfasern im N. statoacusticus des Menschen. Z Mikrosk Anat Forsch 47:448–455

Etemadi AA (1961) The dorsal motor nucleus of the vagus. Acta Anat (Basel) 47:328–332

Garretson HD, Elvidge AR (1963) Glossopharyngeal neuralgia with asystole and seizures. Arch Neurol 8:26–31

Grand W (1980) Microsurgical anatomy of the proximal middle cerebral artery and the internal carotid artery bifurcation. Neurosurgery 7:215–218

Gudmundsson K, Rhoton AL Jr, Rushton JG (1971) Detailed anatomy of the intracranial portion of the trigeminal nerve. J Neurosurg 35:592–600

Harris W (1926) Neuritis and Neuralgia. Oxford University Press, New York

Hayreh SS, Dass R (1962) The Ophthalmic artery. I: Origin and intracranial and intra-canalicular course. Br J Ophthalmol 46:65–98

Hayreh SS, Dass R (1962) The Ophthalmic artery. II. Intraorbital course. Br J Ophthalmol 46:165–185

Henschen F (1961) Zur Histologie und Pathogenese der Kleinhirnbrückenwinkeltumoren. Arch Psychiatr Nervenkr 56:20–122

Jannetta PJ (1977) Observations on the etiology of trigeminal neuralgia, hemifacial spasm, acoustic nerve dysfunction, and glossopharyngeal neuralgia. Definitive microsurgical treatment and results in 117 patients. Neurochirurgica (Stuttg) 20:145–154

Jannetta PJ, Dujovny M, Gendell HM, Segal R, Wolfson S (1981) Neurovascular compression of the left hind brain and the vagus nerve in neurogenic "essential" hypertension. In: Dietz H, Metzel E, Langmaid C (eds) Neurological Surgery, Abstracts of the 7th International Congress of Neurological Surgery München, July 12–18, 1981. Suppl. to Neurochirurgica. Thieme, Stuttgart New York

Jenkins T, Truex RC (1963) Dissection of the human brain. Anat Rec 147:364–365

Kazda S, Putz R (1981) Die Verhältnisse des Nervus trigeminus an seiner Austrittsstelle aus dem Hirnstamm. Morphol Med 1:25–30

Kleiss E (1941/42) Die verschiedenen Formen des Circulus arteriosus cerebralis Willisi. Anat Anz 92:216–230

Konigsmark BU, Kalyanamarama UP, Corey P, Murphy EA (1969) An evaluation of techniques in neuronal population extremales: the sixth nerve nucleus. John Hopkins Hosp Bull 125:146–158

Koos WTh, Spetzler RF, Pendl G, Perneczky A, Lang J (1985) Color Atlas of Microneurosurgery. Thieme, Stuttgart New York

Lang J (1974) Eintritt und Verlauf der Hirnnerven (III, IV, VI) „im" Sinus cavernosus. Z Anat Entwickl Gesch 145:87–99

Lang J (1979) Praktische Anatomie: Ein Lehr- und Hilfsbuch der anatomischen Grundlagen ärztlichen Handelns/begr. von T von Lanz, W Wachsmuth. Fortgef u hrsg von J Lang, W Wachsmuth. Springer, Berlin Heidelberg New York. NE: Lang, Johannes (Hrsg); Lanz, Titus von (Begr) Teil 1: Bd 1 Kopf. Teil B Gehirn- und Augenschädel/von J Lang. In Zsarb mit K-A Bushe, W Buschmann u D Linnert

Lang J (1981) Neuroanatomie der Nn. opticus, trigeminus, facialis, glossopharyngeus, vagus, accessorius und hypoglossus. Arch Otolaryngol 231:1–69 (Kongreßbericht)

Lang J (1981) Neuroanatomie der Nn. opticus, trigeminus, facialis, glossopharyngeus, vagus, accessorius und hypoglossus (Erläuterungen zum Referat). Arch Otorhinolaryngol 231:451–482 (Kongreßbericht)

Lang J (1981) Klinische Anatomie des Kopfes – Neurokranium, Orbita, kraniozervikaler Übergang. Springer, Berlin Heidelberg New York

Lang J (1982) Über Bau, Länge und Gefäßbeziehungen der „zentralen" und „peripheren" Strecken der intrazisternalen Hirnnerven. Ein Beitrag zur vaskulären Hirnnervenschädigung und Dekompressionsbehandlung bei Trigeminusneuralgie, okularer

Neuromyotomie, Spasmus hemifacialis, Tinnitus und Vertigo, Glossopharyngeusneuralgie und Caput obstipum spasticum). Zentralbl Neurochir 43:217–258
Lang J (1983) Clinical Anatomy of the Head. Neurocranium–Orbit–Craniocervical Regions. Translated by RR Wilson and DP Winstanley. Springer, Berlin Heidelberg New York
Lang J (1984) Clinical Anatomy of the Cerebellopontine Angle and internal Acoustic Meatus. Adv Otorhinolaryngol 34:8–24
Lang J (1985) Zur Anatomie und Topographie der A. vertebralis. In: Gutmann G (ed) Arteria vertebralis: Traumatologie und funktionelle Pathologie. Springer, Berlin Heidelberg New York Tokyo, S 3–63
Lang J (1985) Lanz/Wachsmuth, Praktische Anatomie Band I/1 Kopf Teil A: Übergeordnete Systeme. J Lang (Hrsg), in Zsarb mit Jensen H-P, Schröder F. Springer, Berlin Heidelberg New York Tokyo
Lang J, Belz J (1981) Form und Maße der Gyri und Sulci an der Facies superolateralis und Facies inferior hemispherii. J Hirnforsch 22:517–533
Lang J, Brunner FX (1978) Über die Rami centrales der Aa. cerebri anterior und media. Gegenbaurs Morphol Jahrb 124:364–374
Lang J, Brunner FX (1978) Rami diencephalici inferiores anteriores, inferiores, inferiores posteriores und inferiores laterales posteriores – Anzahl, Durchmesser, Ursprungs- und Verlaufsvariationen. Verh Anat Ges 72:429–431
Lang J, Dehling U (1980) A. cerebri media, Abgangszonen und Weiten ihrer Rami corticales. Acta Anat (Basel) 108:419–429
Lang J, Deymann-Bühler B (1984) Über die Größe bestimmter Mittelhirnstrukturen (Messungen an der Außenseite). J Hirnforsch 25:375–384
Lang J, Fischer G (in press) Über die Lagebeziehungen der A. lamina tecti und des R. chorioideus posterior medialis zum N. oculomotorius. Anat. Anz.
Lang H, Häckel HR (1980) Neue Befunde zum Verlauf der A. cerebri anterior (Pars postcommunicalis), zu den Abgangszonen und Weiten ihrer Rami corticales. Acta Anat (Basel) 108:498–509
Lang J, Köth R, Reiss G (1981) Über die Bildung, die Zuflüsse und den Verlauf der V. basalis und der V. cerebri interna. Anat Anz 150:385–423
Lang J, Reiter U (1984) Über den Verlauf der Hirnnerven in der Seitenwand des Sinus cavernosus. Neurochirurgia (Stuttg) 27:93–97
Lang J, Reiter U (1985) Über den Verlauf des N. abducens vor der Austrittszone aus dem zentralnervösen Organ bis zum M. rectus lateralis. Neurochirurgia (Stuttg) 28:1–5
Lang J, Reiter U (in press) Über die intrazisternale Länge der Hirnnerven VII–XII. Neurochirurgia (Stuttg)
Lang J, Schlehan F, Jensen H-P, Lemke J, Klinge H, Muhtaroglu U (1976) Cranio-cerebral topography as a basis for interpreting computed tomograms. In: Lanksch W, Kazner E (eds) Cranial computerized tomography. Springer, Berlin Heidelberg New York, p 24–42
Lang J, Stefanec P, Breitenbach W (1983) Über Form und Maße des Ventriculus tertius, von Sehbahnteilen und des N. oculomotorius. Neurochirurgia (Stuttg) 26:1–5
Larina VN (1965) Der Nucleus n. hypoglossi des Menschen, Topographie, makro- und mikroskopische Beschreibung, Zahl der Ganglienzellen (russ.) Arch Anat 48:77–82
Larsell O (1951) Anatomy of the nervous system. 2nd ed. Appleton-Century-Crofts. Inc., New York. xi, 520 pp
Lazorthes G, Lacomme J, Gaubert I, Planel H (1961) La constitution du nerf auditif. Presse Med 69:1067–1068
Maleci O (1934) Contributo alla conoszenza delle variazioni quantitative delle cellule nervose nella senesenze. Arch Ital Anat Embriol 33:883–901
Mazzoni A (1969) Internal auditory canal arterial relations at the porus acusticus. Ann Otol 78:797–814
McCormick WF (1969) Vascular disorders of nervous tissue: Anomalies, Malformations, and Aneurysms. Biochemistry Disease 3:537–596
Nathan H, Quaknine G, Kosary IZ (1974) The abducens nerve. J Neurosurg 41:561–566
Naufal PM, Schuknecht HF (1972) Vestibular, facial and oculomotor neuropathy in diabetes mellitus. Arch Otolaryngol 96:468–474
Nothnagel H (1884) Anzeiger der KK Gesellsch d Aerzte in Wien, p 92

Olszewski J, Baxter D (1954) Cytoarchitecture of the human brain stem. Lippincott, Philadelphia
Passet J (1883) Über einige Unterschiede des Großhirns nach dem Geschlecht. Arch Anthropol 14:89–141
Ponomarev VS (1958) Die Nuclei vestibulares im Hirnstamm des Menschen (russ.) Vopr Nejrochir (Frag Neurochir) 42–45
Porter JD, Guthrie LB, Sparks DL (1983) Innervation of monkey extraocular muscles: Localization of sensory and motor neurons by retrograde transport of horseradish peroxidase. J Comp Neurol 218:208–219
Renn WH, Rhoton AL (1975) Microsurgical anatomy of the sellar region. J Neurosurg 43:288–298
Ricker K, Mertens HG (1970) Okuläre Neuromyotonie. Klinische Monatsblätter für Augenheilkunde 156/6:837–842
Roche AF (1953) Increase in cranial thickness during growth. Hum Biol 25:81–92
Rosen S (1950) The tympanic plexus. Arch Otolaryngol 52:15–18
Schubert M (1976) Praktisch-anatomische Befunde in der Fossa cranii posterior. Med Diss Würzburg
Shindo K (1959) Prenatal development of the human facial nucleus. Bull Kobe Med Coll 16:168–191
Sjöquist O (1938) Studies on pain conduction in the trigeminal nerve. A contribution to the surgical treatment of facial pain. Acta Psychiatr Neurol Scand [Suppl] 17:9–139
Spiegel EA, Wycis HT (1952) Stereoencephalotomy (Thalamotomy and related procedures). Grune and Stratton, New York
Strobel FJ (1980) Über Lagebeziehungen des Ganglion trigeminale. Med Diss Würzburg
Sunderland S (1945) Arterial Relations of the Internal Auditory Meatus. Brain 68:23–27
Sunderland S (1957/58) The tentorial notch and complications produced by herniation of the brain through that aperture. Br J Surg 45:422–438
Szentàgothai, cited at Blinkov and Glezer (1968)
Tarlov IM (1937) Structure of the nerve root. I. Nature of the junction between the central and the peripheral nervous system. Arch Neurol Psychiatr 37:555–583
Tarlov E (1972) Anatomy of the two vestibulo-oculomotor projection systems. Brain Res 37:471–491
Thorsteindottir K (1982) Über Faserzahlen des N. oculomotorius, N. trochlearis, N. abducens, N. opthalmicus, N. maxillaris und N. mandibularis sowie die Faszikelanzahl des N. maxillaris. Med Diss Würzburg
Torkildsen A (1933/34) The gross anatomy of the lateral ventricles. J Anat 68:480–491
Vidiċ B, Stefanatos J (1969) The roots of the trigeminal nerves and their fiber components. Anat Rec 163:330 (Proc)
Vraa-Jensen G (1942) The motor nucleus of the facial nerve. Ejnar Munksgaard, Kopenhagen
Warwick R (1953) Observations upon certain reputed accessory nuclei of the oculomotor complex. J Anat 87:46–53
Warwick R (1953) Representation of the extra-ocular muscles in the oculomotor nuclei of the monkey. J Comp Neurol 98:449–495
Warwick R (1955) The so-called nucleus of convergence. Brain 78:92–114
Yaşargil MG (1984) In: Smith RD, Young PH, Teddy PJ (eds) Microsurgical Anatomy of the Basal Cisterns and Vessels of the Brain, Diagnostic Studies, General Operative Techniques and Pathological Considerations of the Intracranial Aneurysms. Thieme, Stuttgart New York
Young RF, Stevens R (1979) Unmyelinated Axons in the Trigeminal Motor Root of Human and Cat. J Comp Neurol 183:205–214
Zvorykin (1959) cited by Blinkov and Glezer (1968)

The Three-Dimensional Anatomy of the Fourth Ventricle and Adjacent Structures

F. Afshar, London/England

Introduction

The rapid advances in neuroimaging and stereotaxic neurosurgery now demand a profound knowledge of the precise three-dimensional (3-D) anatomy within the brain stem and IV ventricle as well as within the thalamus and basal ganglia in the treatment of pain [11, 12] and movement disorders.

The increasing use of stereotaxic-CT integrated techniques for tumor biopsy [9], interstitial irradiation [10] and brain stem haematoma evacuation [5], requires information about the position and variability of structures through which an electrode, or cannula, are passed. Furthermore, as increasing microneurosurgery is performed around the brain stem, precise knowledge of the 3-D internal anatomy of the individual tracts and nuclei, with their specific blood supplies, will add to the safety and success of the surgery.

This paper presents the methods and results whereby material from two-dimensional serial sections of the IV ventricular area have been reconstructed into a three-dimensional format.

Materials and Methods

The two-dimensional stereotaxic atlas of Afshar et al. (1978) [2] forms the data base for the 3-D reconstructions. The original atlas was obtained from thirty autopsied human brains after in situ fixation of the posterior fossa contents, using the Corsellis technique [6].

Each specimen was stereotaxically marked and specific steps were obtained in each stage of specimen preparation in order to avoid distortion and shrinkage [1]. Rigid criteria for the choice of reference points and planes took into account the points that could be identified macroscopically for anatomical purposes, as well as being demonstrated radiologically.

Furthermore, a reference system was chosen which, itself, had the least inherent variability from one brain to the next. In this manner, an accurate coordinate system could be constructed as seen in Fig. 1.

The original atlas enabled the precise location of the major nuclei and tracts within the brain stem, together with the variability of their position and a statistically significant composite atlas was thus obtained, with transverse sections at 1 mm apart from the rostral mesencephalon to the cervico-medullary junction. Computer

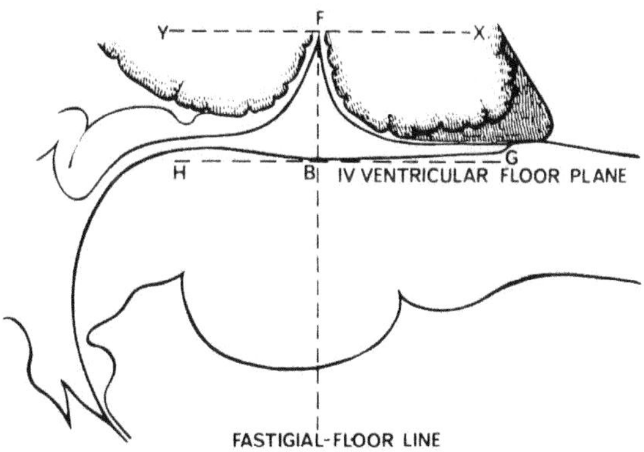

Fig. 1. Schematic representation of the sagittal section of the brain stem, illustrating the reference points and planes used by Afshar et al. F = Fastigium of the fourth ventricle, F–B = Line from the fastigium to the floor of the fourth ventricle, H–B–G = Plane of the floor of the fourth ventricle at right angles to F–B, F–X = Line through fastigium and parallel to the plane of the floor of the fourth ventricle

AT POSITION 5

NUMBER SPECIMENS= 14

POSTERIOR-ANTERIOR PLANE	MEDIAL LATERAL PLANE 4	5	6	7	8	9	10	11
1	0	0	0	0	0	0	0	0
2	0	0	0	0	7	7	0	0
3	0	0	0	7	21	14	0	0
4	0	0	7	29	93	64	14	0
5	0	0	7	21	71	50	14	0
6	0	0	0	7	14	7	0	0
7	0	0	0	0	0	0	0	0

a

SPINAL TRACT V -20

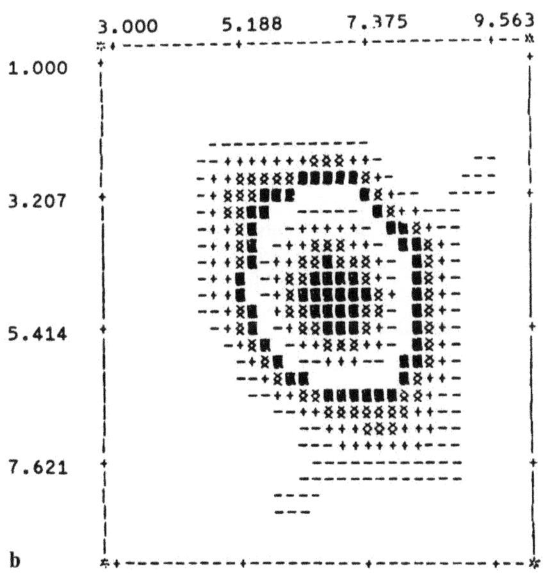

b

Fig. 2. a Probability table of spinothalamic tract 5 mm rostral to the fastigial level. **b** Computer generated map of probability data of the spinal tract of V 20 mm caudal to the fastigial level

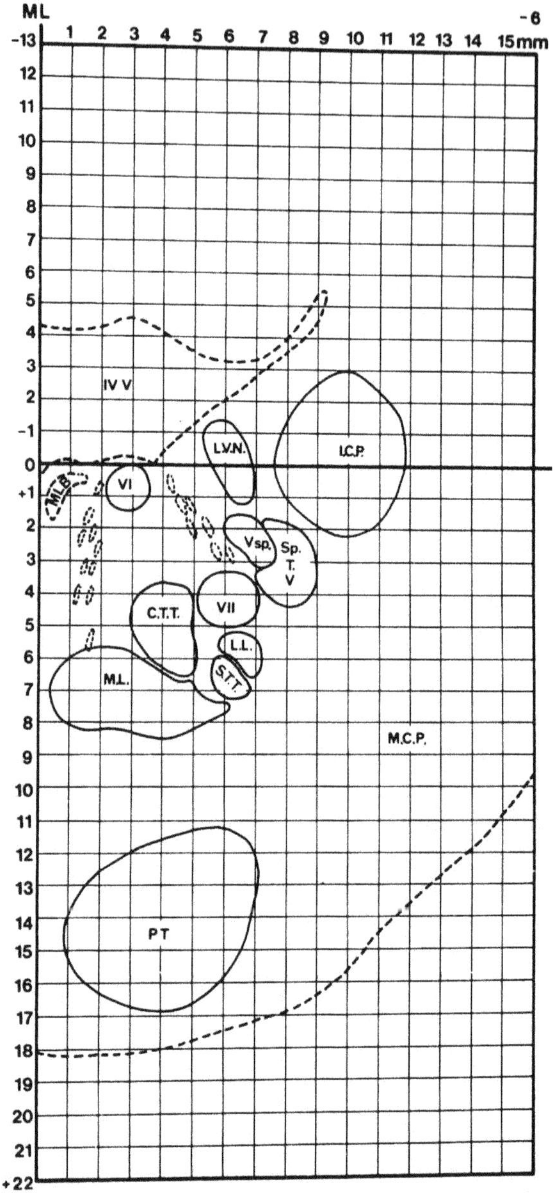

Fig. 3. Composite transverse section through the pons 6 mm caudal to the fastigial level. Drawings are based on calculations of means from data obtained from 70% or more of specimens. *IV V* = Fourth ventricle, *MLB* = Medial longitudinal bundle, *LVN* = Lateral vestibular nucleus, *VI* = VI nerve nucleus, *VSp* = Spinal nucleus of V, *MCP* = Middle cerebellar peduncle, *VII* = VII nerve nucleus, *Sp. T. V.* = Spinal tract of V, *CTT* = Central tegmental tract, *ICP* = Inferior cerebellar peduncle, *ML* = Medial lemniscus, *LL* = Lateral lemniscus, *STT* = Spinothalamic tract, *PT* = Pyramidal tract

generated probability tables for each nucleus and tract, at every 1 mm, was produced, together with a graphic mode (Fig. 2).

The composite atlas drawings, at each 1 mm (Fig. 3), are based on calculations of means from data obtained from 70%, or more, of the specimens. Each structure, at every 1 mm interval, delineated in the two-dimensional atlas, was digitized using an x-y plotting microscope [7], utilizing micrometers connected to potentiometers. This permitted the micrometer stage movement to cause a change in the voltages

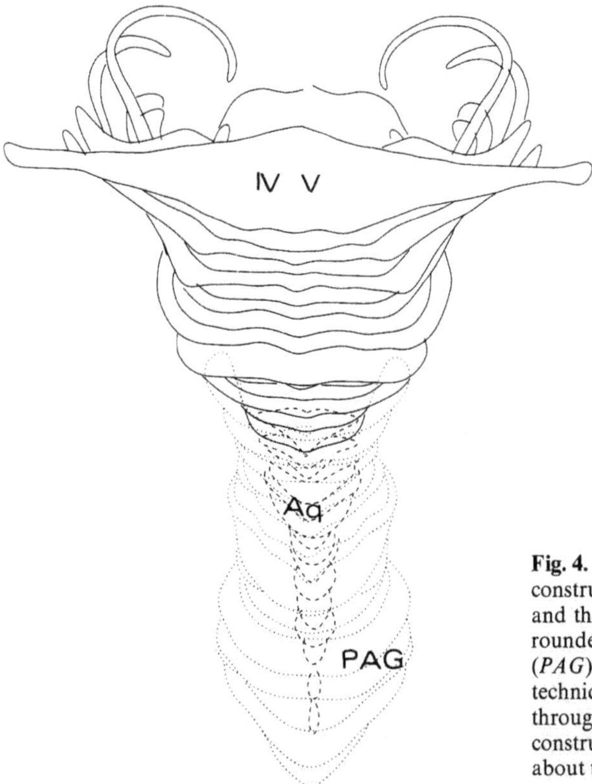

Fig. 4. Computer generated reconstruction of the IV ventricle (*IV V*) and the Aqueduct of Sylvius (*Aq*) surrounded by the periaqueductal grey (*PAG*). Non-hidden line removal technique illustrates the aqueduct through the overlapping PAG. Reconstruction viewed after 30° rotation about the x axis only

generated in both the x and y potentiometers and their subsequent conversion into x and y coordinates by digital voltmeters.

The use of fixed reference points common to all sections, allows scaling and rotation of each section to its adjacent section. Computer programs have been devised, allowing the reconstruction of the tegmental structures in relation to the IV ventricle [8].

Two modes of display are possible [3, 4]. In the first instance, a non-hidden line removal technique allows the reconstruction of one structure to be seen through overlapping structures (Figs. 4 and 6).

In the second reconstruction, the hidden line removal technique allows the display of one structure to be hidden by an overlapping nucleus or tract (Fig. 5).

In the original two-dimensional atlas, all structures are viewed in a transverse plane. Our computer program allows the reconstructed images to be viewed from different angles and permits rotation about any of the three orthogonal axes.

Results

In Fig. 5 the IV ventricle is viewed after 30° rotation about the longitudinal axis in an anti-clockwise direction. Utilizing a non-hidden line removal program, the aque-

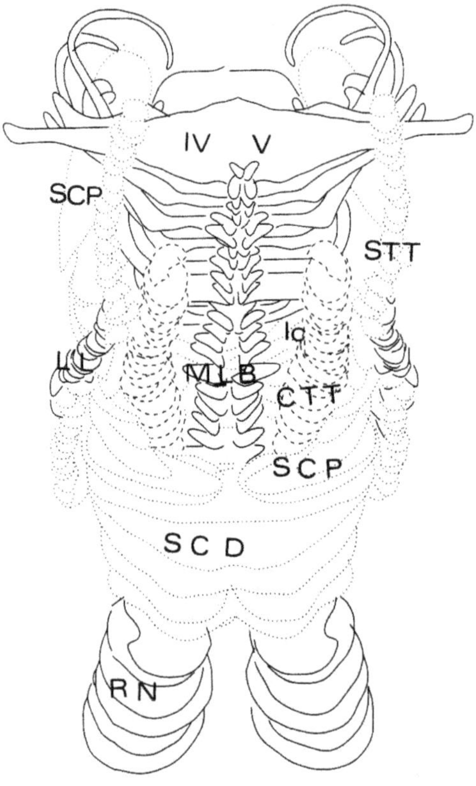

Fig. 5. Computer generated reconstruction of the brain stem tegmentum and IV ventricle (*IV V*) viewed after 30° rotation about the x axis only. *CTT* = Central tegmental tract, *SCP* = Superior cerebellar peduncle, *STT* = Spinothalamic tract, *MLB* = Medial longitudinal bundle, *lc* = Locus coeruleus, *SCD* = Superior cerebellar decussation, *LL* = Lateral lemniscus, *RN* = Red nucleus

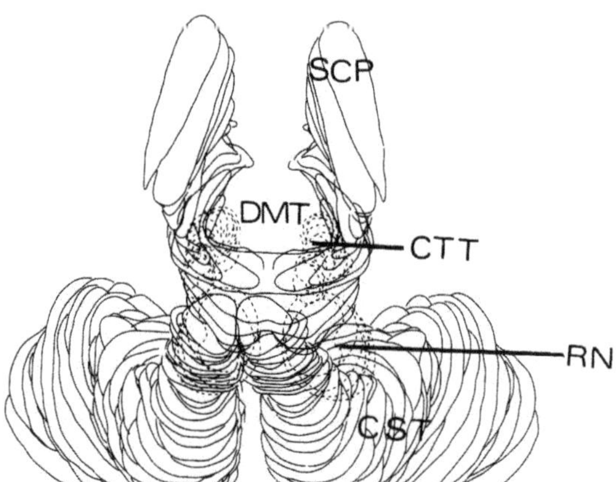

Fig. 6. Computer generated reconstruction of brain stem structures as viewed from caudal to rostral with no rotation about the x, y or z axes. *SCP* = Superior cerebellar peduncle, *CTT* = Central tegmental tract, *CST* = Cortico-spinal tract, *DMT* = Dorsal midbrain tegmentum, *RN* = Red nucleus

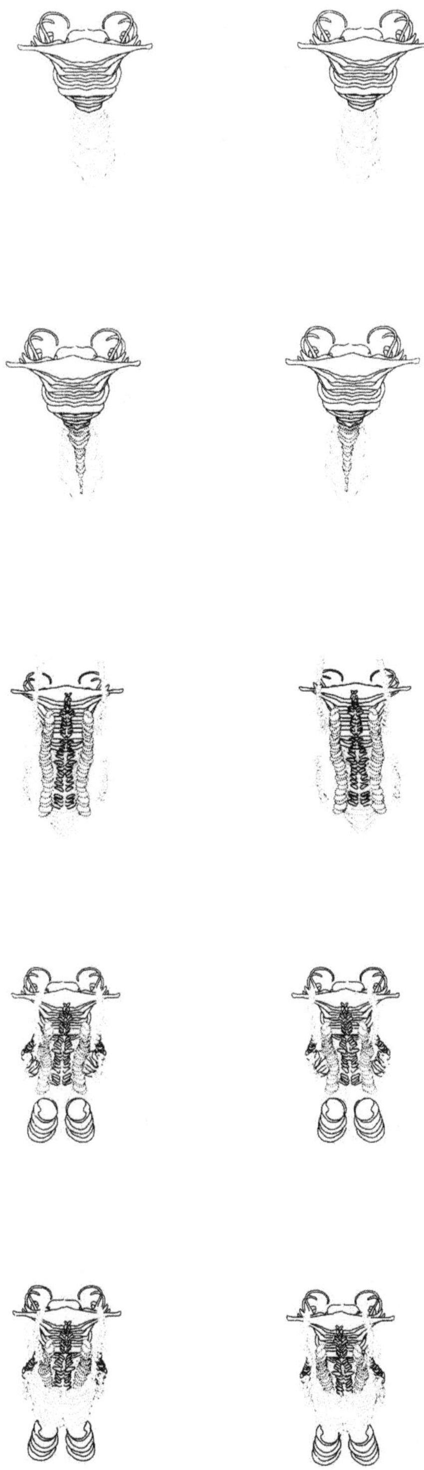

Fig. 7. Computer generated stereopairs of structures shown in Figs. 4 and 5. The use of stereoscopic spectacles will produce true three dimensional visualisation. The interocular angle is 6°

duct is demonstrated within the periaqueductal grey. In Fig. 5, the relationship of the medial longitudinal bundle (MLB) is seen, together with the central tegmental tract (CTT). This forms a well defined tract lying in the dorsal reticular formation and extending from the mesencephalon to the upper medullary region. This tract comprises both ascending and descending pathways. The former originate from the mesencephalic tegmentum, the periaqueductal grey and the red nucleus (Truex and Carpenter 1969) [13]. A large ascending component arises from the medial portion of the medial parts of the brain stem reticular formation.

The locus coeruleus (lc) is immediately medial to the rostral half of the CTT. The spinothalamic tract (STT) is also included and lies lateral to the CTT. At the mid-pontine level this tract becomes totally unrecognizable as a distinct entity, though post-cordotomy degenerative studies (Walker 1940) [14] show it to lie immediately lateral to the medial lemniscus (see also Afshar et al. 1978) [2] and medial to the lateral lemniscus.

In Fig. 5 the superior cerebellar peduncles (SCP) are seen laterally adjacent to the IV ventricle at its caudal end. The peduncle can be followed rostrally to the point in the midbrain where the superior cerebellar decussations (SCD) is encountered. In the same longitudinal plane, and more rostral, are found the red nuclei (RN).

In Fig. 6, the superior cerebellar peduncles (SCP), central tegmental tract and the cortico-spinal tract (CST) are seen in an end on orientation, with no rotation about the x, y or z axes.

The non-hidden line removal technique demonstrates the SCD overlapping the CTT, as well as the portion of the red nuclei. Further programs, utilising colour graphics display, help to improve the delineation of the various tracts and nuclei. Programs for generating stereopairs (Fig. 7), together with the use of shades and hues of colour, have been achieved and give true three-dimensional visualization of these neuro-anatomical structures.

Discussion

Using such techniques, a series of alternative trajectory pathways can be computed and reconstructed for electrode or cannula passage. Furthermore, the computer may be programmed to obtain specific trajectories, obviating any particular structure through which the electrode, or cannula, passage is undesirable.

These techniques allow greater scope for planning and following the electrode passage and can give two-dimensional or three-dimensional maps at every one mm as the target site is approached.

Utilization of similar reference points and planes, with two-dimensional CT and NMR scans, as in the brain stem atlas, will allow the precise three-dimensional anatomical reconstruction of pathological, or normal, tissues and help locate the area of pathology in relation to the nuclei and tracts.

These techniques further add new methods for neuroanatomical teaching purposes, utilizing computer dissections and reconstructions in the complex areas of the brain.

References

1. Afshar R (1977) A Stereotaxic Atlas of the Human Brainstem. Doctoral Thesis. University of London, England
2. Afshar F, Watkins ES, Yap JC (1978) Stereotaxic Atlas of the Human Brainstem and Cerebellar Nuclei (A Variability Study). New York, Raven Press
3. Afshar F, Dykes E (1982) A Three-Dimensional Reconstruction of the Human Brainstem. J Neurosurg 57:491–495
4. Afshar F, Dykes E (1984) Computer-Generated Three-Dimensional Visualization of the Trigeminal Nuclear Complex. Surg Neurol 22:189–196
5. Bosch DA, Beute GN (1985) Successful Stereotaxic Evacuation of an Acute Pontomedullary Haematoma. J Neurosurg 62:153–156
6. Corsellis JAN (1958) Individual Variation in the Size of the Tentorial Opening. J Neurol Neurosurg Psychiatry 2:279–283
7. Dykes E, Clement JG (1980) The Construction and Application of an x-y Coordinate Plotting Microscope. J Dent Res 59:1800
8. Dykes E, Afshar F (1982) Computer Generated Three-Dimensional Reconstructions from Serial Sections. Acta Stereol 82:289–296
9. Gutin PH, Phillips TL, Hosobuchi Y et al. (1981) Permanent and Removable Implants for the Brachytherapy of Brain Tumours. Int J Radiat Oncol Biol Phys 7:1371–1381
10. Gutin PH, Dormandy RH (1982) A Coaxial Catheter System for After Loading Radioactive Sources for the Interstitial Irradiation of Brain Tumours. J Neurosurg 56:734–735
11. Hitchcock ER, Schvarcz JR (1972) Stereotaxic Trigeminal Tractotomy for Post Herpetic Facial Pain. J Neurosurg 37:412–417
12. Schvarcz JR (1977) Functional Exploration of the Spinomedullary Junction. Acta Neurochir [Suppl] (Wien) 24:179–185
13. Truex RC, Carpenter MB (1971) Human Neuroanatomy. Williams & Wilkins Co., Baltimore, Maryland
14. Walker AE (1940) The spinothalamic tract in man. Arch Neurol Psychiat 43:284–298

Trigeminal DREZ for Craniofacial Pain

B. S. NASHOLD, H. LOPES, J. CHODAKIEWITZ, and P. BRONEC, Durham, NC/USA

Introduction

Chronic facial pain continues to challenge the neurosurgeon to use and devise new methods of surgical treatment. This paper describes 13 patients with intractable pain of the face who were treated by coagulation of the trigeminal nucleus caudalis at the cervico-medullary junction. Noxious stimuli from the trigeminal distribution relay via the secondary neurons that make up the nucleus caudalis, and these secondary neurons project directly to the midbrain and thalamic centers associated with nociception. The operation differs from the medullary tractotomy originally described by Sjoquist (6) and others in that the nucleus itself is destroyed by multiple small thermal lesions using the DREZ electrode.

Clinical Materials and Methods

These 13 patients presented with a variety of chronic head and neck pain whose pain had failed to respond to numerous surgical and medical treatments (Table 1). Six patients developed pain in the trigeminal distribution following herpetic infection. The pain was localized to one or all divisions of the trigeminal nerve. In one patient treatment had consisted of a previous stereotactic midbrain lesion while another had had a percutaneous trigeminal coagulation. The remaining three were treated with drugs and TENS. Two patients developed pain after a dental operation (root canal, nerve block). One was treated with drugs while the other had multiple operations (Jannetta procedure ×2, percutaneous coagulation of the trigeminal nerve). None were relieved but developed more extensive pain involving greater areas of the head and neck. One woman suffered from an undiagnosed head pain associated with a long history of psychiatric disturbance which was worsened after posterior fossa operation with manipulation of the trigeminal nerve. Another woman's facial pain came on after the removal of a posterior fossa tumor when the trigeminal nerve was damaged. The man with orbital carcinoma had been treated by exenteration of the eye and radiation and suffered from localized pain deep in the orbit (Table 2).

The surgical technique of the DREZ operation has been described for the spinal cord [5]. The DREZ lesions at the cervico-medullary junction are made using the DREZ electrode designed by Dr. Eric Cosman and made by Radionics Corporation. The lesions are made in the ipsilateral nucleus caudalis of the trigeminus on the side of the pain. A small suboccipital craniectomy and removal of the lamina of C1 and 2 is carried out to expose the surgical site. It is important to visualize the obex of the fourth ventricle as this represents the landmark for the cephalad extent of the lesions. The cervico-medullary junction is visualized using the operating microscope and three important anatomical landmarks are visualized–namely, the obex, dorsal root of C2 and the spinal accessory nerve coursing laterally alongside the spinal cord along with its small filaments which emerge just below the level of the dorsal roots and contribute to the medial portion of the spinal accessory. The lesions are begun just above the most caudal dorsal filaments of the C2 sensory root and slightly ventral to it (1–2 mm) in the region between the exit for the rootlets of the spinal accessory and the dorsal sensory rootlets (Fig. 1). Placing the lesion too dorsally will invade the lateral border of the fasciculus cuteatus and too ventrally will involve the spinal cerebellar pathway. The electrode is angled at about 25° off a horizontal line pointing at right angles to the long axis of the spinal cord. Penetration of the cord is for 2 mm and the lesions are produced at 75 °C for 15 seconds using the Radionics radiofrequency generator. The distance from C2 to the obex is about 10 mm so that at least 10 lesions are made very close together. The line of lesions curves slightly ventrally as one proceeds toward the level of the obex. A small lateral groove can be seen at the cervico-medullary junction which acts as a guide. It is important to extend the lesions to or slightly above the level of the obex (1–2 mm) as failing to do this will result in a post lesion effect with sparing of the medial aspect of the face involving the nose and mouth, as pointed out by Kunz, and may not totally relieve the patient of pain. The post DREZ sensory defect involves the entire three divisions of the trigeminal nerve to the midline of the face and posteriorly over the scalp, ear and jaw. The pain may only involve the first or second division of the trigeminal

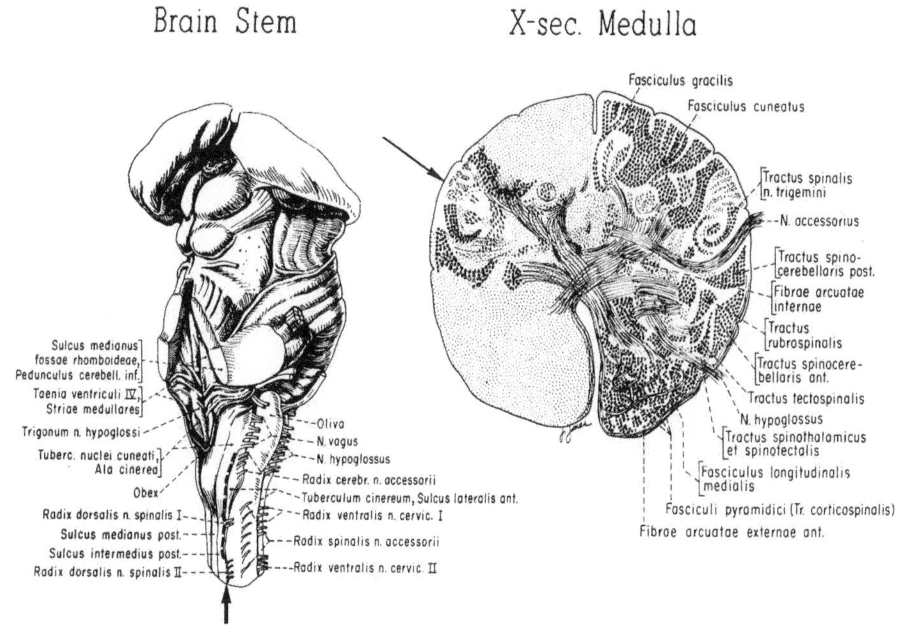

Fig. 1. A Operative site for DREZ lesions of trigeminal nucleus caudalis

Table 1. Clinical information. Trigeminal DREZ

Case	Name Age Sex	History	Neurol. findings Pre-DREZ	Previous treatments	DREZ, date, result		Post-DREZ complications
					Early	Late	
1 1982 Feb	D. P. 76 F	'76 root canal Pain R V_2–V_3 Involves C1–C2 Burning, shooting pain	'82 hypesthesia V_2–V_3 Trigger V_3	Jannetta op ×2 Trigem. coagulation ×2 Dilantin, Tegretol	6 wks Good	Fair	Post-op brainstem stroke with cardiac and pulmonary complication. Gradual improvement
2 1982 Mar	Y. R. 70 F	'70 tic douloureux V_1, V_2, V_3. '77 trigem. op. Burning pain increase entire face	'82 hyperesthesia V_1. Hypesthesia	Trigeminal alcohol injection. Percut. coag. Jannetta op ×1. Stereo mid-brain lesion post. fossa sec. trig.	2 wks Good	8 mos Poor	Pain recurred
3 1982 April	J. C. 30 M	'80 CA orbit Pain onset 6 mos post-op	'82 hyperesthesia V_1. Trigger V_1 rt. eyebrow	Alcohol block sub-temporal trigem. resec. Supraorbital and temp. ar. avulsion	3 wks Good	7 mos Fair	Complaining of orbital discomfort
4 1982 Sept	M. C. 78 F	'78 Post-herpetic pain, V_1	'82 hypesthesia V_1. Hyperalgesia V_1, V_2 to pin prick Skin lesion V_1	Stereo mid-brain lesion. TENS stimulation	Excel-lent	2½ yrs Excel-lent	Post-DREZ somnolent hypotensive episode, L. hemiparesis. Blood in lateral ventricle on CT. Complete recovery
5 1983 March	C. C. 74 M	'82 Post-herpetic pain V_1, V_2.	'83 hypesthesia V_1, V_2.	Percut. coagul. ×2	6 wks V_1 good V_2 fair	1 yr good fair	V_2 pain described as discomfort

6 1983 March	E. K. 48 F	'78 Head, vace and neck pain	'83 hypesthesia V_1, V_3 plus C_3, C_4	Ant. cerv. fusion C_{5-6}, C_{6-7} Ant. discectomy C_{3-4}, C_{4-5}. Occipital neurec. neuroma excised. Rhizotomy C2, C3.	2 wks Excel-lent	1 yr Poor	
7 1983 April	J. G. 60 F	'81 cerebellar hemorrhage, cere-bellar tumor. Resect. tumor and cobalt therapy	'83 Burning facial pain. Cerebellar deficit. Hypesthesia face, C_1, C_2.	TENS stimulation Acupuncture	2 wks Good	1 yr Fair	
8 1983 May	S. M. 68 M	'80 dental surg. and nerve block	'83 Pain since 1980 V_2, V_3. Hypesthesia in V_2, V_3.	Acupuncture, multiple meds	3 wks Good V_2 Fair V_3	1 yr Good Fair	Post-DREZ complication myocardial infarction, meningitis, pneumonia. Resolved
9 1984 Feb	A. A. 52 M	'82 Post-herpetic pain, V_1, severe burning, shooting	'84 skin lesions V_1 Hypesthesia V_1 Hyperalgesia V_2, V_3	C. sympathectomy Multiple meds	2 wks Excel-lent	1 yr Excel-lent	Hyperalgesia disappeared V_2, V_3. Transient weak-ness and incoord. rt. arm.
10 1984 Feb	M. B. 52 F	'78 facial pain V_1 Long history of depression with psych. treatment	Shooting pains V_1 especially eye Numbness lt. ear Mild cerebellar sign	Trigem. coag. post. fossa expl. only	2 wks Good	6 mos Fair	? increase in cerebellar signs
11 1984 May	W. H. 73 M	'80 Post-herpetic pain $V_{1,2,3}$ plus C_{2-5} involvement	Skin lesions face, neck, shoulder	TENS stimulation Multiple meds	1 wk Good	1 yr Poor	Rt. hemiparesis with cerebellar signs that resolved slowly
12 1984 Aug	S. C. 51 F	'83 Post-herpetic V_1, V_2. Burning pain. Electric shocks	Hypesthesia $V_{1,2}$ Decrease corneal reflex	Multiple meds	1 wk Excel-lent	6 mos Good	None
13 1984	T. B. 68 M	'83 Post-herpetic pain $V_{1,2,3}$, Burning & cutting pains	Hypesthesia, $V_{1,2,3}$	Multiple meds	1 wk Excel-lent	3 mos Excel-lent	None

Table 2. Results of DREZ operation

Pain relief Results	13 patients	
Early 3 mos	13	Good–excellent
Late 6 mos–2½ yrs	7	Poor–fair
	5	Good–excellent
Post herpetic pain relief		
Early 3 mos	6	Good–excellent
Late 6 mos–2½ yrs	5	Good–excellent

nerve in some patients, but the lesions will result in a complete analgesia over all three divisions. In future, with the use of evoked potentials from each of the three divisions of the trigeminus, it could be possible to make more selective DREZ lesions that involve only separate or combinations of divisions of the trigeminal nerve.

Discussion

The surgical treatment of atypical facial pain, such as anesthesia dolorosa and post-herpetic pain, has been unsatisfactory. Painful tic involving the trigeminal nerve can be successfully relieved by various surgical techniques. Sjoquist in 1938 published a monograph on pain conduction in the trigeminal nerve and developed the surgical technique of section of the bulbospinal trigeminal pathways in the medulla, the so-called medullary tractotomy, and reported partial relief of pain in patients with atypical facial pain and herpetic neuralgia [6]. The section of the tract at the level of the inferior olive resulted in complete analgesia and thermal anesthesia in the homolateral trigeminal area, as well as reduction of deep pressure pain in the face. Sjoquist commented that the pain of herpes might be nuclear in origin. He went on further to say, "It is, therefore, reasonable to assume that the pathologico-anatomical substrate in herpetic neuralgia is mainly located in the nuclei for the receipt of tactile stimuli, i.e. the nuclei of the dorsal columns and the main sensory fifth nucleus but also in the nuclei for the receipt of pain (substantia gelatinosa Rolandi and spinal fifth nucleus). The relationship between the anesthesia dolorosa in cases of atypical and herpetic facial neuralgia, in which section of the fifth nerve root or bulbospinal tract have failed to give relief is evident and favours the opinion, that even atypical trigeminal neuralgia is nuclear in origin. The evidence provided in Case 11, that herpetic eruption may be produced by lesion of the spinal nucleus in spite of previous interruption of the trigeminal nerve is in good conformity with the view, that herpes zoster may be of nuclear etiology."

Kerr carried out neuroanatomical and physiologic studies of the craniofacial sensory pathways in animals and concluded that there is convergence of descending spinal fibers of the fifth, seventh, ninth and tenth cranial nerves in the pars spinalis of the trigeminal subnucleus (nucleus caudalis) at the medullospinal junction [1, 2, 3]. In 1966 he made lesions with a fine electrode in this nuclear region in cats and concluded that "the destruction of the nucleus (caudalis) itself is not associated with any apparent deficit in the cat" and further recommended the lesion technique could be applied in man with atypical facial pain [4]. We have lesioned the caudalis nucleus of the trigeminal nerve at the medullocervical junction in atypical facial pain, as described above, with relief of pain, particularly in patients with post-herpetic pain of the trigeminal pathways. Post-herpetic trigeminal pain may represent a form of central pain phenomenon in humans involving the trigeminal nucleus caudalis.

References

1. Kerr FWL (1961) Structural relations of the trigeminal spinal tract to upper cervical nerves and solitary nucleus in cat. Exp Neurol 4:131–148
2. Kerr FWL, Oladson RA (1961) Trigeminal and cervical volleys: Convergence or single units in spinal gray at C1 & C2. Arch Neurol 5:161–178
3. Kerr FWL (1962) Facial, vagal and glossopharyngeal nerves in the cat. Arch Neurol 6:261–281
4. Kerr FWL (1966) Spinal V nucleolysis: Intractable craniofacial pain. Surg Forum 17:419–421
5. Nashold BS, Jr (1984) Current status of the DREZ operation: 1984. Proceedings of the First World Conference on Dorsal Root Entry Zone (DREZ). Neurosurgery 15:942–944
6. Sjoquist O (1938) Studies on pain conduction in the trigeminal nerve. A contribution to the surgical treatment of facial pain. Acta Psychiatr Scand [Suppl] 17:1–139

Interpeduncular Fossa Microvascular Anatomy

J. I. Ausman, A. Pedroza, M. Dujovny, F. G. Diaz, J. C. Artero, S. K. Berman, and H. G. Mirchandani, Detroit, MI/USA

Introduction

Knowledge of the microanatomic features of the interpeduncular fossa (IF) is of paramount importance for surgeons approaching vascular lesions of this area, particularly basilar bifurcation aneurysms or vascular reconstruction.

Material and Methods

Twenty-eight unfixed brains were obtained at routine autopsy four to eight hours postmortem from adult individuals without signs of central nervous system disease. After the brains were immersed in Ringer's solution, the basilar arteries were cannulated with 18-gauge polyethylene catheters positioned immediately anterior to the origin of the superior cerebellar arteries (SCAs). The supraclinoid internal carotid arteries, the middle cerebral arteries, and both anterior cerebral arteries were ligated with 3-0 ligatures. The arteries were flushed with 300 cc of normal saline, and then injected with polyester resin according to the previously reported technique (Gomes et al. 1984) until good basal arteries filling was evident. A Zeiss OPMI surgical microscope with a K-1000 Pentax photographic attachment set at 2× magnification was used for the dissections. The brain was placed on its ventral surface and examined from anterior to posterior direction to permit direct view of the interpeduncular fossa.

The IF is defined as the space limited by the mamillary bodies (MB) and the anterior half of the posterior perforated substance (PPS) superiorly, the posterior half of the PPS and the anterior part of the mesencephalic tegmentum posteriorly, the upper part of the pons inferiorly, the cerebral peduncles laterally, and the basilar bifurcation and the proximal segment of the posterior cerebral artery (PCA) anteriorly. The roots of the III cranial nerve converge, and emerge from the midbrain in the posterior part of the IF immediately anterior and lateral to the PPS. The nerve roots transverse the IF, curving ventrolaterally around the medial surface of the cerebral peduncle and passing between the supracerebellar artery (SCA) and the PCA.

The origin, length, outer diameter (OD), course, branching pattern, and point of penetration of the vessels arising from the segment of the PCA proximal to the posterior communicating artery (PCoA) (Pl segments), from the last 5 mm of the basilar artery, and from the proximal 7 mm of the SCA into the IF were studied. Detailed schematic drawings of the findings were made and photographs of the anatomic dissections were taken.

Results

The PPS occupies the superior and dorsal parts of the IF. It is a depressed, punctuated area of gray matter located behind the mamillary bodies. It is shaped like a triangle with the base anterior and the apex posterior. The base was 3.25±0.29 mm long and 8.11±1.19 mm high.

The vessels that course through the IF originate in the posterior part of the circle of Willis. They originate from the Pl segment, from the last 5 mm of the basilar artery, and from the proximal 7 mm of the SCA. These vessels penetrate the PPS, the anterior surface of the mesencephalic tegmentum, the medial surface of the cerebral peduncles, the III cranial nerve, and the mamillary bodies.

The vessels which penetrate the PPS and the anterior mesencephalic tegmentum were classified as paramedian thalamic arteries (PThAs), superior paramedial mesencephalic arteries (SPMAs), and inferior paramedian mesencephalic arteries (IPMAs). The PThAs and the SPMAs originated as a single or common trunk from the Pl segment. These trunks usually run back through the IF, where they branch and follow a sinuous course, entering the parenchyma through the PPS. The PThAs penetrate the anterior half of the PPS, and the SPMAs penetrate the posterior half of the PPS. The PPS was penetrated by 278 arteries, 123 (44%) in the anterior half and 155 (56%) in the posterior half. The arteries in the anterior half were larger (OD: 0.40–1.0 mm) and more lateral than the arteries in the posterior half (0.20–0.50 mm). These penetrating branches originated from 74 trunks (averaging 1.3 trunks for each Pl segment).

We classified these trunks into types based on the pattern of branching and on the distribution of their perforating branches through the PPS (Fig. 1) and into groups based on the patterns of their origin from the P1 segment (Fig. 2). We found seven types of trunks: 22 trunks were exclusive to the anterior half of the PPS, 10 trunks were exclusive to the posterior half, and 42 trunks were common to both halves. The trunks exclusive to the anterior half of the PPS entered the brain without branching (type A) in 77% (17/22) of the cases and branched (type B) in 33% (6/22) of the cases (Fig. 1). The 17 type A trunks (OD: 0.56±0.06 mm) arose 4.99±1.6 mm from the Pl segment origin. The five type B trunks (OD: 0.75±0.10 mm) arose 2.5±1.1 mm from the Pl segment origin. They branched into 11 perforating arteries (2.2±0.4 for each trunk) with an OD of 0.46±0.09 mm. Six of the trunks exclusive to the posterior half of the PPS entered the brain without branching (type C), and four branched before they penetrated the PPS (type D). The six type C trunks (OD: 0.39±0.06 mm) arose 1.4±0.7 mm from the Pl segment origin. The four type D trunks (OD: 0.36±0.08 mm) originated 2.65±0.09 mm from the Pl segment origin and branched into eight perforating arteries. The 42 trunks coursing to both halves of the PPS branched into 236 perforating arteries (5.6±1.6 arteries for each trunk). These trunks had ipsilateral perforating branches (type E), bilateral perforating branches (type F), and contralateral perforating branches (type G). There were 26 type E trunks (OD: 0.69±0.09 mm) which arose 2.76±0.84 mm from the Pl origin. They branched into 123 perforating arteries (4.73±1.06 branches from each trunk) with a diameter of 0.33±0.10 mm. There were 15 type F trunks (OD: 0.83±0.14 mm) which originated 2.35±0.87 mm from the P1 origin. They branched into 109 arteries (averaging 7.26 arteries for each

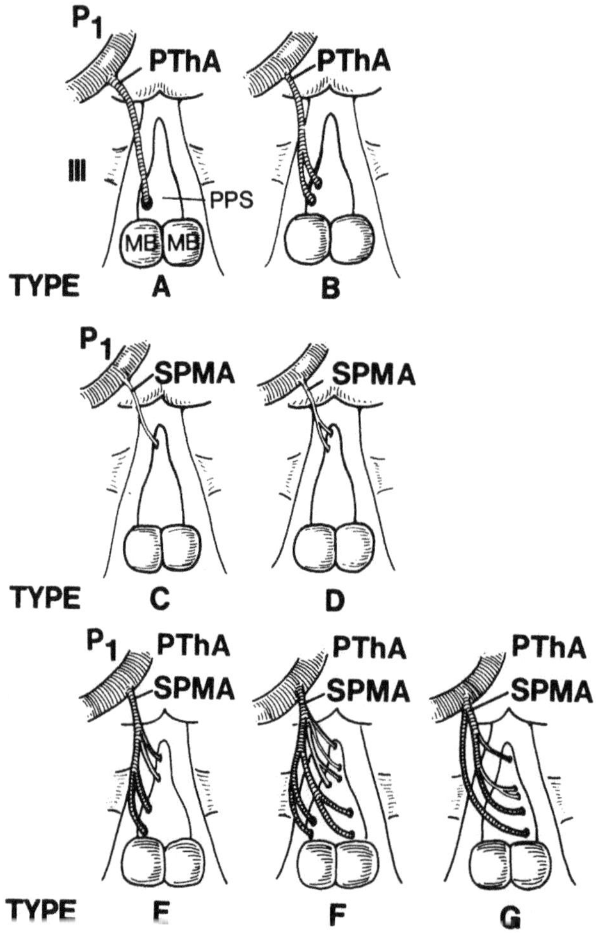

Fig. 1. Types of trunks according to pattern of branching and distribution of their perforating branches through the PPS

trunk) with an OD of 0.39±0.11 mm. Only one type G trunk (diameter: 0.9 mm) arose 2.5 mm from the P1 segment and branched into four perforating arteries.

In brief, 28 PThAs penetrating the anterior half of the PPS originated separately, 14 SPMAs penetrating the posterior half of the PPS originated separately, and 236 PThAs and SPMAs originated as common trunks. In six brains (21.5%), a P1 segment from one side was the parent vessel for ipsilateral, bilateral, and contralateral PThAs and SPMAs for the entire PPS. In addition, in three of these six P1 segments (10.7% of the 28 brains), a single trunk was the origin for all perforating branches that penetrated the PPS.

The second classification of six groups was based on the patterns of origin from the P1 segment (Fig. 2). In group 1, a single trunk arose from the P1 segment, and the PPS was vascularized by a single trunk (three brains). In group 2, two trunks originated from one P1 segment, one from each side (eight brains). In group 3, two

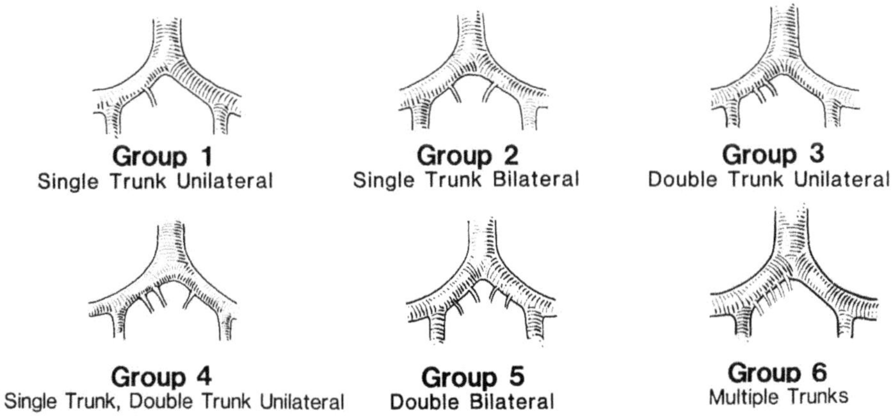

Fig. 2. Showing different groups of trunks based on patterns of their origin

trunks originated from one P1 segment, and none originated from the other P1 segment (three brains). In group 4, two trunks originated from one P1 segment, and one trunk arose from the other P1 segment. This was the most frequently observed pattern, present in 10 brains (35.7%). In group 5, two trunks originated from each P1 segment (two brains). Two other brains, whose pattern of origin did not fit in any of the previous groups (multiple trunks), were grouped together (group 6). Of 74 trunks, 72 arose from the superior and posterior wall, and two arose from the anterior wall of the P1 segment. Most of these trunks had an acute angle of origin, and the initial course was medial, superior and posterior. Forty arteries (OD: 0.15 ± 0.03 mm) arising from the perforating arteries vascularized the III cranial nerve in its course through the IF. These were present in 71% (20/28) of the brains.

In addition, 129 arteries (OD: 0.14 ± 0.03 mm) arising from the perforating arteries penetrated the medial surface of the cerebral peduncles in the IF. These arteries were found in all 28 brains, with an average of 4.6 arteries in each brain. The inferior paramedian mesencephalic arteries (IPMAs) arose from arterial trunks which originated from the P1 segment, from the proximal 7 mm of the SCAs, and from the last 5 mm of the basilar artery. These trunks coursed around the upper part of the pons through the inferior part of the IF, where they branched, producing the IPMAs. The IPMAs coursed dorsalward, reaching their penetration point at the anterior surface of the mesencephalic tegmentum immediately superior to the pontomesencephalic junction. The IPMAs supplied the paramedial territories of the inferior mesencephalon. In 28 brains, 30 trunks originated from the P1 segment, 42 trunks from the SCAs, and 24 trunks from the basilar artery. From the 30 P1 segment trunks, 18 arose from 17 right P1 segments (OD: 0.41 ± 0.09 mm), and 12 (OD: 0.39 ± 0.10 mm) arose from the left P1 segment. Half of the P1 segments did not have an IPMA originating from them, but from the posterior wall 1.34 ± 1.14 mm from the P1 segment origin. The 24 trunks (OD: 0.3 ± 0.08 mm) of the last 5 mm of the basilar artery originated from its posterior wall 2.58 ± 1.53 mm before the basilar bifurcation. Of the 28 basilar arteries, 14 (50%) were the origin of these 24 trunks. The 42 trunks (OD: 0.29 ± 0.10 mm) of the proximal 7 mm of the SCAs arose from the posterior and inferior wall following the same course as the basilar trunks. They originated from 29 SCAs 2.36 ± 1.62 mm from its origin. The remaining 27 SCAs (48.2%) did not have IPMA trunks.

In the 28 brains studied, we found 71 arteries coursing to the MB, with an average of 1.26 ± 0.95 arteries for each mamillary body. They arose from the PCoA, from the P1 segment, and from the perforating arteries. Thirty-two arteries arose from the distal one-third of the PCoA to 2.05 ± 1.39 mm from the junction with the PCA, 13 arose from the medial wall, and 19 from the superior wall, coursing superiorly and medially to supply the MB. Thirteen arteries (OD: 0.17 ± 0.04 mm) arose from the distal one-third of the P1 segment, at a distance of 7.33 ± 2.10 mm from the P1 segment origin. Seven vessels arose from the anterior wall, and six arose from the superior wall, coursing superiorly and medially to reach the MB. The other 26 arteries (OD: 0.14 ± 0.03 mm) arose from the PThAs.

Other vessels arising from the P1 segment are the circumflex arteries, which are divided into long and short circumflex groups. The short circumflex (ShC) arteries course to the geniculate bodies, and the long circumflex arteries (LC) course to the colliculi. We studied only the circumflex arteries arising from the P1 segment. Thirty-four ShC (OD: 0.26 ± 0.06 mm) were present in 46.4% of the hemispheres. The vessels arose from the posterior wall at a distance of 4.2 ± 1.5 mm from the P1 origin. They coursed medially to the PCA around the midbrain, supplying small perforating branches to the cerebral peduncle and substantia nigra. Most of the vessels (74%) terminated at the posterolateral border of the peduncle. Forty-nine LC (OD: 0.65 ± 0.008 mm) arteries were found arising from 49 P1 segments. For each P1 segment an average of 0.84±0.33 LC arteries arose from the posterior wall at a distance of 5.22 ± 1.4 mm from the P1 origin. They encircled the midbrain to reach the quadrigeminal plate, with small branches coming off the trunks and going to the cerebral peduncle, geniculate body, and tegmentum.

In conclusion, the interpeduncular fossa is an important space in the upper and anterior part of the brainstem because of the vascular structures that course through it arising from the posterior part of the circle of Willis. Since these vessels supplying the paramedian territories of the mesencephalon and the thalamus are surgically and clinically significant, the surgeon operating in that area should be aware of their origin and course so that injury from clip placement or other incidental vessel damage which could result in severe neurological deficit can be avoided.

References

Gomes FB, Dujovny M, Umansky F, Ausman JI, Diaz FG, Ray WJ, Mirchandani HG (1984) The recurrent artery of Huebner. J Neurosurg 60: 130–139

Microsurgical Anatomy of the Pineal and Midbrain Region

G. PENDL, Wien/Austria

Introduction

The surgical removal of lesions in the pineal region was and still is considered to be both dangerous and tedious. Even more so are intrinsic lesions within the midbrain. But since microsurgical techniques have renewed the debate, with the aid of technical advances in neuroimaging, anesthesia and postoperative care, it has become necessary to provide a more detailed anatomical knowledge of this region (Pendl 1984, 1985; Quest and Kleriga 1980; Rhoton et al. 1981; Yamamoto et al. 1981). Knowledge of the vascular structures and their microtopographic relationships, and knowledge of the finer anatomical structures for microsurgical dissection must be provided, not only in order to select the proper approach to this region of the pineal gland and the midbrain, but also to avoid further morbidity. Emphasis must be given to the vein of Galen and its tributaries, since they are a key to the success of surgery.

Material and Methods

This study is based on the results obtained from 26 cadaver brains studied under microsurgical operating conditions, as well as 6 human brains fixed in formalin, whose vascular systems were previously injected with acrylate. The characteristics of these findings were compared with the surgical exposures and personal experience in 40 lesions in the pineal region, 15 cases of them with intrinsic lesions within the midbrain, and with a mortality related to surgery in 3 cases (7.5%).

Observations and Discussion

On the basis of clinical and morphological findings the pathology of the pineal gland region includes: its tumors, the invading and intrinsic tumors of the midbrain and those of the posterior part of the third ventricle, as well as the various other lesions of the quadrigeminal cistern like arachnoid cysts, meningeomas and vein of Galen aneurysm. All these lesions are grouped together as pineal and midbrain lesions necessitating the same considerations about the anatomical structures especially the tributaries of the vein of Galen, when surgically approached. The different approaches to this region recommended in the literature (Pendl 1984) will be greatly influenced by the deep veins, not so much by the arteries, and their course will determine the choice of operative approach.

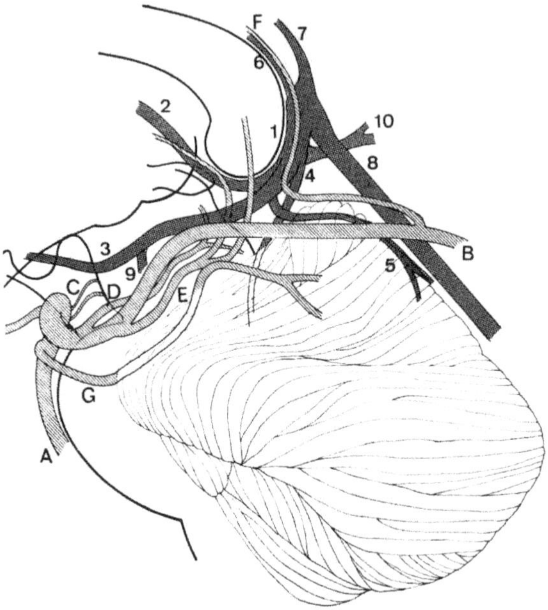

Fig. 1. Common course of arteries and veins of the midbrain and pineal region: *A,* basilar artery; *B,* posterior cerebral artery; *C,* posterior thalamoperforating arteries; *D,* quadrigeminal artery with geniculate artery; *E,* posterior choroidal arteries; *F,* posterior pericallosal artery; *G,* superior cerebellar artery; *1,* vein of Galen; *2,* internal cerebral vein; *3,* basal vein of Rosenthal; *4,* precentral cerebellar vein; *5,* superior cerebellar vein; *6,* posterior pericallosal vein; *7,* inferior sagittal sinus; *8,* straight sinus; *9,* lateral mesencephalic vein; *10,* internal occipital vein

Figure 1 shows the common course of the arteries and veins schematically. Additionally it should be noted that the redundancy of the vascular supply to the midbrain and anastomosis formation explains the rather rare occurrence of infarcts in the mesencephalic area and the remarkable tolerance of the midbrain to direct surgical intervention (Pendl 1976). The deep venous structures of the vein of Galen and its tributaries form a roof-like dense venous network above the pineal gland and the quadrigeminal plate (Fig. 2). Their vulnerability was the main cause of the pessimistic attitude towards surgery of lesions in the pineal region.

Figure 3 demonstrates the 5 most important and experienced approaches to the pineal-midbrain region; the subtemporal route to the cerebral peduncle and interpeduncular cistern should not be discussed further. The historical perspective of the surgery of pineal region lesions is important for understanding the past and still lasting discussion about choosing the most appropriate access but should be studied elsewhere (Pendl 1984; Zülch 1981). Since the various surgical approaches reported in the literature incorporate many personal and individualistic characteristics developed mainly by macrosurgical techniques, one has to compare and reevaluate all these approaches under the light of microsurgical techniques. We will confine our study to the 4 most important approaches: 1. Transcallosal approach, 2. transventricular approach, 3. occipital transtentorial approach, 4. infratentorial supracerebellar approach.

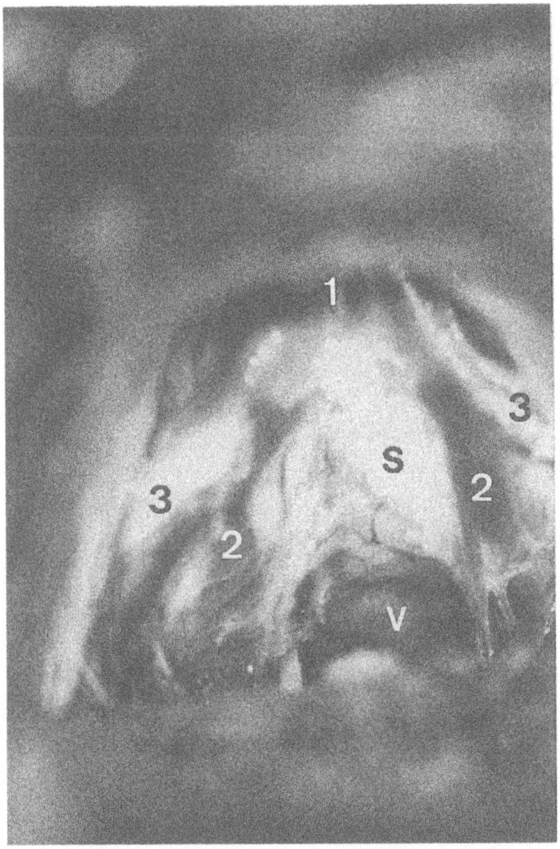

Fig. 2. Infratentorial exposure of the main tributaries of the vein of Galen in the tentorial notch after research of a small pineal tumor: *1*, vein of Galen; *2*, internal cerebral veins; *3*, basal veins of Rosenthal; *S*, splenium; *V*, roof of third ventricle

1. Transcallosal Approach

This approach formerly preferred by most neurosurgeons, was introduced by Dandy in 1921. Figure 4 demonstrates the exposure of a pineal lesion by this approach in a schematic drawing showing how the deep veins block the access to a pineal tumor and even more to the quadrigeminal cistern and plate in case of a midbrain tumor. The site and length of the craniotomy in the parieto-occipital region parallel to the sagittal sinus depends on the location of major bridging veins to the sinus. The dura mater is flapped towards the sinus, evacuation of the CSF from hydrocephalic enlarged ventricles will help to retract the parieto-occipital lobe between draining veins from the falx in order to expose the splenium of the corpus callosum, which has to be transected in a length of 1.5–3 cm according to the extension of the lesion. It may also be necessary to incise the inferior sagittal sinus vertically and the lower part of the falx in order to obtain a better view towards the opposite side. The vein of Galen with both internal cerebral veins and basal veins of Rosenthal, as well as the medial occipital vein will not only hinder the access to a pineal tumor but even more to the quadrigeminal plate or ambient cistern (Fig. 5). Therefore we consider this approach to the pineal region and midbrain as the least feasible except in cases

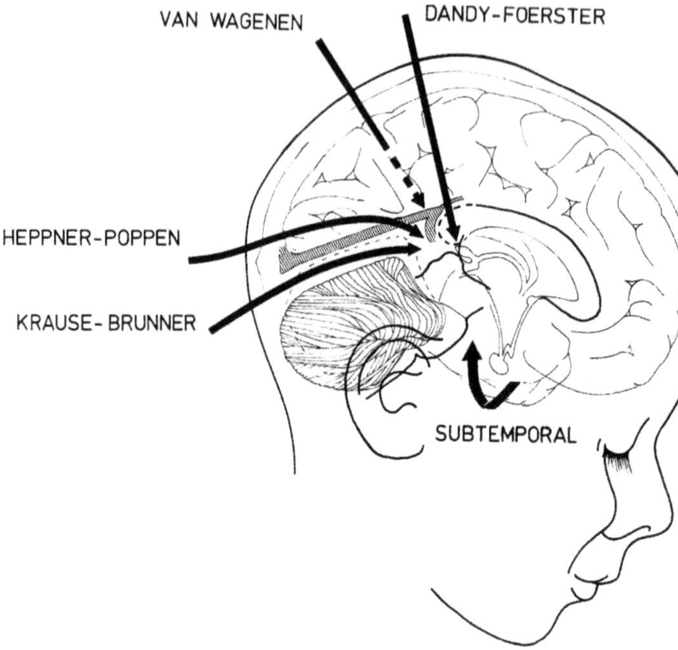

Fig. 3. Schematic presentation of the 5 most important approaches to the pineal and midbrain region

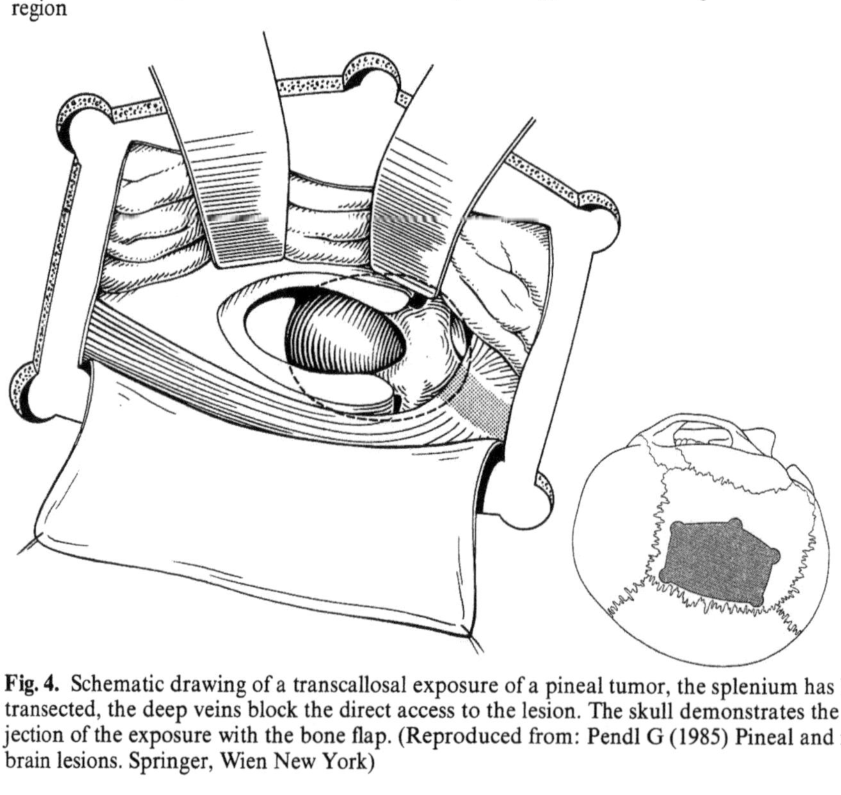

Fig. 4. Schematic drawing of a transcallosal exposure of a pineal tumor, the splenium has been transected, the deep veins block the direct access to the lesion. The skull demonstrates the projection of the exposure with the bone flap. (Reproduced from: Pendl G (1985) Pineal and midbrain lesions. Springer, Wien New York)

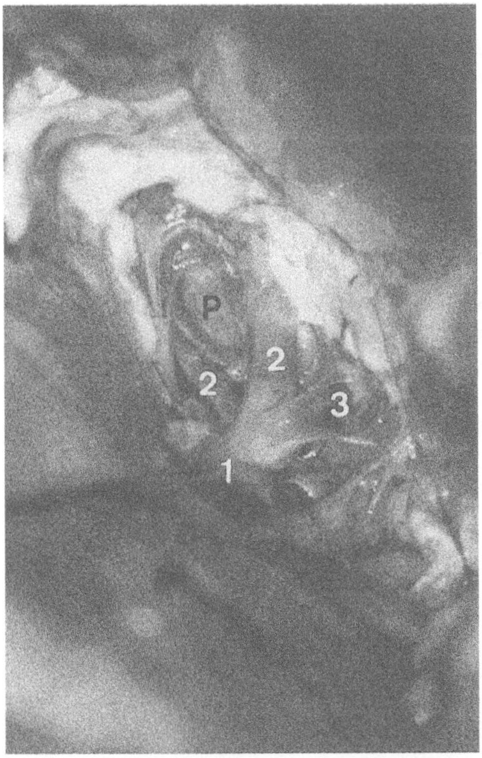

Fig. 5. Exposure of the pineal gland *P,* in a fresh cadaver using the transcallosal approach. The vein of Galen *1,* internal cerebral veins *2,* and the basal vein of Rosenthal *3,* obstruct the access to the quadrigeminal plate

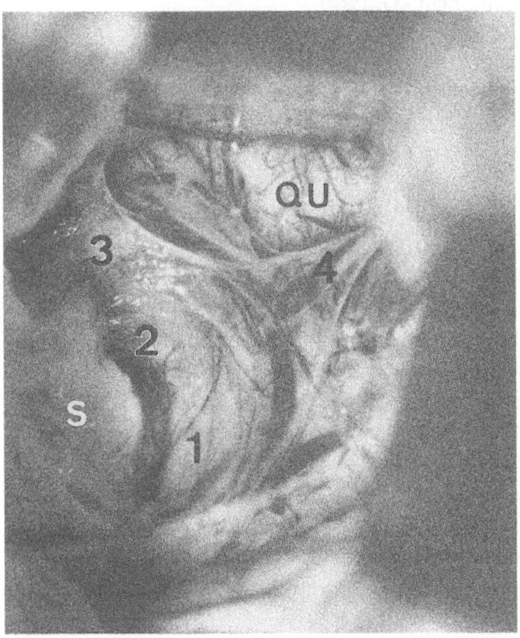

Fig. 6. Exposure of the deep veins by a right transventricular approach: *1,* vein of Galen; *2,* internal cerebral vein; *3,* basal vein of Rosenthal; *4,* precentral cerebellar vein; *QU,* quadrigeminal plate; *S,* splenium

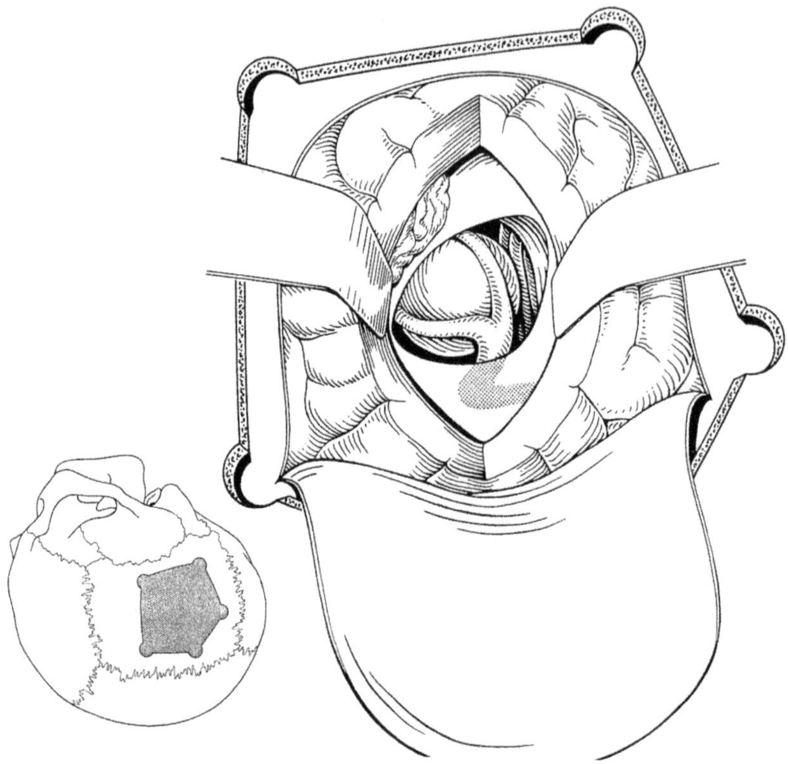

Fig. 7. Schematic drawing of a right transventricular exposure of a pineal tumor, the deep veins block the direct access to the lesion. The skull demonstrates the projection of the exposure with the bone flap. (Reproduced from: Pendl G, 1985)

of vein of Galen aneurysms, where the feeding arteries are best exposed by this approach.

2. Transventricular Approach

This approach, published by Van Wagenen in 1931, uses the hydrocephalic enlarged lateral ventricles as an access. After an L-shaped cortical incision in the superior temporal gyrus towards the parietal region of the trigonal area of the lateral ventricle, the ventricle is reached close behind the choroid plexus. The expansive lesion will be localized under the thinned wall of the ventricle and after incision of the ventricular wall the lesion is enucleated by sparing the deep lying structures. Although in small lesions of the midline in the pineal region the tributaries to the vein of Galen will not allow an easy dissection, also in cases of intrinsic lesions of the midbrain the exposure of the quadrigeminal plate will be obstructed by these veins (Fig. 6). Figure 7 shows schematically the exposure of a pineal lesion by a transventricular approach with the vein of Galen and even more the basal vein of Rosenthal obstructing the access, the variable internal occipital vein being not included in the drawing.

3. Occipital Transtentorial Approach

This approach described by Heppner in 1959 became popular through Poppen (1966), although this version is far too narrow and technically difficult. In this approach now much preferred, the patient is usually placed in a semisitting position and the craniotomy is placed close to the sagittal and right transverse sinus over the occipital pole. The dura mater is incised in a T-shaped or stellate fashion and the occipital lobe is retracted superiorly and laterally. Bridging veins have to be sacrificed, also occasionally bridging veins from the inferior aspect of the occipital lobe to the transverse sinus and tentorium. When the tentorial edge is reached it is incised parallel to the straight sinus and eventually both edges retracted with sutures thus exposing the arachnoid folds of the quadrigeminal cistern if not the lesion itself. A good view of the splenium with the Galenic venous system, also of the quadrigeminal plate is provided. Care has to be taken not to injure the posterior cerebral artery within the calcarine fissure and the internal occipital vein from the retraction, although the precentral cerebellar vein can be sacrificed without having to expect any unfavourable reaction. Figure 8 schematically demonstrates the exposure of a pineal lesion by this approach with the venous architecture rooflike on top of the lesion except for the precentral cerebellar vein. Also in cases of midbrain lesions the access to the quadrigeminal plate will not be hampered by the vein of Galen and its tributaries (Fig. 9). Reid and Clark (1978) have compared this approach to the infratentorial approach and they believe that the occipital transtentorial approach gives a broader range of exposure.

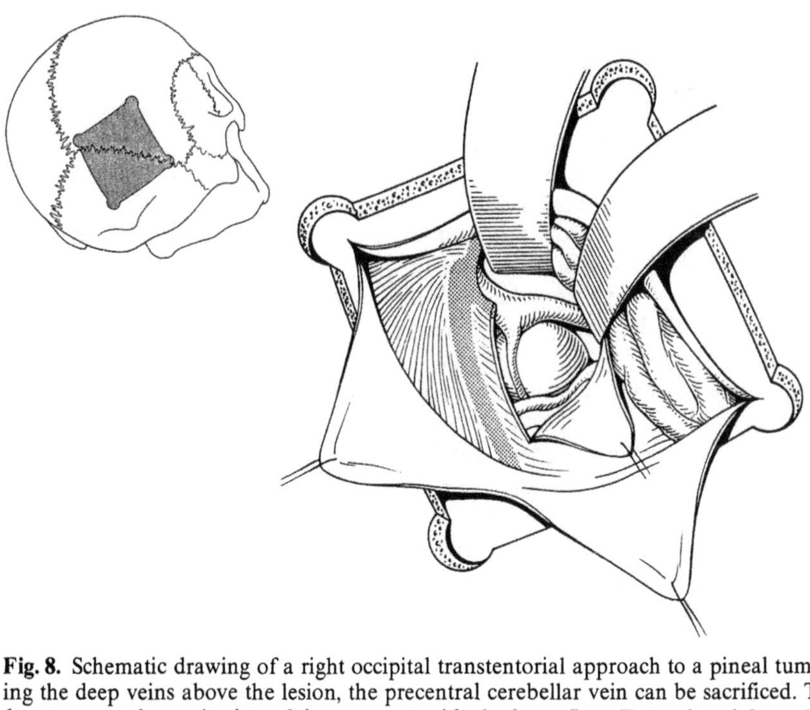

Fig. 8. Schematic drawing of a right occipital transtentorial approach to a pineal tumor keeping the deep veins above the lesion, the precentral cerebellar vein can be sacrificed. The skull demonstrates the projection of the exposure with the bone flap. (Reproduced from: Pendl G, 1985)

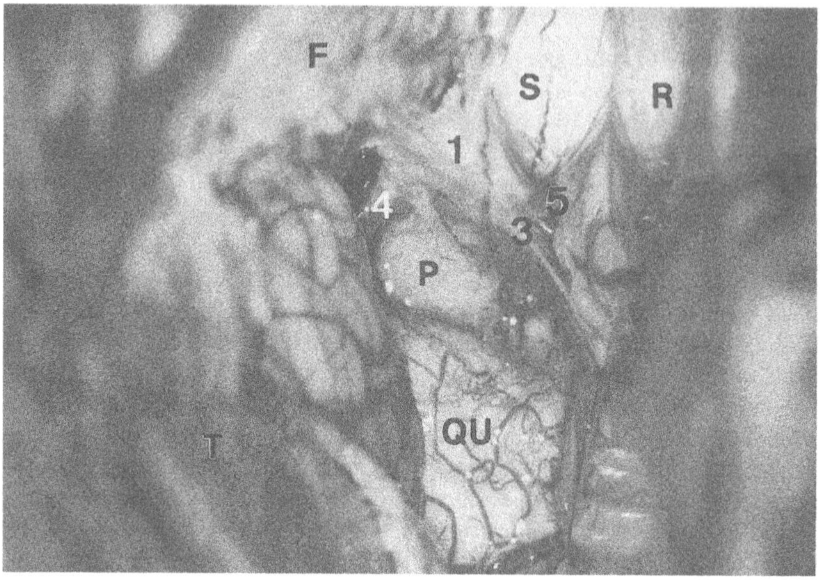

Fig. 9. Oblique view from the right into the quadrigeminal cistern using the occipital transtentorial approach in a fresh cadaver: *1,* vein of Galen; *3,* basal vein of Rosenthal; *4,* precentral cerebellar vein; *5,* internal occipital vein; *P,* pineal gland; *S,* splenium; *QU,* quadrigeminal plate; *F,* falx; *T,* tentorium (incised); *R,* retractor

4. Infratentorial-Supracerebellar Approach

Special credit must be given to Stein (1971) for reviving this surgical approach to the pineal region first described by Krause in 1911. In this approach, a suboccipital craniectomy with exposure of the torcula, and extension well above the transverse sinus bilaterally in order to allow upward retraction of the tentorium if necessary, is performed with the patient usually in a sitting position. It is possible to spare the arch of the atlas and also the foramen must not be reached. After the dura is opened Y-shaped and bridging veins from the cerebellar hemispheres and vermis to the tentorium are sacrificed, the cerebellum sinks well down and reveals a wide enough gap under the tentorium to the quadrigeminal cistern. Almost no further displacement downward with a retractor is necessary. The dense opalescent arachnoid folds of the quadrigeminal cistern obstruct the topography of the quadrigeminal cistern and must be parted with sharp dissection in order not to tear the vascular structures (Fig. 10). After the dissection, the quadrigeminal plate with the pineal gland and veins is sufficiently exposed. The deeper venous structures are well exposed, rooflike above the surgical field, occasionally only the precentral cerebellar vein must be sacrificed without producing any adverse effects (Fig. 11). Usually after a lesion of the pineal region has been removed a large opening to the posterior third ventricle will result (Fig. 12). In the lateral parts of the quadrigeminal cistern, small branches of the median posterior choroidal artery will be encountered and may be sacrificed without adverse effects. Figure 13 shows this approach schematically with a pineal mass lesion.

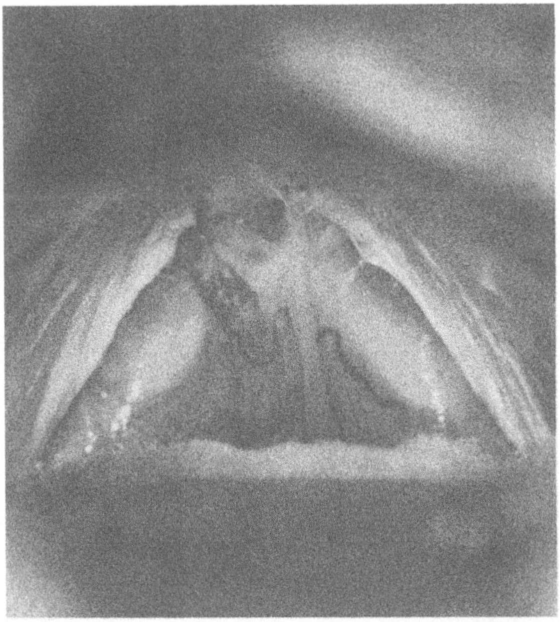

Fig. 10. The dense opalescent arachnoid folds of the quadrigeminal cistern in the tentorial notch by an infratentorial supracerebellar exposure

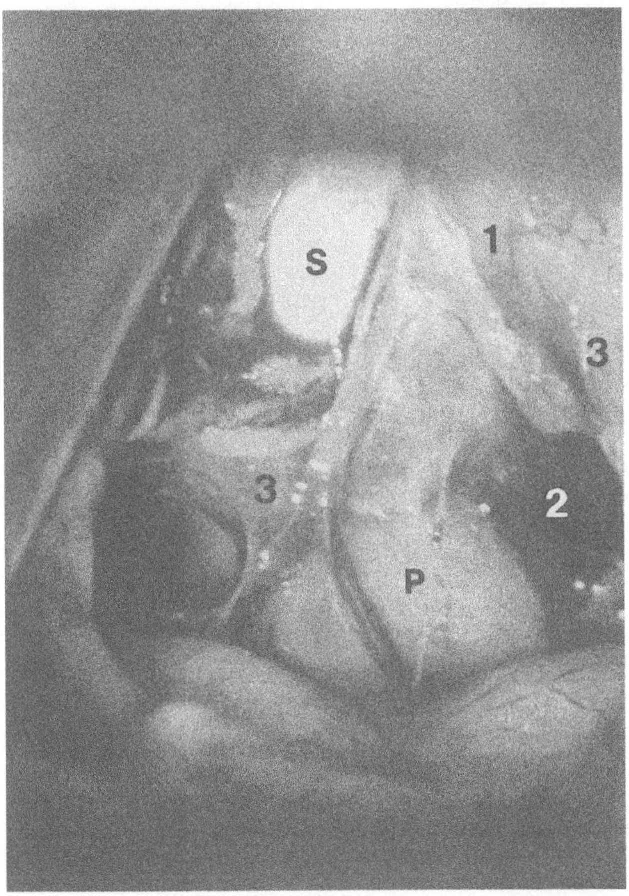

Fig. 11. Exposure of the quadrigeminal cistern with pineal gland in a fresh cadaver by an infratentorial supracerebellar approach: *1*, vein of Galen; *2*, right internal cerebral vein; *3*, basal veins of Rosenthal; *P*, pineal gland nestling between the upper colliculi; *S*, splenium

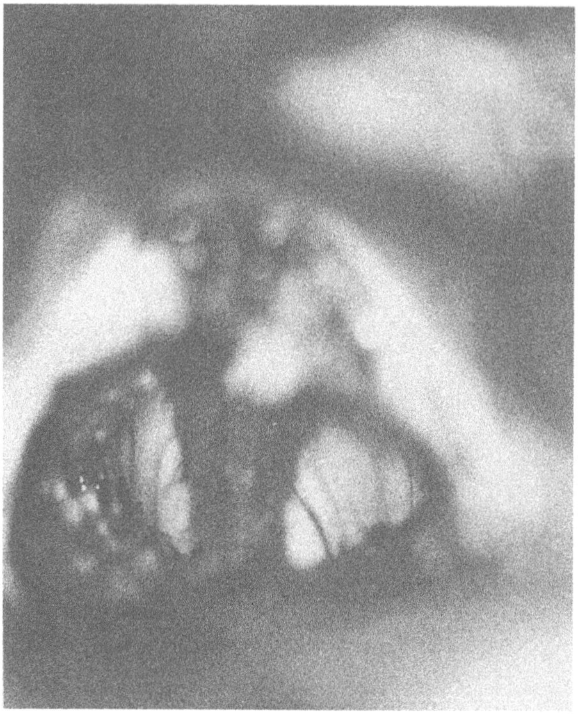

Fig. 12. Large opening into the third ventricle after removal of a pineal tumor by an infratentorial approach. Note the choroid plexus on the roof of the ventricle

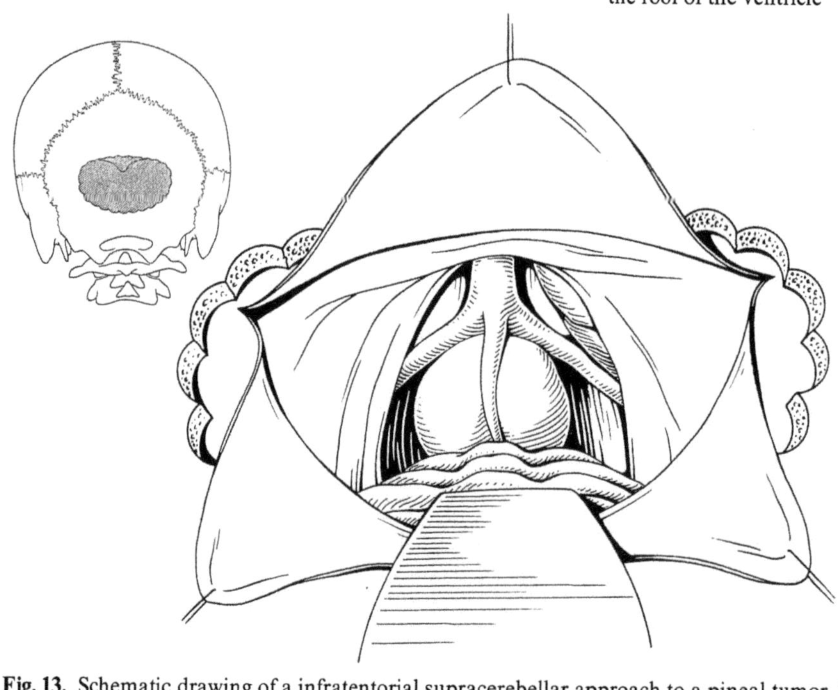

Fig. 13. Schematic drawing of a infratentorial supracerebellar approach to a pineal tumor. The skull demonstrates the projection of the exposure with the craniectomy. (Reproduced from: Pendl G, 1985)

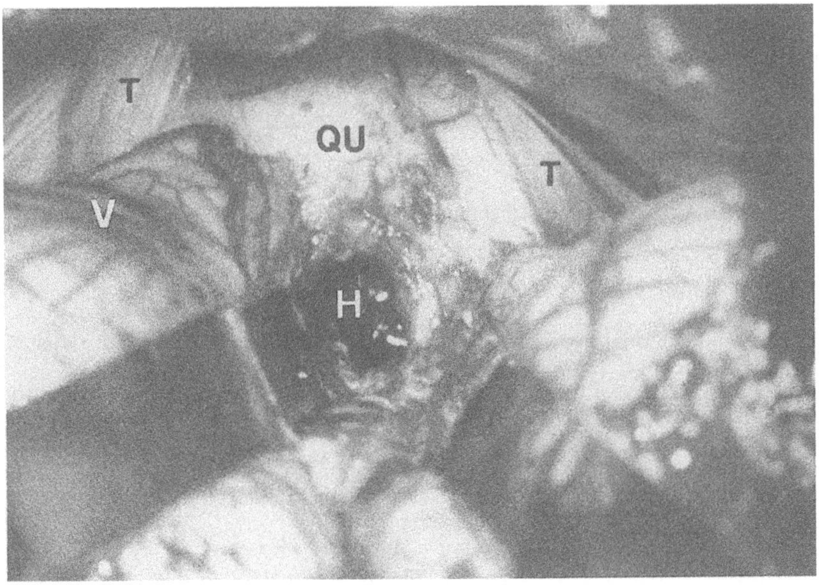

Fig. 14. Exposure of the quadrigeminal plate *QU*, in case of a hematoma of the midbrain *H*, by an infratentorial approach, the right hemisphere is incised at the anterior margin close to the vermis *V*; *T*, tentorium

In order to expose the quadrigeminal plate and reach the ambient cistern the anterior margin of the cerebellar hemisphere close to the vermis is incised for 1 or 2 cm (Fig. 14). The incision of the quadrigeminal plate in 15 of our cases of intrinsic lesions of the midbrain was either performed in the trigonum lemnisci or just below the trochlear nerve on either side, also the lesion was followed right from the cerebellar region well into the midbrain and often as far as into the posterior third ventricle. If dissection is confined to the pathological tissue no further mortality is to be expected.

Conclusion

The feasibility for direct surgical attack upon lesions of the pineal and midbrain region depends on the angioarchitecture of the pineal region. The most important factors for which approach to choose are the vascular course of the vein of Galen and its tributaries as well as achieving an access to intrinsic lesions of the midbrain through the quadrigeminal plate. Therefore the infratentorial approach is recommended, an alternative route is the occipital transtentorial approach, both techniques are most suitable to protect the deep veins and explore the pineal region in all respects. Either approach provides a safe, adequate exposure of the pineal region, although in cases of intrinsic midbrain lesions, the infratentorial approach with additional partial transection of the cerebellar hemisphere should be preferred. The transcallosal approach is considered as the most inadequate, which for many years was preferred but was burdened with greater surgical risk. Microtopographic studies and surgical experience in the past 12 years seem to support this attitude.

References

Dandy WE (1921) An operation for the removal of pineal tumors. Surg Gynecol Obstet 33:113–119

Heppner F (1959) Zur Operationstechnik bei Pinealomen. Zentralbl Neurochir 19:219–224

Krause F (1911) Chirurgie des Gehirns und Rückenmarks. Vol. 1. Urban & Schwarzenberg, Berlin Wien

Pendl G (1976) Infratentorial approach to mesencephalic tumors. In: Koos WTh, Böck F, Spetzler FR (eds) Clinical microneurosurgery. Thieme, Stuttgart, pp 143–150

Pendl G (1984) The surgery of pineal lesions – historical perspectives. In: Neuwelt EA (ed) Diagnosis and treatment of pineal region tumors. Williams & Wilkins, Baltimore London, p 139–154

Pendl G (1984) Microsurgical anatomy of the pineal region. In: Neuwelt EA (ed) Diagnosis and treatment of pineal region tumors. Williams & Wilkins, Baltimore London, pp 155–207

Pendl G (1985) Pineal and midbrain lesions. Springer, Wien New York

Poppen JL (1966) The right occipital approach to a pinealoma. J Neurosurg 25:706–710

Quest DO, Kleriga E (1980) Microsurgical anatomy of the pineal region. Neurosurgery 6:385–390

Reid WS, Clark WK (1978) Comparison of the infratentorial and transtentorial approaches to the pineal region. Neurosurgery 3:1–8

Rhoton AL, Yamamoto I, Peace DA (1981) Microsurgery of the third ventricle: Part 2. Operative approaches. Neurosurgery 8:357–373

Stein BM (1971) The infratentorial supracerebellar approach to pineal lesions. J Neurosurg 35:197–202

Van Wagenen WP (1931) A surgical approach for the removal of certain pineal tumors. Surg Gynecol Obstet 53:216–220

Yamamoto I, Rhoton AL, Peace DA (1981) Microsurgery of the third ventricle: Part 1. Microsurgical anatomy. Neurosurgery 8:334–356

Zülch KJ (1981) Reflections on the surgery of the pineal gland. Neurosurg Rev 4:152–162

Pathology, Metabolic Disturbances

Neuropathology of the Processes in the Third Ventricle and the Brain Stem

K. J. Zülch, Köln/FRG

It is exactly 75 years now that Fedor Krause in Berlin opened the way to surgery of the cranial base, first in 1900 by removing through the transfrontal approach a pistol bullet from the chiasm and later in 1904 by the hemilateral flap to the posterior fossa the way to the cerebellopontine angle for the removal of the acoustic neurilemmoma (Krause 1909–1912). Both ways became the routine technique for the following century and are still for today.

The very subject of my paper is the illustration of the pathological processes by demonstrating both, either the most important or very rare lesions (Fig. 1).

Eight topographic subdivisions shall be discussed:

1. The sella
2. The parasellar region
3. The third ventricle, basal section
4. The third ventricle, oral and anterior section
5. The third ventricle, caudal/posterior section or the quadrigeminal region
6. The cranial basis
7. The posterior fossa
8. The cranial spinal outlet.

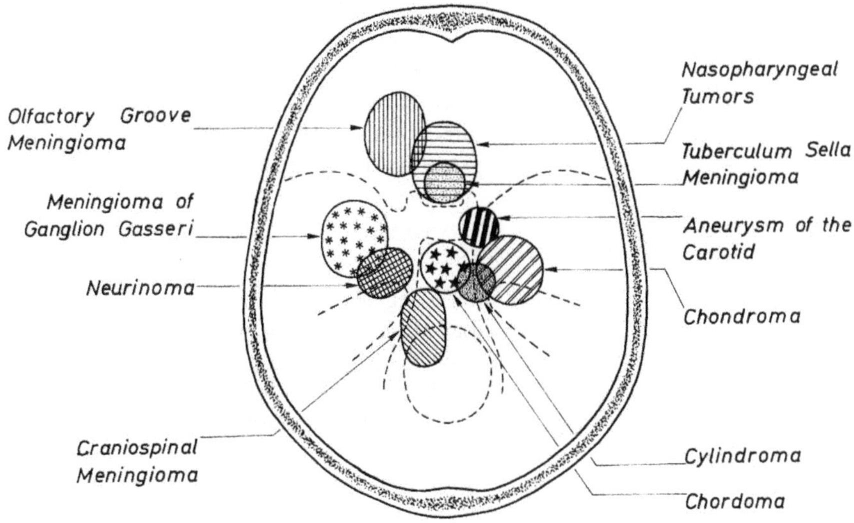

Fig. 1. Picture showing main pathological processes in the skull base that can affect the third ventricle

The Sella Region

This region has been broadly discussed in Hannover in 1981 (Samii and Jannetta 1981). I recall only the subclassification of the tumors for the neuropathologist and general pathologist. The terminology of the pituitary adenomas is still the conventional one, e.g., the subdivision into chromophilic (acido- and basophilic) chromophobe and the oncocytic varieties and the "mixed" tumors. Earlier we have shown that by special sophisticated methods the endocrinological properties of the aforementioned tumors can be further analyzed and subclassified. It has to be remembered that many endocrinological active tumors are in fact either mixed tumors or microadenomas, such as commonly the prolactinomas.

Even if these have not been localized in the CT exactly, they may be removed by the transnasal approach to the sella, a technique I had the opportunity to admire in the skillful hands of Dr. Norman Dott in Edinburgh as a student already in 1933. The progress in the diagnostic methods has been of great advantage for the neurosurgeons, namely, that the adenomas are detected far earlier, e.g., when they are still of a smaller size; the large lesions with extensions into the frontal and temporal lobe as well as with growth toward the third ventricle or clivus are now getting rarer. Very infrequent or almost only occurring as a rarity are subdural extensions of an adenoma into the diploe of the base from where the tumor may turn up into the intracranial cavity around the vessels or nerves after piercing the basal dura.

The different growth of the second frequent tumor in the sellar region, the craniopharyngioma, is well-known intrasellar, intra-/suprasellar, whereas such lesions located entirely within the lumen of the third ventricle and without any macroscopic pedicle to the sellar region are less well known.

Parasellar Tumors

Among the parasellar tumors the meningiomas of tuberculum anterius are probably the best known and most frequent although even olfactory meningiomas and adenoid cystic adenomas (cylindromas) may extend posteriorly. The same is true for other "nasopharyngeal" tumors: fibromas, sarcomas, lymphomas (reticular sarcomas), carcinomas etc. The parasellar tumors sensu strictiori are the teratomas and epidermoids as well as the infra- and suprasellar aneurysms of the carotid artery.

Tumors of the Basis of the Third Ventricle

A few tumor entities are particularly interesting because of their neurological syndrome, amongst these the gangliocytomas (pubertas praecox, macrogenitosomia) and the ectopic pinealomas. The former have been analyzed by the endocrinological studies of Spatz (1951, 1958) and E. and B. Scharrer (1954) on the secreting properties of some of the autonomic cell groups in the hypothalamus, which explained this syndrome (nucleus Cajal).

The latter form is a most important infundibular or suprasellar tumor now usually recorded by some authorities as a germinoma. Here the inanition, polydipsia and polyurea and other autonomic symptoms apart from a loss of consciousness are prominent symptoms, as also lesions of the optic system are.

Amongst the "infundibular tumors" metastases from pinealomas/germinomas and from cerebellar medulloblastomas by the CSF spread must be mentioned, as well as the primary tumors of this region, the granular cell myoblastoma or pituicytoma.

Oral/Anterior Section of the Third Ventricle

Chorioid plexus papillomas, the ependymal cyst of the foramen Monro, epidermoids, and the already mentioned rare intraventricular type of craniopharyngioma are prominent. However, it is less well-known that even real ependymomas occur in that region.

Paramedian tumors of the ventricles as the typical ventricular tumors in tuberous sclerosis (subependymal giant cell astrocytomas) can extend into that part of the ventricle.

It is most rational to consider here also the septum pellucidum neoplasms which may be either members of the oligodendroglioma or the glioblastoma group. Some of the frontal astrocytomas, namely, the frontomedial type, can blow up the septum by infiltration and thus may appear also as a genuine septal tumor.

Caudal or Posterior Segment of Third Ventricle – The Quadrigeminal Region

It is interesting to see that quadrigeminal tumors here play the most important role and can be of a very similar outer appearance. Amongst the pineal tumors according to the WHO classification the benign pinealocytoma and the malignant pineoblastoma (which correspond to the medulloblastomas elsewhere in malignancy) have to be distinguished. Moreover, ependymomas of the posterior part of the third ventricle can act as quadrigeminal tumors as well as the usually pilocytic astrocytomas of the quadrigeminal plate itself. Also to be mentioned are the ependymal and arachnoid cysts of the quadrigeminal region as real space-occupying tumors, yet we should not forget the genuine teratomas of this region. These teratomas were particularly thouroughly studied at the beginning of the century because of the not infrequent occurrence of pubertas praecox in these cases. Lastly, also the meningioma of the hiatus tentorii can act as a typical quadrigeminal tumor.

Historically important is the last mentioned tumor of this region, namely, the meningioma of the hiatus tentorii which was the first "quadrigeminal" tumor to be successfully operated already in 1913, again by Fedor Krause after a neurological diagnosis by Oppenheim (see Zülch 1981).

The neuropathologists of today are very satisfied by the issue of the World Health Organization (Histological Typing of tumors of the Central Nervous System), the new classification of the brain tumors (Zülch 1979). I may characterize the importance of this new classification by the following points:

1. The entities are well characterized
2. They provide biological information by grades of malignancy
3. In dubious cases there are still two interpretations possible
4. Anaplastic variants are foreseen for most groups

However, in spite of this statement I will discuss here one important point, the pathology of the pineal tumors, where we could not come to a consent and did not foresee two possible different classifications: This was the problem of the pinealoma of Krabbe (1923), the two-cell tumor.

In Europe since the classic descriptions of Krabbe of the "pinealoma" this term has been predominant till our time and only in the last years it has been partly or totally replaced by the concept that this type of a two-cell type tumor would actually correspond to the germinoma (seminoma) in the sense of Friedman (1947).

It has been my personal opinion (Riverson and Zülch 1979) from the beginning that there are two types of two-cell pineal tumors, which may be histologically similar in the pattern yet different in origin. I am not of the opinion that all of the two-cell type tumors (which we called anisomorphous in former editions) were in fact germinomas. Our special studies (see Riverson and Zülch 1979; Federmann 1983) proved that actually two types could be distinguished by more accurate histological investigations.

One of the typical two-cell pattern tumors could be impregnated by the method of Girolami, where the elements mimicked the pineal parenchymal cells of Del Rio Hortega; on the other side they were negative when stained with PAS.

The second type was characterized by greater polymorphism containing usually even large polynuclear cells, which did not show any trend to impregnation according to Girolami, however, were stained heavily by PAS.

The former was the pinealoma type of Krabbe, the second the germinoma type.

I have listed all my arguments in 1986, but shall repeat here only a few ones: In one of our cases of a small quadrigeminal tumor with a large ectopic seeding, probably a secondary, we found in the CSF cells with long processes, which were almost identical with those Del Rio Hortega has described in his normal anatomy (see Riverson and Zülch 1979, Figs. 3, 4). Furthermore, Dr. Matsutani, a co-worker of Dr. Sano, has proved immunologically that the large tumor cells were derivative from the pineal parenchyma (Matsutani 1976).

The last point in my arguments is the trend to calcification of many of these quadrigeminal two-cell type tumors, a characteristic which is certainly infrequent in germinomas. Meanwhile in 1985 Dr. Sano also shared my opinion of the twofold nature of these tumors.

Tumors of the Posterior Fossa

Here I shall briefly demonstrate the midline cerebellar tumors, the large pilocytic astrocytomas, mostly cystic with small mural nodules, and the medulloblastomas, both not only be encountered at the vermis but rarely also in the pons. If the medulloblastomas occur in the lateral cerebellar hemisphere and in an older age group, they usually belong to the type which has been described as the desmoplastic type of medulloblastoma by Rubinstein and Northfield (1964), however, had been earlier described as arachnoidal cerebellar sarcoma by Foerster and Gagel (1939). Berghorn (1982) has recently confirmed the arguments of Foerster and Gagel.

Another common tumor of the cerebellum is the hemangioblastoma Lindau, sited either in the hemisphere or else within the fourth ventricle itself, extending then from the posterior roof. It may occur single or multiple. The angioblastoma of the roof of the fourth ventricle may be in our appearance very similar to the more common ependymoma, which, however, sticks firmly to the ventricular floor. In both cases, however, the anterior part of the fourth ventricle is usually enlarged.

Ependymomas rarely occur also in the cerebellopontine angle and extend only with a small tongue into the fourth ventricle. In the angle also choroid plexus papillomas are encountered, similarly located as the meningiomas which start growth at the tip of the pyramid.

However, the most frequent representative angle tumor is the neurilemmoma, which should be detected today – if possible – when still very small and growing within the meatus. Sometimes the larger representatives can have gross arachnoidal cysts at the caudal end of the tumor, and this adds much volume so that a remarkable cerebellar pressure cone may result. In the cerebellopontine angle also chondromas may be encountered as well as adenoid cystic carcinomas (cylindromas). Glomus tumors (chemodectomas) are characterized because of their large extension with projection not infrequently to the outer ear, and also by their extreme vascularity. Epidermoids also occur in the cerebellopontine angle as sometimes also saccular aneurysms do.

Tumors at the "Cranial Outlet"

The most frequent tumors in the medulla oblongata and upper spinal cord are probably the pilocytic astrocytomas, which we have recorded also already in the vermis and in the pons. Here they sometimes form great nodules at the outer side, and this is the more favorable appearance compared to the other type diffusely infiltrating the pontine parenchyma. On the ventral side of the medulla oblongata large saccular aneurysms may occur at the basilar artery besides the more common fusiform type, which, however, has no surgical importance.

At the cranial outlet, the foramen magnum meningiomas and neurilemmomas are the two most common tumors. Meningiomas are found in two forms, either called craniospinal, when the bulk of the tumor mass lies within the posterior fossa, or spinocranial, when only the smaller part is located in the posterior fossa and the larger part of the volume beyond the foramen magnum.

The neurilemmomas on the other part have a predilection for lying outside the foramen magnum, where Fields, Zülch et al. have described in 1972 a prominent type of neurilemmoma at the second and third cervical roots. One can count that one-tenth of the cervical neurilemmomas are sited at the roots C 1–4.

The Cranial Base

The tumors of the base of the skull should be subdivided according to three different localizations (a) anterior part, (b) middle part, (c) posterior part.

a) The important representatives of the anterior part have been described above as the sellar and parasellar tumors.
b) In the middle part the sellar and parasellar tumors were discussed as well as the tumors extending from above downwards.
c) In the posterior part the glomus jugulare tumors have to be more broadly described. They appear at the anterior part of the petrous bone and may extend to the outer meatus of the ear as a polyp or in the contrary direction down to the

mastoid process. They can destroy the bony outlets of cranial nerves or penetrate even into the jugular vein or the neighboring dural sinuses.

Adenoid cystic carcinomas (cylindromas) were already mentioned in the anterior third, however, may also have their origin near the tuba Eustachii, e.g., the tip of the petrous bone.

Chondromas, extra- or intradural osteochondromas, if large, may destroy the tip of the pyramid and the clivus, but may also extend forwards to the nasopharynx. Lipomas in the cerebellopontine angle are rare as well as ceruminal adenocarcinomas are, which invade the petrous bone and may be histologically mistaken at first sight for choroid plexus papillomas.

The midline tumors of the clivus, preferentially chordomas, can have the size of a head of a pin and discovered incidentally (Ribbert et Steiner 1894, in 2% of autopsies) or may attain any other size. Their extensions may be either in the direction of the nasopharynx and chiasm or toward the foramen magnum.

Finally we have to mention the arachnitic, usually cystic lesions around the cisterns of the base, particularly the chiasm and foramen magnum. These cysts are usually formed in the large cisterns, mainly cisterna magna, or cause a closure of the foramen Magendi or the foramina Luschka. Near the foramen Magendi they can appear as a close sac filling the cisterna magna and extending toward the fourth ventricle (Zülch 1950).

Other tumors of the cranial base may have as an origin bone, cartilage, connective tissue, vascular tissue, or they may belong to the family of the lymphomas.

Giant cell tumors (fibroma, epulis) and bone cysts are rare in the base of the skull (sphenoid, sellar region, petrous bone), they may be included into the group of the semibenign osteoclastomas.

Finally I would like to emphasize that neuropathology of today is familiar with the location, form and growth behavior of the pathological lesions around the brainstem and the third ventricle. With a good knowledge of the pathology it is possible to recognize and define almost all of these lesions preoperatively by radiologic pictures and good computer-assisted tomograms (eventually taken by the bone window) and often even better in NMR pictures (posterior fossa and cranial basis). Therefore a good knowledge of pathology will be of paramount importance for diagnosis and surgery of this region.

References

Berghorn WJ (1982) Untersuchungen zur biologischen Wertigkeit des klassischen und des desmoplastischen Medulloblastoms. Med. Dissertation, Universität Düsseldorf

Federmann M (1983) Die klinische Symptomatik der Tumoren der Pinealisregion. Med. Dissertation, Universität Köln

Fields WS, Zülch KJ, Maslenikov V (1972) High cervical neurinoma. Special neurologic and radiologic features. Zentralbl Neurochir 33:89–102

Foerster O, Gagel O (1939) Das umschriebene Arachnoidalsarkom des Kleinhirns. Z Gesamte Neurol Psychiatr 164:565–580

Friedman NB (1947) Germinoma of the pineal. Its identity with germinoma ("seminoma") of the testis. Cancer Res 7:363–368

Krabbe KH (1923) The pineal gland, especially in relation to the problem of its supposed significance in sexual development. Endocrinology 7:374–414

Krause F (1909–1912) Surgery of the brain and spinal cord on personal experiences. 3 vols. Rebman, New York

Matsutani M (1976) Ultrastructural study of pinealoma in view of its histogenesis. No To Shinkei 28:41–56

Ribbert H, Steiner H (1894) Über die Ecchondrosis physalifora sphenooccipitalis, nach Untersuchungen von Hermann Steiner. Zentralbl Allg Pathol 5:457–461

Riverson EA, Zülch KJ (1979) Pineal parenchymal tumours and germinomas (the problem of the so-called pinealomas). Neurosurg Rev 1:3–11

Rubinstein LJ, Northfield DWC (1964) The medulloblastoma and the so-called "arachnoidal cerebellar sarcoma". A critical re-examination of a nosological problem. Brain 87:379–410

Samii M, Jannetta PJ (1981) The cranial nerves. Springer, Berlin Heidelberg New York

Scharrer E, Scharrer B (1954) Neurosekretion. Von Möllendorffs Handbuch der mikroskopischen Anatomie des Menschen VI/5. Springer, Berlin Göttingen Heidelberg

Spatz H (1951) Neues über die Verknüpfung von Hypophyse und Hypothalamus. Acta Neuroveg (Wien) 3:5–49

Spatz H (1958) Die proximale (supraselläre) Hypophyse, ihre Beziehungen zum Diencephalon und ihre Regenerationspotenz. Pathophysiologia et diencephalica. Mailand 1956. Springer, Wien, S 53–77

Zülch KJ (1950) Zur Pathologie der äußeren Liquorräume: Beobachtungen über die Entstehung der Arachnoidalcysten und der liquormechanischen Vorgänge beim Hydrocephalus occlusus. Zentralbl Neurochir 10:25–38

Zülch KJ (1979) Histological typing of tumors of the central nervous system. WHO, Geneva

Zülch KJ (1981) Reflections on the surgery of the pineal gland. (A glimpse into the past.) Gleanings from Medical History. Neurosurg Rev 4:123–127

Zülch KJ (1986) Brain tumors. Their biology and pathology. Springer, Berlin Heidelberg New York, 3rd edn, revised and enlarged

Clinical and Pathological Findings in Brain Stem Gliomas

J. Artigas, J. Cervós-Navarro, M. Brock, and Cristina Aruffo, Berlin/FRG

Traditionally, gliomas of the brain stem were regarded as malignant, inoperable, resistant to radiotherapy and responseless to chemotherapy. Their prognosis was almost invariably bad. However, it has been suggested that some BSG are amenable to partial surgical resection and compatible with long term survival (Pool 1968; Lassiter et al. 1971). Thus, a more aggressive treatment was advocated (Hoffman et al. 1980). We have studied, clinically and pathologically, 39 cases of brain stem gliomas in an attempt to solve this controversy.

Material and Methods

All material which was filed between 1969 and 1984 under the heading 'glial neoplasm' of the brain stem was collected. Two cases were excluded because of the lack of adequate follow-up, and another case because it corresponded to a phacomatosis. Thus, 24 biopsies and 26 autopsies remained, which corresponded to 39 cases. Routine light microscopic stains, silver impregnations, and immunohistochemistry using antibodies against the main components of CNS tissue (neurofilaments (NF), glial fibrillary acidic protein (GFAP), and myelin basic protein (MBP)) were performed.

Results

There were 24 males and 15 females in the group. A trimodal distribution of ages was seen (Table 1); children had a mean age of 8.5 years (2 to 15 years); adults of 37.8 years (24 to 54 years), and elderly of 68.3 years (60 to 78 years). As initial symptomatology, 18 patients presented the characteristic clinical picture of progressive multiple bilateral cranial nerve palsies, pyramidal tract signs, and ataxia; 12 patients complained of headaches and vomiting; 6 presented signs depicting mental alterations, whilst in 2 patients the first and unique symptoms were those of a subarachnoidal hemorrhage. One patient was symptomless and the tumor was only a casual finding at autopsy. As the disease progressed these symptoms appeared intermingled. Increased intracranial pressure in 15 cases and signs of hydrocephalus in 16 cases were present sometime during the evolution of the tumor.

Radiologic Diagnosis

In 11 cases the diagnosis of brain stem occupying mass was made with angiography and pneumoencephalography. In 25 cases the CT revealed a brain stem tumoral

Table 1. Age and sex distribution of patients with BSG. A trimodal age distribution is seen, in which the age groups between 1–16, 30–40, and 60–70 predominate. Women (dotted areas) are distributed in every age group except between 16 and 50 years of age, period in which interestingly only one woman is seen

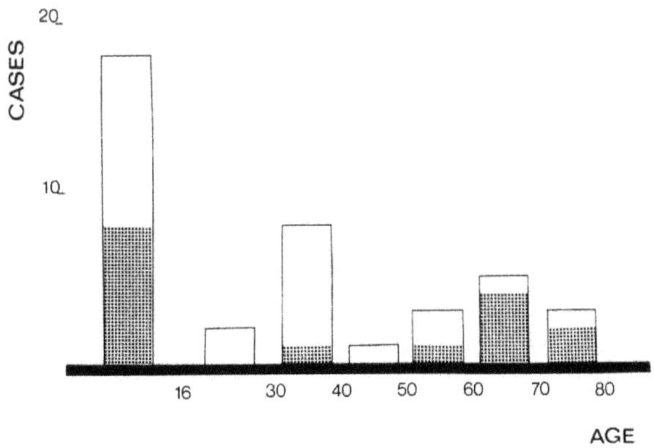

Table 2. Precise histological diagnosis of the cases studied

11 Pilocytic astrocytomas	3 Protoplasmic astrocytomas
8 Glioblastomas	2 Ganglioglioma
7 Gliomatosis	1 Angioglioma
4 Subependymomas	3 Gliomas

mass in the fourth ventricle or in the posterior fossa. The precise diagnosis of BSG was made with CT and NMR (Fig. 1) in three cases.

Pathological Classification

A precise histological diagnosis was attained in 36 cases (Table 2). However, in 3 cases the material was so scanty that despite special techniques we could only identify it as a glioma.

Pilocytic astrocytomas are made-up of fibrillary astrocytes. These cells are fasciculated and elongated as they conform to the polarity of the fiber pathways, although they assume their typical configuration when they escape this confinement. In *protoplasmic astrocytomas* the cells have round to oval nuclei, the cytoplasm extends into short radial processes. *Gangliogliomas* are made up of neurons arising from neuroblasts and glial cells, mainly astrocytes in various stages of development. Glial cells show anaplastic differentiation. Microcalcifications are frequent, as well as some degree of microcystic degeneration. Glial cells were strongly GFAP positive, whilst many neurons were NF positive. *Gliomatosis* is made up of a wide infiltration of glial cells in all stages of differentiation. Normal tissue is infiltrated

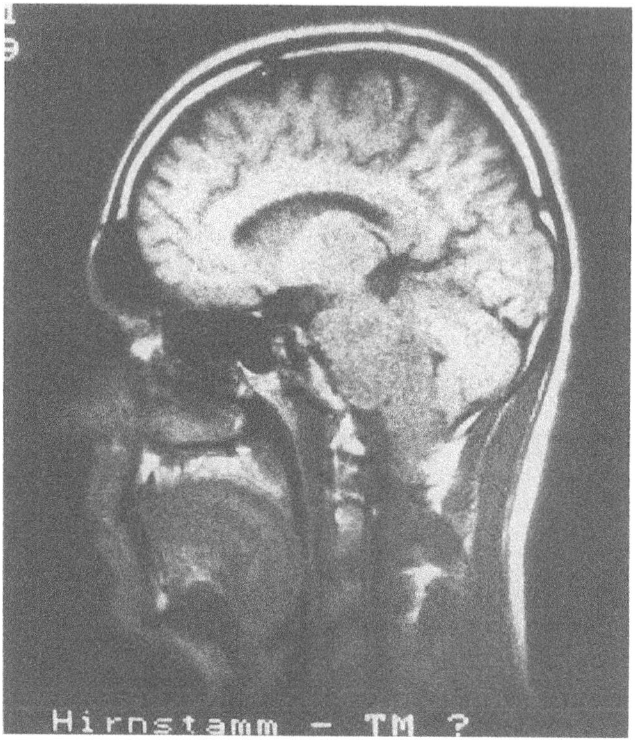

Fig. 1. Direct sagittal NMR section shows enlargement of the brain stem due to a mass having decreased signal

but preserved. Malignization signs are not seen. Neoplastic cells are irregularly positive to GFAP, MBP and NF stains, but GFAP positive cells predominate. In *glioblastomas*, the cells range from fibrillary or protoplasmic astrocytes to undifferentiated bizarre forms. We have found two types of glioblastomas. The first is well delimited (Fig. 2). It originates and restricts its growth to the brain stem area. Histologically hemorrhages, necroses and pseudopalisadings are evident. The second type of glioblastoma grows diffusely, infiltrates not only the brain stem but also the peduncles and often the cerebellum (Fig. 3). Histologically this type seems to arise from a malignized pilocytic or fibrocytic astrocytoma. *Subependymomas* are highly fibrillar tumors of low cellularity in which nests of typical astrocytic nuclei are separated by broad bands of neuroglial fibers. Many tumoral cells in *angiogliomas* (Bonnin et al. 1983) are fibrillary while others are more gemistocytic in nature. Vascular proliferation is conspicuous throughout, as confirmed by the presence of an abundant reticulin fiber network highlightening the vascular pattern. Most of the fibrillary and gemistocytic astrocytes are GFAP positive.

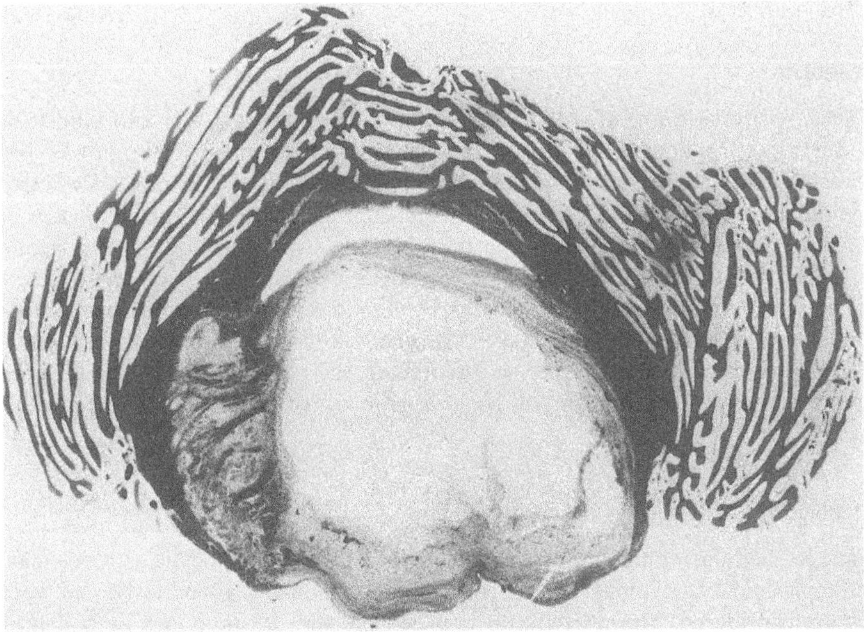

Fig. 2. Well delimited glioblastoma of the brain stem. (Celloidin preparation. Myelin stain ×1)

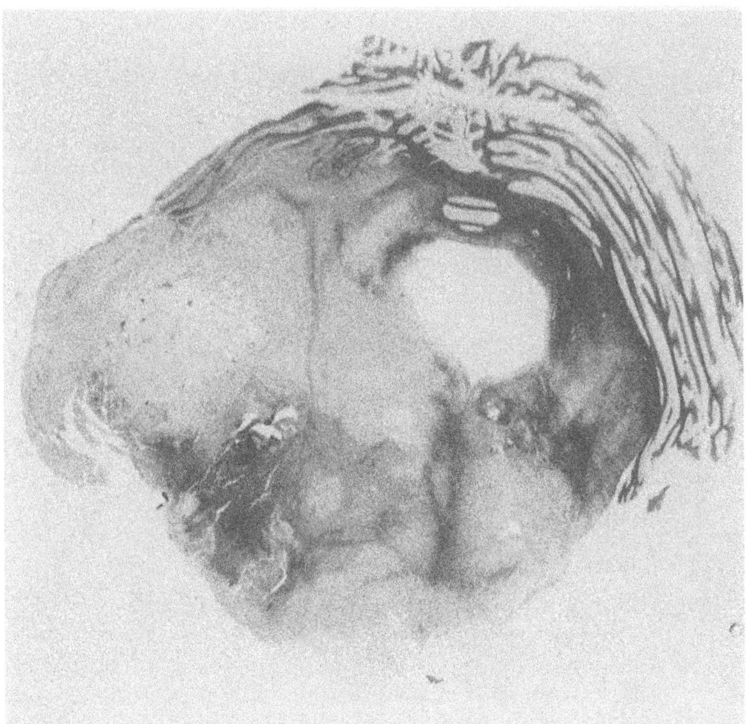

Fig. 3. Infiltrating glioblastoma of the brain stem. (Celloidin preparation. Myelin stain ×1)

Treatment

Surgical operation was performed in 20 cases, either for exploration and biopsy, or for partial extirpation of the tumor. 9 cases (4 glioblastomas, 3 gliomatosis and 2 gangliogliomas) underwent *radiotherapy* (total dose, 4000 to 6000 rads). Two cases of glioblastoma received *chemotherapy* in addition to radiotherapy. In two cases of pilocytic astrocytoma and one case of protoplasmic astrocytoma, an *iridium needle* was implanted after the diagnosis was established by means of a stereotactic biopsy (Fig. 4). *Palliative treatment:* in 11 cases Holter's drainage for symptomatic treatment of occlusive hydrocephalus was performed. *Conservative treatment:* only medical symptomatic treatment or no treatment at all was given in 6 cases (3 glioblastomas, 1 gliomatosis, 1 protoplasmic astrocytoma and 1 subependymoma).

Pathological Classification and Survival Time

7 patients died during the postoperative course (2 exophytic pilocytic astrocytomas, 1 protoplasmic astrocytoma, 1 subependymoma, 1 glioma, 2 gliomatosis) and were thus not considered. The relationship between the survival time and pathological diagnosis is depicted in Table 3. Glioblastomas showed a survival time of approximately 5 months, with or without radiotherapy. Only two patients with glioblastomas treated with both, radiotherapy and chemotherapy, survived longer, 1

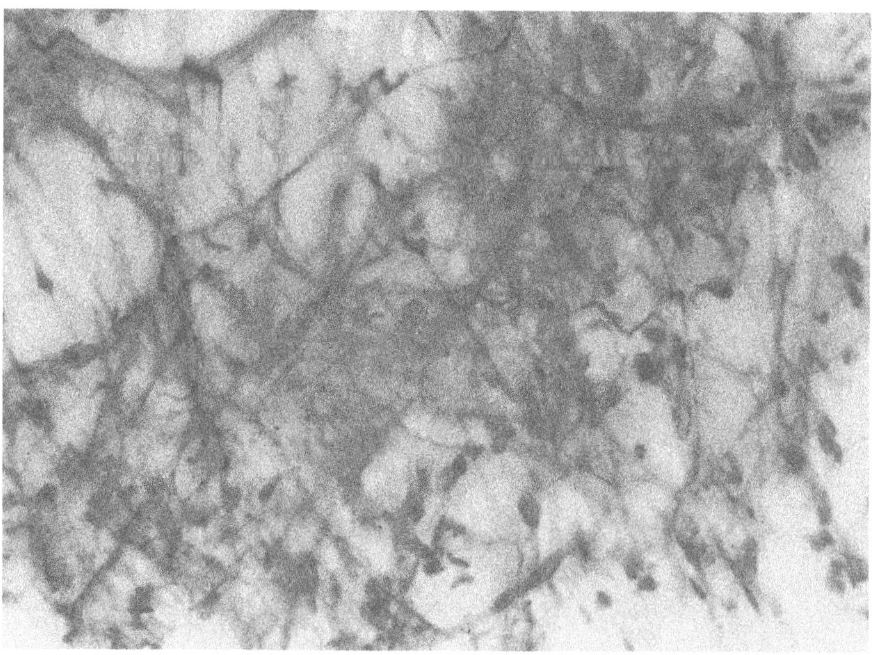

Fig. 4. Stereotactic biopsy. Typical picture of a pilocytic astrocytoma. Notice the fibrillary astrocytes with well delimited processes. (HE, ×250)

year and 2 years. Gangliogliomas showed a survival time of 7 months after radiotherapy. The mean survival time of gliomatosis was 18 months with great individual variations ranging from a minimum of 3 months to a maximum of 10 years. The patient with the angioglioma showed no recurrence after extirpation and is still alive after 12 years. Of the two patients with subependymoma which survived operation,

Table 3. The mean survival time varies from one type of BSG to another. Glioblastomas have a very short survival time and subependymomas a very long one, gangliogliomas, gliomatosis and pilocytic astrocytomas having intermediary survival times. (For more itemized survival times see text)

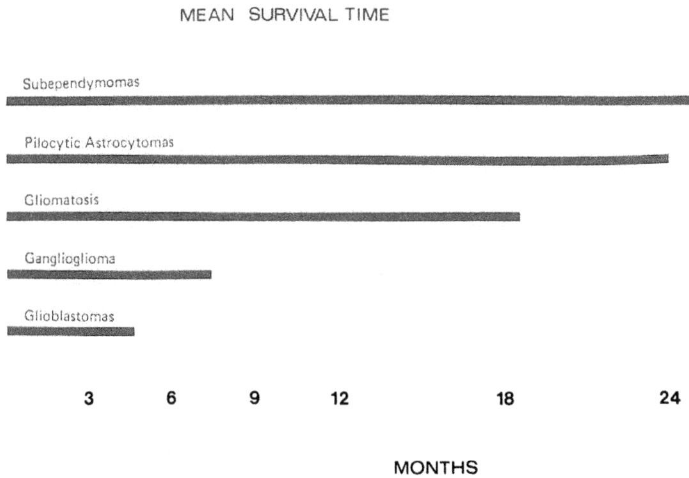

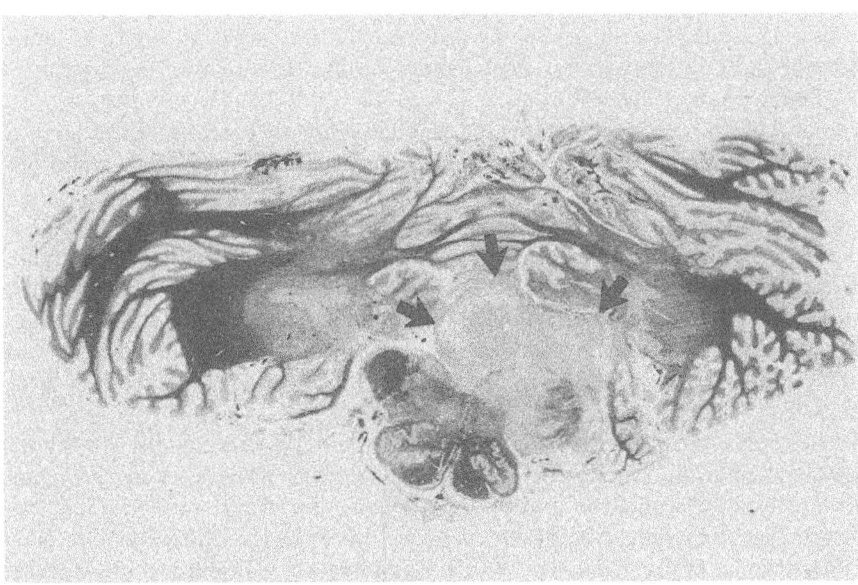

Fig. 5. Typical case of exophytic tumor (*arrows*). The patient survived 15 years after onset of the symptoms. (Celloidin preparation. Myelin stain × 1)

one survived 15 years, the other is still alive after 8 years. 5 of the pilocytic astrocytomas were exophytic (Fig. 5) and one cystic. Two of these patients died after operation, one survived 15, one 7 and one is still alive after 4 years. The patient with the cystic pilocytic astrocytoma survived 3 years.

Discussion

We have found brain stem gliomas (BSG) in every age group except from 16 to 24 years. They predominate in children, as is classically known (Cervós-Navarro and Schwartzman 1981). Also conspicuous is the fact that between 24 and 50 years of age there was only one woman with a BSG. Unfortunately, previously reported series either lack a complete histological diagnosis or the specification of sex in relation to age. We believe this finding calls for a more detailed revision of age and sex distribution with relation to tumor type in future studies.

The signs and symptoms of BSG and gliomatosis are well known (Renier and Grabreels 1980; Schoenmayr and Agnoli 1983; Artigas et al. 1985). It has already been reported that subependymomas may present as unique symptoms those characteristic of a subarachnoid hemorrhage (Changaris et al. 1981), as seen in 2 of our subependymomas.

Radiological Diagnosis

Even CT, which nowadays dominates the radiological diagnosis, has its problems because many BSG are isodense regardless of the injection of contrast material. Hence, in these cases the CT depicted an occupying mass lesion with narrowing of the cisterns, the aqueduct or the fourth ventricle, and occlusive hydrocephalus, without allowing a differential diagnosis (Weisberg 1979; Littman et al. 1980). In future NMR will be the diagnostic test of preference for the evaluation of brain stem tumors (Zimmerman et al. 1985).

Surgical treatment, radiotherapy and chemotherapy of BSG are well described (Pool 1968; Lassiter et al. 1971; Hara and Takeuchi 1977; Littman et al. 1980; Fulton et al. 1981; Mantravadi et al. 1982; Levin et al. 1984). Probably because in the past BSG were inoperable, efforts to correlate pathological anatomy and cellular behavior with treatment and clinical course are lacking. Gangliogliomas of the brain stem are rare and have a longer survival time than other gliomas of the brain stem (Garcia et al. 1984). The two gangliogliomas of this series were histologically malignant and had a bad outcome. We believe that a precise histological diagnosis can open new horizons as to the outcome of the BSG, since a correlation between them seems to exist (Table 3).

Interesting is to consider the histogenesis of some brain stem tumors. We believe that some gliomatosis, particularly the craniospinal form (Kawano et al. 1978) may originate from those pilocytic astrocytomas which grow continuously without becoming malignized, infiltrating healthy nervous tissue. Thus, a diffuse benign pilocytic astrocytoma of the brain stem can be considered as the origin of a gliomatosis. On the other hand, when a pilocytic astrocytoma is malignized it gives origin to that type of glioblastomas which are infiltrative, these last ones being clearly distinguish-

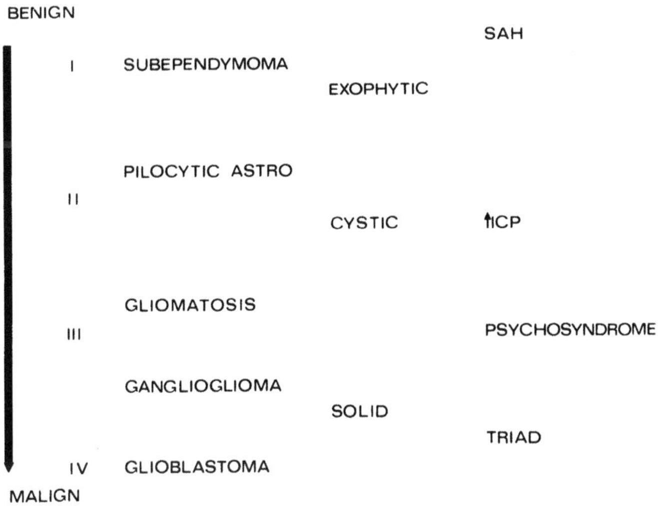

Fig. 6. Diagram depicting the factors contributing to the evolution of a given brain stem glioma as observed in our series. The direct relationship between degree of malignancy, precise histologic diagnosis, texture of the tumor and symptomatology is clearly seen. (For a more detailed explanation see text)

able from the well delimited glioblastomas of the brain stem which do not originate from pilocytic astrocytomas.

A detailed analysis of our series has led us to the finding that there are several factors which determine the outcome of a given BSG (Fig. 6). The grading is undoubtedly important. The precise histological diagnosis is important since the biological behavior is different in every type of glioma. The texture of the tumors is related to the histological type and can be seen on CT and NMR. We have found that subependymomas and exophytic pilocytic astrocytomas can be considered as benign BSG. Finally the clinical features could give us a hint as to the outcome.

It is a fact, that different histological categories of BSG exist. It is important to distinguish them because their biological behavior and thus the therapy to be followed and the outcome vary from tumor to tumor. As an example we can see that subependymomas and exophytic astrocytomas are benign in nature, being their symptomatology, treatment and outcome different from that of other BSG which are more malignant.

References

Artigas J, Cervós-Navarro J, Iglesias J, Ebhart G (1985) Clinico-pathological findings in gliomatosis cerebri. Clin Neuropathol 4: 135–148

Bonnin JM, Pena CA, Rubinstein LJ (1983) Mixed capillary hemangioblastoma and glioma. A redefinition of the "angioglioma". J Neuropathol Exp Neurol 42: 504–516

Cervós-Navarro J, Schwartzman A (1981) Pathologie der kindlichen Hirntumoren. Neuropediatrics [Suppl] 13–43

Changaris DG, Powers JM, Perot PL, Hungerford, Neal GB (1981) Subependymoma presenting as subarachnoid hemorrhage. J Neurosurg 55:643–645
Fulton DS, Levin VA, Wara WM, Edwards MS, Wilson CB (1981) Chemotherapy of pediatric brain-stem tumors. J Neurosurg 54:721–725
Garcia CA, McGarryu PA, Collada M (1984) Ganglioglioma of the brain stem. J Neurosurg 60:431–434
Hara M, Takeuchi K (1977) A temporal study of survival of patients with pontine gliomas. J Neurol 216:189–196
Hoffman HJ, Becker L, Craven MA (1980) A clinical and pathological distinct group of benign brain stem gliomas. Neurosurgery 7:243–248
Kawano N, Miyasaka Y, Yada K, Atari H, Sasaki K (1978) Diffuse cerebrospinal gliomatosis. J Neurosurg 49:303–307
Lassiter KRL, Alexander E, Davis CH, Kelly DL (1971) Surgical treatment of brain stem gliomas. J Neurosurg 34:719–725
Levin VA, Edwards M, Wara WM, Allen J, Ortega J, Vestnys P (1984) CCNU followed by hydroxyurea, misonidazole, and irradiation for brain stem gliomas. Neurosurgery 14:679–681
Littman P, Jarret P, Bilaniuk LT, Rorke LB, Zimmerman RA, Bruce DA, Carabell SC, Schut L (1980) Pediatric brain stem gliomas. Cancer 45:2787–2792
Mantravadi RVP, Phatak R, Bellur S, Liebner EJ, Haas R (1982) Brain Stem Gliomas: an autopsy study of 25 cases. Cancer 49:1294–1296
Pool JL (1968) Gliomas in the region of the brain stem. J Neurosurg 29:164–167
Renier WO, Gabreels FJM (1980) Evaluation of diagnosis and non-surgical therapy in 24 children with a pontine tumor. Neuropediatrics 11:262–273
Schoenmayr R, Agnoli AL (1983) Brain stem tumors. Diagnosis and surgical treatment. Neurosurg Rev 6:57–65
Weisberg LA (1979) Computed tomography in the diagnosis of brain stem gliomas. Computertomographie 3:145–153
Zimmerman RA, Bilaniuk LT, Packer R, Sutton L, Samuel L, Johnson MH, Grossman RI, Goldberg HI (1985) Resistive NMR of brain stem gliomas. Neuroradiology 27:21–25

Blood Flow and Metabolism in Brain Stem – Pathophysiological Implications

A. BAETHMANN, München/FRG

Not only the neurosurgeon but also neurochemists and -physiologists have an increasing exploratory access to the brain including brain stem structures with an ever better resolution for functional and metabolic studies. Purpose of this discussion is to compare and relate blood flow and metabolic findings in brain stem with other cerebral areas under normal and various pathophysiological situations, such as hypotension, anesthesia, etc. and to analyze metabolic aspects of brain stem injury.

Table 1 is a survey of flow data on brain stem obtained in experimental animals, e.g. cat, dog, monkey and rat under control conditions. Medulla and pons are compared with cortex and white matter. As seen, blood flow in brain stem and pons is not significantly different from the levels found in cortex during anesthesia. With consciousness maintained differences between cortex and brain stem may become visible, however, this may as well result from the respective CBF method employed.

Table 2 summarizes findings on regional cerebral metabolism of Sokoloff et al. (1977) using ^{14}C-deoxyglucose in rats. Consciousness and thiopental anesthesia were compared in these studies. Brain stem, e.g. medulla or lateral lemniscus had

Table 1. Regional blood flow in different cerebral tissues under control conditions (ml/100 g min)

Species	Cortex	Brain stem Medulla	Pons	White matter	Anesthesia	CBF-method	Author
Cat	37± 4	34± 4	26± 4	19±2	Chloralose-urethan	15 μm microspheres	D. D. Heistad et al., Am. J. Physiol. 235, 1978
Dog	50± 0	40± 5	32± 3	27±4	Chloralose-urethan	15 μm microspheres	D. D. Heistad et al., Am. J. Physiol. 235, 1978
Dog	41± 6	36± 5	30± 5	24±3	Pento-barbital	16 μm microspheres	R. Chen et al., Stroke 14, 1983
Monkey (cynomolgus)	89±13	85±16	76±11	35±5	Chloralose-urethan	15 μm microspheres	D. D. Heistad et al., Am. J. Physiol. 235, 1978
Rat (3 mo)	166± 8	82± 2	86± 3	54±4	Awake	^{14}C-iodo-antipyrine	M. Ohata et al., Brain 104, 1981
Cat	109± 4	95±11	65± 3	21±2	Awake	^{14}C-antipyrine	M. Reivich et al., J. Appl. Physiol. 27, 1969

Table 2. Effect of thiopental on LCGU (^{14}C-DG) in rats in μM/100 g min (compiled from Sokoloff et al. 1977)

	Conscious	Thiopental*	% Change
Sens. mot. cortex	118±3	67±2	−43
Medulla, vest. n.	133±4	81±4	−39
Pons, GM	69±3	46±3	−33
Lat. lemn.	114±7	75±4	−34
Corpus call.	42±2	30±2	−29

* Dosis: Disapp. of corneal reflex

Table 3. LCGU (^{14}C-DG) in conscious rats in hypo- and hyperthermia in μM/100 g min (compiled from McCulloch et al. 1982)

	Normo-thermia	Hypo-thermia	% Change	Hyperthermia	% Change
Sens. mot. cortex	111± 4	86±6	−23	125±13	+12
Medulla, vestib. nucl.	103± 8	77±6	−25	114± 4	+11
Pons, GM	50± 5	34±5	−32	57± 2	+14
Lemn. lat.	119±11	82±7	−31	101± 7	−15
Corpus call.	21± 1	10±3	−52	30± 2	+42

higher, or equal metabolic rates as compared to cerebral cortex. Pontine grey matter and corpus callosum were less active. Thiopental led to a homogenous decrease of local cerebral glucose uptake between 29% in white matter and 43% in cortex. Depression of metabolism in brain stem by thiopental was in a similar range as in cortex. Corresponding studies on hypo-, or hyperthermia were conducted in conscious rats by McCulloch and coworkers (1982). As shown in Table 3, normothermic medulla or pontine areas had equal, or even higher metabolic rates than cortex. The depression of glucose uptake by hypothermia to 31.8 °C was mostly pronounced in white matter, while moderate in cortex and medulla. Pons was in between. Conversely, hyperthermia of 40.2 °C caused the most extensive increase of glucose uptake in white matter, while only marginal changes in cerebral cortex and medulla. The findings on regional flow and metabolism make obvious a considerable metabolic activity in brain stem areas being equal or even higher than in cerebral cortex. This is indicative of a similar level of function of brain stem tissue. A major point is the blood flow response of brain stem vs. supratentorial brain during severe arterial hypotension. Mueller et al. (1977) studied rCBF by using radioactively labelled microspheres in brain stem, cerebrum, cerebellum and grey, or white matter, respectively. Lowering of blood pressure below the autoregulatory threshold of 50 mmHg led to a significant reduction of blood flow in all tissue areas. However, brain stem as well as cortical grey matter suffered the least as compared to cerebellum, or white matter. Studies of Kassell et al. (1983) arrive at the same conclusions. The authors infused adenosine intravenously until blood pressure fell to 40 mmHg. Blood flow in brain stem remained almost normal, while corpus callosum, cerebral cortex, or the total hemispheres had significant reductions. Such findings may support the contention that brain stem enjoys particular protection against the development of ischemia.

A pertinent subject in this context is traumatic injury of the brain stem and the subsequent changes of regional blood flow and metabolism. Since traumatic brain stem lesions in isolation are rare in patients, respective informations have to te extracted from experimental studies. A suitable model is fluid percussion of the skull as devised by Rinder and Olsson (1968 a) and further developed by Sullivan et al. (1976). Acute damage is largely limited to the brain stem in various modifications of this model. Figure 1 shows schematically in serial sections of the brain the localization of changes induced by fluid percussion. The graph demonstrates restriction of tissue damage to pons, medulla and upper cervical cord. The hemispheres are not affected. Traumatized tissue was recognized in these studies by uptake of Evans-blue albumin. Opening of the barrier to albumin was present for 12 hours, but disappeared 24 hours later. Fluid percussion to the skull induces intermittent changes of various autonomic functions, such as respiration, or the general circulation (Rinder and Olsson 1968 a; Sullivan et al. 1976). The respiration may transiently stop, while the systemic blood pressure is liable to increase abruptly by 100 mmHg, or more. The response of these vegetative functions may indicate a primarily involvement of brain stem centers. The extent of mechanical loading by fluid percussion to the skull can be experimentally adjusted allowing for dose-response studies of the formation of stem lesions. E.g. macroscopical lesions of brain stem were only detected, if the peak pressure during impact exceeded 2.2 atmospheres (Sullivan et al. 1976). Higher peak pressures were associated with extensive subarachnoid and mesencephalic hemorrhage.

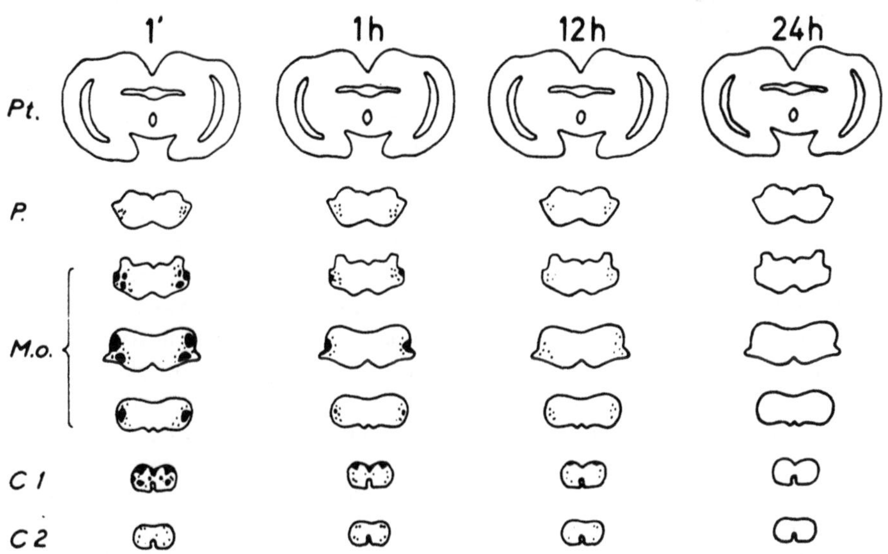

Fig. 1. Schematic drawing of rabbit brain serial sections exposed to fluid percussion of 1.7 atmospheres peak pressure. Damage to the tissue was assessed by uptake of Evans-blue. Note exclusive involvement of pons, medulla and cervical spinal cord. Opening of the barrier persisted for 12 hours only (From: L. Rinder and Y. Olsson 1968 b)

Acute injury to the brain stem induces distinct metabolic and hemodynamic effects involving also remote areas of the cerebral periphery, such as cerebral cortex. Respective findings of Duckrow et al. (1981) on fluid percussion of the skull demonstrate immediate vascular dilation and increase of blood volume in cortical vessels together with an enhancement of the oxidative activity in the tissue. This was concluded, e.g. from a prompt deflection of the cytochrome a, a_3 at the cerebral surface in vivo. Thus, enhancement rather than depression of cerebral metabolism seems to be evoked by acute traumatic insults to the brain stem provided respiration functions properly or is mechanically supported, as in the current studies (Duckrow et al. 1981).

Metabolic changes evolving in brain stem were analyzed by Nilsson and Nordström (1977) in rats in a model closely related to fluid percussion also leading to injury largely confined to brain stem. Table 4 compares energy-rich phosphate-concentrations, such as phosphocreatine and ATP of cortical and brain stem areas. Energy utilization was determined as the decrease of phosphocreatine, or adenosinephosphate-concentrations, respectively as:

$$\Delta{\sim}P = 2\,\Delta\,ATP + \Delta ADP + \Delta PCr + \Delta Lactate \qquad (I)$$

during a 10 sec period of ischemia in animals with and without brain stem injury. Concussion led to a significant increase of energy utilization in both, brain stem and cortex over cerebral ischemia alone. However, energy consumption was substantially higher in brain stem than in cerebral cortex after traumatic exposure. Ischemia led to a more rapid depletion of the energy-rich phosphate compounds in brain stem as compared to the cortex. This would again support the conclusion that energy metabolism in brain stem is enhanced and not depressed immediately after injury. This view is in agreement with observations on extracellular release of potassium in this area, or on the electrical response, respectively indicative of a regional stimulation of the functional activity (Takahashi et al. 1981; Hayes et al. 1984). However, the EEG as a global measure of cerebral function is initially depressed rather than stimulated under these circumstances (Sullivan et al. 1976; Duckrow et al. 1981).

Obviously, respective informations on the metabolic state in acute brain stem lesions can only be obtained with difficulties in patients. One reason is that injury restricted to brain stem is a rare event, another that the metabolic response can hardly be studied under acute conditions, since the patient is not available. Clinical approaches towards the problem have been made, nevertheless. Enevoldsen et al. (1976) studied CSF-lactate levels in severely head injured patients in relation to the CSF-pH. Three groups were distinguished: patients with primarily cortical, primarily brain stem lesions, and with the combination of both. Patients with predominant brain stem injuries had significantly higher CSF lactate levels than patients with cortical lacerations only. This result could not be attributed to a decrease of cerebral blood flow, since CBF was equally reduced in both groups of patients. As expected, outcome was less favorable in patients with brain stem injury than in patients with cortical lesions only. The combination of both made outcome even worse, as well as the metabolic abnormalities. It should be mentioned that these studies were not performed acutely, but only within days after trauma.

Table 4. Energy utilization (ischemic depletion) in cortex and brain stem after acceleration concussion in rats (compiled from Nilsson and Nordström 1977)

	PCr	ATP	Lac	Energy utilization $\Delta \sim P$
Control				
Cortex	4.76	2.96	1.49	
Brain stem	4.25	2.52	1.22	
Cortex				
Ischemia only	2.74	2.83	3.14	3.89
Ischemia + trauma (9 m/sec)	1.71*	2.44*	3.47	5.77*
Brain stem				
Ischemia only	1.71	2.25	4.80	6.54
Ischemia + trauma (9 m/sec)	0.71*	1.65*	5.10	8.60*

* Significantly different from ischemia only

Table 5. CBF, ICP, CPP and $CMRO_2$ in patients with traumatic hemorrhage in diencephalon and brain stem (no mass lesion) (compiled from Bruce et al. 1973)

	Pat. 11	Pat. 12	Normal
CBF [ml/100 g min]	31	36	50
ICP [mm Hg]	22	9	15
CPP [mm Hg]	50	88	75
$CMRO_2$ [ml/100 g min]	1.46	2.44	3.50
SAP [mm Hg]	72	97	85

Table 5 is extracted from data of Bruce et al. (1973) on cerebral blood flow and metabolism in severe head injury, where two patients are shown with predominant injury of the diencephalon and brain stem. Blood flow as well as cerebral oxygen uptake was decreased, although the intracranial pressure was only slightly increased, or even normal. However, the flow data do not differ significantly from findings of head injured patients without exclusive involvement of these central brain structures (Bruce et al. 1973). This underlines again that in severe head injury brain stem tissue is rarely damaged in isolation.

The current analysis of brain stem injury and metabolism is concluded by an interesting experimental observation on fluid percussion concerning the mechanism of immediate unconsciousness. Hayes and coworker (1984) using this model in cats reported a selective increase of the local ^{14}C-deoxyglucose uptake in specific pontine areas indicative of functional activation. Other tissue areas were depressed. The animals were in coma and did not respond to noxious stimulation. An almost identical "clinical" response could be obtained, if the cholinergic compound carbachol was injected in awake cats into the very same area of the pons which was found activated by fluid percussion. The animals became unresponsive and fell into deep coma upon injection. This could be blocked by intravenous, or focal administration of atropine into the same tissue area. Injection of tetracain or saline into pons had no effect (Hayes et al. 1984). The observations suggest coma secondary to brain stem injury to result from an overwhelming activation of cholinergic pontine areas. Such a mechanism may have interesting therapeutical implications.

Summary and Conclusions

Cerebral tissue of brain stem and adjacent areas is metabolically, and thus functionally as active as the peripheral brain. Depression or enhancement by anesthesia, or hyperthermia, respectively induce quantitative changes in brain stem which are similar to those of other brain tissue areas. Blood flow of brain stem seems to be better maintained in critical situations, e.g. severe arterial hypotension than in white matter, or cerebellum indicative of specific protection. Acute traumatic lesions with predominant involvement of the brain stem can be experimentally induced by fluid percussion of the skull in a dose-dependent manner. Valuable informations have been obtained by this model on blood-brain barrier function, hemodynamics, and metabolism of brain stem and on the remote effects in the peripheral brain. Acutely, enhancement rather than depression of metabolism, and consequently function may be assumed. Clinical studies on head injury with preferential involvement of brain stem provide evidence for a specific enhancement of tissue acidosis and metabolic depression, which may be independent of the actual quality of the cerebral perfusion. Finally, acute coma in brain stem injury without mechanical destruction of the tissue may result from an excessive cholinergic activation in pons and adjacent areas. Such a mechanism may have specific therapeutical implications. Further progress in cerebral imaging techniques together with a refinement of non-invasive analytical methods can be expected to enhance our understanding of the pathophysiology of acute brain stem disorders in man.

Acknowledgements: Valuable support during the preparation of the manuscript was provided by Ruth Demmer, Ulrike Goerke and Isolde Juna.

References

Bruce DA, Langfitt TW, Miller JD, Schutz H, Vapalahti MP, Stanek A, Goldberg HI (1973) Regional cerebral blood flow, intracranial pressure, and brain metabolism in comatose patients. J Neurosurg 38: 131–144

Chen RYZ, Fan FC, Schuessler GB, Usami S, Chien S (1983) Effects of sphere size and injection site on regional cerebral blood flow measurements. Stroke 14: 769–776

Duckrow RB, LaManna JC, Rosenthal M, Levasseur JE, Patterson JL, Jr (1981) Oxidative metabolic activity of cerebral cortex after fluid-percussion head injury in the cat. J Neurosurg 54: 607–614

Enevoldsen EM, Cold G, Jensen FT, Malmros R (1976) Dynamic changes in regional CBF, intraventricular pressure, CSF pH and lactate levels during the acute phase of head injury. J Neurosurg 44: 191–214

Hayes RL, Pechura CM, Katayama Y, Povlishock JT, Giebel ML, Becker DP (1984) Activation of pontine cholinergic sites implicated in unconsciousness following cerebral concussion in the cat. Science 223: 301–303

Heistad DD, Marcus ML, Gross PM (1978) Effects of sympathetic nerves on cerebral vessels in dog, cat, and monkey. Am J Physiol 235(5):544–552

Kassell NF, Boarini DJ, Olin JJ, Sprowell JA (1983) Cerebral and systemic circulatory effects of arterial hypotension induced by adenosine. J Neurosurg 58:69–76

McCulloch J, Savaki HE, Jehle J, Sokoloff L (1982) Local cerebral glucose utilization in hypothermic and hyperthermic rats. J Neurochem 39:255–258

Mueller SM, Heistad DD, Marcus ML (1977) Total and regional cerebral blood flow during hypotension, hypertension, and hypocapnia. Effect of sympathetic denervation in dogs. Circ Res 41:350–356

Nilsson B, Nordström CH (1977) Rate of cerebral energy consumption in concussive head injury in the rat. J Neurosurg 47:274–281

Ohata M, Sundaram U, Fredericks WR, London ED, Rapoport SI (1981) Regional cerebral blood flow during development and aging of the rat brain. Brain 104:319–332

Reivich M, Jehle J, Sokoloff L, Kety SS (1969) Measurement of regional cerebral blood flow with antipyrine-^{14}C in awake cats. J Appl Physiol 27:296–300

Rinder L, Olsson Y (1968a) Studies on vascular permeability changes in experimental brain concussion. I. Distribution of circulating fluorescent indicators in brain and cervical cord after sudden mechanical loading of the brain. Acta Neuropathol (Berl) 11:183–200

Rinder L, Olsson Y (1968b) Studies on vascular permeability changes in experimental brain concussion. II. Duration of altered permeability. Acta Neuropathol (Berl) 11:201–209

Sokoloff L, Reivich M, Kennedy C, Des Rosiers MH, Patlak CS, Pettigrew KD, Sakurada O, Shinohara M (1977) The ^{14}C-deoxyglucose method for the measurement of local cerebral glucose utilization: theory, procedure, and normal values in the conscious and anesthetized albino rat. J Neurochem 28:897–916

Sullivan HG, Martinez J, Becker DP, Miller JD, Griffith R, Wist AO (1976) Fluid-percussion model of mechanical brain injury in the cat. J Neurosurg 45:520–534

Takahashi H, Manaka S, Sano K (1981) Changes in extracellular potassium concentration in cortex and brain stem during the acute phase of experimental closed head injury. J Neurosurg 55:708–717

Neurology, Neurophysiology

Topographic Analysis of Neurologic Symptoms in Brain Stem Diseases

A. HARTMANN and J. WAPPENSCHMIDT, Bonn/FRG

In cases of large space-occupying or destructive lesions the topographic assignment of brain stem processes is easily made using cranial computerized tomography (CCT) or nuclear magnetic resonance. However, these technical tools often fail if the tissue alteration is small or does not contrast to the surrounding tissue. In these cases and when technical procedures cannot be performed the topographic assignment must be done only with the clinical examination. F.i. in Wernicke's encephalopathy a positive CCT is an exception (Fig. 1). Usually the diagnosis is made by clinical examination.

This article will summarize some principles of anatomic arrangement in the brain stem. The brain stem consists of medulla oblongata, pons and mesencephalon. The unique structural organization of the brain stem in respect to its longitudinal axis and to its transverse sections often permits an accurate three-dimensional assignment. Functions arising in structures of the brain stem may be affected even by diseases outside the brain stem (3rd ventricle, corpus pinealis etc.).

Two topics will be discussed here:

1. The exact topographic diagnosis using examination of the cranial nerves (CN) and other parts of the brain stem.
2. The topographic value of some symptoms arising from the brain stem.

Symptoms due to CN-involvement in their run outside the brain stem but inside the cranium are not dealt with.

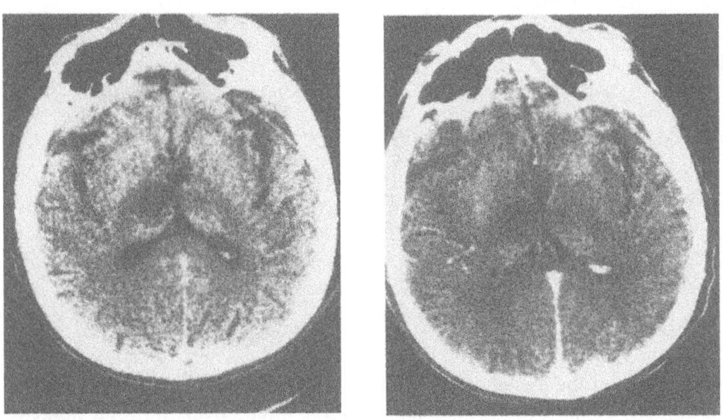

Fig. 1. Wernicke Encephalopathy: Cranial computerized tomography (CCT) with and without (right) contrast administration. Bilateral symmetric hypodensic areas do not indicate enhancement of contrast medium. CT-alterations like this are not typical for Wernicke's Encephalopathy

1. Topographic Assignment Using the Cranial Nerves

1.1 Mesencephalon

1.1.1 Anatomy

In respect to the CN the mesencephalon contains the 3rd and the 4th CN. Both nuclear areas are located in the periaqueductal grey matter, that of the oculomotor nerve at the level of the superior and that of the trochlear nerve at the level of the inferior colliculi. The former is incorporated into optic, the latter into acustic processes.

The nuclear column of the 3rd CN is organized in a particular way: The median part contains parasympathetic fibers from the accessorius nuclei (Edinger-Westphal), the lateral part contains the nuclei for the eye movement. According to Warwick's studies in the monkey the nuclei for the levator palpebrae muscle are positioned like a rucksack on the median dorsal part of the 3rd CN nuclear column (Fig. 2).

The fibers of the 3rd CN run crossed and uncrossed through the mesencephalon, penetrate the red nucleus and leave the brain stem medial to the crus cerebri in the interpeduncular fossa. The nuclear area of the 4th CN is located directly below the 3rd CN column. All fibers cross in the superior medullary velum and leave the brain stem at the *dorsal* aspect of the brain stem. It is the only CN that has such a course and exit from brain stem. Further relevant structures may be seen in Fig. 3.

1.1.2 Vascular Supply

The mesencephalon is supplied by the following arteries: Superior cerebellar artery, posterior cerebral artery, posterior communicating artery, posterior choroideal artery and interpeduncular branches from the basilar artery (Figs. 3, 4).

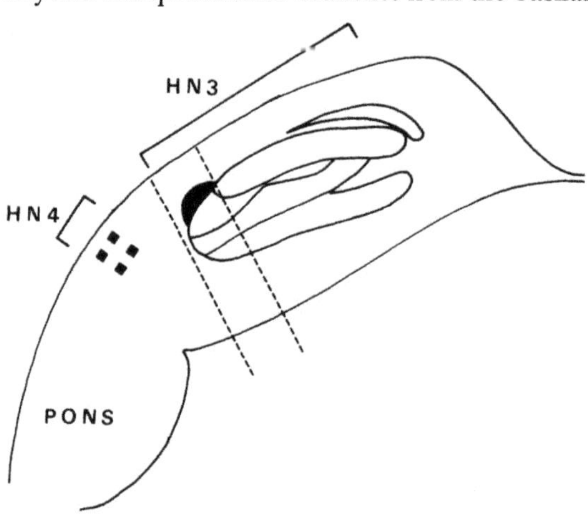

Fig. 2. Schematic arrangement of the nuclei of the 3rd and 4th cranial nerve within the mesencephalon. Actually, the nuclei of the oculomotor nerve do not spread over the total range of the mesencephalon. The "rucksack" position of the nuclei of the nerve fibers for the levator palpebrae muscle is indicated in black (between the *dotted lines*). HN 3 and HN 4: 3rd and 4th cranial nerve

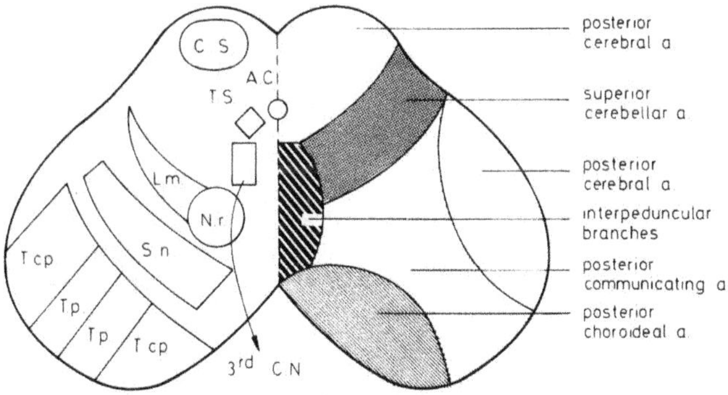

Fig. 3. Anatomical structures and vascular supply within the mesencephalon *C.S.* = Colliculus superior, *A.C.* = Acquaeduct cerebri, *T.S.* = Tractus sympathicus, *L.m.* = Lemniscus medialis, *N.r.* = Nucleus ruber, *S.n.* = Substantia nigra, *T.cp./T.p.* = Tractus pyramidalis, *3rd C.N.* = Nuclei and fibers of the oculomotor nerve

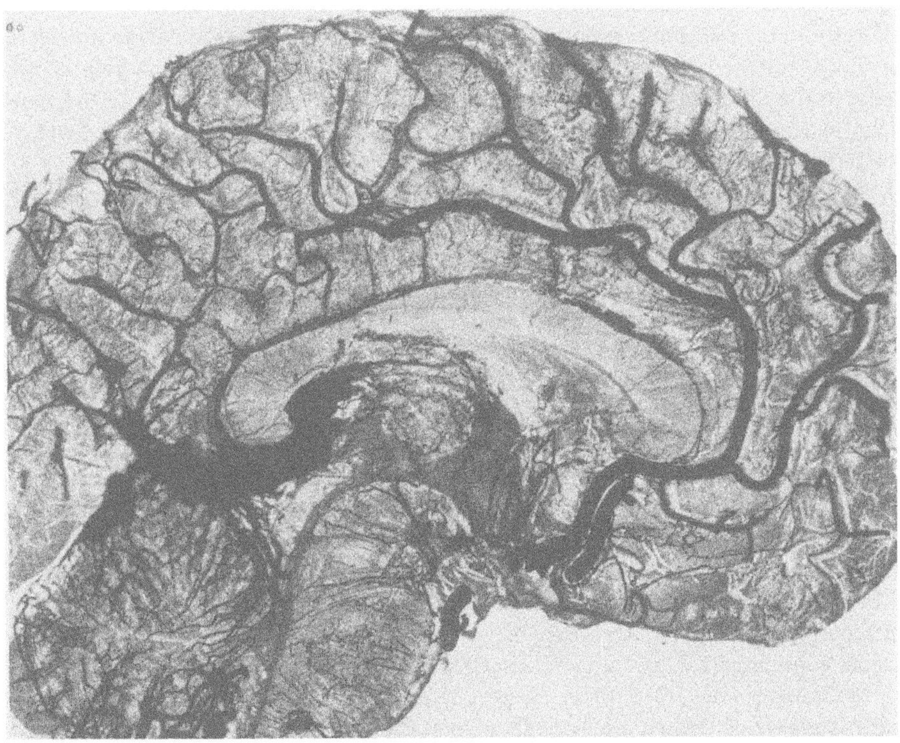

Fig. 4. Vascular supply of the brain stem. The median cut indicates postmortem angiograms of the arterial system in brain stem, supratentorial and cerebellar tissue. Pons and mesencephalon are located at the lower edge of the picture. At the border of pons and mesencephalon the oral part of the basilar artery is indicated with its branches which penetrate the midbrain. (Picture from: Salomon 1971, with permission)

1.1.3 Clinical Topography

The nuclear area of the 3rd and 4th CN is so small that space-occupying lesions almost never cause solely symptoms from these structures. Neighboring structures (central sympathetic tract, reticular formation, aquaeduct cerebri) are often involved as well. Vascular syndromes, however, may affect only very small areas of the brain. We have seen patients with unilateral isolated 3rd CN palsy, where all peripheral processes (neuritis, diabetes, polyneuropathy) were ruled out. However, it is not possible to distinguish a nuclear ischemia from an ischemic polyneuropathy on clinical grounds.

The nuclear area of the CN in the mesencephalon is supplied by the interpeduncular branches of the basilar artery running parallel to the nuclear fibers throughout the brain stem cut. If both, the 3rd and the 4th CN are involved by an ischemic process both eyes deviate to the side and the pupils are dilated due to ischemia of the Edinger-Westphal nucleus. We have never seen a case with isolated trochlear paralysis due to cerebral ischemia. However, this may occur, and then results in an upward-inward movement of the eye contralateral to the regional brain stem ischemia. A central ptosis due to deficiency of the nuclear part (the "rucksack part" of the 3rd CN column) is also possible but should be differentiated from the central ptosis (sometimes inborn) due to deficiency of the sympathetic tract (first neuron). In most of the cases other signs of the 3rd CN (eye ball movement defect, mydriasis) or the sympathetic tract (miosis, enophthalmus, anhydrosis) help in respect to the differential diagnosis. A Horner syndrome due to damage to the first neurons (central Horner) cannot be assigned to any particular brain stem level if there is no other clinical symptom.

In case the center of ischemia is close to the interpeduncular fossa contralateral hyperkinesia (tremor, chorea, athetosis) or contralateral Parkinsonian features (predominantly rigor) might be the clinical symptoms. They are due to involvement of the red nucleus or the substantia nigra respectively (Fig. 3). Since the fibers of the 3rd CN have to transverse this area an ipsilateral 3rd nerve palsy might accompany the contralateral symptoms. If the medial lemniscus is involved one depicts contralateral hyposensitivity to touch, vibration and position only. The tractus spinothalamicus lateralis, responsible for pain and temperature, runs more dorsally.

The combination of an ipsilateral paresis of the oculomotor nerve and a contralateral hemiparesis (Weber syndrome) is one of the so-called crossed motor syndromes (see chapter pons and medullae). Dependent on additional symptoms (hemiparesis or hemihypesthesia on the contralateral side) different neurologic syndromes may be collected which are indicated in Fig. 5 and Table 1.

It is not necessarily only a vascular syndrome which causes symptoms from the mesencephalon. Any space-occupying process (Fig. 6) and any other destructive lesion, e.g. caused by disseminated encephalomyelitic diseases, may be responsible. Since the latter ones often affect the periaquaeductal grey matter the medial longitudinal fasciculus (MLF) might be involved. The MLF runs from the mesencephalon down to the cervical medulla, combining inputs from cervical muscles, vestibular system, reticular formation, brain stem gaze centers, cortex and basal ganglia with the 3rd, 4th and 6th CN. The MLF is located directly ventral to the periaquaeductal grey matter and decussates in the pons directly above the 6th CN nucleus (Cogan et al. 1950).

Table 1.

Syndrome	Possible symptoms	Involved structure	Supplying artery (individual variations)
Benedikt-syndrome	*Contralateral:*		
	– Hyposensitivity to touch, position, vibration	– Medial lemniscus	Interpeduncular branches of the basilar artery
	– Tremor, chorea, athetosis – Rigor	– Red nucleus – Substantia nigra	Penetrating branches of the posterior communicating and posterior choroideal artery
	Homolateral:		
	– 3rd cranial nerve (CN)-palsy	– Fibers of oculomotor nerve	
Weber-syndrome	*Contralateral:*		
	– Spastic hemiparesis – Rigor – Dystaxia – Central paresis of 7th and caudal CNs	– Corticospinal fibers – Substantia nigra – Corticopontine fibers – Corticonuclear fibers	Interpeduncular branches of basilar artery Penetrating branches of the posterior communicating, posterior choroideal and posterior cerebral artery
	Homolateral:		
	– 3rd CN palsy	– Fibers of oculomotor nerve	
Paramedian mesencephalic syndrome	Decreased level of consciousness	– Ascending reticular activating system (ARAS) (reticular formation)	Circumferenting branches of the superior cerebelli artery
	Contralateral:		
	– Hyposensitivity to touch, position and vibration	– Medial lemniscus	
Central mesencephalic syndrome	*Contralateral:*		
	4th CN palsy	– Nucleus of the trochlear nerve	Interpeduncular branches of the basilar artery
	Homolateral:		
	– 3rd CN palsy	– Nucleus of the oculomotor nerve	
Parinaud-syndrome	Gaze palsy upward with convergence deficit	– Colliculi superior – 3rd CN nucleus	Posterior cerebral artery
Chiray-Foix-Nicolescu-syndrome	*Contralateral:*		
	– Hemiataxia – Tremor, chorea, athetosis – Hemiparesis – Hyposensitivity to touch, position, vibration	– Anterior spinocerebellar tract (?) – Red nucleus – Pyramidal tract – Medial lemniscus	

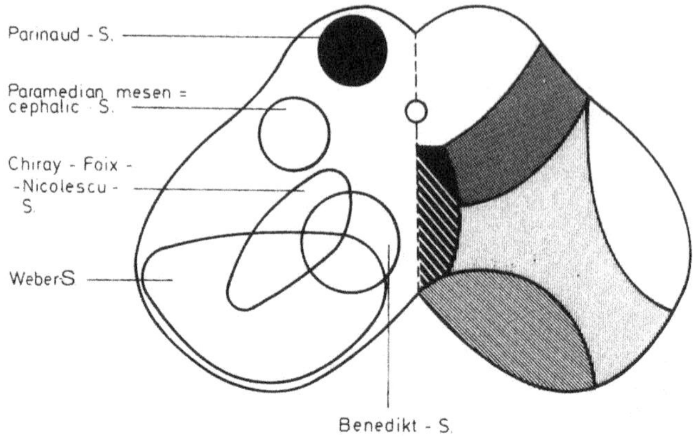

Fig. 5. Vascular supply and anatomical localization of ischemia in certain vascular midbrain syndromes

A left-sided MLF-lesion affects the innervation of the right medial muscle. Reactions to convergence remain preserved. If this patient tries to look to the left side, the right eye will not move inwards, and the left eye presents with a monocular nystagmus. In case both MLF are involved (they are located very close to each other), adduction for both eyes are insufficient and abduction of both eyes are associated with nystagmoid movements. Optokinetic, vestibular and oculocephalic stimulations lead to the identical reactions, called the internuclear ophthalmoplegia. Vertical saccades are unaffected (King et al. 1976; Smith and David 1964).

The examination of the MLF has some localizing signs in respect to the level between the mesencephalon and the pons: A lower lesion is always associated with nystagmus of the abducting eye, a rostral lesion (close to the 3rd CN nucleus) might affect the convergence reaction in addition to the adducting gaze deficit whereas nystagmus is less prominent.

A further peculiarity should be mentioned: Some of the syndromes arising in the mesencephalon are associated with symptoms from the coordinative system. The Claude-syndrome e.g. combines an ipsilateral 3rd nerve palsy with contralateral hemiparesis and hemiataxia (lower red nucleus-syndrome). These coordinative disturbances might be due to impairment of the anterior spinocerebellar tract which comes from the spinal cord and reaches the cerebellum via an uncrossed and crossed way, in the brain stem (up to the mesencephalon) and superior cerebellar peduncle. The Nothnagel-syndrome combines ipsilateral 3rd nerve palsy with contralateral hemiataxia only.

If a tumor – e.g. a pinealoma (Figs. 7, 8) – compresses the mesencephalic tectum with the superior colliculi the patient develops a positive doll's head phenomenon: With anteflexion of the head both eyes will automatically elevate. If the tumor compresses or invades the mesencephalic tegmentum, this might be indicated by an additional paresis of the 3rd and 4th CN. Certainly this will also result in compression of the aquaeduct and development of occlusive hydrocephalus (Fig. 7). The classical Parinaud-syndrome consists of impairment of conjugated upward-gaze with convergence deficit and negative reaction of the pupils to light.

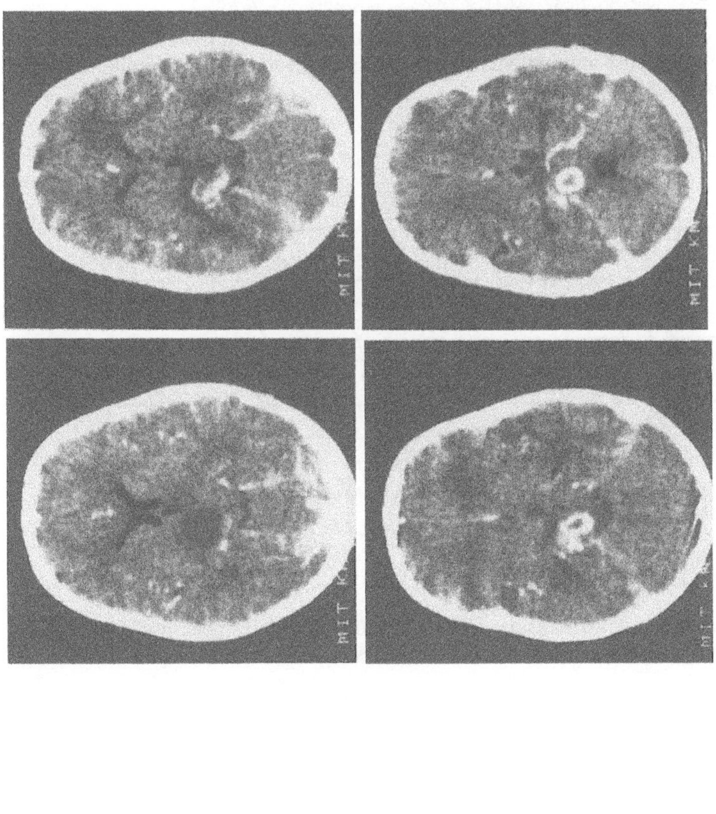

a

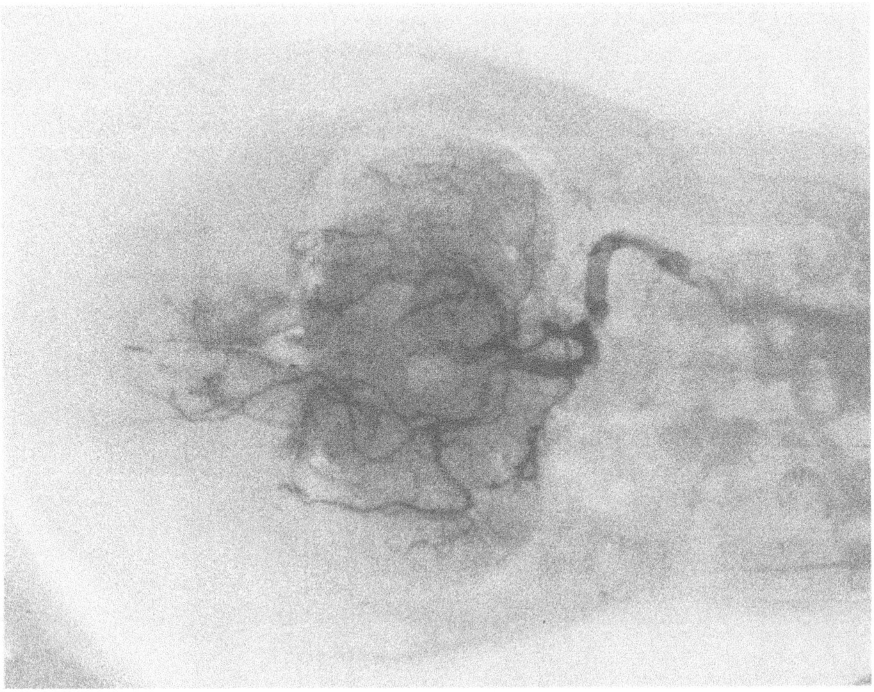

b

Fig. 6a,b. Midbrain tumor (spongioblastoma, confirmed by biopsy). **a** CCT, indicating a hypodense area (*upper left*), which shows intensive contrast enhancement. The 3rd ventricle is shifted to the right side. **b** Vertebral angiogram (AP-view), indicating a vascular tumor in the mesencephalon

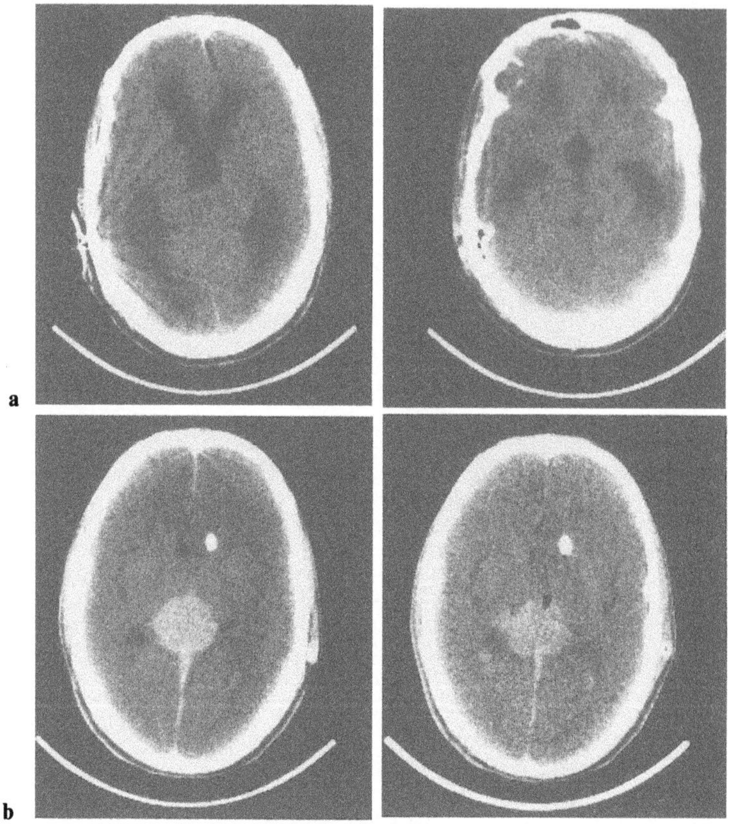

Fig. 7 a, b. Germinoma **a** Hydrocephalus of the 3rd and both lateral ventricles. Posterior to the 3rd ventricle one sees isodense and hypodense tissue. **b** Homogenous contrast enhancement in the area of the pineal gland

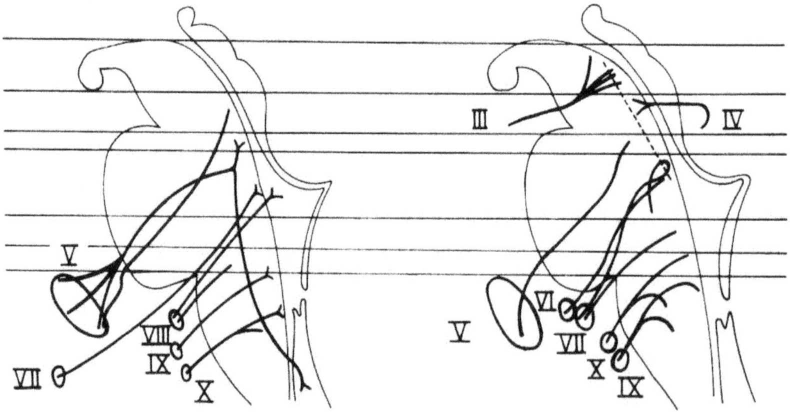

Fig. 8. Schematic arrangement of sensoric (*left*) and motoric (*right*) nuclei and fibers within the brain stem. Only the trochlear nerve leaves the brain stem on the dorsal aspect

1.2 Pons

1.2.1 Anatomy

The dorsal part of the pons is covered by the roof of the 4th ventricle. In the upper half of the pons the motor nuclei of the 5th CN are located, in the most upper part of the lower half the nuclei of the 6th CN. An exact topographic diagnosis in respect to the longitudinal axis of the pons is possible by examination of both nerves (Fig. 8). The fibers of the 6th CN pass the transverse cut of the pons and – after having crossed the corticospinal tract – leave the brain stem just at the border between the pons and the medulla oblongata. At this level but more laterally the fibers of the 7th CN leave the pons. Since the nuclear area of the 7th CN is located below that of the 6th CN they have to run upward to form the so-called "inner knee" at the area of the 6th CN.

The motor nuclei of the 5th CN are located in the lateral part of the pontine tegmentum. Supranuclear impulses are coming from both hemispheres, so that any supranuclear disease must affect both sides to result in a motor deficit of the trigeminal nerve.

The sensoric fibers of the 5th CN end in the nucleus sensorius principalis (pons), nucleus tractus mesencephalicus and nucleus tractus spinalis respectively, stretching from the mesencephalon to the upper cervical part of the spinal cord. The nucleus sensorius principalis in the pons is responsible for touch, tactile discrimination and pressure, and due to its location in a limited area in the dorsal aspect of the pons it is helpful in topographic analysis. The sensitivity for pain and temperature – represented by the nucleus tractus spinalis – is of less topographic value in respect to the longitudinal axis due to its extension downwards to the spinal cord. The nucleus tractus mesencephalicus is responsible for pressure sensitivity of the chewing muscles. In its ventral part the pons contains corticopontine fibers, which then cross at the pontine level and run to the cerebellum (pontocerebellar fibers) via the medial cerebellar peduncle. Otherwise the pons contains the medial lemniscus, lateral to that is the tractus spinothalamicus lateralis and ventral is the trapezoid body, continuing as lateral lemniscus to reach the inferior colliculi in the mesencephalon.

At the most lateral aspect of the bottom of the 4th ventricle one finds the nuclei of the vestibular complex.

1.2.2 Vascular Supply

The pons is supplied by the basilar artery: The median ventral part, where the tractus corticopontocerebelli decussates and intermingles with the corticospinal fibers, is supplied by penetrating paramedian branches. The lateral part (medial cerebellar peduncle, the bottom of the 4th ventricle and the superior medullary velum) is supplied by long circumferenting branches and the area around the nuclei of the 5th, 6th and 7th CN by short circumferenting branches. Since the basilar artery runs close to the clivus extrapontine space-occupying lesions might be recognized by displacement of the artery (Figs. 9, 10).

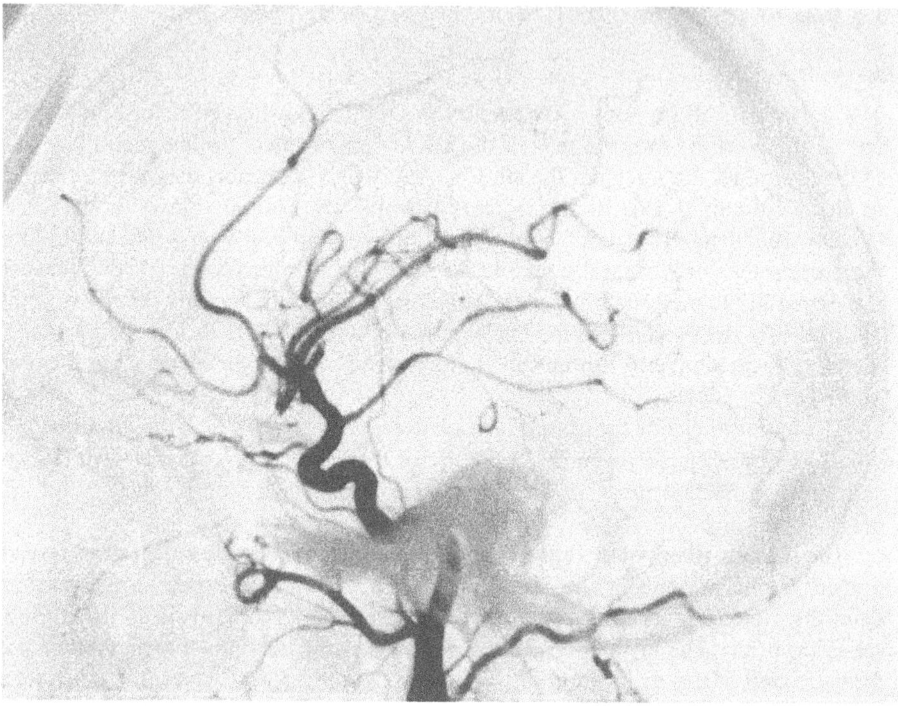

a

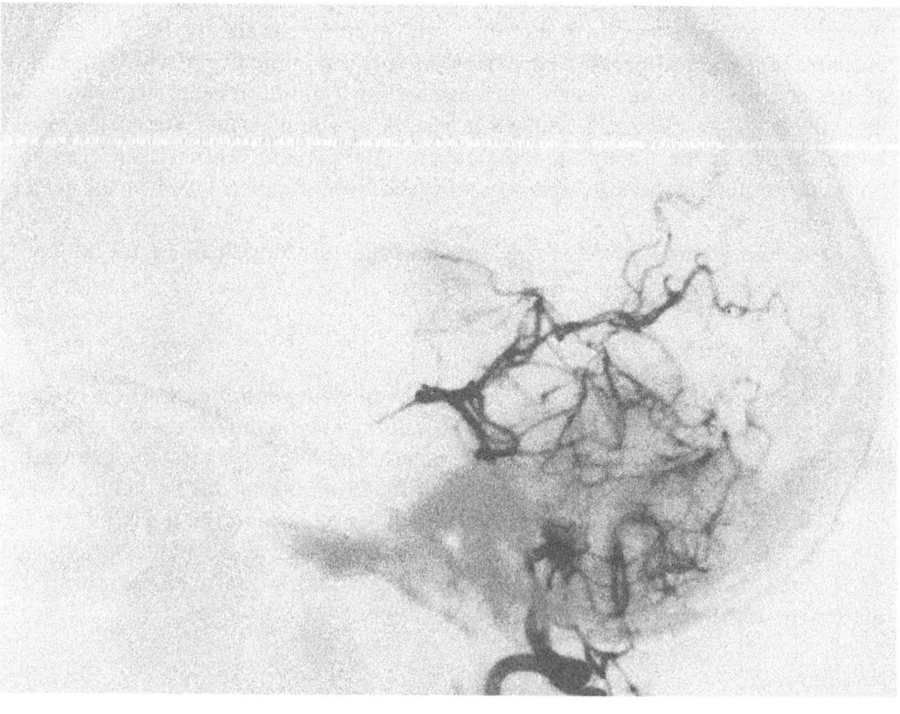

b

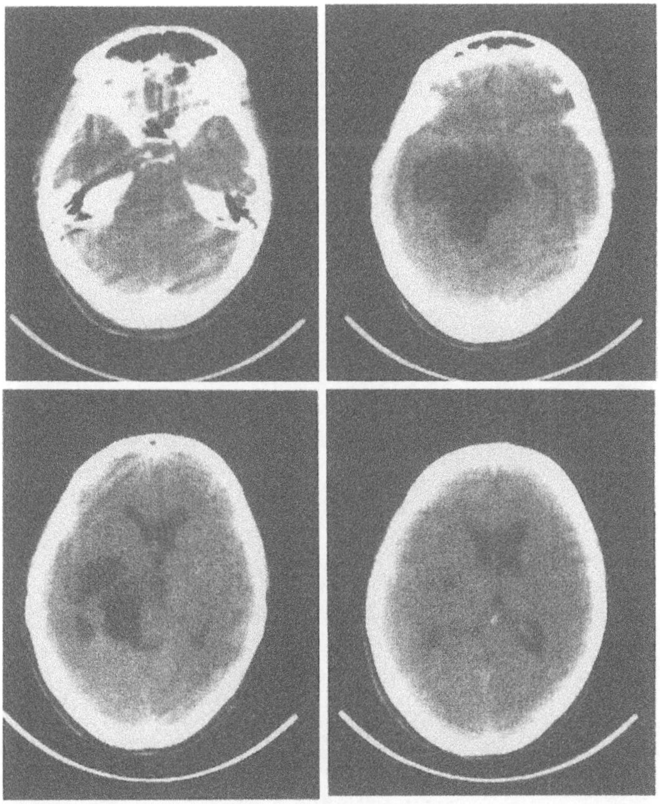

c

Fig. 9a–c. Epidermoid, located in the parasellar region and extending from the temporal lobe to the posterior fossa with compression of the brain stem from the left side. **a** Elevation of the Sylvian vascular group in the left-sided carotid-angiogram (*lateral view*). **b** Posterior displacement of basilar and intracranial part of the vertebral artery in the vertebral angiogram (*lateral view*). **c** Localization of the tumor in CCT. The hypodense tissue spreads from the temporal lobe to the posterior fossa and compresses the left-sided ventricular system

1.2.3 Clinical Topography

Table 2 lists some of the pontine syndromes mostly known from ischemic processes. However, space-occupying processes might cause the same syndromes (Figs. 11–13). If the upper pons is involved one is confronted with symptoms from the 5th CN, whereas with damage to the lower pons the 6th and 7th CN are presenting with pathologic signs. In case the ventral part of the pons is involved one detects symptoms from the pyramidal tract (hemiparesis), the tractus spinothalamicus lateralis (analgesia and thermanesthesia contralaterally) and possibly the medial lemniscus (Fig. 13). With involvement of more dorsally located structures (tegmentum) one misses signs from the pyramidal tract but might see signs from the coordinative and vestibular system (Fig. 13). Again the medial lemniscus which separates the ventral from the dorsal part might be involved.

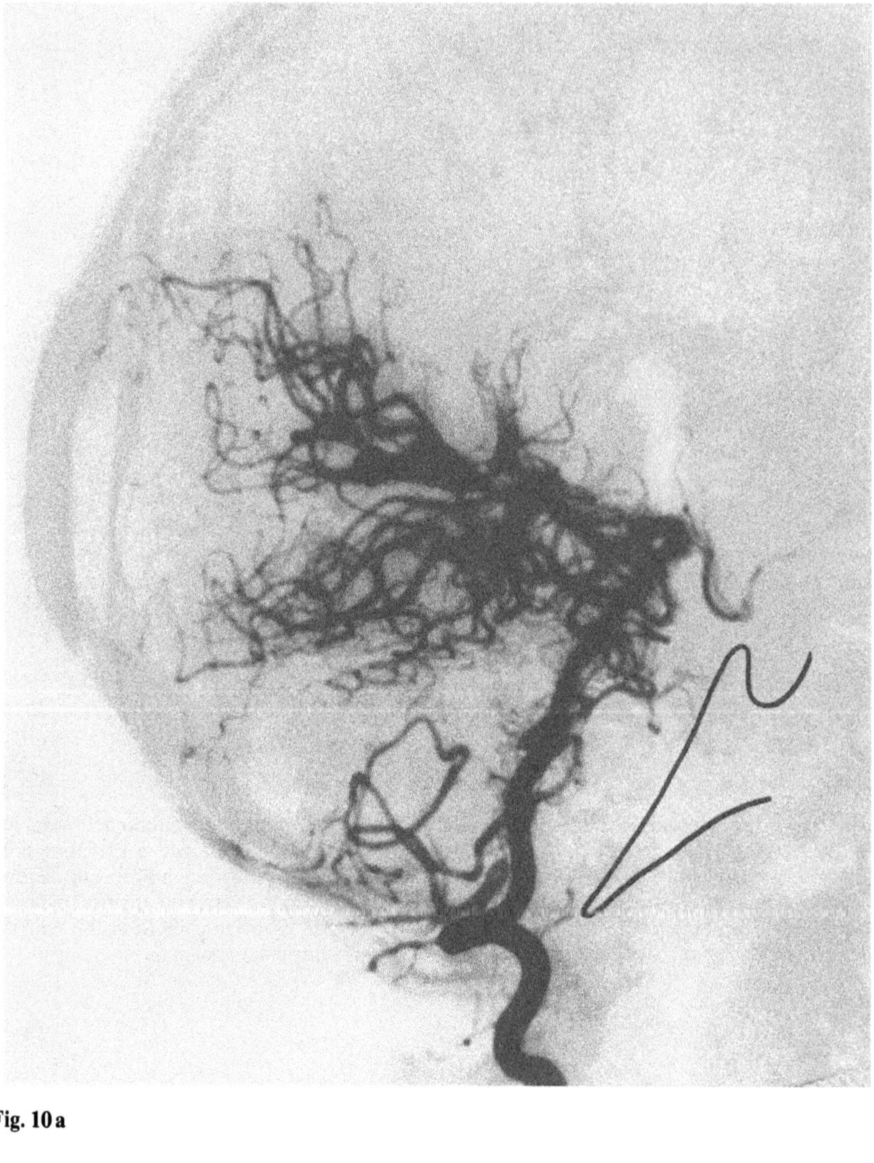

Fig. 10 a

1.3 Medulla Oblongata

1.3.1 Anatomy

The upper end of the medulla oblongata is at the level of the lower part of the middle cerebellar peduncle. The nucleus nervi cochlearis characterizes this level. The lower end of the medulla oblongata (foramen magnum) is characterized by the decussation of the corticospinal fibers which continue as lateral pyramidal tract in the spinal cord. At the transverse section of the pyramidal decussation one finds in

b

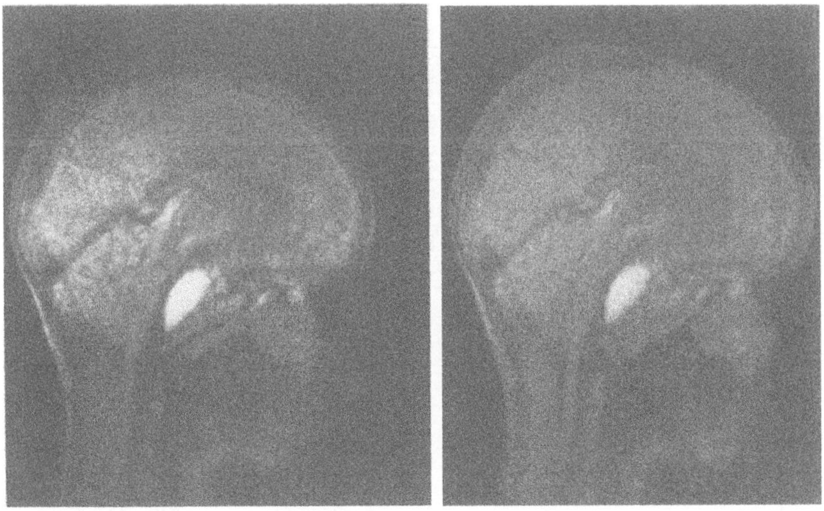

Fig. 10a,b. Chordoma (confirmed by operation). **a** Vertebral angiogram, lateral view. Basilar and vertebral artery are displaced dorsally away from the clivus (*marked by line*). **b** Nuclear magnetic resonance: Extrapontine localization of the tumor, compressing the pons (we wish to thank Prof. Hünermann and Dr. v. Einem, Cologne, for this picture)

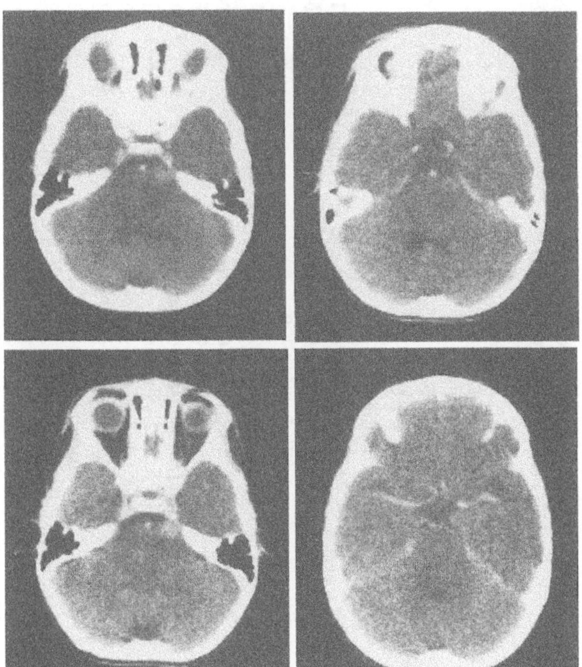

Fig. 11. Glioma of the pons. Compression and dorsal displacement of the 4th ventricle by the hypodense mass

Table 2.

Syndrome	Possible symptoms	Involved structure	Supplying artery (individual variations)
Foville-S. or Millard-Gubler-S. (caudal part of pons, *ventral*)	*Contralateral:*		
	– Hyposensitivity to touch position, vibration	– Medial lemniscus	Paramedian and circumferenting branches of the basilar artery
	– Analgesia, thermanesthesia at the body	– Tractus spinothalamicus lateralis	
	– Spastic hemiparesis	– Pyramidal tract	
	Ipsilateral:		
	– Peripheral 7th CN paresis	– Nucleus or fibers of 7th CN	
	– Peripheral 6th CN paresis	– Fibers of 6th CN	
	Others:		
	– Hypakusis	– Lateral lemniscus	
Caudal part of pons, *dorsal*	– Nystagmus	– Vestibular nuclei	Circumferenting branches of the basilar artery
	– Hypakusis	– Lateral lemniscus	
	Contralateral:		
	– Analgesia, thermanesthesia at the body	– Tractus spinothalamicus lateralis	
	– Hyposensitivity to touch, position, vibration	– Medial lemniscus	
	Ipsilateral:		
	– Peripheral 6th CN paresis	– Nucleus of 6th CN	
	– Peripheral 7th CN paresis	– Fibers of 7th CN	
	– Hemiataxia, intention tremor	– Medial cerebellar peduncle	
	– Horner-syndrome	– Tractus sympathicus	
	– Analgesia, thermanesthesia in the face	– Nucleus tractus spinalis of 5th CN	
	– Myorhythmia of soft palate	– Tractus tegmentalis centralis	
	– Muscular hypotonia	– Tractus spinocerebellaris anterior	

Oral part of pons, *dorsal*	– Hypakusis	– Lateral lemniscus	Circumferenting branches of basilar artery
	Contralateral:		
	– Analgesia, thermanesthesia at the body	– Tractus spinothalamicus lateralis	
	– Hyposensitivity to touch, position, vibration	– Medial lemniscus	
	Ipsilateral:		
	– Hemiataxia, intention tremor	– Superior cerebellar peduncle	
	– Loss of sensitivity to touch in the face	– Nucleus sensorius principalis 5th CN	
	– Analgesia, thermanesthesia in the face	– Nucleus tractus spinalis 5th CN	
	– Nuclear paresis of 5th CN	– Nucleus motorius 5th CN	
	– Myorhythmia of the soft palate	– Tractus tegmentalis centralis	
Middle part of pons, *ventral*	*Contralateral:*		
	– Spastic hemiparesis	– Pyramidal tract	Paramedian and short circumferenting branches of basilar artery
	Ipsilateral:		
	– Hyposensitivity for all qualities in the face	– Fibers of 5th CN	
	– Hemiataxia, hypotonia	– Medial cerebellar peduncle	
	– Motor paresis of 5th CN	– Fibers of 5th CN	

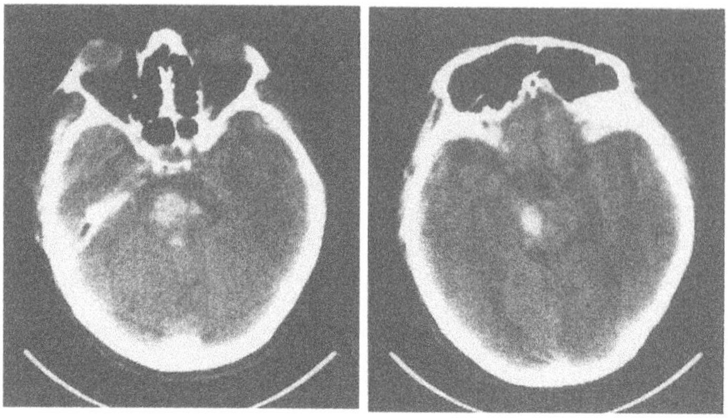

Fig. 12. Pons-angioma, reaching the mesencephalon

the posterior part the nuclei cuneatus and gracilis. From here the afferent impulses run via the medial lemniscus to the thalamus. Both the tractus spinothalamicus anterior (touch, pressure) and lateralis (pain, temperature) keep their lateral position throughout their course through the medulla oblongata but come close to the medial lemniscus (position, vibration, discrimination) at the lower level of the pons. Therefore ischemic processes in the medulla oblongata might be associated more often with selected signs of sensitivity than ischemic processes in the pons.

Except for the lower part of the medulla oblongata the nucleus olivarius is located between the ventral part (pyramidal tract) and central (medial lemniscus) and dorsal part. Functional impairment of the nucleus olivarius leads to myorhythmic movements (myoclonus) of the soft palate, pharynx and diaphragm (singultus). At the cranial part of the medulla oblongata one finds the upper part of the nuclei of

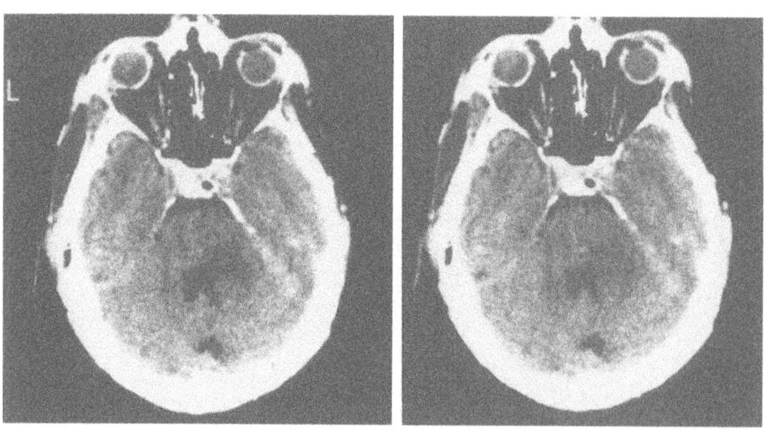

a

Fig. 13a–c. Right-sided tumor of the pons. **a** Displacement of the 4th ventricle dorsally, hypodense area in the anterior right, aspect of the pons. **b** Vertebral angiogram, *lateral view.* Vascular tumor inside the pons. **c** Nuclear magnetic resonance. Huge intrapontine space occupying mass (picture by courtesy of Prof. Hünermann and Dr. v. Einem, Cologne)

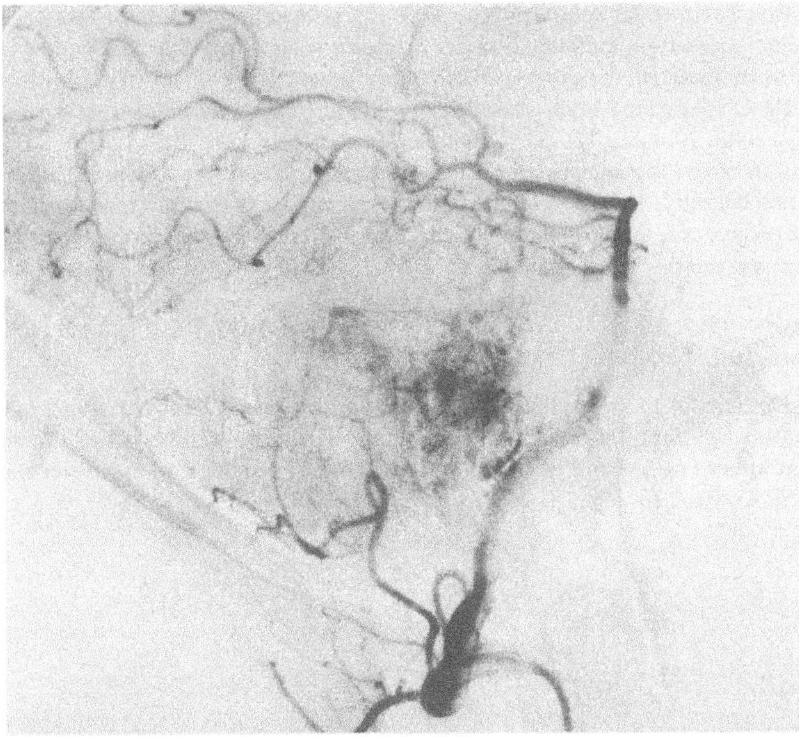

b

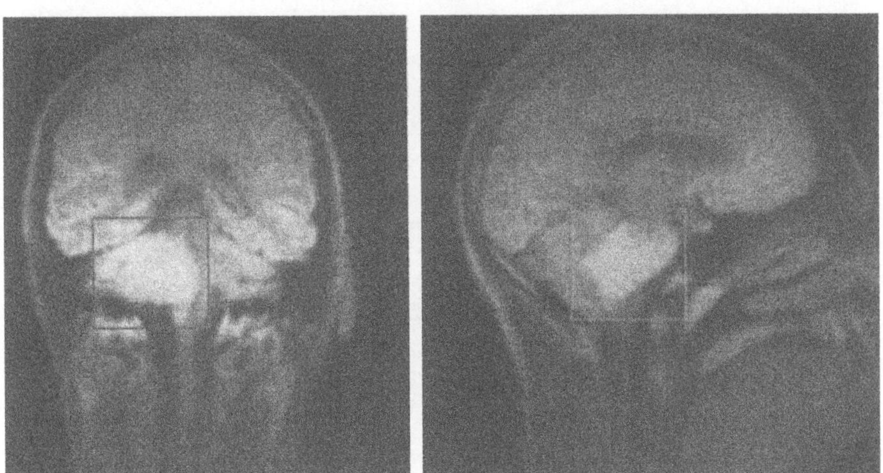

c

Fig. 13b, c

the 9th CN. The nuclear column of the 12th CN also covers more than 50% of the longitudinal axis of the medulla. Sensory or motor signs of these caudal nerves are not able to characterize the exact level of the brain stem process. However, the fibers of the 12th CN leave the brain stem directly lateral to the pyramidal tract whereas those of the 9th, 10th and 11th CN (the latter ones coming from the six upper spinal segments and from the nucleus ambiguus in the medulla oblongata) leave the brain stem more laterally, ventrally to the nucleus olivarius. Therefore signs from the caudal CN have less topographic significance in respect to the longitudinal axis but more in respect to the transverse cut.

1.3.2 Vascular Supply

The median part of the medulla oblongata is supplied by paramedian branches of the spinal and vertebral arteries, the paramedian territory by the anterior inferior cerebellar artery (AICA) and the lateral territory by the posterior inferior cerebellar artery (PICA) (Figs. 10, 14).

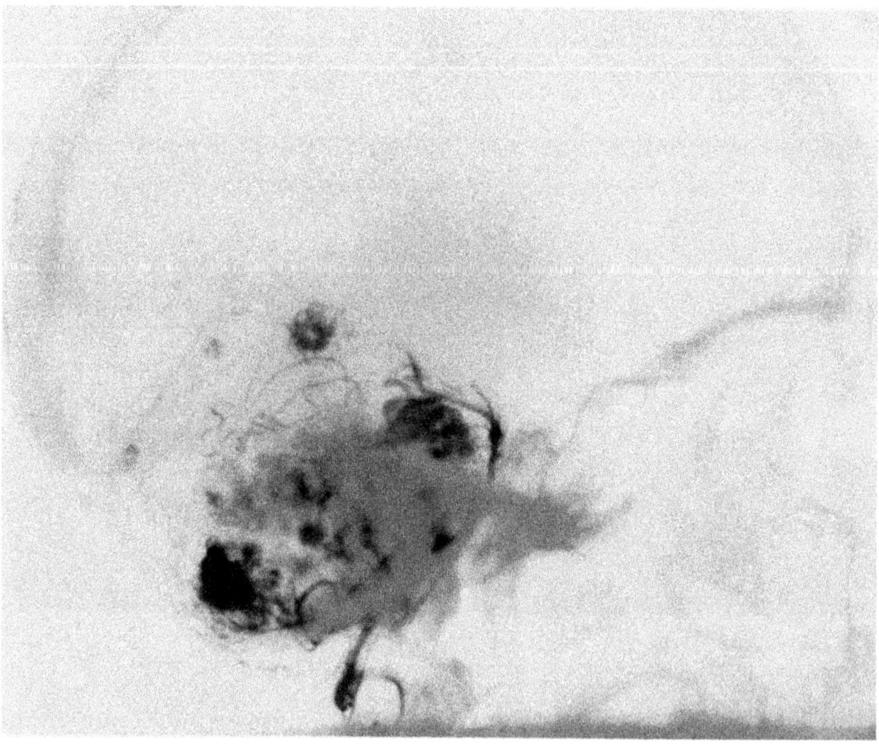

Fig. 14. Lindau-syndrome. The vertebral angiogram (*lateral view*) indicates several vascular tumors, one fed by the posterior inferior cerebellar artery. The tumors are located inside the cerebellum and the pons

1.3.3 Clinical Topography

The best known of all vascular syndromes of the brain stem are those of the Weber-syndrome (midbrain level) and the Wallenberg-syndrome, the latter resulting from ischemia in the area supplied by the PICA (Fig. 10a). In most of the cases the Wallenberg-syndrome shows fast recovery within a few days or weeks. However, since the initial symptoms also concern the nuclear columns of the 9th and 10th CN the patients may experience sudden aspiration. This and other potentially hazardous symptoms, like vomiting (by damage to area postrema) or singultus (reticular formation) request intensive care in all patients for some days.

In respect to topography three so-called crossed paralysis should be mentioned: That of the Weber-syndrome combines an ipsilateral 3rd CN palsy with a contralateral hemiparesis. The Millard-Gubler- or the Foville-syndrome are indicated by ipsilateral nuclear 7th CN palsy plus contralateral hemiparesis due to damage of the ventral part of the lower pons. The Déjérine- or Jackson-syndrome (medial medulla oblongata-syndrome) affects the pyramidal tract and the fibers of the 12th CN. The hemiparesis is contralateral to the tongue paresis.

All brain stem symptoms may appear transiently – then indicating ischemia in the basilar territory. They and others arising from vascular supply of the basilar artery (cortical visual disturbances, drop attack) might be due to a basilar stenosis. Therefore patients with a so-called vertebro-basilar insufficiency should be thoroughly investigated with noninvasive and invasive procedures. Space-occupying tumors, vascular malformations and infectious processes mostly do not produce vertebrobasilar insufficiency (Fig. 15).

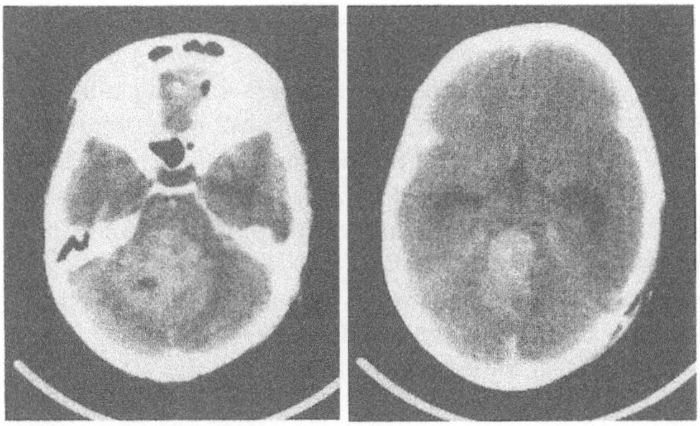

Fig. 15. Medullablastoma of the cerebellum. The CCT indicates a contrast medium enhancing mass with some cystic degeneration in the midline of the cerebellum, located in the vermis and both cerebellar hemispheres. The 4th ventricle is almost filled up

2. Neurologic Symptoms with Localizing Value in the Brain Stem

Many symptoms arising in the brain stem have high localizing value: e.g. the pyramidal tract and the MLF in respect to the transverse section and the fibers of the cranial nerves in respect to the height of lesions along the axis of the brain stem (Fig. 8). Other signs, however, have a less exact topographic meaning but are important in respect to indication of involvement of the brain stem. A few of them will be mentioned here.

2.1 Ventilatory Disturbances

The respiratory centers are located in the reticular formation of the medulla oblongata.

A periodic rhythmic alteration of the ventilation frequency between apnea and hyperpnea is called *Cheyne-Stokes-Respiration* (CSR). It results from an abnormal response to CO_2 causing hyperpnea and in addition from an abnormal forebrain stimulation to hyperpnea thus causing apnea (Cherniack et al. 1979). The possible lesion has to be located in the diencephalon or mesencephalon, rarely in the superior part of the pons (North and Jennett 1974). Disease where CSR has been described are bilateral cerebral infarction, uremic encephalopathy, hypoxia due to heart failure, hypertensive encephalopathy and increased intracranial pressure.

If the lesion is located close to the paramedian reticular formation between the lower mesencephalon and the middle part of the pons a sustained continuous *central neurogenic hyperventilation* (CNH) may be observed. Lactic acidosis in blood and CSF and pulmonary diseases must be ruled out to establish the diagnosis.

The patient may stop breathing for several seconds after a full inspiration. This occurs in extensive pontine damage (mid- and lower part) arising probably from the nucleus parabrachialis close to the motor nucleus of the 5th CN. Meningitis, pontine infarction and hypoglycemia have been described with this apnea.

If the disease affects directly the respiratory centers *ataxic breathing* (AB) may result. Respiration rate as well as depth of ventilation alternate unpredictably. Any space-occupying lesion in the posterior fossa can cause AB. It has been observed in bilateral vertebrobasilar insufficiency, poliomyelitis and demyelinating diseases. A subtype of AB with clusters of ventilation followed by irregular pauses might occur in diseases of the lower pons. AB has to be differentiated from alteration of respiration caused by overdoses of sedation.

Hiccup may be observed with lower brain stem lesions but also by thoracoabdominal or psychogenic diseases (Souadjian and Cain 1938). Vomiting due to central neurogenic processes have been observed mostly with diseases affecting the vestibular nuclei or the area close to the bottom of the 4th ventricle. Increased ICP is associated with projectile-like vomiting without nausea.

2.2 Gaze Abnormalities

If one observes constant monocular eye deviation in resting position one has to assume first injury to the nuclear, nervous or muscular part of the cranial nerves. Deviation of both eyes, however, might be due to damage to the gaze centers.

2.2.1 *Horizontal Gaze Abnormalities*

Under physiologic circumstances both eye axis are straight ahead. However, if the supranuclear oculomotoric pathway is affected on one side or asymmetrically a conjugate gaze deficit will appear. Metabolic diseases are unlikely to do that but any focal process like vascular diseases, tumors or infectious disease of the brain stem. A destructive process of one hemisphere leads to horizontal conjugate gaze deviation to the side of the lesion since the contralateral center is in function. Brain stem diseases with their focus below the decussation of the supranuclear oculomotoric pathways at the level of the 6th CN nucleus cause a deviation of both eyes away from the lesion. The uncertainty of this sign becomes obvious if one realizes that supratentorial thalamic hemorrhage with rupture into the 3rd ventricle may result into conjugate deviation of the eyes to the "wrong" side, i.e. they deviate to the healthy side (Fisher 1969).

2.2.2 *Vertical Gaze Abnormalities*

Usually an upward gaze palsy indicates a brain stem process, mostly at the midbrain level or midbrain-diencephalic junction. Bilateral MLF-lesions can cause a lack of upward gaze (Parinaud-syndrome). Conjugate downward deviation in resting position may be caused by large brain stem lesions or metabolic processes (Keane et al. 1976). If one eye deviates down and the other one up in resting position without preexisting strabismus or paresis of the eye ball muscles this indicates a lesion in the pons or medulla on the side of the downward deviating eye or the MLF on the side where the eye elevates. This skew deviation is diagnostic of brain stem disease (Smith et al. 1964).

2.2.3 *Dysconjugate Eye Movements in Brain Stem Diseases*

Particularly in comatose patients one might observe spontaneous or evoked eye movements which are not conjugate and furtheron not due to involvement of the nuclear, nervous or muscular part of the respective cranial nerve. Signs, possible lesions and diseases causing these spontaneous and evoked eye movements are listed in Table 3.

2.3 Ocular Motility

2.3.1 *Oculocephalic Reflex*

In comatose patients with intact brain stem and normal ocular motor function a brisk rotation of the head to the right (left) leads to fast movement of both eyes to the left (right). Flexion (extension) of the head results in conjugate movement of both eyes upward (downward). This sign is called a positive doll's head phenomenon.

2.3.2 *Oculovestibular Reflex*

With the head elevated for about 30 degree (to put the lateral semicircular canal into vertical position) one irrigates the right (left) ear with cold water (30 degree C°). Both eyes will present with nystagmus to the (left) right side (fast component). This

Table 3. Spontaneous eye movements in brain stem diseases

Type	Description	Disease and topography	Literature
Roving eye movements	Spontaneous slow roving of eyes. Conjugate or dysconjugate. Horizontal, only rarely vertical. Cannot be mimicked voluntarily	Coma with intact oculomotor function. If brain stem function becomes impaired, they disappear	Fisher 1969
Ping-Pong gaze	Conjugate fast rhythmic movements to extreme lateral position, resting for several seconds and followed by movements to the other side	Coma with involvement of hemispheres brain stem or cerebellum	Stewart et al. 1979
Retractory nystagmus	Eye movements back into eyes, often induced by voluntary upward gaze	Mesencephalic lesions	Daroff and Hoyt 1971 Elschnig 1913
Convergence nystagmus	Spontaneous slow diverging movements of both eyes followed by fast convergence	Mesencephalic lesions	Ochs et al. 1979
Ocular bobbing	Conjugate fast eye movements, followed by bobbing-like return to resting position	Pontine lesions or functional impairment of pons by remote lesions (cerebellum, hydrocephalus)	Fisher 1964 Braems and Dehaene 1975
Nystagmoid jerking of one eye	Jerking movements in all directions	Midpontine and lower pontine lesions	
Seesaw nystagmus	Rapid, pendular upward-inward movements of one eye and downward-outward movement of the other eye. Fixation impairs seesaw nystagmus	Area of 3rd ventricle, rostral mesencephalon, rarely pons or medulla	Lourie 1963

will last for about 2 min. If both eyes are irrigated at the same time with cold (hot) water, they will show downward (upward) nystagmus.

2.3.3 Ocular Motility in Brain Stem Disease

Metabolic coma or coma due to supratentorial diseases abolish the fast component and makes the slow component persistent for about 2–3 min, which means the eye will deviate tonically. Severe brain stem injury abolishes caloric response. Structural brain stem lesion may alter caloric response, e.g. the ipsilateral eye in unilateral stimulation may move downward.

Lesion of both MLF lead to the following phenomenon: The ocular reflex to horizontal head movement provokes the physiological abduction of one eye whereas the adduction of the other eye will move the eye only till the midline. Flexion-/extension-reaction is not impaired. Unilateral cold water irrigation provokes nystagmoid movements of the ipsilateral eye to lateral but adduction of the contralateral eye will not occur. In case of lower brain stem damage with interruption of the pathway between the vestibular nucleus and the abducens nucleus both abducting and adducting movements will be missed. In contrast to bilateral MLF-lesions which do not impair eye movements following bilateral simultaneous ear irrigation or flexion/extension of the head in lower brain stem lesion vertical movements of the eyes are inhibited.

Pretectal lesion in the midbrain abolish all upward movements of the eye (like in Parinaud syndrome). Certain drugs, like gentamicin, barbiturates, tricyclic antidepressants or succinylcholine, influence the oculovestibular reflex.

2.4 Pupillary Abnormalities in Brain Stem Coma

Whereas a cervical sympathetic blockade results in ipsilateral miosis, ptosis and hemianhidrosis of neck, face and arm a hypothalamic lesion might cause miosis, ptosis and hemianhidrosis of the total body. This might be the very first sign of transtentorial herniation.

Midbrain lesions may preserve accommodation but impair light reflex if the lesion is located in the pretectal area. The pupils are light-fixed in midposition and may show hippus. The ciliospinal reflex of which the synapse is located in the spinal cord is preserved.

Midposition fixed pupils are also caused by transtentorial herniation or any other space-occupying disease in the midbrain.

Pontine lesion causes pinpoint pupils due to interruption of the sympathetic signal. The light reflex might be seen with a magnifying glass. The same is true for lateral medullary lesion or lesions of the ventrolateral cervical spinal cord.

References

Braems M, Dehaene I (1975) Ocular bobbing: clinical significance. Clin Neurol Neurosurg 78:99–106

Cherniack NS, von Euler C, Homma I et al. (1979) Experimentally induced Cheyne-Stokes breathing. Respir Physiol 37:185–200

Cogan DG, Kubik CS, Smith WL (1950) Unilateral internuclear ophthalmoplegia: report of 8 clinical cases with one post-mortem study. Arch Ophthalmol 44:783–796
Daroff RB, Hoyt WF (1971) Supranuclear disorders of ocular control system in man: clinical and physiological correlations. In: Bach-y-Rita P, Collins CC, Hyde JE (eds) The Control of Eye Movements. Academic Press, New York, 17/5
Elschnig A (1913) Nystagmus retractorius: Ein zerebrales Herdsymptom. Med Klin 9:8–11
Fisher CM (1964) Ocular bobbing. Arch Neurol 11:543–546
Fisher CM (1969) The neurological examination of the comatose patients. Acta Neurol Scand [Suppl 36] 45:1–56
Keane JR, Rawlinson DG, Lu AT (1976) Sustained downward deviation. Two cases without structural pretectal lesions. Neurology (NY) 26:594–595
King WM, Lisberger AG, Fuchs AF (1976) Response of fibers in medial longitudinal fasciculus (MLF) of alert monkeys during horizontal and vertical conjugate eye movements evoked by vestibular or visuli stimuli. J Neurophysiol 65:135–1149
Lourie H (1963) Seesaw nystagmus. Arch Neurol 9:531–533
North JB, Jennett S (1974) Abnormal breathing patterns associated with acute brain damage. Arch Neurol 31:338–344
Ochs A, Stark L, Hoyt WF et al. (1979) Opposed adducting saccades in convergence-retraction nystagmus: a patient with Sylvian aqueduct syndrome. Brain 102:497–508
Salomon J (1971) Atlas de la vascularisation arterielle du cerveau chez l'homme. Sandoz Editions, Paris
Smith JL, David NJ (1964) Internuclear ophthalmoplegia. Two new clinical signs. Neurology (NY) 14:307–309
Smith JL, David NJ, Klintworth G (1964) Skew deviation. Neurology (NY) 14:96–105
Souadjian JV, Cain JC (1938) Intractable hiccup. Etiologic factors in 220 cases. Postgrad Med 43:72–77
Stewart JD, Kirkham TH, Mathieson G (1979) Periodic alternating gaze. Neurology (NY) 29.222–224

Symptoms of Tumors of the Brain Stem and the Third Ventricle

M. SCHIRMER, Düsseldorf/FRG

Between 1963 and 1982 2553 patients with intracranial tumors were treated in the Neurosurgical Department of Düsseldorf University. The case histories of these patients have been evaluated by electronic data processing. Overall 28 symptoms were recorded according to the informations obtained by the patients' admission.

Headaches were the most frequent *symptom* in 60.1% of the patients followed by deterioration of vision in 30.8%, vomiting in 27.4%, vertigo in 25.6%, and epileptic attacks in 23,5%.

Among these 2553 patients were 103 in which the tumors were located in the brain stem and the third ventricle. All data of the patients were coded according to the code-guide of the German Societies of Neurology and Neurosurgery. So we had different possibilities to code the localizations of the tumors.

For our study tumors of the corpus striatum, the globus pallidus, the thalamus, and the entire diencephalon were summarized as tumors of the *diencephalon.* Among 32 of the tumors of the diencephalon were 22 gliomas, 2 ependymomas, 1 craniopharyngioma, 1 metastasis and 6 unknown tumors (Table 1).

Tumors of the foramen of Monro and the entire third ventricle were comprised as tumors of the *third ventricle;* these 28 tumors consisted of 7 gliomas, 6 ependymomas, 4 craniopharyngiomas, 4 pinealomas and 7 others (listed in Table 1).

Among the 28 tumors of the *midbrain* we reckoned tumors of the entire mesencephalon, the pineal gland, the aqueduct, and the quadrigeminal bodies. In this region 12 gliomas, 5 pinealomas, 2 teratomas, and 9 other tumors were found.

In the *pons* 5 gliomas and 10 other tumors existed (Table 1).

The *duration of case history* differed in these groups: In average, tumors of the third ventricle and especially of the pons had a longer anamnesis than tumors of the diencephalon and the midbrain. Of the former over one third had a history exceeding one year, of the latter one third of 1 month only (Table 2).

The symptoms produced by the different tumors were divided in 3 groups:

i. general symptoms,
ii. functional disturbances
iii. mental changes.

As in all other intracranial tumors *headaches* were the most frequent symptom also in tumors of the brain stem and the third ventricle. Nevertheless only one half of the tumors of the diencephalon and the pons, but 71.4% of the tumors of the third ventricle and 67.8% of the tumors of the midbrain caused headaches (Table 3).

Vomiting is a very common symptom in patients with tumors of the third ventricle, midbrain, and the pons, but not with tumors of the diencephalon. The rate of

Table 1. Distribution of tumors in the brain stem and the 3rd ventricle in 103 patients and in 2450 other patients harboring intracranial tumors in other localizations

	Diencephalon n = 32	3rd ventricle n = 28	Midbrain n = 28	Pons n = 15	% Total n = 103	n = 2450 (%)
Medulloblastoma	–	–	1	–	1.0	2.7
Spongioblastoma	–	2	–	–	1.9	0.9
Oligodendroglioma	3	2	–	–	4.9	6.0
Astrocytoma	5	2	3	2	11.7	12.9
Glioblastoma	10	1	1	–	11.7	13.5
Other glioma	4	–	8	3	14.6	3.4
Ependymoma	2	6	1	–	8.7	1.8
Papilloma of chorioid plexus	–	1	–	–	1.0	0.4
Neurinoma	–	–	1	1	1.9	4.8
Gangliocytoma	–	1	–	–	1.0	0.04
Meningioma	–	1	–	1	1.9	18.9
Craniopharyngioma	1	4	–	–	4.9	2.0
Pituitary adenoma	–	1	–	–	1.0	8.9
Epidermoid cyst	–	1	–	–	1.0	0.7
Teratoma	–	1	2	–	2.9	0.4
Malignant lymphoma	–	1	–	–	1.0	0.5
Metastasis	1	–	1	1	2.9	11.3
Unknown tumor	6	–	5	7	17.5	2.5
Pinealoma	–	4	5	–	8.7	0.04

vomiting in patients of the former three groups of tumors exceeds the rate of all other intracranial tumors considerably (Table 3).

The overall rate of *vertigo* caused by tumors of the brain stem and the third ventricle is nearly the same as in other intracranial tumors with a clear preponderance of tumors of the midbrain and the pons.

Fatigue is especially caused by tumors of the diencephalon and the third ventricle in nearly one third of the cases. The overall rate of fatigue in tumors of the brain stem and the third ventricle is double the rate of fatigue in all other intracranial tumors (Table 3). The same relation may be seen in *loss of weight, thirst,* and *incontinence.*

Among functional disturbances (Table 4) *deterioration of vision* and *gait disturbances* were more frequent in tumors of the third ventricle and the brain stem than in intracranial tumors located elsewhere. Especially tumors of the third ventricle produced marked deterioration of vision in 39.3%. 60% of the tumors of the pons caused gait disturbances, and one third of the tumors of the diencephalon and the midbrain, while only 10.7% of the patients harboring tumors of the third ventricle complained of disturbances of gait. All other functional disturbances were more common in other intracranial tumors.

Table 2. Duration of history in 103 patients harboring tumors of the brain stem and the third ventricle

	Dien-cephalon n=32 (%)	3rd ventricle n=28 (%)	Midbrain n=28 (%)	Pons n=15 (%)	n=103 (%)
Until 1 week	–	3.6	3.6	–	1.9
Until 1 month	31.3	17.9	32.1	–	23.3
Until 3 months	21.9	17.9	28.6	6.7	20.4
Until 6 months	15.6	7.1	10.7	33.3	14.6
Until 1 year	15.6	10.7	7.1	20.0	12.6
Over 1 year	9.4	35.7	17.9	40.0	23.3
Unknown	6.3	7.1	–	–	3.9

Table 3. General symptoms in 103 patients harboring tumors of the brain stem and the third ventricle and in 2450 other intracranial tumors

	Dien-cephalon n=32 (%)	3rd ven-tricle n=28 (%)	Mid-brain n=28 (%)	Pons n=15 (%)	n=103 (%)	n=2450 (%)
Headaches	46.9	71.4	67.8	46.7	59.2	60.1
Vomiting	18.8	46.4	60.7	53.3	42.7	26.7
Vertigo	15.6	17.9	35.7	40.0	25.2	23.1
Fatigue	31.3	28.6	14.3	13.3	23.3	11.5
Nausea	3.1	14.3	21.4	6.7	11.7	10.4
Loss of weight	9.4	17.9	–	6.7	8.7	4.6
Incontinence	6.3	10.7	–	13.3	6.8	3.1
Thirst	3.1	10.7	–	–	3.9	1.6
Hormonal disturbances	3.1	3.6	7.1	–	3.9	4.7
Hypersalivation	–	–	–	13.3	1.9	0.2
Increase in weight	–	7.1	–	–	1.9	1.8
Tremor	–	–	–	13.3	1.9	2.1
Fever	–	–	–	6.7	1.0	1.3

Table 4. Functional disturbances in 103 patients harboring tumors of the brain stem and third ventricle and in 2450 other patients with intracranial tumors

	Dien-cephalon n=32 (%)	3rd ven-tricle n=28 (%)	Mid-brain n=28 (%)	Pons n=15 (%)	n=103 (%)	n=2450 (%)
Gait disturbances	31.3	10.7	35.7	60.0	31.1	22.6
Deterioration of vision	21.9	39.3	32.1	33.3	35.0	30.6
Speech disorders	21.9	3.6	10.7	20.0	13.6	14.1
Epileptic attacks	9.4	17.9	–	6.7	8.7	24.1
Tinnitus	–	3.6	–	13.4	2.9	3.4
Olfactory disturbances	3.1	7.1	–	–	2.9	3.1
Deterioration of hearing	–	–	–	20.0	2.9	7.7
Dysgraphia	3.1	–	–	–	1.0	3.2

Table 5. Mental changes in 103 patients harboring tumors of the brain stem and third ventricle and in 2450 patients with intracranial tumors of other localizations

	Dien-cephalon n=32 (%)	3rd ven-tricle n=28 (%)	Mid-brain n=28 (%)	Pons n=15 (%)	n=103 (%)	n=2450 (%)
Personality changes	37.5	32.1	14.3	6.7	25.2	19.6
Lack of motivation	25.0	25.0	7.1	13.3	18.4	11.1
Retardation	18.8	28.6	14.3	6.7	18.4	15.3
Disturbances of memory	18.8	14.3	10.7	6.7	13.6	16.1
Confusion	12.5	7.1	3.6	–	6.8	9.2
Depression	3.1	3.6	–	20.0	4.9	3.8

Mental changes (Table 5) like confusion, depression and euphoria are rare symptoms of tumors of the brain stem and the third ventricle. One quarter of the patients developed *personality changes,* especially patients harboring tumors of the third ventricle (32.1%) and the diencephalon (37.5%). Also *retardation, lack of motivation,* and *disturbances of memory* were much more frequent in patients with tumors in the rostral parts of the brain stem than in those with tumors in other areas of the brain.

5.8% of our patients harboring tumors of the brain stem and the third ventricle were *unconscious* at admission, especially patients with tumors of the midbrain (7.1%), third ventricle (7.1%), and diencephalon (6.3%). The ratio of unconsciousness at admission in all other patients was 2.8%, the ratio of clouding of consciousness 21.2%, in patients with tumors of the brain stem and the third ventricle 27.2%.

Conclusions

There are no special symptoms or a special pattern of symptoms which characterize tumors of the third ventricle and the brain stem.

In the distribution of symptoms the midbrain seems to be a borderline between the rostral parts of the brain stem and the pontine area. Tumors of the rostral parts tend to cause more mental changes and typical "diencephalic" disorders. Tumors of the midbrain and pons produce more often functional disturbances.

All symptoms depend on subjective informations and may not be misinterpreted as objective findings. Nevertheless the results of our study confirm practical experiences by objective data.

Functional Anatomy of Sensory Motor Afferences of the Thalamus

A. STRUPPLER and P. BIRK, München/FRG

The target point in the human ventrolateral thalamus for the treatment of Parkinsonian tremor was found empirically in the last decades. Fundamental work was done by Hassler, who established a model of functional anatomy of the human ventrolateral thalamus (Fig. 1) [6, 7]. Nowadays, the target point for the abolition of Parkinsonian tremor is well established, but the functional anatomy of the target area is still a subject of research. Some of our findings will be presented and compared to findings from recent animal studies.

Postoperatively, a hypotonia contralateral to the operated thalamus occurs, which the patient can compensate by visual control. The tremor is abolished, but no loss of force, epicritic sensitivity or an ataxia is observed, and the phasic stretch reflexes remain unchanged [15, 16]. In accordance with these postoperative findings we suggest that a system involved in the control of muscle tone might be affected by the lesion in a rather selective way [4].

Intraoperatively, a facilitatory effect in the periphery, concerning muscle tone and tremor, is observed during electrical stimulation of the target area. Additionally, evoked potentials with short onset latency can be recorded within the target area, following electrical stimulation of contralateral peripheral mixed nerves (Fig. 2). In contrast, no significant evoked potentials were recorded in the same thalamic area following selective stimulation of skin afference (Fig. 3).

The stimulation of the mixed nerves was done with bipolar surface electrodes, skin afference was stimulated by using two pairs of wire electrodes wound around fingers II to IV. The stimulus strength was 2 to 3 times that of the motoric and sensitive threshold, respectively, consisting of square pulses of 0.1–0.3 ms duration. The stimulus frequency was 2–3 Hz. For the monopolar recording a tungsten semimicroelectrode was used, with it's reference to the frame. The filter range was 0.5 to 2 kHz, 400–500 sweeps were averaged.

The target area, where recording and stimulation were done, is within the nucleus v.im., and the adjacent subthalamus as mentioned in Fig. 2. The anatomical calculations are based on positive ventriculograms (3rd ventricle), the transfer to the stereotaxic atlas was in reference to CACP length (Fig. 4a + b) [4].

The findings so far presented lead to the suggestion that fast conducting muscle afference may project to the v.im. and the adjacent subthalamus, via direct ascending spinal input. No information about the anatomy of the projecting tracts is provided from these data.

A direct correlation of these findings with data from animal studies is problematic. This has several reasons, methodical ones, as well as phylo- and ontogenetic ones. However, a comparison of functional anatomy between humans and animals,

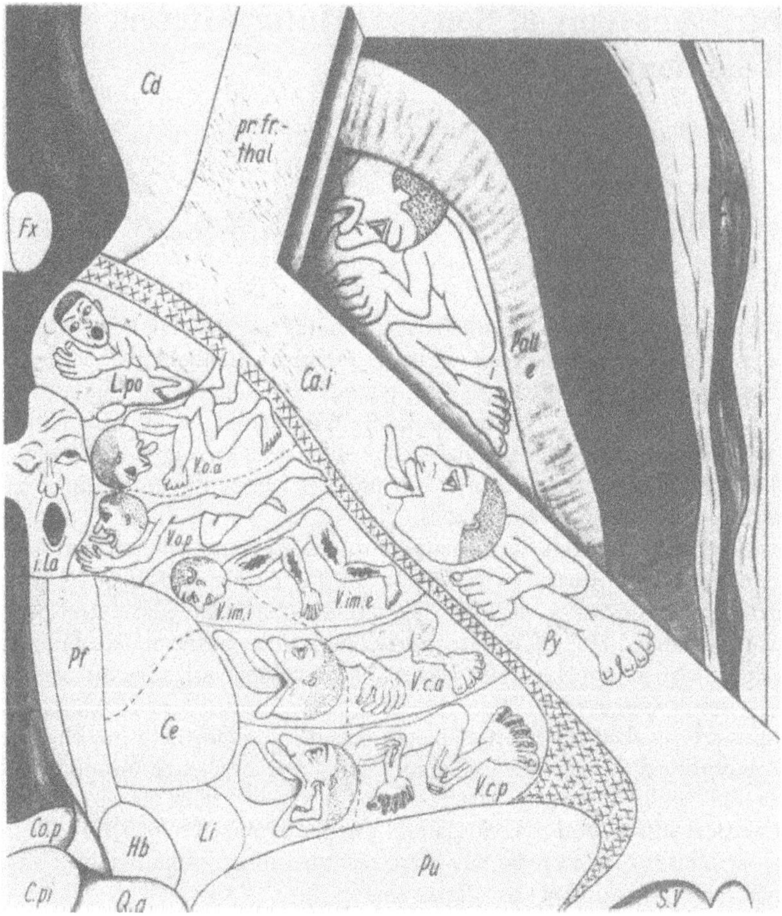

Fig. 1. Diagram of the right human thalamus (from Kunc [11]). The horizontal section shows the functional anatomy of the six ventral thalamic nuclei. From dorsal to frontal follow the homunculi of joint sensitivity (*V.c.p.*), tactile sensitivity (*V.c.a.*), and of muscle spindles (*V.im.e*) and labyrinth (*V.im.i.*). Then the homunculus of the cerebellar input (*V.o.p.*) follows, and more frontal the homunculus of the turning to the contralateral side, the raising of the contralateral area, and vocalization is shown

especially primates, may be helpful for the development of models. Oversimplified, the lateral ventrobasal thalamus in primates can be divided into three parts according to their respective afferent input. A more oral part (VLo), where pallidothalamic, and a more caudal part (VPLo, VLc), where cerebellothalamic afference terminate. Third, a caudal part (VPLc), which receives spinothalamic and lemniscal input [1, 2, 5, 8]. A certain overlap of cerebellothalamic and spinal afference in the VPLo is discussed (Fig. 5) [3, 10]. According to Jones and Friedman, the VPLc is divided into a shell and a core region depending on the respective afferent input. "Deep" input (joint and muscle afferents) is represented in the shell region, "cutaneous" input in the core region (Fig. 6) [9].

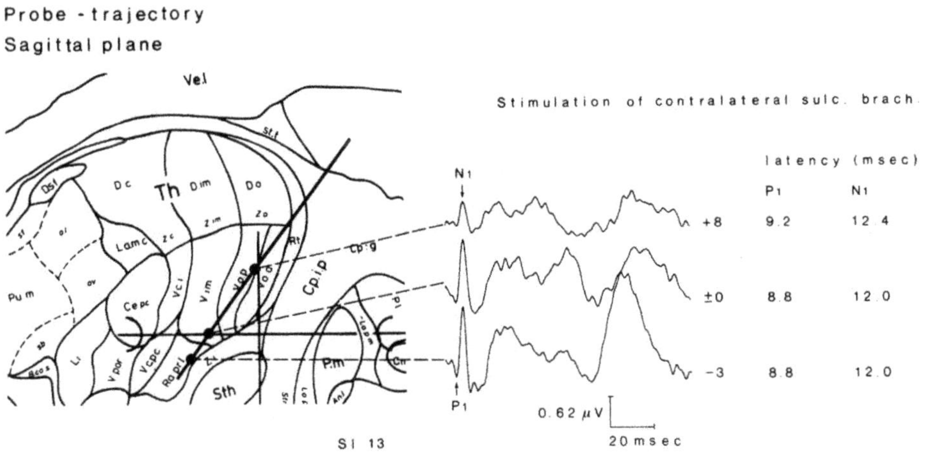

Fig. 2. Evoked potentials following mixed nerve stimulation in reference to the stereotaxic atlas of Schaltenbrand-Wahren (plane sagittal lateral 13 [14]). The evoked potentials initially are triphasic. The latencies of the first positivity (*P1*) and the first negativity (*N1*) show a slight decrease with depth (9.2 ms to 8.8 ms, 12.4 ms to 12.0 ms, respectively), whereas the amplitudes show a slight increase. The probe passes *V.o.p.*, *V.im.* on the way to subthalamus (*Ra.prl*). The target point is situated in the *V.im.* and *Ra.prl.* border region (depth 0 to −3)

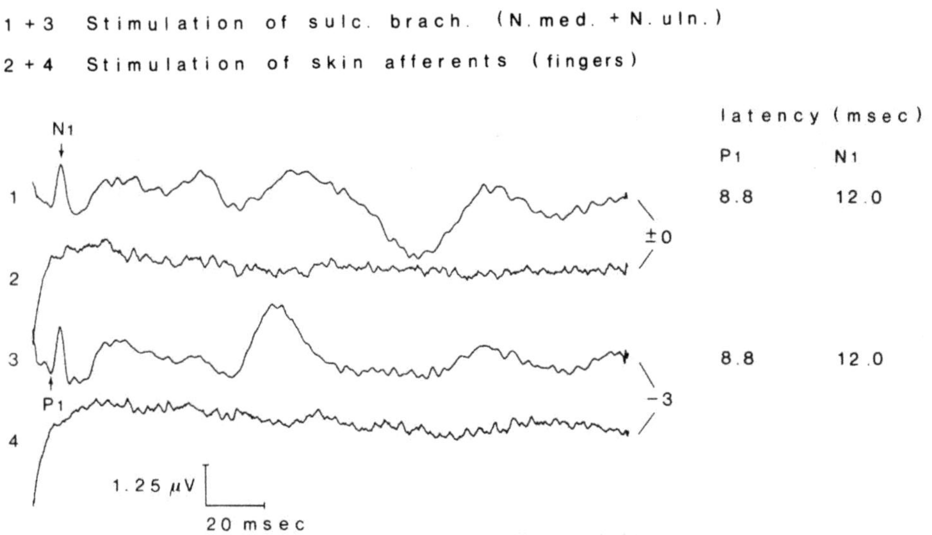

Fig. 3. In contrast to stimulation of mixed nerves, stimulation of skin afferents evokes no significant potential within the target region

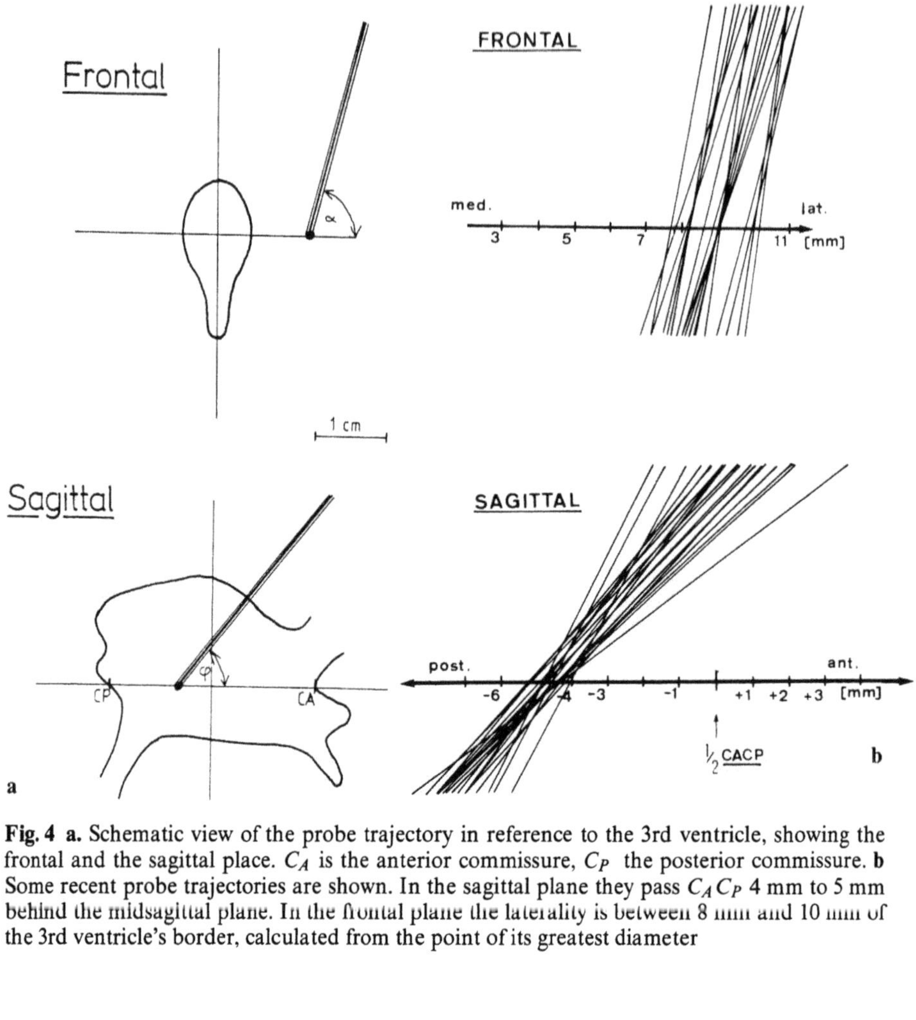

Fig. 4 **a.** Schematic view of the probe trajectory in reference to the 3rd ventricle, showing the frontal and the sagittal place. C_A is the anterior commissure, C_P the posterior commissure. **b** Some recent probe trajectories are shown. In the sagittal plane they pass $C_A C_P$ 4 mm to 5 mm behind the midsagittal plane. In the frontal plane the laterality is between 8 mm and 10 mm of the 3rd ventricle's border, calculated from the point of its greatest diameter

Fig. 6. The VPLc is divided into a shell and a core region (according to Jones and Friedman [9]). In the shell region single units react to "deep" stimuli (*vertical bars*), as movement of joints and pressing the muscle belly. In the core region single units reacting to cutaneous stimuli (slight touch of the skin, movement of hair) are represented by *horizontal bars*

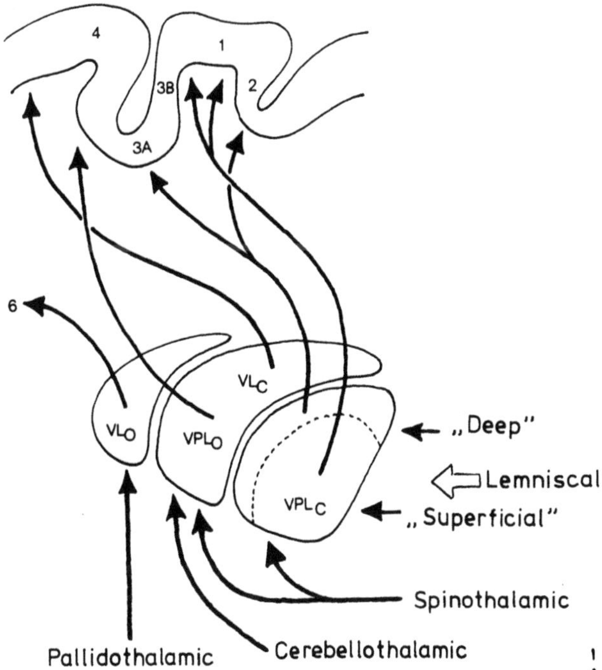

Fig. 5. The afferent projection to the ventrolateral thalamus and the cortex of primates (according to Jones [10]). For further explanation see text

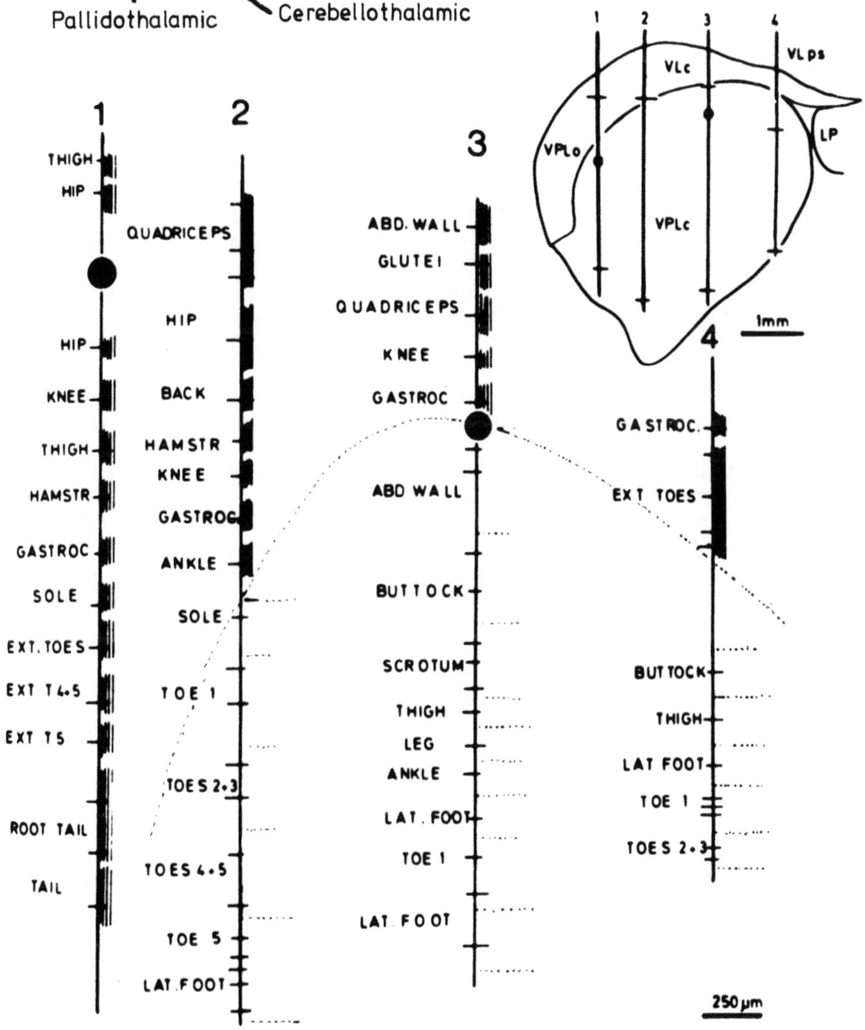

Comparing this functional anatomic organisation with our results, the target area for the abolition of tremor could be in that region where direct spinal input terminates, but so-called cutaneous qualities are of less importance. According to the overlap between cerebellar and spinal input in the VPLo and the intermediate position of v.im. (see Hassler's scheme in Fig. 1), this could be in between the spinal and cerebellar termination area, according to the nomenclature of Olszewski, the border of VPLo adjacent to VPLc [12, 13]. One might argue that an interruption of muscle afference directly ascending from the spinal level plays a role for the abolition of tremor. Additionally, an interruption of cerebellothalamic afference as well must be taken into account for the mechanism of tremor abolition.

References

1. Asanuma H (1981) Functional role of sensory inputs to the motor cortex. Prog Neurobiol 16:241–262
2. Asanuma H, Thach WF, Jones EG (1983) Distribution of cerebellar terminations and their relation to other afferent terminations in the ventral lateral thalamic region of the monkey. Brain Res Rev 5:237–265
3. Berkley KJ (1983) Spatial relationship between the terminations of somatic sensory and motor pathways in the rostral brainstem of cats and monkeys. II. Cerebellar projections compared with those of the ascending somatic sensory pathways in lateral diencephalon. J Comp Neurol 220:229–251
4. Birk P, Struppler A, Riescher H, Keidel M (in press) Somatosensory evoked potentials in the human ventrolateral thalamus. Symposion on Evoked Potentials, Tübingen 1984
5. Gless P (1945) The interrelation of the striopallidum and the thalamus in the macaque monkey. Brain 68:331–346
6. Hassler R (1949) Über die afferenten Bahnen und Thalamuskerne des motorischen Systems des Großhirns. II. Mitteilung. Weitere Bahnen aus Pallidum, Ruber, vestibulären System zum Thalamus. Übersicht und Besprechung der Ergebnisse. Arch Psychiatr. Z Neurol 182:786, 818
7. Hassler R, Mundinger F, Riechert T (1979) Stereotaxis in parkinson syndrome. In: Hassler R (ed) With an atlas of the basal ganglia in parkinsonism. Springer, Berlin Heidelberg New York
8. Ilinsky JA, Kultas-Ilinsky K (1982) Comparative study of pallidothalamic projections in the cat and monkey. Neurosci Lett 10:248–249
9. Jones EG, Friedman DP (1982) Projection pattern of functional components of thalamic ventrobasal complex on monkey somatosensory cortex. J Neurophys 48:521–544
10. Jones EG (1983) The nature of the afferent pathways conveying short latency inputs to primate motor cortex. In: Desmedt JE (ed) Motor Control Mechanisms in Health and Disease. Raven Press, New York, pp 263–285
11. Kunc Z (1970) Significant factors pertaining to the results of trigeminal tractotomy. In: Hassler R, Walker AE (eds) Trigeminal Neuralgia. Thieme, Stuttgart, pp 90–100
12. Olszewski J (1952) The thalamus of the macaca mulatta. Basel New York
13. Olszewski J, Baxter C (1954) Cytoarchitecture of the human brain stem. S.B. Lippincott Company, Philadelphia
14. Schaltenbrand G, Wahren W (1971) Atlas for stereotaxy of the human brain. Ed 2, Thieme, Stuttgart
15. Struppler A (1982) Contribution of electromyography to stereotaxy. In: Schaltenbrand G, Walker AE (eds) Stereotaxy of the human brain. Thieme, Stuttgart New York, pp 436–448
16. Struppler A (1985) Stereoencephalotomy and motor control. In: Struppler A, Weindl A (eds) Electromyography and evoked potentials. Springer, Berlin Heidelberg New York Tokyo, pp 37–44

Intracranial Pressure, Neurological Condition and Operative Management in Relation to the Outcome of Patients with Supratentorial Midline Tumors

K.-E. RICHARD, R. KNIPPRATH, P. SANKER, P. VAN DEN BERGH*, and R. A. FROWEIN, Köln/FRG and *Boston, MA/USA

Summary

In 199 children, juveniles and adults operated on for supratentorial midline tumors, the clinical neurological factors important for the determination of the disease course were analysed. In 68 patients the importance of the intracranial pressure was examined.

When ranking clinical indicators for the disease course and for the outcome of patients, pre- and postoperative disturbances of consciousness, respiratory function and cranial nerve function are listed first.

Pathological increases of intracranial pressure correlate well with simultaneously persisting disturbances of consciousness in determining the disease course.

In 5 cases, anisocoria or mydriasis associated with coma after surgery of a tumor in the hypothalamic area, especially craniopharyngiomas, was not a sign of irreversible mesencephalic or brainstem herniation, but a reversible symptom related to functional alterations of nervous structures near the hypothalamus. Intracranial pressure monitoring in these cases facilitates the interpretation of this finding.

The extent of tumor resection was decisive for the postoperative ventricular fluid pressure. In all cases with subtotal resection of a midline tumor, acute rises of the intracranial pressure because of predictable CSF circulation disturbances, should be prevented by implanting an internal shunt. Implantation of a ventricular-peritoneal shunt is most appropriate for this purpose.

Introduction

Supratentorial midline tumors particularly lead to CSF circulation disturbances causing increased ventricular fluid pressure. Incomplete removal of these tumors is a frequent cause of problems because of pressure differences building up in the ventricular compartments, separated from each other by the tumor [1–3].

The aim of this study is to examine the importance of the intracranial pressure as related to other factors essential for the determination of the disease outcome: preoperative neurological condition, size of ventricles, postoperative state of consciousness and pupillary behavior, and surgical management of the tumor.

Patient Material (Table 1)

199 patients with a supratentorial midline tumor were treated between 1973 and 1983.

In 68 patients (34%) the ventricular fluid pressure (VFP) was perioperatively measured with a mean duration of 6 days.

From the relatively high mortality rate in the pressure monitored patients, that is 41% as compared to 21%, it is clear that pressure monitoring was performed only in those patients endangered by severe neurological deficits.

Results

1. Preoperative Neurological Findings and Outcome (Fig. 1)

When preoperatively *unconscious* the mortality rate in patients was 57–100%. The outcome was also unfavorable in patients admitted with respiratory problems, the operative mortality rate being 60–100%.

Preoperative *palsies* and *abnormalities of the third and the sixth cranial nerves* correlated with a 25–75% mortality. In the absence of the above mentioned disturbances of consciousness and neurological functions the operative mortality rate at most was 28%.

2. Degree of Ventricular Enlargement and Outcome

The operative mortality rate for all patients was 32–37% when ventricular enlargement was present before surgery, whereas it was only 17% when radiological signs of CSF circulation disturbances were absent.

The mortality rate was slightly higher in second and third degree ventricular enlargement as compared to first degree enlargement.

When an increase of VFP was measured, a relatively high mortality rate in patients with still a normal-sized ventricular system was noticed.

3. Postoperative State of Consciousness, Pupillary Behavior, Intracranial Pressure, and Outcome (Figs. 2–5)

A general review of the state of consciousness and the mean intracranial pressure measured in separate pre- and postoperative days shows that in conscious as well as in semiconscious patients, especially in children and juveniles, very high mean VFPs up to 50 mm Hg in the *preoperative course* may survive (Fig. 2).

In the *postoperative course* the outcome was favorable only in those patients in whom no severe disturbances of consciousness were present with pressures higher than 20 mm Hg and in comatose patients in whom the mean VFP was not higher than 20 mm Hg (Fig. 2). Young patients have survived regardless their state of consciousness if the maximum postoperative VFP did not exceed 20 mm Hg.

With VFP's higher than 20 mm Hg, the rate of survival of the semiconscious and comatose patients dropped to 57% and 33%, respectively.

Table 1. Patient material: Location of midline tumors and mortality rate of all patients and of patients with VFP-measurement

	Supratentorial midline tumors 1973–1983 (N=199)														
	N			Mortality %			With VFP-measurement								
	Σ	Adults >20 yrs	Youths <20 yrs	Σ	Adults >20 yrs	Youths <20 yrs	Σ	%	Adults		Youths		Σ	Mortal. %	
									N	%	N	%		Adu.	Youths
Craniopharyngioma	68	29	39	10	17	5	8	12	1	3	7	18	12	0	14
Thalamus, hypothalamus	14	5	9	29	20	33	8	57	3	60	5	56	37	33	40
Third ventricle	64	16	48	20	19	20	26	41	6	39	20	42	27	33	25
Pineal region	19	6	13	39	50	33	7	39	3	50	4	33	57	67	50
Basal ganglia	34	16	18	44	44	44	19	56	11	69	8	44	63	55	75
	199	72	127	21	20	21	68	34	24	33	44	35	41	47	36

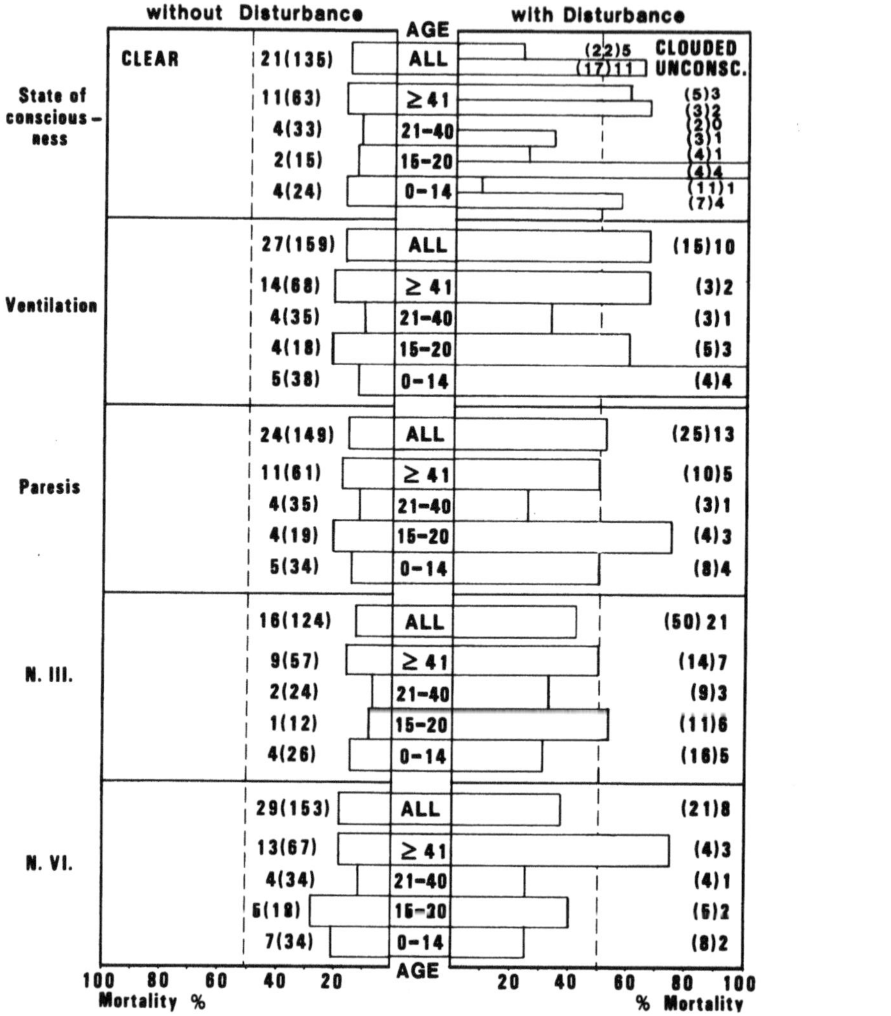

Fig. 1. Age of patients at surgery, preoperative neurological state and mortality rate. The figures represent patients with or without neurological disturbances in each group; the figures within parentheses represent the total number of patients

Unconscious patients with *complete absence of motor and pupillary reactions* – Coma IV – did not survive, irrespective of the intracranial pressure level.

The presence of *non-reactive pupils* in comatose patients after surgery of a tumor near the hypothalamus does not have definitely prognostic significance (Fig. 3). From 40 juveniles with a craniopharyngioma, 7 children, aged 3–15, were found to have had non-reactive dilated pupils in the early postoperative course. This finding persisted for a less or more prolonged time period and was associated with coma in 4 children and with semicoma in 3 children. Two of the patients died at 10 days and 3 weeks after surgery, respectively, whereas 5 children completely recovered, inclusive pupillary function.

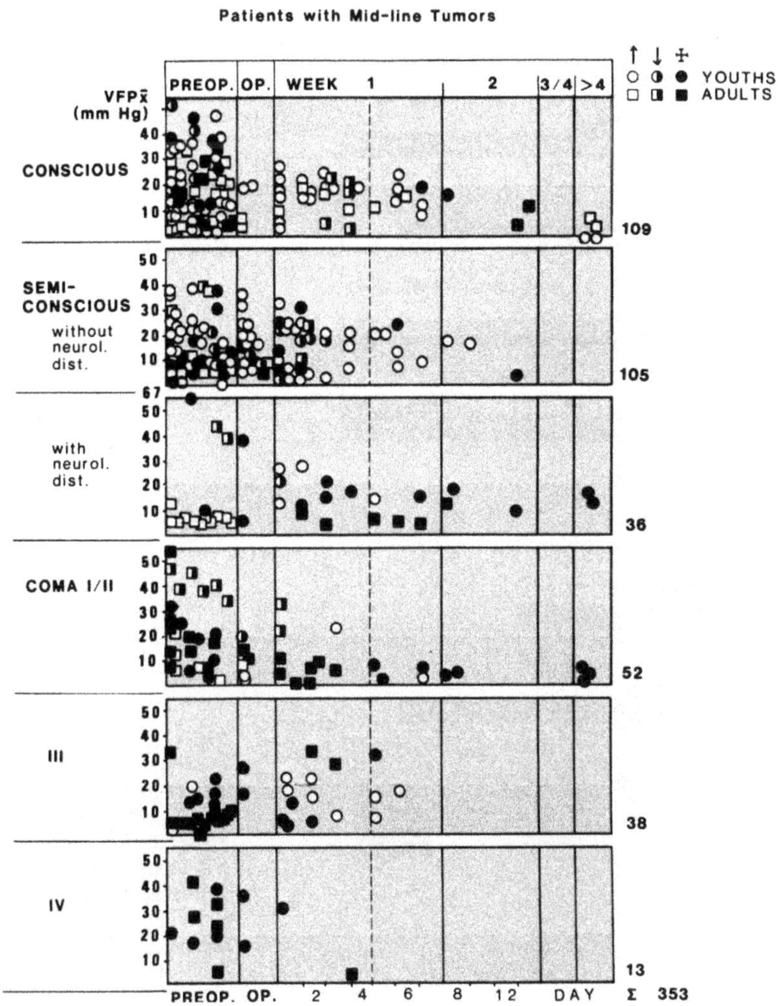

Fig. 2. Mean intracranial pressure (VFPx̄) and neurological state, pre- and postoperatively, in relation to the outcome (↑: full recovery; ↓: disabled; † postoperatively deceased)

During the period of mydriasis and coma normal VFPs were measured in 2 children.

The last patient was a 6-year-old girl with a large cystic craniopharyngioma. From the day of surgery till the 2nd day she was in coma; till the 3rd day she presented with non-reactive pupils. VFP was normal with external drainage and the patient recovered rapidly (Fig. 4).

Coma with mydriasis after surgery of a cystic tumor regrowth 10 months later. No evidence of hemorrhage or reactive brain swelling at immediate second look operation (Fig. 5).

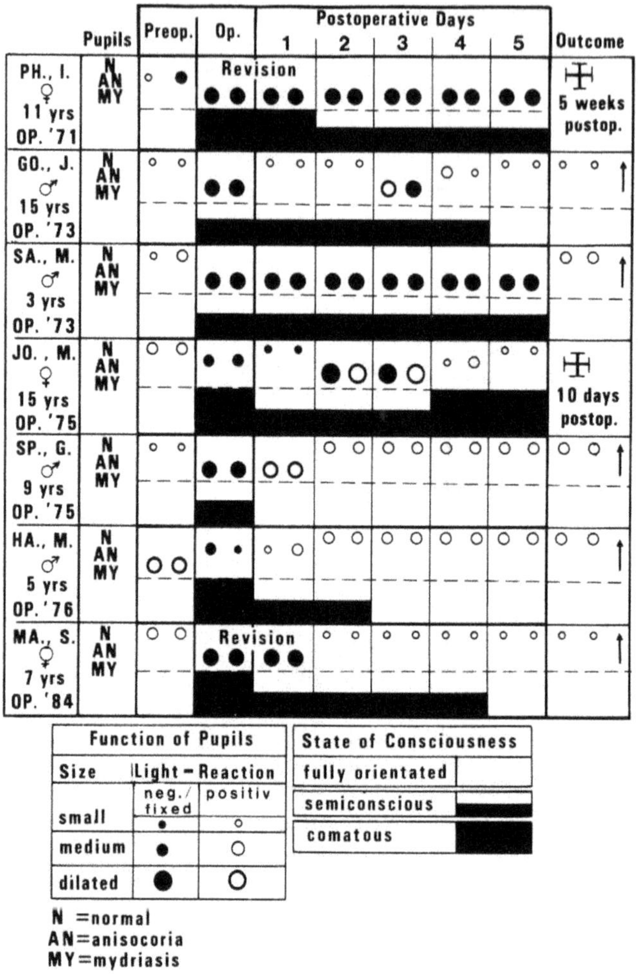

Fig. 3. Outcome of 7 children with craniopharyngioma after severe postoperative pupillary dysfunction (Anisocoria, fixed and/or dilated pupils) and disturbance of consciousness (Coma, Semicoma)

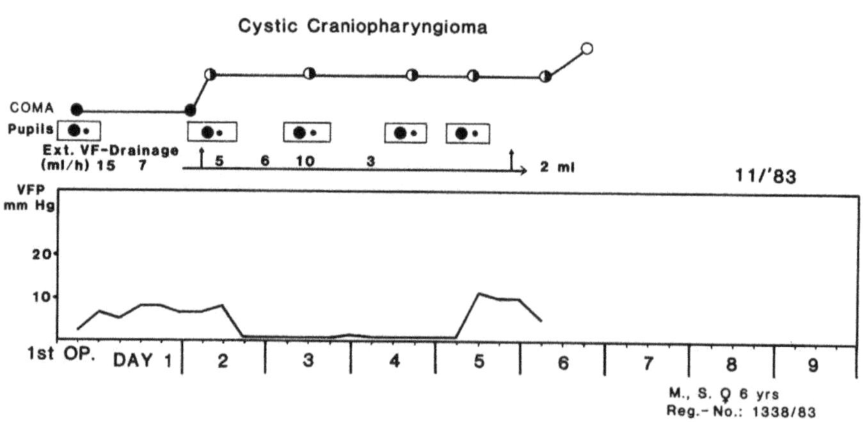

Fig. 4. Postoperative pupillary dysfunction and intracranial pressure in a child following surgery of a cystic craniopharyngioma: After the first operation (11/'83) coma II with anisocoria

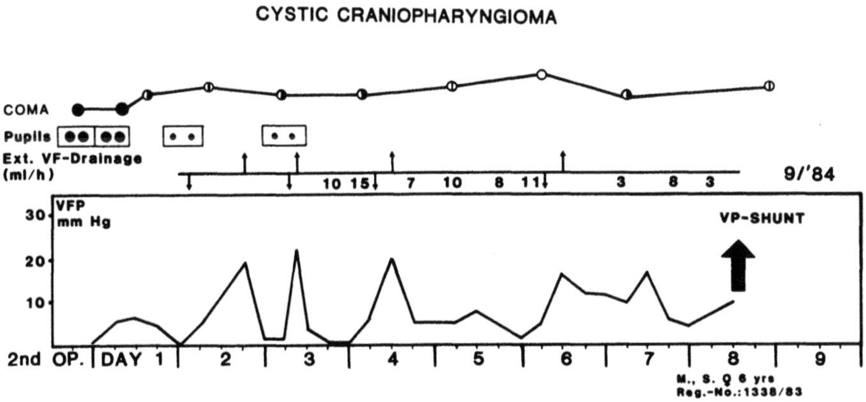

Fig. 5. Same case: After the second operation (9/'84) coma IV with bilaterally dilated and fixed pupils without reaction to pain stimuli. In both postoperative courses the VFP was not pathologically elevated. The child survived and fully recovered after both operations

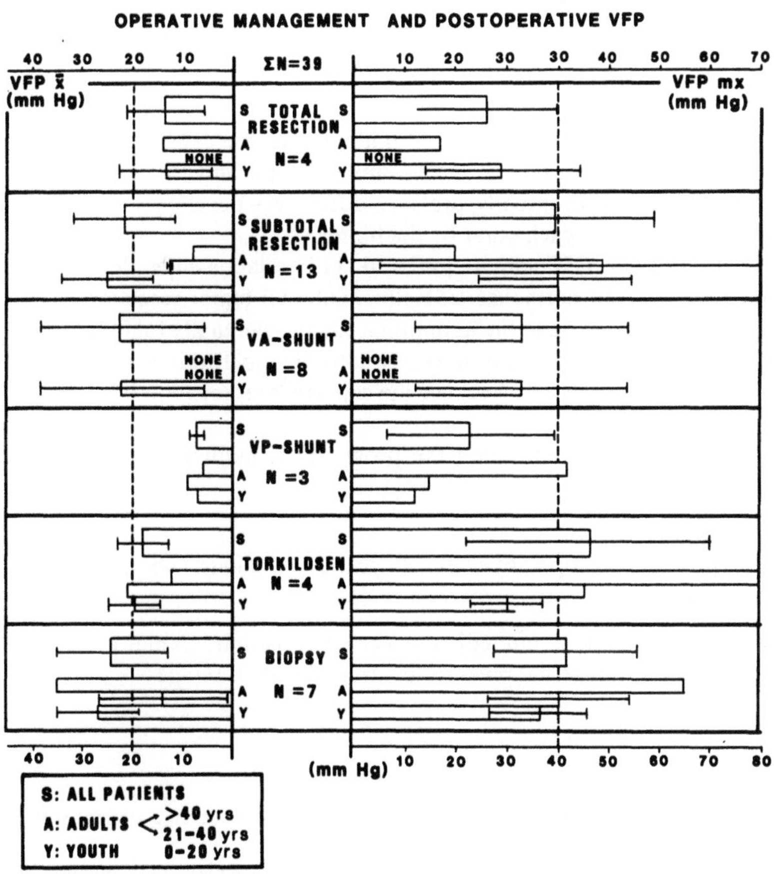

Fig. 6. Relation of operative management and mean (VFPx̄) and maximum (VFPmx) postoperative intracranial pressure. Nature of operative management: Total or subtotal tumor resection, VA-shunt, VP-shunt, Torkildsen-shunt, biopsy

VFP was 10 mm Hg. Increasing pressure, but only after recovery of consciousness and pupillary function from the first day on. Persisting CSF circulation disturbances with increasing VFP during further course. Implantation of a ventricular-peritoneal shunt system on the 8th day.

4. Operative Management and Intracranial Pressure Level (Fig. 6)

Finally, the postoperative VFP was related to the nature and the extent of the operative management:

- after complete tumor removal the mean and maximum postoperative pressures were within normal or nearly normal limits;
- they also were after implantation of a VP-shunt system;
- subtotal tumor resection as well as implantation of a ventricular-atrial shunt system or a Torkildsen shunt were less effective in lowering the VFP;
- limitation to tumor biopsy was particularly problematic with regard to postoperative pressure relationships.

Conclusion

Space-occupying lesions of the supratentorial midline area are causing obstruction of the CSF circulation by occlusion of the foramina Monro and the 3rd ventricle. The VFP abruptly rises and eventually pressure differences develop in ventricular compartments separated from each other by the tumor.

Restoration of normal CSF circulation and VFP relationships depends on whether tumor resection can normalize CSF flow. Subtotal tumor resection should be completed with CSF-shunting to the abdominal cavity, eventually bilaterally.

The earlier popular ventricular cisternostomy according to Torkildsen frequently fails to restore normal CSF pressure, because the capacity of resorption of the spinal CSF space is not large enough.

In summary, the factors determining the prognosis of midline tumor patients are:

- the extent of tumor resection;
- the severity of pre- and postoperative neurological dysfunctions, especially disturbance of consciousness.

Hence, in a comatose patient, immediate lowering of the intracranial pressure is mandatory, above all by an external pressure-controlled CSF drainage.

References

1. Crockard HA, Hanlon K, Ganz E (1976) Intracranial pressure gradients in a patient with a thalamic tumor. Surg Neurol 5: 151–155
2. Lundberg N (1960) Continuous recording and control of ventricular fluid pressure in neurosurgical practice. Acta Psychiatr Neurol Scand 40: 1–147
3. Richard KE (1981) Long-term monitoring of ventricular fluid pressure in intracranial space-occupying lesions. Fortschr Neurol Psychiatr 49: 1–33

Neurophysiological Results (Brain Stem Reflexes and Evoked Potentials) in Primary and Secondary Brain Stem Disorders

N. KLUG, Giessen/FRG

The recording of evoked potentials (EPs) has become one of the most useful functional diagnostic techniques in the neurosciences during recent years. In combination with the neurophysiological investigation of brain stem reflexes (BSRs) they provide good information concerning circumscribed and diffuse brain and brain stem lesions. In this paper alterations of the brain stem acoustic evoked potentials and the electrically elicited blink reflex will be discussed with regard to space-occupying lesions of the posterior fossa.

Brain Stem Acoustic Evoked Potentials

Within the first 10 ms after a brief auditory stimulus one can see a series of 7 vertex positive potentials corresponding to the successive activation of the peripheral,

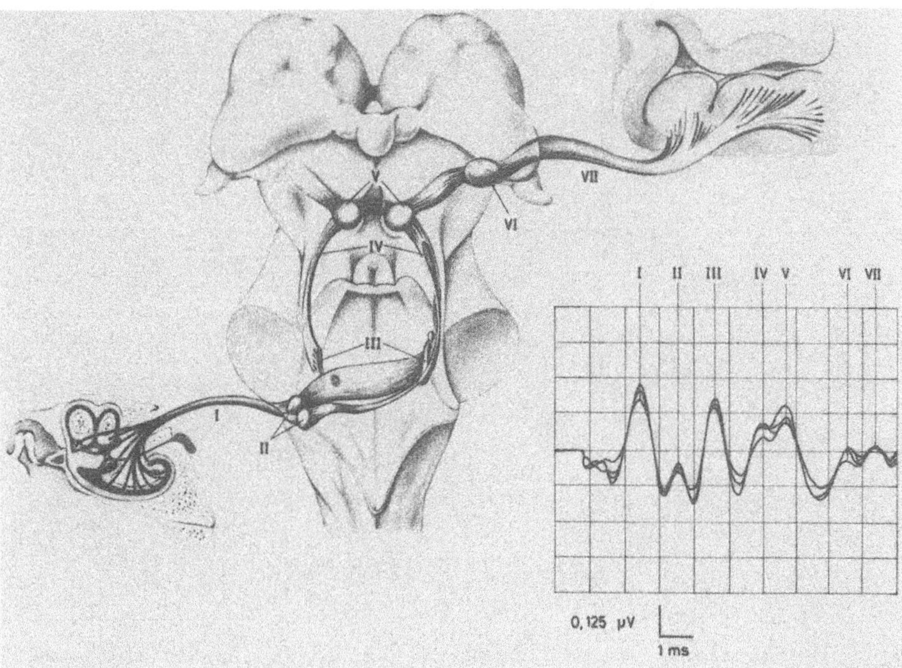

Fig. 1. Original BAEP recording and diagram of BAEP generators. Anatomical drawings after Tandler (1929) and Nieuwenhuys et al. (1981)

medullary, pontine and mesencephalic portions of the auditory pathway (Fig. 1). Wave I is likely to be the nerve action potential of the cochlear nerve, II is generated in the nucleus of the cochlear nerve (medulla oblongata), III in the superior olivary complex (lower pons), IV in the nucleus of the lateral lemniscus (rostral part of the pons), V in the inferior colliculi (mesencephalon), VI in the medial geniculate body and VII in the acoustic radiation.

Blink Reflex

Among brain stem reflexes the blink reflex (BR) (Fig. 2) is the most important. It is generally regarded as a trigemino-facial reflex, which can be elicited for example by electrical stimulation of the supraorbital nerve. The reflex consists of an early ipsilateral (R_1) and a late bilateral (R_2) reflex. R_1 is an oligosynaptic reflex which enters the pons in the sensory root of the trigeminal nerve. It is transmitted through the pons and relayed via neurones at the level of the principle sensory nucleus of the fifth nerve. R_2 is polysynaptic. It is also transmitted through the sensory root and reaches the facial nuclei via medial parts of the reticular formation (Fig. 3). R_2 corresponds with the visible closure of the eye lids. The common efferent pathway of both is represented by the motor facial fibres of the lateral, ventral inferior part of the facial nucleus.

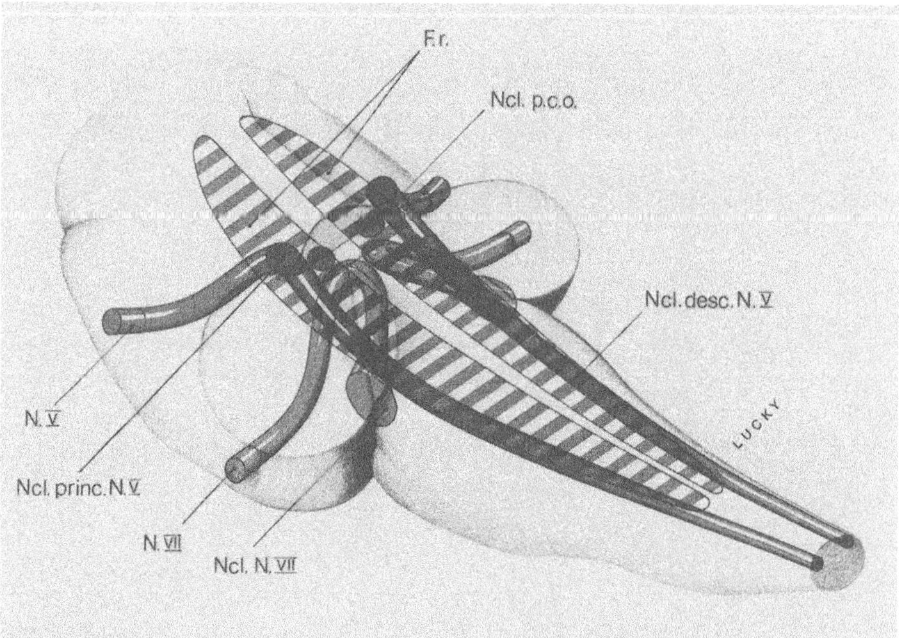

Fig. 2. Threedimensional schematic drawing of BR pathways in the brain stem. *NV* = trigeminal nerve, *N VII* = facial nerve, *Ncl. princ. NV* = main trigeminal nucleus, *Ncl. desc. NV* = descending trigeminal tract and nucleus, *Ncl. p.c.o.* = nucleus centralis pontis oralis, *F.r.* = reticular formation

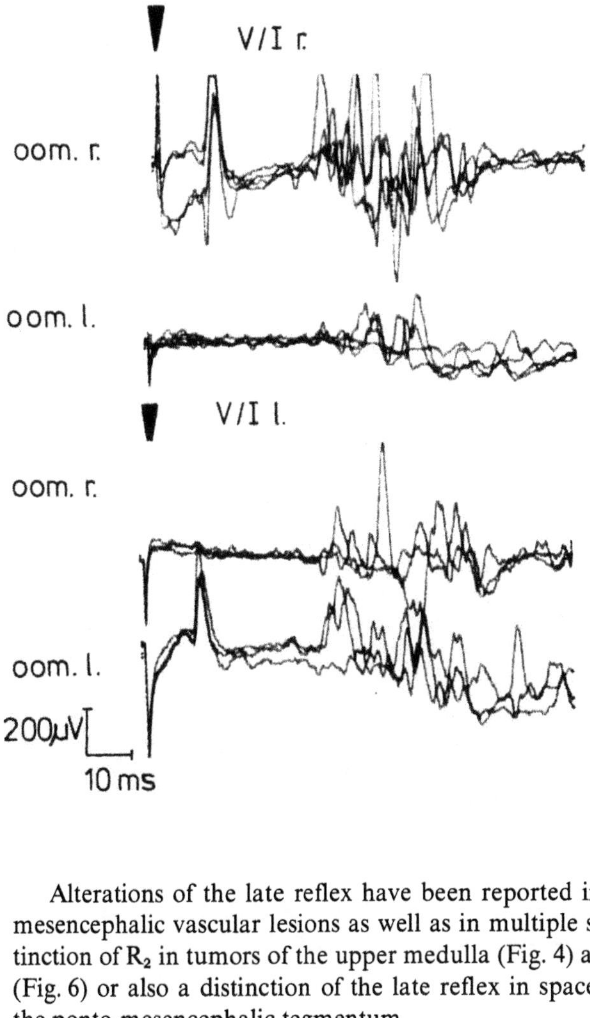

Fig. 3. Normal blink reflex after stimulation of the supraorbital nerve on the right (*V/I r.*) and left (*V/I l.*) side. Recording of the early ipsilateral and late bilateral responses of orbicularis oculi muscles (*oom*)

Alterations of the late reflex have been reported in localized medullary and in mesencephalic vascular lesions as well as in multiple sclerosis. We have seen a distinction of R_2 in tumors of the upper medulla (Fig. 4) and an increased latency of R_2 (Fig. 6) or also a distinction of the late reflex in space-occupying lesions involving the ponto-mesencephalic tegmentum.

Primary Brain Stem Tumors

Primary brain stem tumors of the midline are characterized by "symmetrical" alterations of BAEP and BR (Figs. 4 and 6). The additional investigation of somato-sensory (SEP) and visual (VEP) evoked potentials as well as the registration of the masseter reflex (MR) provide information concerning size and location of brain stem lesions (Fig. 6): The preserved medullary function is indicated by the normal SEP over the dorsal collum nuclei. Additionally the preserved BAEP wave II on both sides and the normal early blink reflex indicate the lower pons function, although the interpeak latency I–III is somewhat increased. The absence of the BAEP complex IV/V on both sides coincides with the pathologically altered masseter reflex and the extremely increased latency or missing late blink reflex indicating a severe

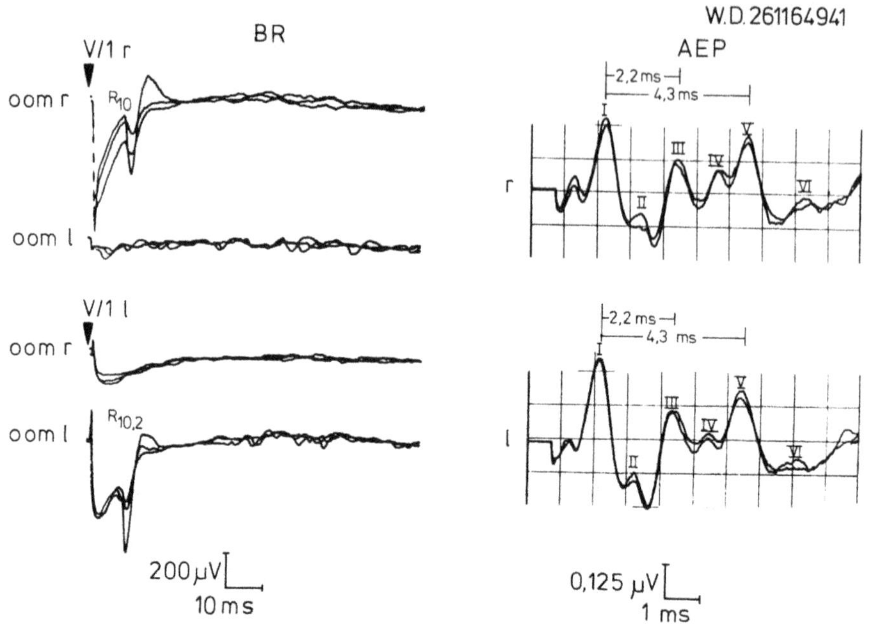

Fig. 4. BR and BAEP findings in a patient with a malignant glioma of the upper medulla. The distinction of the late blink reflex on both sides indicates the functional disturbance of the descending trigeminal tract and nucleus. BAEP waves on both sides are nearly normal. Autopsy revealed that the cochlear nuclei on both sides were spared by the tumor

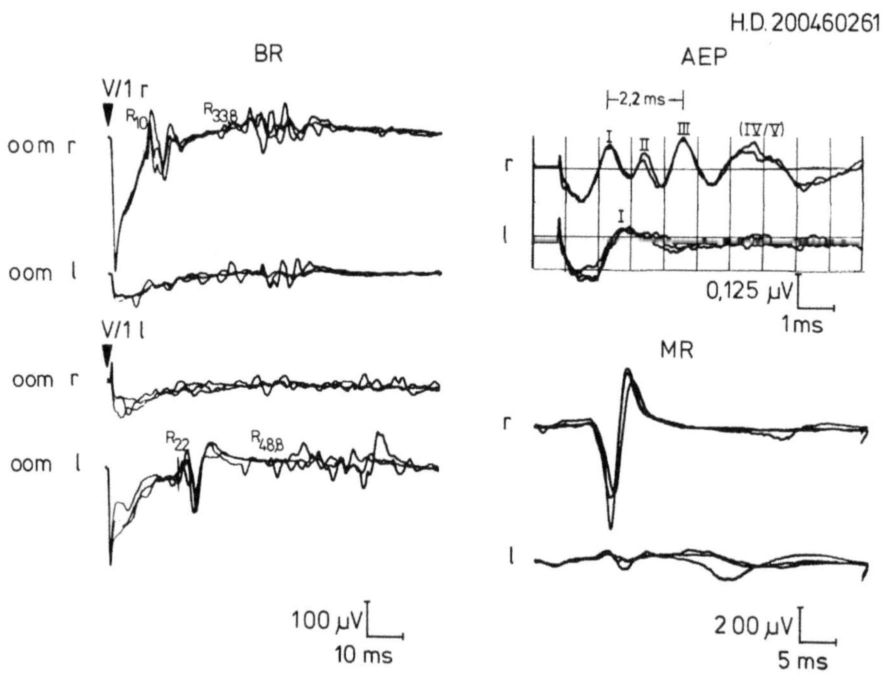

Fig. 5. BR and BAEP in a patient with a left-sided acoustic neurinoma. The impaired function of the pons is indicated by the extremely increased latency of the early blink reflex. AEP recording on the tumor side shows only wave I but no wave thereafter. Yet the functional brain stem disturbance is to be seen in the severely altered IV/V-complex on the contralateral side, which means a ponto-mesencephalic lesion. This latter finding is supported by the distinction of the masseter reflex on the side of the tumor

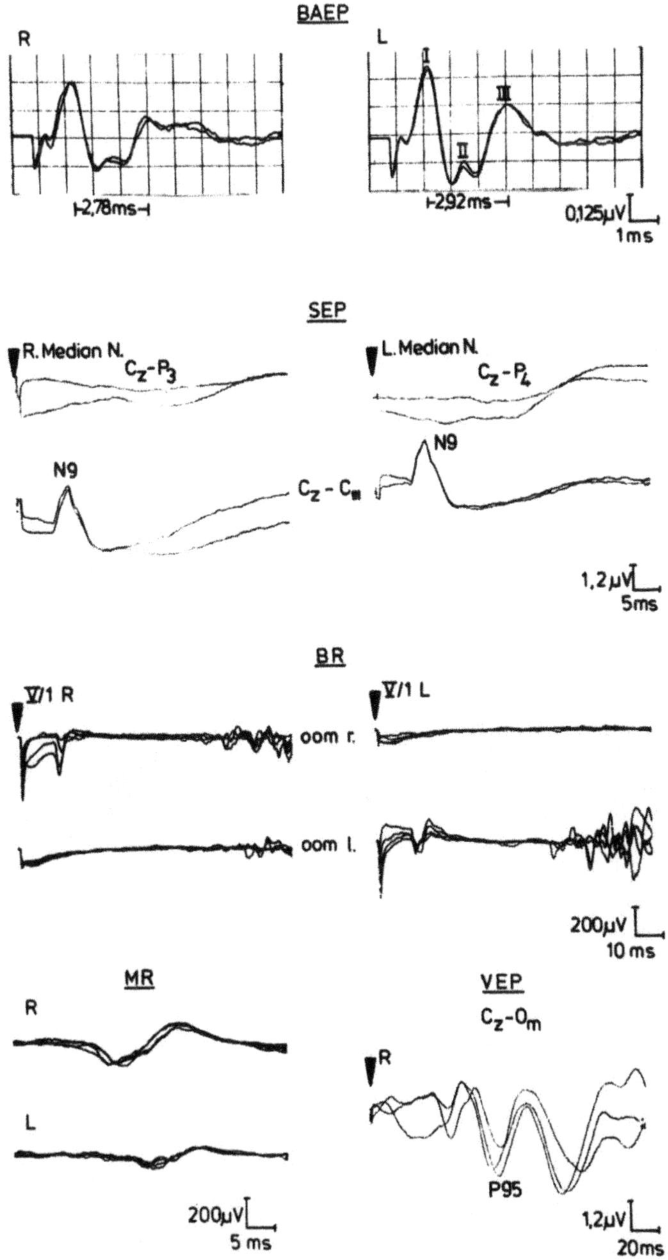

Fig. 6. H. J. 110379282. BR and AEP findings in a 5-year-old child with a ponto-mesencephalic spongioblastoma. The early (pontine) reflex is preserved on both sides, yet the latency is a little bit increased, indicating some functional disturbance. This finding coincides with the alteration of wave III on both sides. The bilateral involvement of the ponto-mesencephalic segments is indicated also by the extremely increased latencies of the late blink reflex on the side of the stimulation and the missing R_2 contralaterally. Additionally all waves rostral from wave III are extremely altered or missing on both sides

ponto-mesencephalic functional lesion. Together with the normal VEP these findings allow the conclusion that the missing SEP on both sides is due to a lemniscal functional disturbance. Space-occupying lesions with predominant unilateral invasion of the brain stem lead to asymmetrical BR- and BAEP-findings.

Extracerebral Tumors with Secondary Brain Stem Involvement

Extracerebral space-occupying lesions of the posterior fossa with secondary brain stem involvement are characterized by asymmetrical alterations of brain stem acoustic evoked potentials and brain stem reflexes (Fig. 5).

Conclusion

The registration of EPs and BSRs allow to differentiate between intra- and extracerebral tumors affecting the brain stem. By its use it is also possible to lateralize brain stem disturbances and to define the functionally affected segments of the brain stem in the rostral-caudal direction.

References

Nieuwenhuys R, Voogd J, Huijzen C v (1981) The human central nervous system. 2nd ed. Springer, Berlin Heidelberg New York
Tandler J (1929) Lehrbuch der systematischen Anatomie, Bd IV. Vogel, Leipzig

Intraoperative Monitoring of Evoked Potentials for Surgery in and around the Third Ventricle and the Brain Stem

J. SCHRAMM, C. CEDZICH, R. FAHLBUSCH, T. MOKRUSCH, and H. HOCHSTETTER,
Erlangen/FRG

Monitoring central nervous system function intraoperatively using evoked potentials is applied with the hope that impairment of afferent function is noted before the damage to nervous structures has become irreversible, thus giving the surgeon a chance to change his mode of working. Flash-evoked visual potentials (VEP) and acoustic evoked brain stem potentials (BAEP) have been used to monitor the acoustic pathway in the brain stem and the visual pathway encircling the hypothalamus. (Ojeman et al. 1984; Grundy et al. 1982; Raudzens 1982; Allen et al. 1981; Feinsod et al. 1976).

We are reporting here on 45 monitoring procedures, 25 with BAEP and 20 using VEP.

Methods

Routinely pre- and postoperative recordings are performed using a CA-1000 averager (Nicolet). Silver cup electrodes are used with adhesive electrolyte paste, impedance usually is below 1 kΩ. Operative recordings are started after intubation and positioning. First recordings are performed before skin preparation and draping.

Control values are obtained during draping. A protocol is maintained in which anesthetic data, the surgeon's remarks, time and floppy disc memory numbers are put down.

BAEP: With a band pass of 150–3000 Hz, at a frequency of 11.3 Hz 1500 responses are averaged with an analysis time of 10 ms, in some cases with delayed peaks with 20 ms. Recording position is C_Z–$A_{1,2}$, vertex positivity is shown upward. Contralateral masking with 35 dB. Alternating rarefaction and condensation clicks at 85 dB over hearing level.

VEP: Flashing diode goggels are used at a frequency of 1.9 Hz. Band pass 5–100 Hz, 100 recordings per average, analysis time 250 ms. Recording electrodes: O_Z–F_Z. EP's are continuously recorded throughout the operation. A dual floppy disc drive is used for data storage and retrieval.

Materials

BAEP Cases: 25 procedures in 20 patients, with 22 procedures in the cerebellopontine angle (CPA): 7 acoustic neurinomas, 3 CPA-meningeomas, 1 CPA-craniopharyngeoma, 2 CPA-epidermoids, 1 basilar artery aneurysm, 1 astrocytoma in the CPA, 3 neurovascular decompressions, 2 hemispheric tumors. In 2 large tumors with diameter over 6 cm removal was subtotal: one huge cystic craniopharyngeoma and one large tentorial meningeoma; these patients were operated on several times.

Acoustic Neurinomas: They were 2 cm in size in 1 case, between 2 and 2.5 cm in 2 cases, and above 2.5 cm in 4 cases. 4 patients were deaf, 1 showed minimal residual hearing and 2 patients demonstrated impaired hearing (20 and 40 db loss). At surgery in 3 acoustic neurinomas the 8th nerves were kept *anatomically* intact, in 1 of these the patient demonstrated normal hearing postoperatively. The other patients with normal hearing and with residual hearing were deaf after the operation. Tumor size in the other cases varied between 1.5 and 6 cm. In no patient brain stem related morbidity was seen, although one patient died after 10 days from pulmonary embolus.

VEP Cases: 1 skull base-meningeoma with compression of the optic foramen, 2 intraventricular meningeomas and 17 perisellar tumors: 4 craniopharyngeomas, 11 pituitary adenomas, 1 meningeoma and 1 germinoma. Only 2 patients had a normal visual field and 3 a normal visual acuity. Bitemporal heminopia was found in 8 cases and a visual acuity between 0.1 and 0.5 in 8 cases. The other patients showed less severe defects in various combinations.

The acoustic neurinomas and neurovascular decompressions were performed in the lateral decubitus position. The transsphenoidal route was used in 1 of 4 craniopharyngeomas and 10 of 11 pituitary adenomas. These operations were performed by the two senior authors (R. F und J. S).

Results

BAEP Cases: In 21 of 24 cases recordings were of a quality to allow monitoring. No BAEP were obtained in 4 out of 25 cases: one technical failure and in 3 cases the reason remained unclear. In 11 procedures stable BAEP were obtained, in 10 cases temporary BAEP changes or minor alterations occurred but did not impair with monitoring.

Intraoperative BAEP Changes: Interpeak latency (IPL) increases are commonly found for I/III and I/V IPL's (Fig. 1). The wave I latency increases often in a slight degree, sometimes after dura opening. These latency increases are usually within the two-standard-deviation range (Table 1).

Significant BAEP changes occurred in 9 patients. In 5 patients there was improvement with appearance of waves in 4 cases (wave II; wave II and III; wave IV and V; wave V) and a latency decrease in 1 case (Fig. 1). The potential deteriorated 6 times, either by showing a partial reversible loss (wave II, IV + V; wave II–V; wave IV + V) or a latency increase (3×), occasionally in the same patient. In no case a complete loss of BAEP's was seen. Commonest reason for a latency increase was positioning of the spatula, the second most common reason was dissection of

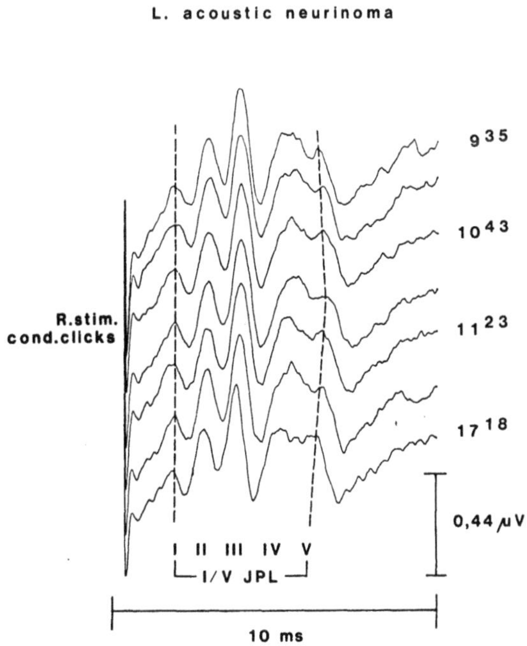

Fig. 1. BAEP changes often seen during monitoring without clinical sequelae. The right ear was stimulated with condensation clicks at 85 dB. The I/V interpeak latency (*IPL*) increases, as does the I/III IPL. These changes do not indicate damage to the brain stem

Table 1. Intraoperative interpeak latency (IPL) increases in BAEP monitoring

	Ipsilateral	Contralateral	Developing
Wave I/III IPL	0,3 ms	0,2 ms	Within 30 min.
	0,5 ms	0,2 ms	Till end of surgery
Wave I/V IPL	0,5 ms	0,4 ms	Within 30 min.
	0,8 ms	0,4 ms	Till end of surgery

the tumor. In 1 case latency increased during air embolism, in another during dissection of the 8th nerve. Reasons for improvement of BAEP's were repositioning of retractor, end of tumor preparation, opening of dura and puncture of tumor cyst (Figs. 2–4).

The 2 cases with postoperative hearing loss demonstrated atypical BAEP-findings. One patient with residual hearing (60 dB loss) and acoustic neurinoma had no detectable preoperative and intraoperative BAEP. Another acoustic neurinoma patient with 40 dB loss had poor BAEP's preoperatively, much better BAEP's intraoperatively with well reproducible BAEP's at 1 week – just to be deaf and without BAEP 3 months after the operation (Fig. 3).

VEP Cases: In 20 monitoring procedures technical problems made monitoring impossible in 4 cases due to the use of halogenated anesthetics, in another case a cable break temporarily hindered monitoring. These problems, which are principally avoidable, were outnumbered by the number of cases in which VEP were lost.

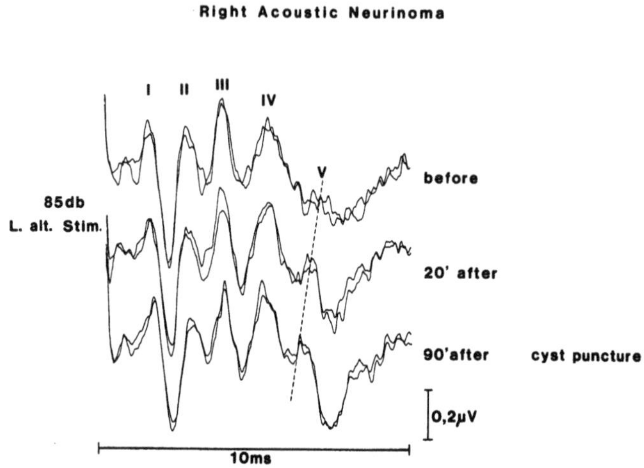

Fig. 2. Intraoperative improvement in BAEP. The left ear was stimulated at 85 dB with alternating clicks. After puncture of a tumor cyst the pressure on the brain stem was relieved and a wave V, which had been absent, reappeared and its latency decreased towards normal values

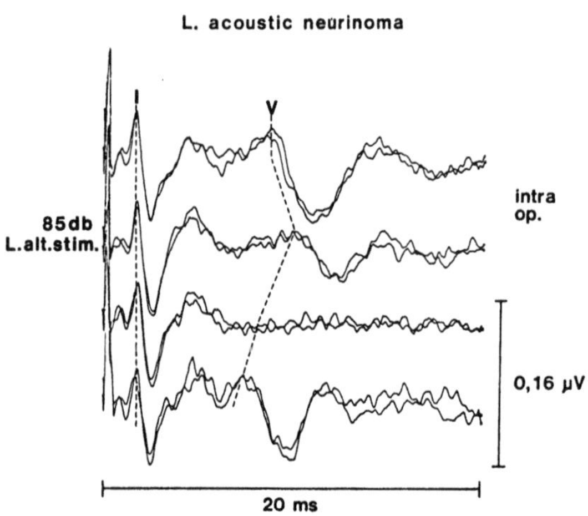

Fig. 3. Temporary deterioration and recovery of BAEP with ipsilateral stimulation. The abnormal BAEP, with wave II to wave IV not reproducible, deteriorates temporarily with a loss of waves IV/V and normalizes during the same operation with reappearance of wave II–V. Hearing in this patient was nearly normal pre- and postoperatively (20 dB loss) with a delayed hearing loss

In 9 cases VEP disappeared when tumor dissection or chiasma manipulation was begun (Fig. 5). In another 4 cases the potential loss occurred even earlier, before any manipulation at the visual pathways had begun. In all these cases VEP reappeared towards the end of the operation. From these 13 cases a further increase in visual function impairment would have been theoretically possible in 11 cases, but clinical deterioration was not detected postoperatively despite temporary intraoperative VEP loss (2 cases with complete homonymous hemianopia excluded). No monitoring problems were found in 2 cases only.

VEP overall showed marked variability, both in amplitude and latency. The wave configuration in some cases was also variable, with peaks sometimes being bi-

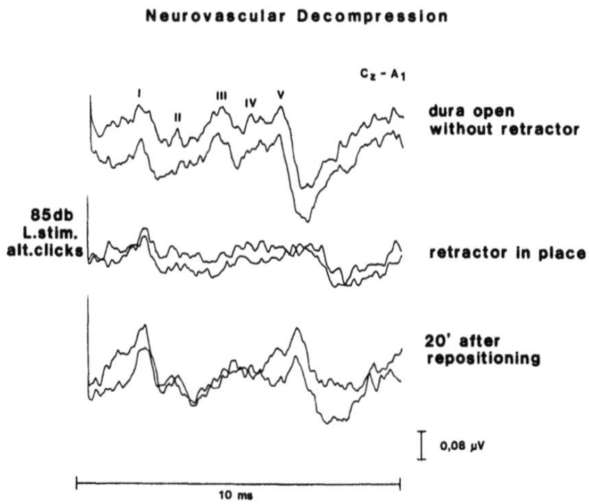

Fig. 4. BAEP deterioration during neurovascular decompression for trigeminal neuralgia. Ipsilateral stimulation (alternating clicks) evoked normal BAEP at the beginning of surgery. After cerebellar retraction waves II to IV disappeared and wave V was delayed. After repositioning of the retractor the BAEP reappeared within 20 minutes. No neurological deficits postoperatively

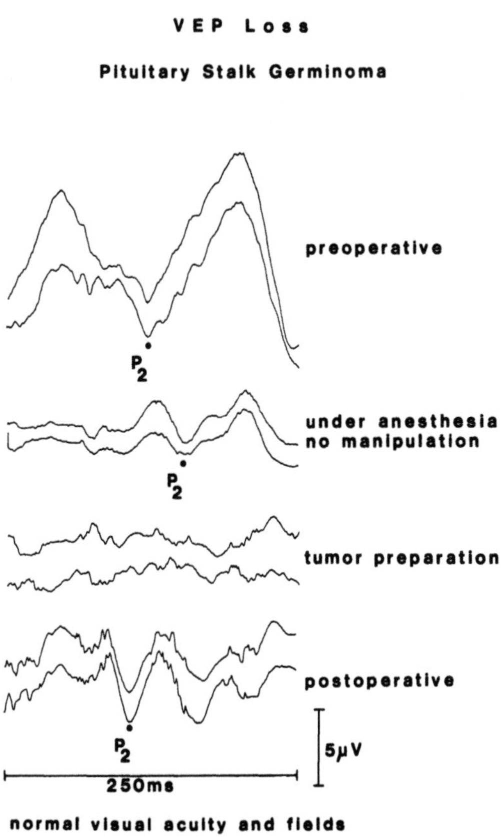

Fig. 5. VEP loss without clinical sequelae. The typical postinduction changes in VEP are demonstrated with amplitude reduction and latency increase. During tumor dissection with manipulation of the chiasm the potential is lost whereas postoperatively visual function remained normal

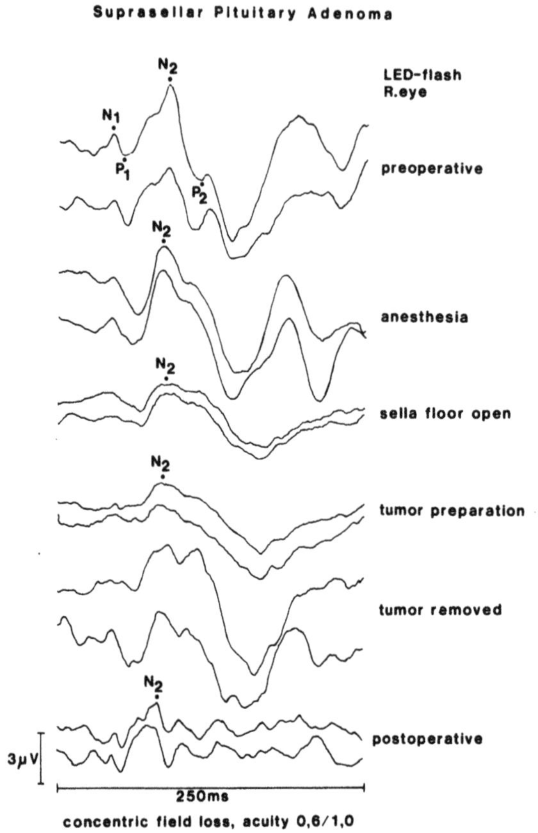

Fig. 6. Transsphenoidal surgery for intra- and suprasellar pituitary adenoma. The typical variability and postinduction changes are demonstrated. Although traces are fairly well reproducible a wide degree of variation is obvious. Postoperatively visual fields normalized and visual acuity had slightly improved

lobed temporarily (Fig. 6). There were also typical changes after induction of anesthesia with latency increases for $\overline{N2}$ between 5 and 15 ms with a maximum value of 38 ms. $\overline{P2}$ latency increased between 5 and 20 ms with a maximum value of 24 ms (Fig. 5). In nearly all cases amplitude decreased. In 7 cases the amplitude decrease after induction was over 50% of control values.

No patient in this series demonstrated significant visual function impairment after the operation, postoperatively visual fields improved in 13 cases, visual acuity improved in 8 cases and in 1 case there was an insignificant change from 0.8 to 0.7.

The influence of enflurane onto VEP is marked. In 4 cases the VEP were virtually abolished due to enflurane concentrations up to 1.5 vol.-%, thus rendering monitoring impossible.

Discussion

Our results and those of others (Ojeman et al. 1984; Raudzens 1982; Allen et al. 1981) have demonstrated that the technical feasibility of BAEP-recording in the operating theatre is given. The quality of signals in the majority of cases is good enough as to permit monitoring of brain stem function. Temporary changes are usually found with BAEP and VEP after induction of anesthesia which do not indicate morphological injury. VEP changes which may be surprisingly large pertaining to amplitude and latency have been very common in our material and in others (Raudzens 1982) without proving damage to visual pathways. The variability in VEP is also great under normal circumstances and even more so in monitoring (Raudzens 1982). We have no certain explanation for the high frequency of VEP loss not associated with clinical deterioration of visual function postoperatively. Sometimes VEP's were lost after opening the dura, possibly due to shifting of cerebral mass after air under atmospheric pressure was able to enter the subarachnoid space. Similar observations have been observed with BAEP after dura opening, but then changes were minimal.

The high percentage of lost VEP's in our cases does not allow the conclusion that flash-VEP may routinely be used for monitoring visual function, although early reports demonstrated that rapid change of optic nerve function is possible and can be monitored by flash-VEP (Feinsod et al. 1976).

In BAEP monitoring cases no true brain stem morbidity occurred although mild reversible facial weakness was observed in 2 cases. In the 4 cases in which significant change in hearing function was observed, changes in intraoperative BAEP's were variable and did not allow conclusions to predict postoperative hearing function from intraoperative BAEP alterations (Allen et al. 1981; Grundy et al. 1982). For example in 1 case with a preoperative hearing loss of 40 dB BAEP's showed only temporary wave component loss with fairly normal BAEP's at the end of the operation (Fig. 3). Three months after the operation the patient was deaf, however, and had no BAEP. In one patient with severe preoperative hearing impairment, who was deaf immediately after the operation, no preoperative BAEP was obtainable from the diseased but still hearing ear and therefore monitoring on the ipsilateral side was impossible. Only the brain stem could be monitored by using the input by the contralateral ear. There were, however, no true "false-positives" with BAEP monitoring – these are cases which demonstrated complete potential loss but normal hearing postoperatively, as described by Allen et al. (1981). There were also no true "false-negatives" – i.e. patients who demonstrated good BAEP's intraoperatively and hearing loss postoperatively, provided only the immediate postoperative period is considered. The immediate postoperative existence of hearing and BAEP's does not exclude a new hearing loss, occurring in the following weeks, most likely due to scarring. This is an important conclusion from our findings.

On numerous occasions during the operations monitored, we were able to demonstrate that the brain stem reacts sensitively to retraction after retractor positioning and reacted promptly to repositioning of the retractor, as has been seen by Grundy et al. (1982). Therefore it might be hypothetized that without monitoring BAEP's and the resulting retractor repositioning longer lasting impairment of brain stem function would have occurred with possible postoperative deficits. Therefore, by reacting to BAEP changes intraoperatively and thus relieving adverse brain stem effects, this small series likely represents a series which already should have benefitted from monitoring.

The high incidence of VEP loss without clinical sequelae seems to make routine use of this method unlikely. Monitoring BAEP, however, seems to be sensitive in demonstrating brain stem function impairment and larger series will increase our knowledge about the value of this method.

References

Allen A, Starr A, Nudleman K (1981) Assessment of sensory function in the operating room utilizing cerebral evoked potentials: A study of fifty-six surgically anesthetized patients. Clin Neurosurg 28:457–481

Feinsod M, Selhorst SB, Hoyt WF, Wilson C (1976) Monitoring optic nerve function during craniotomy. J Neurosurg 44:29–31

Grundy BL, Jannetta PJ, Procopio PT, Lina A, Boston R, Doyle E (1982) Intraoperative monitoring of brain stem auditory evoked potentials. J Neurosurg 57:674–681

Ojeman RG, Levine R, Montgomery WM, McGaffigan P (1984) Use of intraoperative auditory evoked potentials to preserve hearing in unilateral acoustic neuroma removal. J Neurosurg 61:938–948

Raudzens PA (1982) Intraoperative monitoring of evoked potentials. Ann NJ Acad Sci 388:308–326

Stimulation Mapping of the Periventricular-Periaqueductal Gray (PVG-PAG) in Man – an Autopsy Study

R. R. TASKER, M. YOSHIDA, A. A. F. SIMA, and J. DECK, Toronto/Canada

Chronic stimulation of PVG-PAG, introduced by Richardson and Akil (1977 a, b), is commonly used for pain control. The present autopsy study localizes anatomically for the first time a variety of stimulation-induced effects frequently reported in the literature during the stimulation of PVG-PAG as an aid to future electrode localization.

Clinical Details

A 34-year-old man clinically with a total quadriplegia below C6 developed disabling pain as if his "blood was boiling", "skin freezing", three months after his accident, affecting chiefly left buttock and foot. Conservative therapy including dorsal epidural cord stimulation failed and brain stimulation was attempted. Following stereotactic stimulation mapping (Tasker et al. 1982) two quadripolar electrodes (5 mm pole separation) were inserted, one in PVG-PAG, and the other in the leg area of ventrocaudal nucleus (Vc) June 26, 1978 along two of the explored trajectories. Postoperatively the patient developed meningitis, refused electrode removal, and died July 21, 1978 despite aggressive therapy.

Methods

Two trajectories were explored in Vc (17.0 mm from midline), five in medial brainstem 2.5 mm lateral to the third ventricular wall (ventricular width 8.0 mm) and therefore in the 5.0 mm sagittal plane in the atlas by Schaltenbrand and Bailey (1959).

Serial coronal sections 1.0 mm apart were cut perpendicular to the anterior-posterior commissure (ACPC) line whose location was marked on the block. Electrode artifacts identified by a "blinded" observer (AS) were marked on 4X photomicrographs arranged in sequence. These were correlated (Tasker et al. 1982) with acute stimulation data plotted on sagittal diagrams in the operating room, on which locations of the serial sections were marked, by knowing ACPC distance in fixed and living brain, noting trajectory interrelationships, plotting coronal planes of passage and termination for each trajectory, noting trajectory height above ACPC line, distance from PC anteroposteriorly, and responses identified with discrete easily localized anatomical features.

One of the two trajectories in the 17.0 mm lateral and two of the five in the 5.0 mm lateral sagittal planes were identified and the stimulation sites every 2.0 mm along them allocated to the appropriate artifact in the appropriate photomicrograph. The remaining stimulation sites were then marked by extrapolation.

Results

Figures 1, 2 and 3 plot the acute stimulation data obtained in the operating room by stimulating every 2.0 mm along the five parasagittal trajectories 2.0 mm apart in the medial brainstem. Similar data in lateral thalamus (not figured) consisted of con-

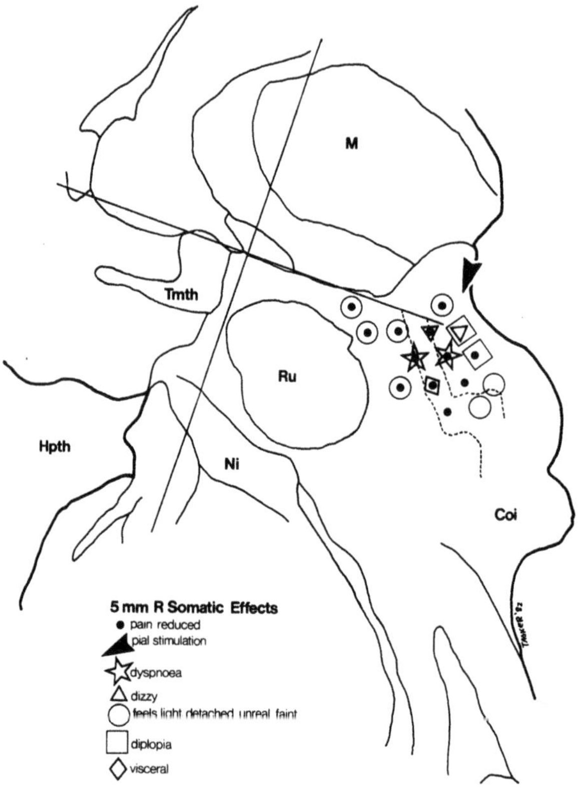

Fig. 1. Miscellaneous effects (symbols as per legend) elicited by threshold 60 Hz stimulation with trains of 3.0 msec damped square waves (maximum 1.5 mA) delivered with a 1.1 mm (0.5 mm pole separation) concentric bipolar electrode relative to sites of acute pain reduction (small filled circles) plotted on a computer-generated diagram adjusted from the 5.0 mm lateral sagittal plate (Schaltenbrand and Bailey 1959) to the patient's 27.5 mm ACPC distance in life. Lines at right angles represent ACPC line and a vertical through its center. Dotted lines mark the location of aqueduct extrapolated back to the stimulation map. Psychic effects (large hollow circles in trajectories 1 to 4 from left to right, lettered from a to c from above to below): 1 (a) felt "light", "neutral", 1 (b) "loose", 1 (c) "unreal", 2 (a) "detached", had to tell date, where he was "to be sure of himself", 3 (a) "Is that really my imagination", "not really clear it is happening", 4 (a) "lightheaded, partly drunk", 4 (b) "Unreal". The arrow marks where stimulation of pia produced ipsilateral eye pain

Explanation of Symbols, Figs. 1–6
Ce = centre median, *Coi* = inferior colliculus, *Cp* = *PC*, *Cpi* = internal capsule, *Dbc* = decussation of brachium conjunctivum, *Gl* = lateral geniculate nucleus, *Gm* or *Mg* = medial geniculate nucleus, *Hpth* = hypothalamus, *Lm* = medial lemniscus, *M* = dorsomedian nucleus, *Ni* = substantia nigra, *Pf* = parafascicular nucleus, *Pspd* = cerebral peduncle, *Ru* = red nucleus, *Tmth* = mamillothalamic tract, *Vc* = ventrocaudal nucleus.

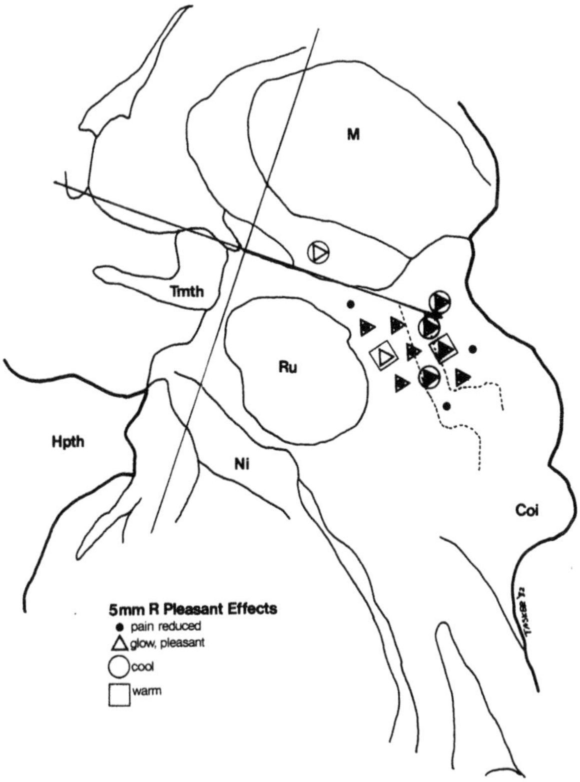

Fig. 2. As for Fig. 1. Pleasant effects relative to sites of pain reduction. The "glow" was generalized and likened to the effects of alcohol. Coolness was referred to ears, neck, back and shoulders. These diffuse warm and cool effects are very different from the contralateral discretely somatotopographically organized effects elicited in spinothalamic tract more laterally (Tasker et al. 1982)

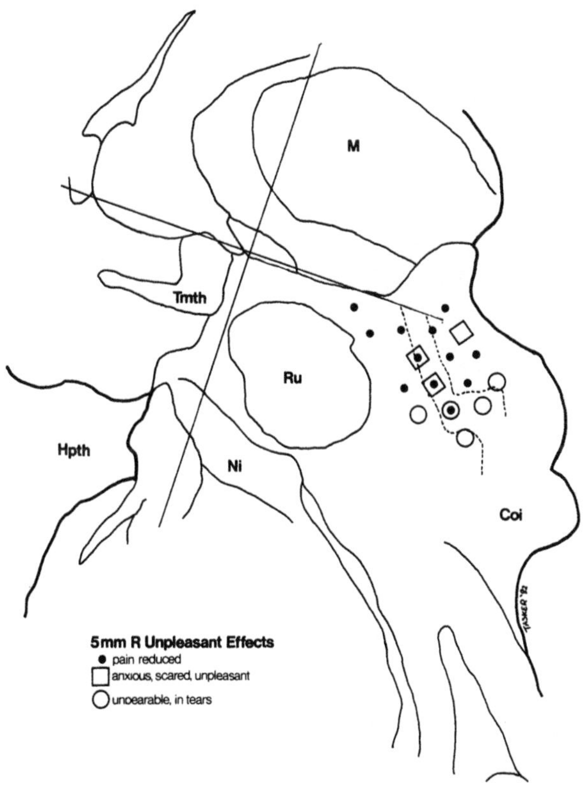

Fig. 3. As for Fig. 1. Unpleasant effects relative to sites of pain reduction. Unbearable effects (open large circles) were identical: voice in tears, unwilling to permit further stimulation, reticent about what was felt

tralateral paresthetic responses in Vc, low-pitched contralateral ear buzzing near medial geniculate, and mechanically induced ipsilateral eye pain as the electrode pressed against the dorsal midbrain pia.

Though medial stimulation was begun about halfway down the dorsal height of dorsomedian nucleus covering its entire rostral two-thirds, and was continued to the level of the rostral-caudal middle of superior colliculus, no responses occurred up to 1.5 mA till the level of 1 to 2 mm above ACPC was reached.

The sites of pain relief, marked with small filled circles, are widely distributed through posterior PVG-PAG, usually accompanied by a variety of bizarre psychic, pleasant, and visceral effects. More caudally in PAG, unpleasant effects stopped further exploration. Oculomotor effects occurred in dorsal superior colliculus.

Figures 4, 5 and 6 display representative physiological-anatomical reconstructions at 8.0, 11.0 and 11.5 mm behind the middle of the ACPC line.

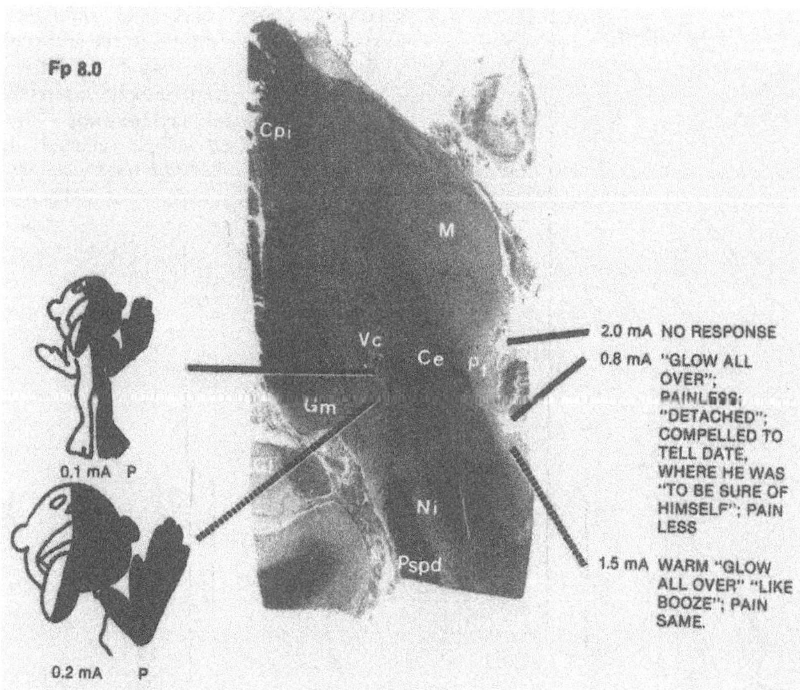

Fig. 4. Two identified electrode artifacts in dorsal PAG and medial Pf; extrapolated response in PAG; two contralateral paresthetic responses in Vc

Fig. 4–6. Coronal sections ×3.0 (Heidenhain myelin stain) 8.0, 11.0 and 11.5 mm behind middle of ACPC measured in fixed brain (ACPC = 20 mm). PC occurred at Fp 10.0. Identified electrode artifacts where stimulation was done (often visible in the sections) indicated by solid lines, extrapolated sites by dotted lines. At left, somatosensory responses in lateral thalamus shown in figurine charts (threshold in mA, quality indicated by symbol such as P for paresthetic). At right, responses elicited in medial brain stem

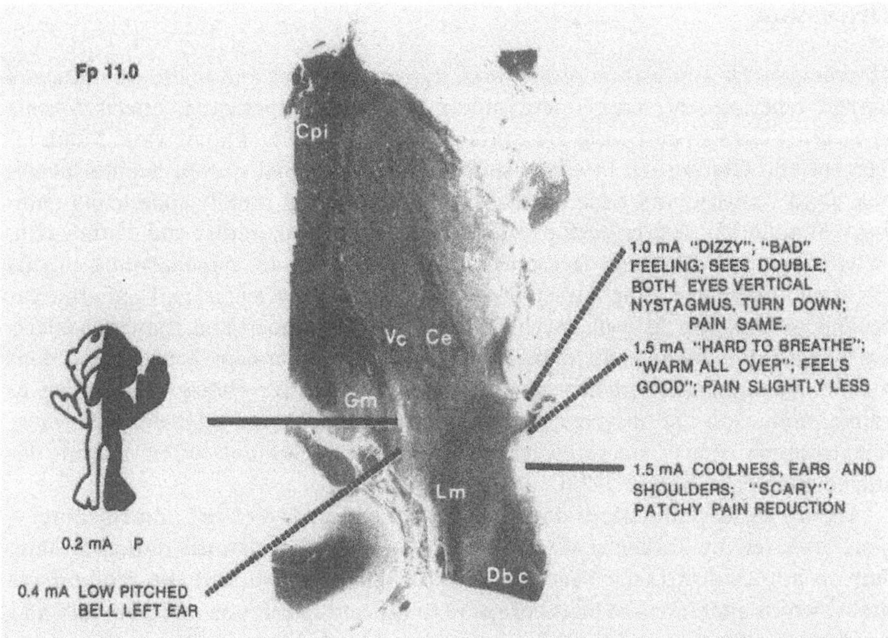

Fig. 5. Responses at one visualized and two extrapolated sites in PAG, just inferomedial to Pf; a lateral paresthetic response in Vc and an auditory one near Mg

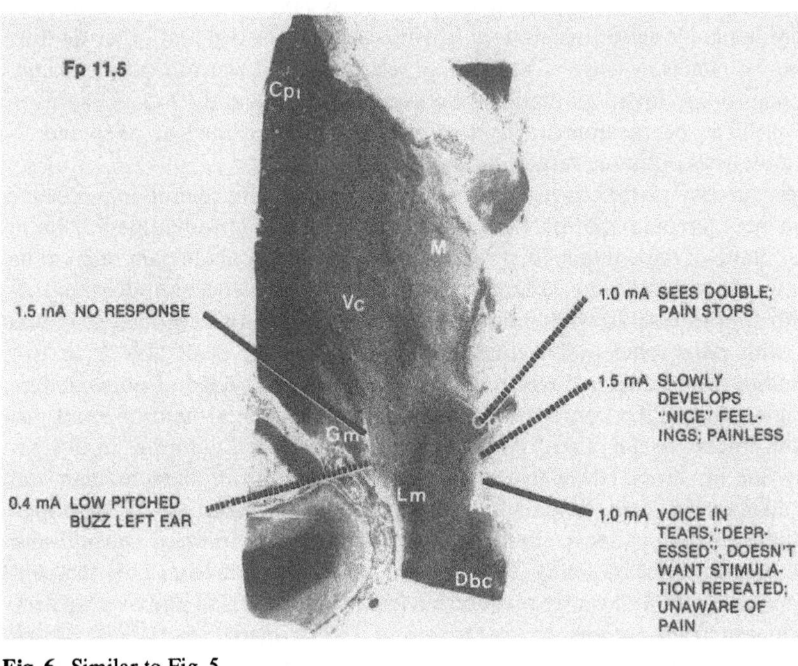

Fig. 6. Similar to Fig. 5

Discussion

Threshold 60 Hz stimulation of the wake human thalamus and midbrain induces a limited repertoire of sensory and motor but rarely experiential effects (Tasker et al. 1977). Sensory responses are confined to primary afferent pathways. Motor effects include tetanization in corticospinal tract and cranial nerves. Sagittal planes near third ventricle and aqueduct lack recently acquired rapidly conducting pathways. Stimulation here induces pupillary, oculomotor, respiratory and cardiovascular effects, head tilting and face movement, presumably in hypothalamus, medial forebrain bundle, tectospinal tract, medial longitudinal fasciculus, and supranuclear oculomotor systems. As well, psychic, visceral sensory, mood and conscious effects are induced. Finally, in some patients with deafferentation pain, contralateral non-somatotopographically organized, monotonously repetitive feelings of burning or pain reproduction are observed in medial mesencephalic and thalamic sites where somatosensory effects are rarely encountered in patients not suffering from deafferentation pain (Tasker 1982).

Though many publications describe stimulation-induced effects in medial brainstem, reviewed by Tasker et al. (1982, Chapter 13), who mapped responses here, they do not localize them. Sano et al. (1970), however, mapped the presumptive sites at which alterations of blood pressure, pulse and respiration and pupillary and oculomotor effects were induced in posterior hypothalamus under general anesthesia, stimulation in the awake patient inducing a feeling of horror. Schaltenbrand and Wahren's (1977) atlas figures depicting a large area of rostral diencephalon, where pupillary dilatation and a feeling of warmth were induced, do not cover PVG-PAG. Nashold et al. (1969), Richardson and Akil (1977a, b), Richardson (1982), Hosobuchi et al. (1977), Cosyns and Gybels (1979), and Meyerson et al. (1978) recorded oculomotor, respiratory, cardiovascular, visceral and other midline and autonomic effects, a sense of well-being, relaxation and warmth, startle, fright, and apprehension, nausea and dizziness between septal area and PAG. Richardson and Akil (1977a, b) recommended medial parafascicular nucleus (Pf) and N medialis caudalis as optimum targets for pain relief.

Previous autopsy studies have been mostly concerned with identifying effective stimulation sites for pain control. Richardson and Akil (1977b) identified a site in the coronal plane of habenula medial to Pf where stimulation made pain seem to be "floating away", with startling, dizziness, nystagmus, fright, and apprehension occurring with suprathreshold stimulation. In another patient, a site in medial Pf was identified with pain relief and feelings of heat. Hosobuchi et al. (1977), in two autopsy studies found effective electrode locations in medial edge of dorsomedian nucleus against habenular commissure in one and in tegmental field of Forel just dorsal to third nerve in the other. Gybels et al. (1980) reviewed autopsies in five patients, only one of whom, stimulated at the junction between Pf, dorsomedian and centre median nuclei, enjoyed pain relief. Boivie and Meyerson (1982) described autopsy studies in five patients, stimulation in four of whom induced warmth and pain relief, anatomical data being displayed for three. The optimum area for pain relief was medial to Pf and centre median nuclei above the ACPC line over an area measuring 6 mm from anterior to posterior and 3 from medial to lateral. Baskin et al. (1980) reviewing seven autopsies from various centers correlated optimum pain relief with sites in ventrobasal PAG at the level of PC, most often dorsal to the third nerve nucleus, medial to mesencephalic reticular formation and dorsal and rostral to the dorsal tegmental nucleus of Gudden in the region of the periventricular bundle.

Conclusion

Acute stimulation of PVG-PAG in a quadriplegic patient with deafferentation pain induced pain relief and various other effects similar to those frequently reported in the literature. The sites at which these effects were elicited have been plotted on serial coronal sections of the brain prepared at autopsy.

References

Baskin DS, Mehler W, Hosobuchi Y, Richardson D, Adams JE, Flitter MA (1980) Cartography of periaqueductal gray stimulation in humans. Presented AANS, New York, April 22

Boivie J, Meyerson BA (1982) A correlative anatomical and clinical study of pain suppression by deep brain stimulation. Pain 13: 113–126

Cosyns P, Gybels J (1979) Electrical central gray stimulation for pain in man. In Bonica JJ et al. (eds) Advances in Pain Research and Therapy, Vol 3. Raven, New York, pp 511–514

Gybels J, Dom R, Cosyns P (1980) Electrical stimulation of the central gray for pain relief in human: autopsy data. Acta Neurochir [Suppl] (Wien) 20: 259–268

Hosobuchi Y, Adams JE, Linchitz R (1977) Pain relief by electrical stimulation of the central gray matter in humans and its reversal by naloxone. Science 179: 183–186

Meyerson BA, Boëthius J, Carlsson AM (1978) Percutaneous gray stimulation in cancer pain. Appl Neurophysiol 41: 57–65

Nashold BS, Wilson WP, Slaughter DG (1969) Sensations evoked by stimulation in the midbrain of man. J Neurosurg 30: 14–24

Richardson DE (1982) Analgesia produced by stimulation of various sites in the human beta endorphin system. Appl Neurophysiol 45: 116–122

Richardson DE, Akil H (1977a) Pain reduction by electrical brain stimulation in man. Part 1. Acute administration in periaqueductal and periventricular sites. J Neurosurg 47: 178–183

Richardson DE, Akil H (1977b) Pain reduction by electrical brain stimulation in man. Part II. Chronic self-administration in the periventricular grey matter. J Neurosurg 47: 184–194

Sano K, Mayanagi Y, Sekino H, Ogashiwa M, Ishijima B (1970) Results of stimulation and destruction of the posterior hypothalamus in man. J Neurosurg 33: 689–707

Schaltenbrand G, Bailey P (1959) An Introduction to Stereotaxis with an Atlas of the Human Brain. Thieme, Stuttgart

Schaltenbrand G, Wahren W (1977) Atlas for Stereotaxy of the Human Brain. Thieme, Stuttgart

Tasker RR, Organ LW, Hawrylyshyn P (1977) The sensory organization of the human thalamus. Appl Neurophysiol 39: 139–153

Tasker RR (1982) Identification of pain processing systems by electrical stimulation of the brain. Hum Neurobiol 1: 261–272

Tasker RR, Organ LW, Hawrylyshyn PA (1982) The Thalamus and Midbrain of Man. A Physiological Atlas Using Electrical Stimulation. In: Wilkins RH (ed) A monograph in the Bannerstone Division of American Lectures in Neurosurgery. Thomas, Springfield

Monitoring of Brain Stem Function by Brain Stem Auditory Evoked Potentials (BAEP)

C. B. LUMENTA, M. KRÄMER, and W. J. BOCK, Düsseldorf/FRG

Introduction

The application of microneurosurgical technique permits surgery in and around the brain stem, but the rate of mortality and morbidity of such operations is still high because of compression and/or ischemia of the brain stem following surgery. The continuous measurements of the Brain Stem Auditory Evoked Potentials (BAEP) open a new possibility for the neurosurgeon to monitor brain stem function during and after the operation, although the hypothesis of the brain stem generators of the BAEP by Jewett and Williston [3] and Buchwald and Huang [1] is increasingly disputed.

To control the value of BAEP as a parameter for brain stem function the data of 59 patients with posterior fossa operations in the time between July 1, 1982 and June 30, 1984 was analysed.

Patient Population and Methods

34 patients had an acoustic neuroma, eight a meningioma of the cerebello-pontine angle, five a medulloblastoma, three a hemangioblastoma, three an intracerebellar metastatic tumor, three an intracerebellar hemorrhage, two an intracerebellar cyst and one an ectopic pinealoma (Fig. 1).

There were 33 female and 26 male patients between 5 and 73 years of age (mean value: 46.3 years). The BAEPs were recorded from conventional surface electrodes, the technical data were the same as previously described [5, 6].

The data were analysed by the computer and visually by a technician and a physician. The statistical analysis of our data was based on mean values of the BAEP of each patient before, during and after surgery.

Five categories for assessment of BAEP were selected: *1.* normal (less than 1 SD) *2.* possible pathologic (1–2 SD) *3.* sure pathologic (more than 2 SD) *4.* not defined and *5.* not present. Undefined wave configurations, mostly because of artefacts, were not analysed for this study. Unpresent BAEPs were determined as sure pathologic changes.

The outcome of the patients was estimated as follows:

1. good recovery
2. moderate disability (without brain stem function impairment)
3. severe disability (with impairment of brain stem function)
4. death

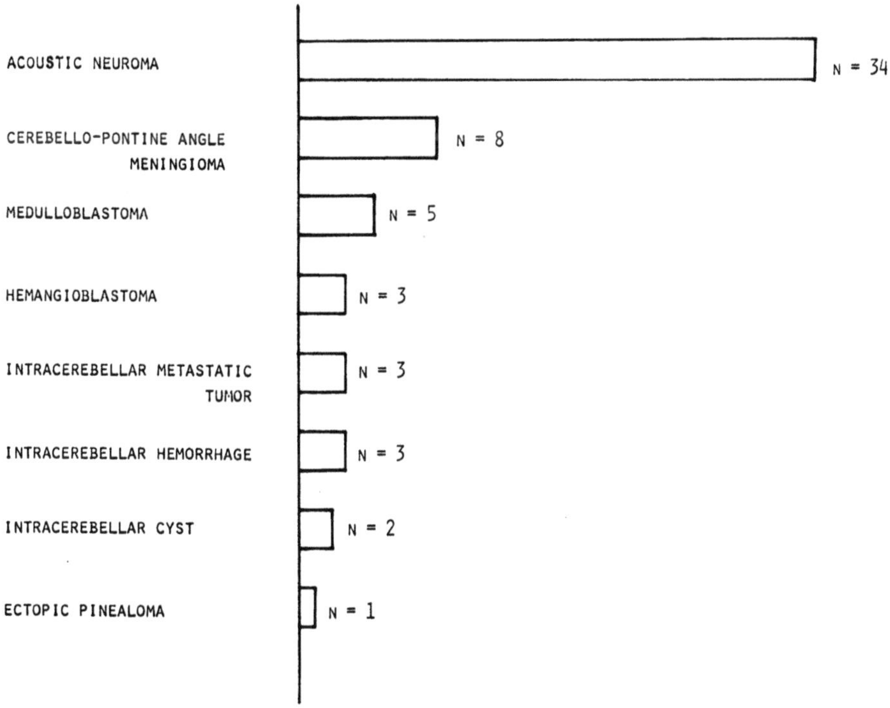

Fig. 1. Distribution of posterior fossa operations (n=59) (July 1st, 1982 till June 30th, 1984) in the Neurosurgical Clinic of the University of Düsseldorf

Results

Nearly all the patients with acoustic neuroma were deaf on the side of the tumor, consequently the ipsilateral BAEP were not present or showed sure pathologic changes. Therefore if BAEP was pathologic from wave I and the patient had a tumor in the cerebello-pontine angle the probability of acoustic neuroma was 98.5%. Intraoperatively the BAEP could only be recorded on the contralateral side to the tumor. Analysing the BAEP in patients with acoustic neuroma showed that only half of the patients had normal BAEP during surgery. A recovery after the operations could be seen in nearly all the patients (Fig. 2). None of them had severe disability 6 months after the operation. About a quarter of the BAEP could not be defined because the artefact was too high. Analysing the data of the ipsilateral side of patients with meningioma of the cerebello-pontine angle showed that about 20% of them had normal BAEP. Recovery could only be assessed in half of these patients (Fig. 3). On the contralateral side the BAEP demonstrated normal and possible pathologic wave configurations in 50% of the cases. Postoperative recovery could not be established with certainty (Fig. 4). Half of these patients died, another half was dismissed with severe disability. Analysing the data of another 17 patients with posterior fossa tumors showed the same result.

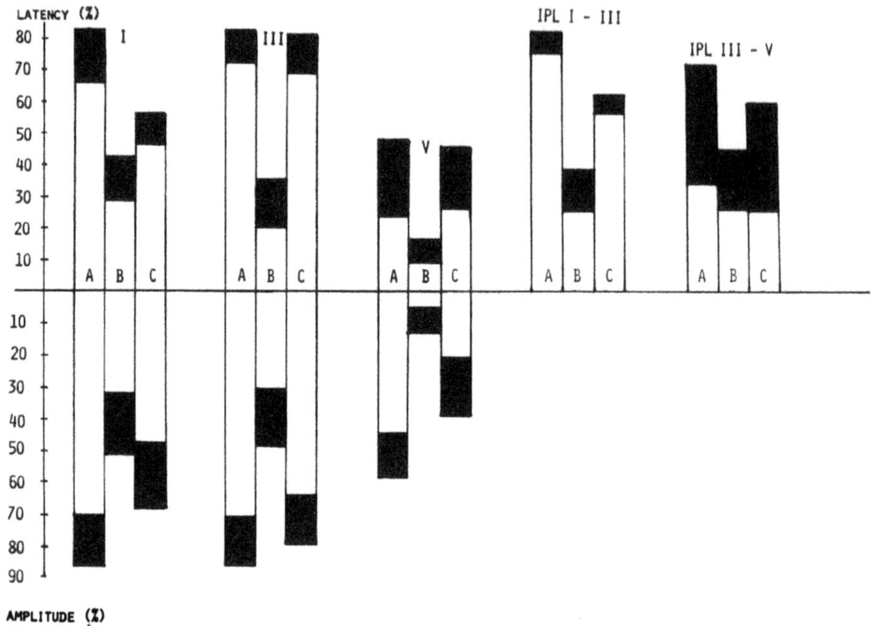

Fig. 2. Average BAEP findings (in %) of 34 patients with acoustic neuroma (contralateral)

Figs. 2–4. □: normal (less than one standard deviation). ■: possible pathologic (one to two standard deviations). A: preoperative findings, B: intraoperative findings, C: postoperative findings. I: wave I, III: wave III, V: wave V, IPL I–III: interpeak latency of waves I–III, IPL III–V: interpeak latency of waves III–V

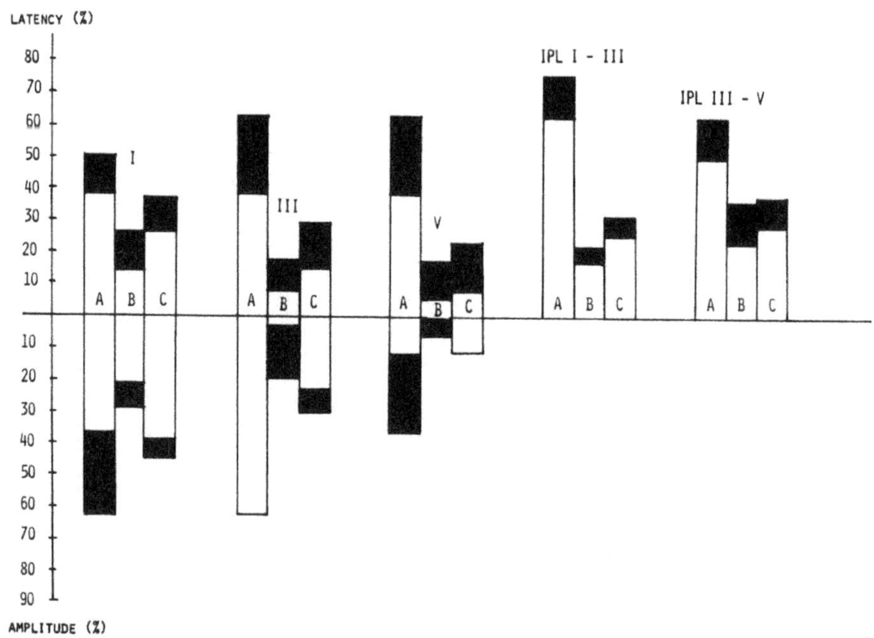

Fig. 3. Average BAEP findings (in %) of 8 patients with meningioma of the cerebello-pontine angle (ipsilateral)

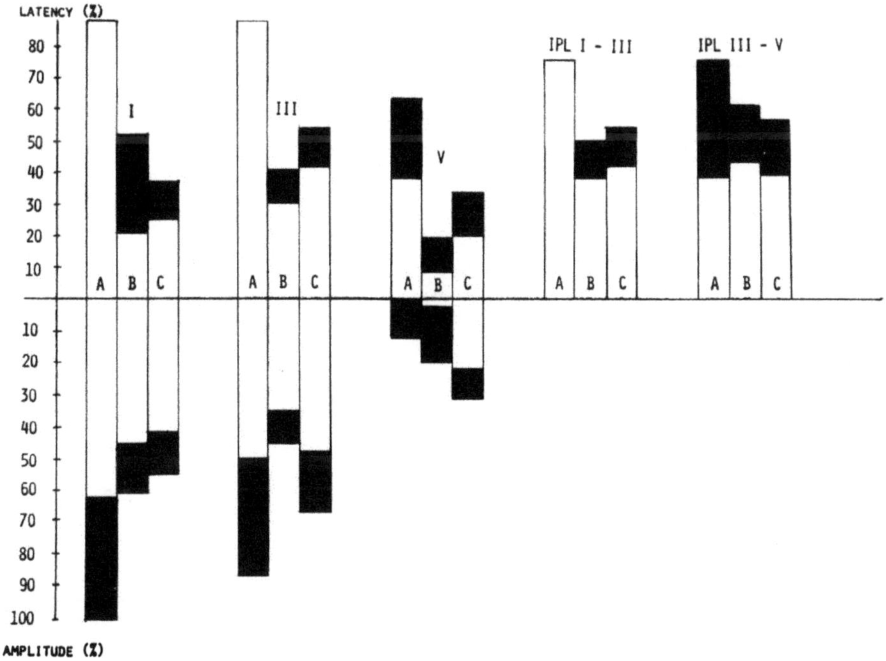

Fig. 4. Average BAEP findings (in %) of 8 patients with meningioma of the cerebello-pontine angle (contralateral)

Illustrative Case Reports

1. Patient D. M., a 27-year-old woman with an acoustic neuroma on the right side (Fig. 5).

Before surgery (stage A) the ipsilateral BAEP was not present and the contralateral one was normal. Stage B indicated the beginning of surgery. Neuroleptanesthesia induced insignificant prolonged latency of waves I till V. No BAEP-changes could be established till stage C, marked as the beginning of tumor dissection. The latency of wave V began to increase till the end of the dissection (stage D). At the end of the operation (E) the BAEP showed prolonged latency of wave V again but the latency of waves I and III was normal. We supposed that unspecific reaction of the brain stem to the surgery developed at this time. The BAEP registration 6 hours after the operation already indicated complete recovery. The patient was well on dismissal.

2. Patient E. W., a 49-year-old woman with a recurrence of hemangioblastoma (Fig. 6).

The preoperative BAEP showed a normal value (A). At the beginning of surgery (B) the amplitude of all waves was reduced (reaction of neuroleptanesthesia?). No significant BAEP changes could be established up to stage C, marked as the beginning of tumor dissection. At 12.30 p.m. a major midline bleeding occurred; several arteries (of the brain stem?) had to be coagulated. Hemostasis was attained at 12.55 p.m. However, BAEP already showed sure pathologic changes at 12.45 p.m. and at

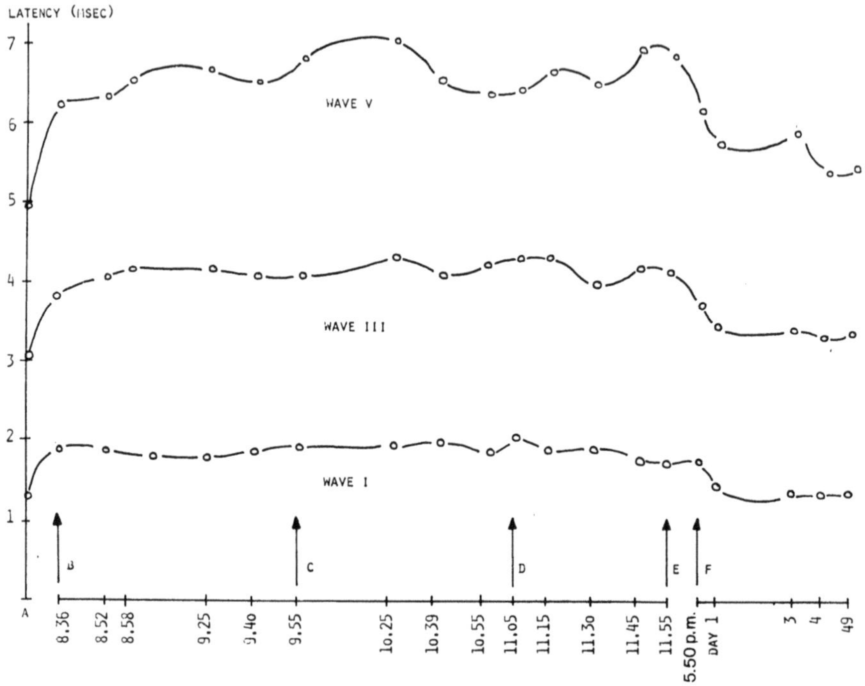

Fig. 5. The course of the latency of waves I, III and V on the left side before, during and after surgery on a 27-year-old woman with an acoustic neuroma on the right side (text). *A* = preoperative stage, *B* = beginning of the operation, *C* = tumor dissection, *D* = end of the dissection, *E* = end of the operation, *F* = after surgery (on ICU)

12.55 p.m. were not present any more. At 1 p.m. the patient developed bradycardia; between 1.08 p.m. and 1.25 p.m. a resuscitation was made but without response.

Discussion

Under the unshielded conditions of the operating theatre and the ICU we decided that the BAEP was abnormal (= sure pathologic), if it differed from the normal value obtained under shielded conditions by more than two standard deviations (SD). Transient intraoperative alteration of BAEP was seen in 50% of the patients with acoustic neuroma and up to 80% of those with meningioma of the cerebello-pontine angle. Follow-up recording of BAEP showed a complete recovery in all patients with acoustic neuroma and only in half of the patients with meningioma of the cerebello-pontine angle, who had abnormal intraoperative BAEP. The last patient group died or was dismissed with severe disability in a relation of fifty to fifty. The mean time for recovery of transient BAEP changes in our study was about 2 hours. This, however, depended on the age of the patients, the size and biology of the tumor and last not least on the technique of the tumor dissection. The older the patients were, the shorter was the required time for recovery, and the higher the probability to be

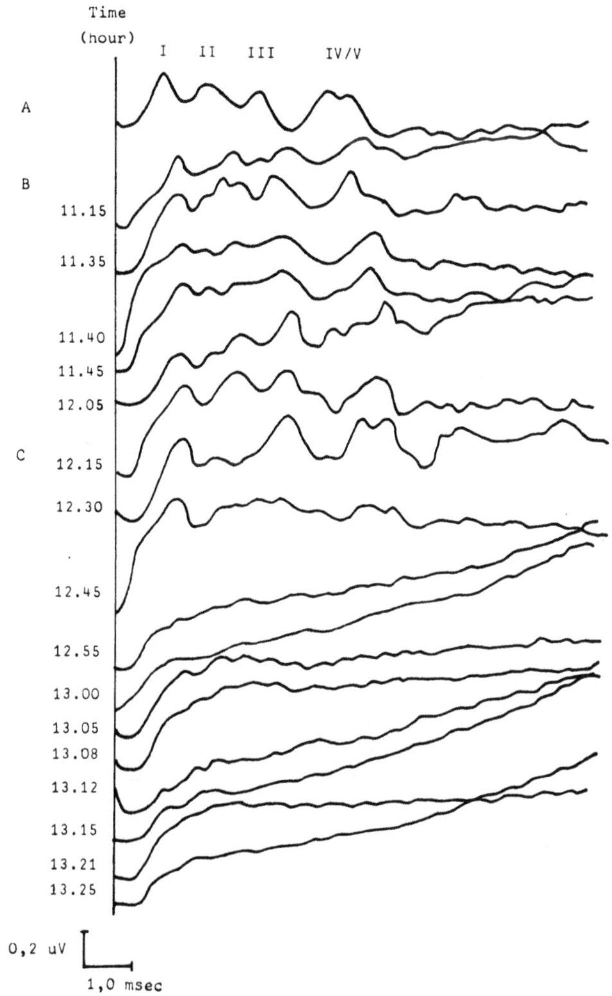

Fig. 6. Contralateral BAEP measurements during surgery on a 49-year-old woman with a recurrence of hemangioblastoma (text).
A = preoperative BAEP,
B = beginning of surgery,
C = tumor dissection

dismissed well or with moderate disability. Younger patients tend to be more resistant.

As demonstrated in case report No. 1, BAEP changes were associated with operative retraction and manipulation. Grundy and Jannetta [2] monitored BAEP in 54 patients during posterior fossa operations and found if BAEP were stable, or if they returned to normal in the operating room, hearing was preserved. In all the patients with transient BAEP changes normal values returned before 177 minutes. Little and Lesser [4] found a good correlation of BAEP abnormalities with the neurological findings before and after operations. Three of ten patients in their group, in whom the BAEP was lost during surgery, died. The same result was found by Raudzens and Shetter [7].

Case report No. 2 showed that BAEP was lost a short time before cardiac arrest. Such a result could only be gained by continuous measurements.

Summary

Analysing the data of 59 patients with posterior fossa operations demonstrated that pathological BAEP changes for longer than two hours caused an ipsilateral hearing deficit and brain stem function impairment. Contralateral BAEP changes were normally followed by impairment of brain stem function only. The outcome of these patients is severe disability or death in a relation of fifty to fifty. Jewett and Williston [3] and Buchwald and Huang [1] made a hypothesis about the brain stem generators of the BAEP. This theory is increasingly disputed, though our results showed that continuous registration of the BAEP is very helpful as a guide during surgery in and around the brain stem.

References

1. Buchwald JS, Huang CM (1975) Far-field acoustic response origin in cats. Science 189:382
2. Grundy BL, Jannetta PJ et al. (1982) Intraoperative monitoring of brain-stem auditory evoked potentials. J Neurosurg 57:674–681
3. Jewett DL, Williston JS (1971) Auditory evoked far-fields averaged from the scalp of human. Brain 94:681–696
4. Little JR, Lesser RP et al. (1983) Brain-stem auditory evoked potentials in posterior circulation surgery. Neurosurgery 12/5:496–502
5. Lumenta CB, Krämer M et al. (1984) Brain-stem auditory evoked potentials (BAEP) during and after posterior fossa operations. Adv Neurosurg 12:247–252
6. Lumenta CB (1984) Measurement of brain-stem auditory evoked potentials in patients with spontaneous intracerebral hemorrhage. J Neurosurg 60:548–552
7. Raudzens PA, Shetter AG (1982) Intraoperative monitoring of brain stem auditory evoked potentials. J Neurosurg 57:341–348

The Perioperative Monitoring of Brain Stem Auditory Evoked Potentials (BAEP)

P. GÜRTNER, E. KOHMURA, R. RAMINA, R. LORENZ, and M. SAMII, Hannover/RFG

Introduction

Recently BAEP have been used as a diagnostic tool in the operating room [1–4]. Patients undergoing surgery around the brain stem or in the posterior fossa are at a high risk of damage to the brain stem. While operating on large tumors or arteriovenous malformations it is of advantage to inform the surgeon intraoperatively on brain stem function. Postoperatively we try to safeguard these patients by a routine check-up including BAEPs. Besides that, we use the prognostic value of BAEPs in severely head injured patients (Tables 1 and 2).

Table 1. Indications for intraoperative monitoring of BAEP

1) Surgery within the posterior fossa
2) Surgery around the brain stem

Table 2. Indications for postoperative monitoring of BAEP

1) Surgery within the posterior fossa
2) Surgery around the brain stem
3) Severe head injuries

Method

All our recordings we did with a Nicolet CA 1000. Plate electrodes were placed over the mastoid processes, the vertex and the midline. We stimulated with 90 dB clicks, a duration of 150 microseconds at a rate of 11.3/s with 1000 repetitions. Usually we measured latencies of the peaks I to V.

BAEP 'C A 1000' – normal values
n=69 ears

I–V:	$\bar{x}=4.02$, s= 19 msec+2.5 s	≦4.50 msec
I–III:	$\bar{x}=2.15$, s= 15 msec+2.5 s	≦2.53 msec
III–V:	$\bar{x}=1.84$, s= 15 msec+2.5 s	≦2.22 msec

(By courtesy of R. Lorenz, Neurological Dept., Nordstadt Krankenhaus, Hannover/FRG)

Amplitudes were not measured since we found them highly variable.

Table 3. Postoperative flow chart

The neurological function is evaluated at 15 minutes intervals

↓

If abnormal after 60 minutes

↓

Reversal of neuroleptoanalgesia

If failing

↓

CT-SCAN

If normal or non-surgical abnormal

↓

BAEP

If continuously abnormal

↓

Antiedematous therapy → repeat CT-scan

Table 4. BAEPs are of diagnostic value

	CT	CT and BAEP
Edema	?	+
Brain stem infarction (early phase)	–	+

The outline of the diagnostic evaluation of a postoperative complication is shown on the Flow Chart. If the patient presents with an abnormal neurological status 60 minutes after his arrival at the ICU, a reversal of neuroleptanalgesia is done. If the patient doesn't improve we do a CT-scan. If by the CT-scan there is no need for an immediate surgical intervention, we do BAEPs. If these are altered while the CT-scan is normal we suspect brain stem edema or infarction. Then anti-edematous therapy is begun. On deterioration of the neurological status or BAEP latencies the CT-scan is repeated (Tables 3 and 4).

Case 1: Illustrating our postoperative monitoring we would like to present the case of a middle-aged lady, who was operated on an acoustic neurinoma of medium size. One hour postoperatively her pupils didn't react to light, a corneal or a coughing reflex could not be elicited. We did a reversal of neuroleptanalgesia. There was no change in her neurological status.

Next we did a CT-scan. Besides the pneumocephalus we couldn't find any major pathology. We did BAEPs and found them normal in latencies except that there was a severe hearing loss on the right side (Fig. 1). Regarding this we felt that the explanation for the poor neurological status was not within the operating site. The patient was known to suffer from a psychiatric disorder in the past. Further examinations revealed an acute catatonic state. After receiving Haloperidol, within 48 hours she was alert and moving her limbs on command.

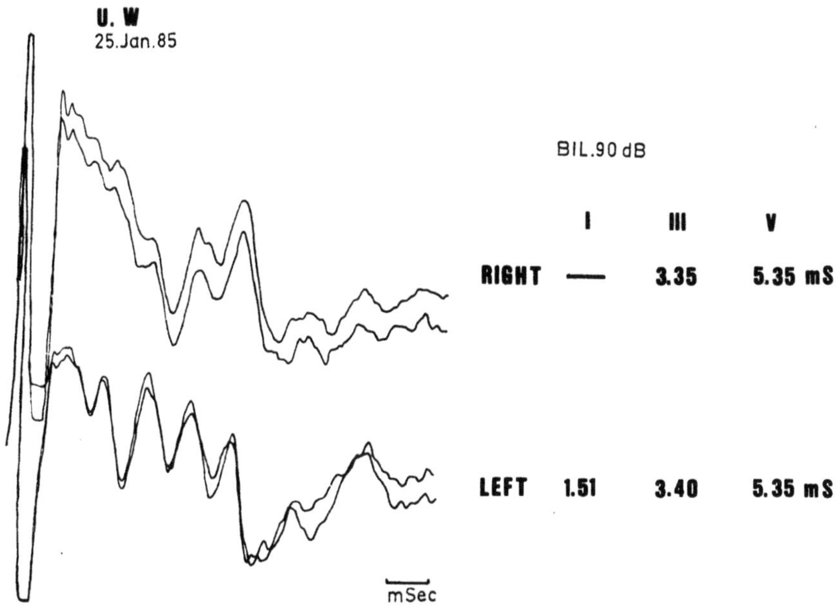

Fig. 1. Normal BAEPs in a comatose patient U. W. operated on an acoustic neurinoma of the right side

As I already mentioned we also appreciate the prognostic value of BAEPs in severe head injuries.

Case 2: This patient was operated on a very large epidural hematoma of the left side. Preoperatively he clinically presented with signs of transtentorial herniation.

Postoperatively he remained deeply comatose. His pupils did not react to light, and to painful stimulus he showed decerebrated posture. We did BAEPs on him, which were of low amplitude on the left side, despite that latencies were only slightly prolonged on both sides (Fig. 2). Within six weeks he made a slow recovery and is reading newspapers now.

Next we'll give an exemplary case for intraoperative monitoring of BAEPs.

Case 3: Intraoperative BAEPs were done in a young patient who had an AVM around the brain stem. He complained of a right homonymous hemianopsia and of a weakness of his right side. The AVM was fed by the posterior cerebral artery, the superior cerebellar artery, the anterior and posterior choroidal arteries of the left side. Preoperatively his BAEPs were normal.

Surgery was performed by a subtemporal approach, the tentorium was incised to reach down to the AVM. As expected BAEPs were abnormal in latencies I–V and III–V as soon as coagulation around the brain stem started (Fig. 3). Still we were very much reassured when the temporary clipping of a presumably pathological vessel did not disturb the pattern of the BAEP. After eight hours of operating time

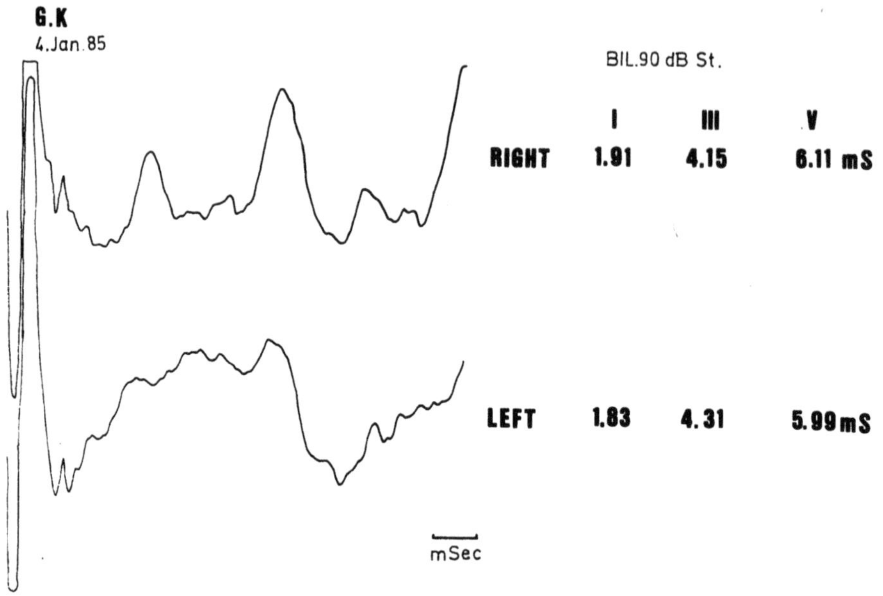

Fig. 2. Slightly abnormal BAEPs in a comatose patient G. K. operated on a very large epidural hematoma on the left side

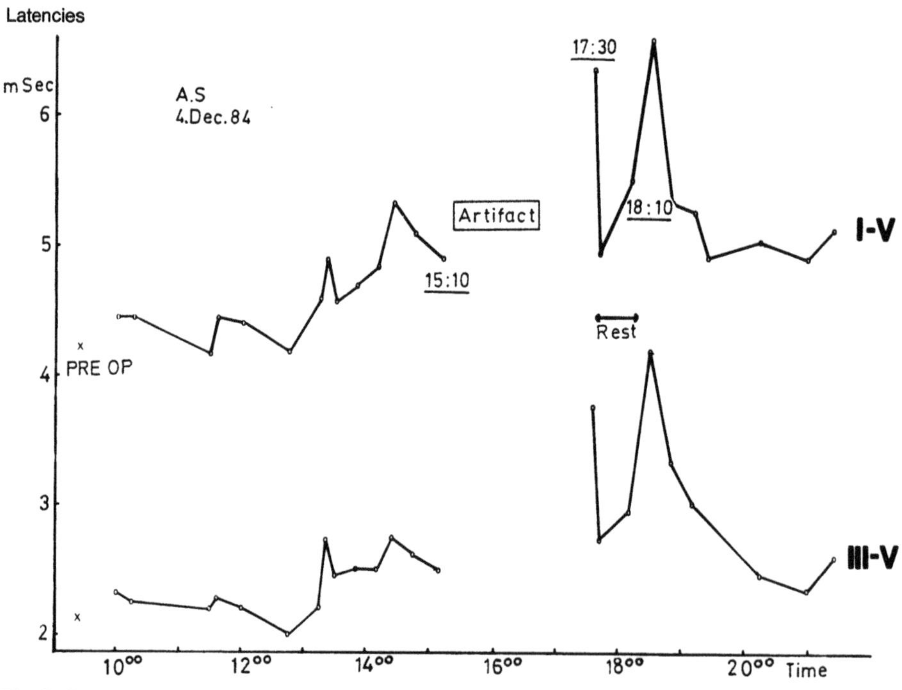

Fig. 3. Intraoperative change of BAEP latencies

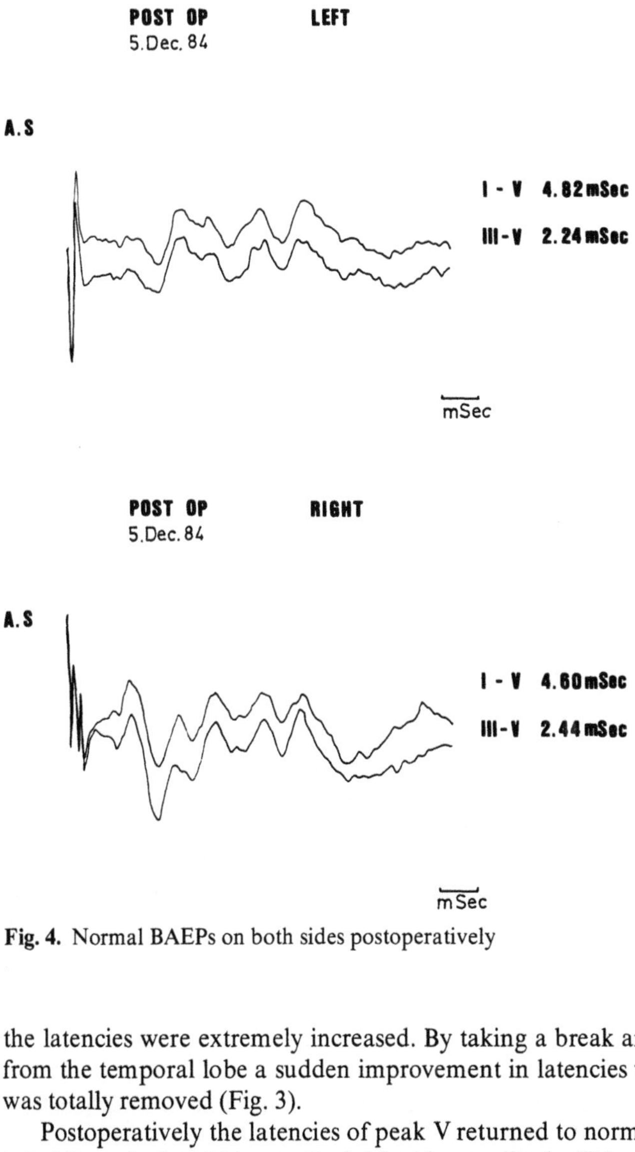

Fig. 4. Normal BAEPs on both sides postoperatively

the latencies were extremely increased. By taking a break and removing the spatula from the temporal lobe a sudden improvement in latencies was observed. The AVM was totally removed (Fig. 3).

Postoperatively the latencies of peak V returned to normal on both sides. On the left side peaks I and II were diminished in amplitude. This severe hearing loss might be due to impaired vascular supply of the internal auditory artery or due to local edema or coagulation injury (Fig. 4).

Discussion

In our clinic we found BAEPs useful for every day routine. Intraoperatively we learnt that latencies increase with the length of the operating time. By prolonged latencies the surgeon is cautioned against continuing retracting structures [1–4]. The

Table 5. Conclusions (in our clinic we found BAEPs are useful)

Intraoperatively	Postoperatively
a) As a warning signal	a) In diagnosing surgical complications
b) In guiding the surgeon in coagulation and retraction	b) In monitoring the course of reversible brain stem damage
	c) In predicting the outcome of severe head injuries
Problems	
a) Elongation of the operating time	
b) Impaired interpretation due to artifacts	

temporary occlusion of a vessel resulting in deteriorating BAEPs should advise the surgeon to remove the clip and to abstain from coagulation.

Postoperatively patients with a dissatisfactory neurological status were subjected to BAEPs. In addition to the CT-scan BAEPs were of special diagnostic value for brain stem infarction or edema. Also BAEPs are especially valuable in monitoring the course of comatose patients and predicting the outcome of severe head injuries [5].

The problems we encountered in monitoring BAEPs are artifacts due to all kinds of electrical noise at the OR and at the ICU. It hampers the interpretation a lot. We also felt that obtaining BAEPs is elongating the operating time (Table 5).

There are still many questions about BAEPs, f.e.: Is there a critical point in prolonged latencies? When do intraoperatively prolonged latencies signal permanent damage? What is the exact origin of BAEPs in humans?

Nowadays we have many diagnostic tools, f.e. CT, NMR, angiography etc. BAEPs are a breakthrough in evaluating brain stem function. But we mustn't forget the limitations. It is to be regretted that there still is a discrepancy between BAEP changes and brain stem lesions. We hope further clinical and experimental data will settle this problem.

References

1. Grundy BL (1983) Intraoperative Monitoring of Sensory Evoked Potentials. Anesthesiology 58:72–87
2. Moller AR, Jannetta PJ (1983) Monitoring auditory functions during cranial nerve microvascular decompression operations by direct recording from the eighth nerve. J Neurosurg 59:493–499
3. Raudzens PA, Shetter AG (1982) Intraoperative monitoring of brain stem auditory evoked potentials. J Neurosurg 57:341–348
4. Warnke PC, Lorenz R, Samii M, Ramina R (1984) Evozierte Hirnstammpotentiale zur Therapiekontrolle bei Operationen am Tentoriumrand. Adv in Neurosurg, vol 13 (in print)
5. Warnke PC, Lorenz R, Ramina R, Samii M (1984) Akustische und somatosensible Potentiale im klinischen Verlauf bei Hirnstammkontusion. Adv in Neurosurg, vol 13 (in print)

Neuroradiology

Artificial Intelligence in Radiology

A. WACKENHEIM, Strasbourg/France

The present time is characterized by a tremendous increasing of knowledge. The traditional ways of stocking and transmission of this knowledge (oral transmission, traditions, books) are unable to organize the patrimony of knowledge and of new ways of thinking. This is particularly true in radiology which is one of the most explosive disciplines in the present time. We propose to develop our equipment and to improve our way of professional life and general competence in adopting the so-called artificial intelligence among our computer programs in the future.

It is very hard work to realize a computer program of reading and interpreting radiologic images. We try to do it with an experimental program concerning only three identical cervical vertebrae. In previous papers, we discussed the phenomenology of perception of the cervical triplet i.e. the three proximal and identical vertebrae C_3, C_4 and C_5 [1]. Figure 1 illustrates schematically these three vertebrae. For an expert system capable to read the image, we need to give heuristic rules of going through the picture. These rules are the essence of our practical competence in the matter. Our theme concerning three identical vertebrae simplifies the practical approach because we only take one theoretical vertebra into account which represents each of the three components of the triplet.

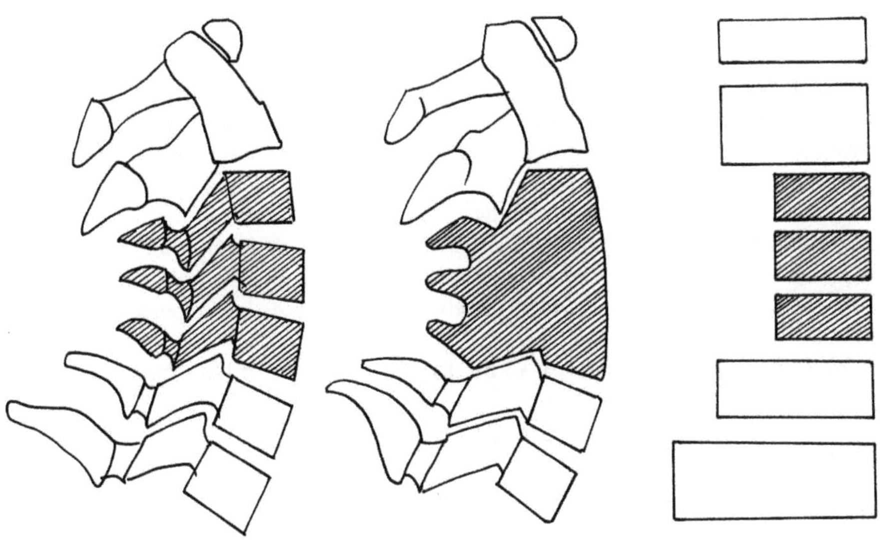

Fig. 1. Three identical and proximal vertebrae form together a phenomenological unit of perception. Our program concerns these three vertebrae

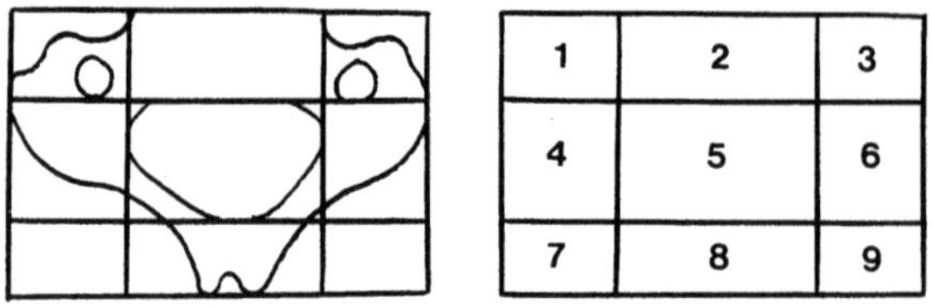

Fig. 2. Diagram dividing the axial view of a vertebra into 9 sectors. The main line is tangent to the posterior margin of the vertebral body, the others are perpendicular or parallel

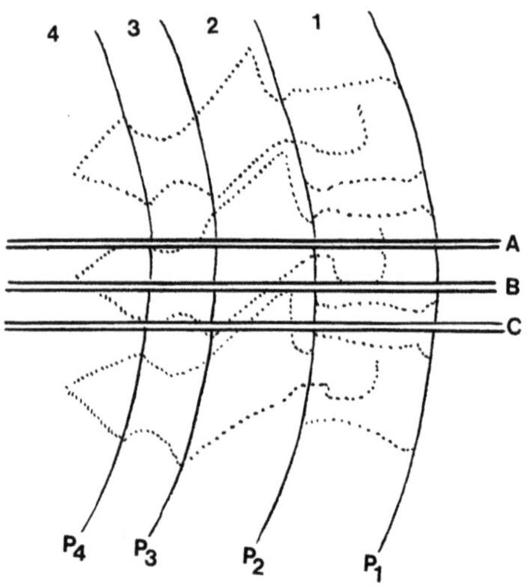

Fig. 3. Division of the lateral projection, P_1 = line of the anterior wall of the vertebral body, P_2 = line of the posterior wall of the vertebral body, P_3 = line of the posterior aspects of the articular processes, P_4 = line of the anterior limit of the spinous process, *1* = sector of the vertebral bodies, *2* = sector of the articular processes, *3* = sector of the laminae, *4* = sector of the spinous processes

For the first steps, we propose to work on two images: a lateral roentgenographic plain film (radiograph or scout view) and one of the three levels of the axial view. It is easy to understand that by eliminating the frontal view we simplify the first steps of creating an intelligent program.

For the first approach of automatic reading of the image, we believe that it is necessary to divide it into sectors. Figure 2 illustrates this division in an axial view of one of the three vertebrae. The division is based on a main line which is tangent to the posterior margin of the vertebral body, the other lines being perpendicular or parallel.

The lateral projection has also to be divided by means of lines in different sectors, as in the drawing of Fig. 3.

Thus, we may distinguish four images:

- a lateral projection
- three axial cuts: A, B and C.

The correlation between these images are schematized in Fig. 4. With these preparations of the image material, the computer program has to verify many heuristic

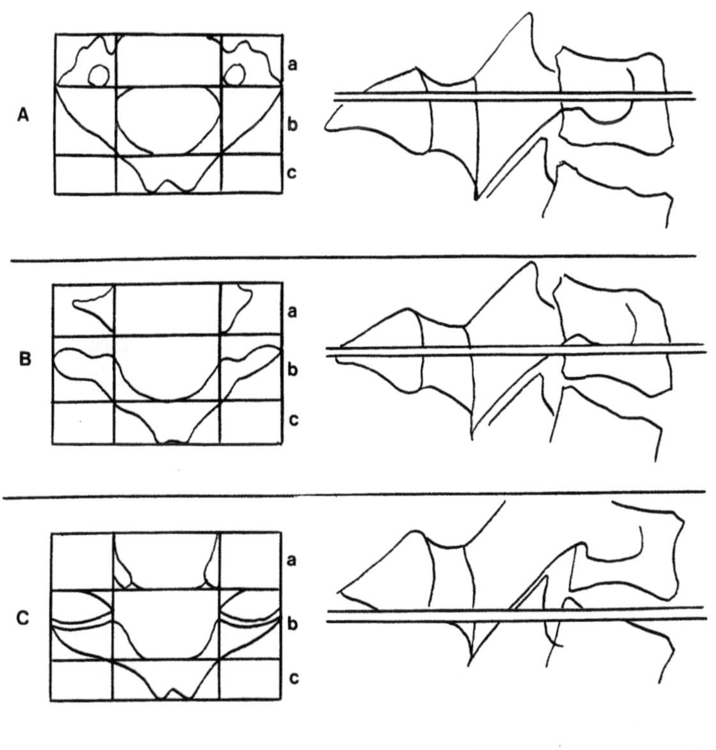

Fig. 4. Correlation between the lateral image and the axial cuts *a, b* and *c*

rules. Let us see some examples of this kind of rules:

AP diameter: $a \leqq b$ (Fig. 4)
sagittal diameter: $1 < 2 + 3$ (Fig. 3)
normal lamina: $3 \approx 1/2\ 2$ (Fig. 3)
AP diameter $a > 12$ mm (Fig. 4)
sagittal diameter $2 + 3 > 12$ mm (Fig. 3)

The list of this kind of verifications is to be established by a group of experts of the cervical spine, including radiologists, neurosurgeons as well as orthopedists.

Let us see four examples of pathologic situations which have to be solved by the program:

1. the diagnosis of constitutional stenosis of the vertebral canal at the level of C_3–C_4–C_5.
2. the diagnosis of hypertrophy of the articular processes in cases of arthrosis
3. the pathology of the transverse canal (foramen transversarium)
4. the diagnosis of the variety of spondylolisthesis.

1. Diagnosis of Constitutional Stenosis of the Vertebral Canal at the Level of C_3–C_4–C_5

In previous papers [2, 3], we demonstrated the very easy and rapid way to recognize a cervical canal stenosis as a phenomenologic perception. We do not insist on the

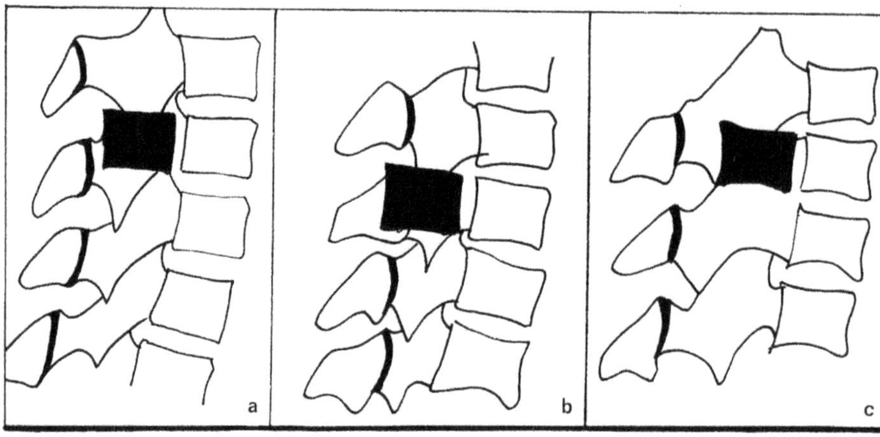

Fig. 5a–c. Visual palpation of the A. P. diameter of the cervical spine. **a** normally there is space enough for the corresponding vertebral body, **b** in canal stenosis, there is not enough space for it, **c** in canal dilatation, there is too much space for it

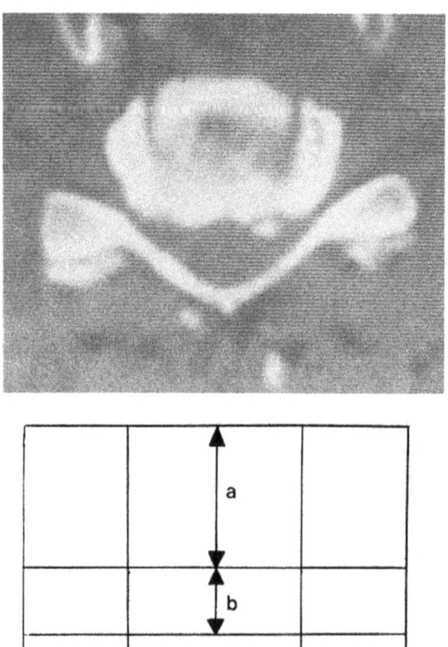

Fig. 6. Constitutional stenosis of the cervical canal (there in not enough space for the body in the canal, $a > b$)

psychologic implications of the relationships between "to see" and "to perceive". In his routine work, the radiologist perceives an anomaly. He only afterwards analyses the details of the anomalous image. An experienced radiologist, seeing a lateral view of the cervical spine, perceives the eventual canal stenosis. In a second step, he indicates tomographies and measurements. We have to find out the way of the thoughts leading to the perception of the stenosis. This question is generally answered by "it is the experience". What is experience? We find out a way of thinking in this precise question of the constitutional canal stenosis and we try to include it in the computer program. Indeed, it is very easy to displace mentally the vertebral body in the corresponding canal on a lateral view, as illustrated in Fig. 5 (visual palpation). Normally, there is enough space in the canal for the corresponding vertebral body. If not, we have to suspect either a canal stenosis (the most frequent hypothesis) or a hypertrophy of the vertebral body (hyperostosis, Paget, tumor). If there is clearly too much space for the vertebral body in the canal, we suspect a canal dilatation (syringomyelia, hydromyelia).

This mental displacement can be performed by the computer as well in a lateral view as in an axial view. The latter is illustrated in Fig. 6 in which you recognize very easily that there is not enough space for the body in the canal (constitutional stenosis of the cervical canal). A large program of logico-mathematical procedure then measures and calculates diameters, surfaces for evaluation of size, shape . . .

2. The Diagnosis of Hypertrophy of the Articular Processes in Cases of Arthrosis

The sector 4 and 6 (Fig. 2) is normally divided in two parts by a diagonale. The antero-medial part of the sector is normally occupied by the articular process (Fig. 7).

Schematically, we have to distinguish the situations of frontal, medial, external, posterior and combined hypertrophies. We have also to check the density of the hypertrophied bone, the thickness of the corticalis . . . (Figs. 8, 14). It is also possible to check the posterior displacement of post-traumatic fragments, as demonstrated in Fig. 9.

3. The Pathology of the Foramen Transversarium

As schematized in Fig. 10, the foramen transversarium is located in the postero-medial quarter of sector 1 or 3.

Our program has to distinguish four pathologic situations in a first attempt of automatic reading:

- the asymmetry. One foramen is very much smaller. We have to suspect a hypoplasia or agenesis of the vertebral artery (Figs. 15, 16)
- the location in front of the normal position, i.e. in the antero-medial quarter. This case corresponds to a canal stenosis. We illustrated this anomaly in Fig. 11 (achondroplasia)

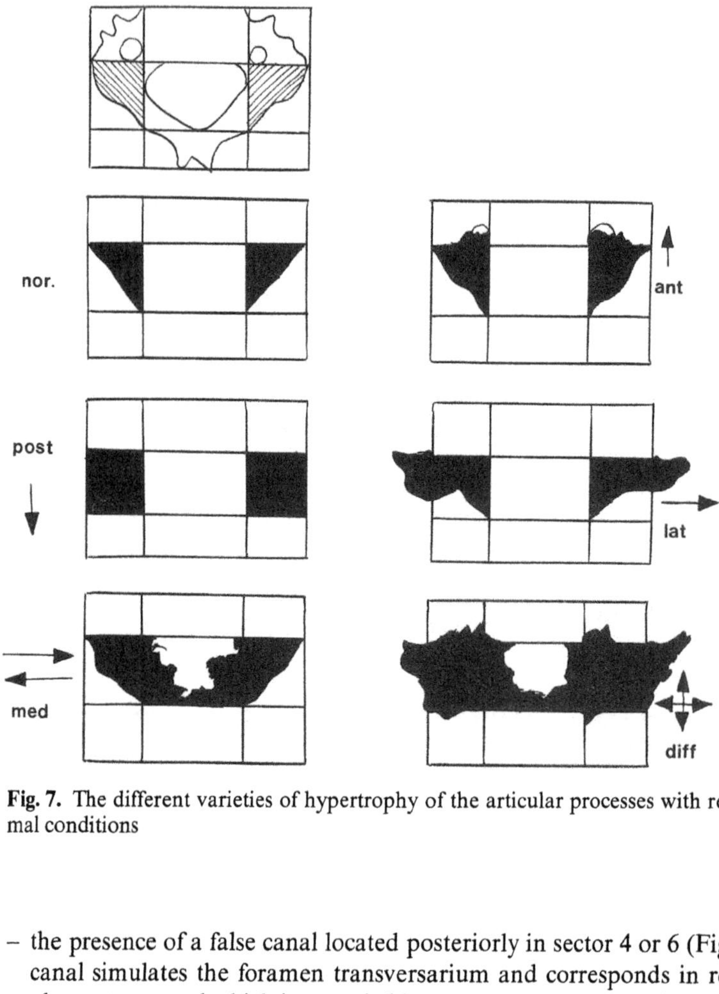

Fig. 7. The different varieties of hypertrophy of the articular processes with respect to the normal conditions

- the presence of a false canal located posteriorly in sector 4 or 6 (Figs. 12, 13). This canal simulates the foramen transversarium and corresponds in reality to a supplementary canal which is occupied by nervous anastomoses between the roots
- the deformation of the foramen transversarium by the hypertrophy and the increased density of the articular processes (Figs. 14–16). In this case, we suspect a compression of the vertebral artery and have to go over to the special program of this question.

Fig. 8. Hypertrophy of the anterior part of the articular processes. Posteriorly, the hypertrophy is very moderate (this hypertrophy narrows the intervertebral foramen and eventually compresses the vertebral artery)

Fig. 9. Fracture (*1*) of the articular pillar of C_4 with schematic demonstration of the posterior displacement in the whole sector 4 (*2*)

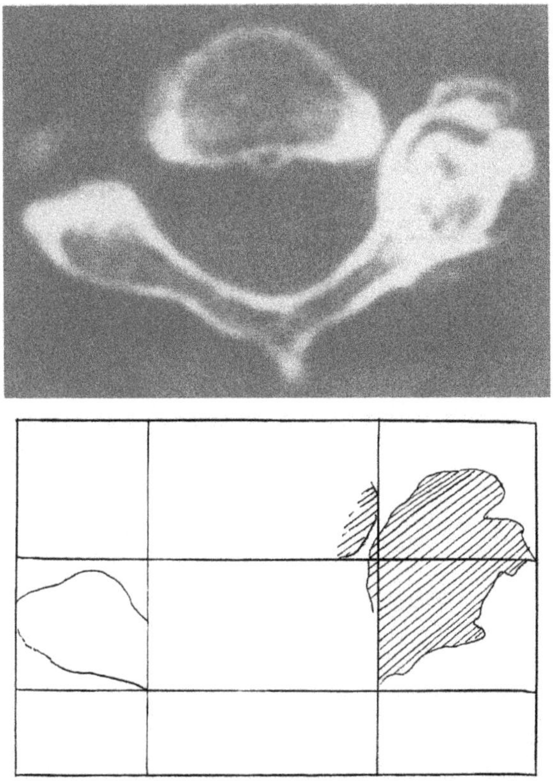

Fig. 8

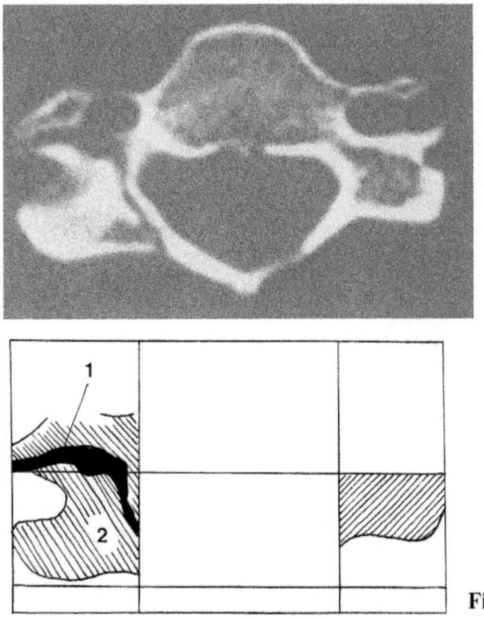

Fig. 9

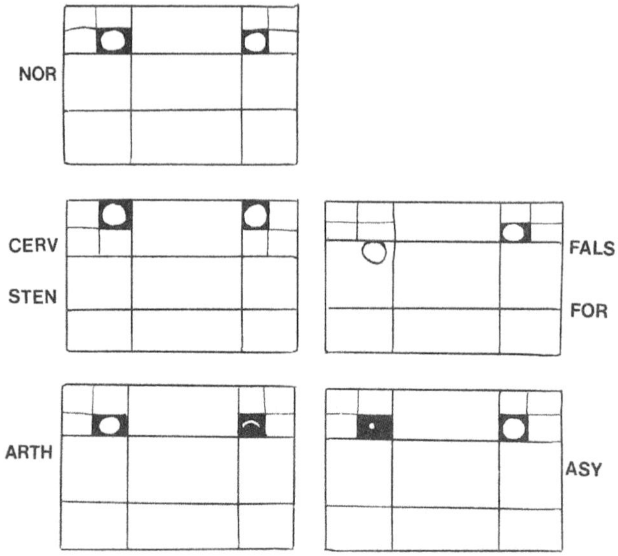

Fig. 10. Example of normal, abnormal and pathologic locations and configurations of the foramen transversarium (cervical stenosis, false foramen, arthrosis, asymmetry)

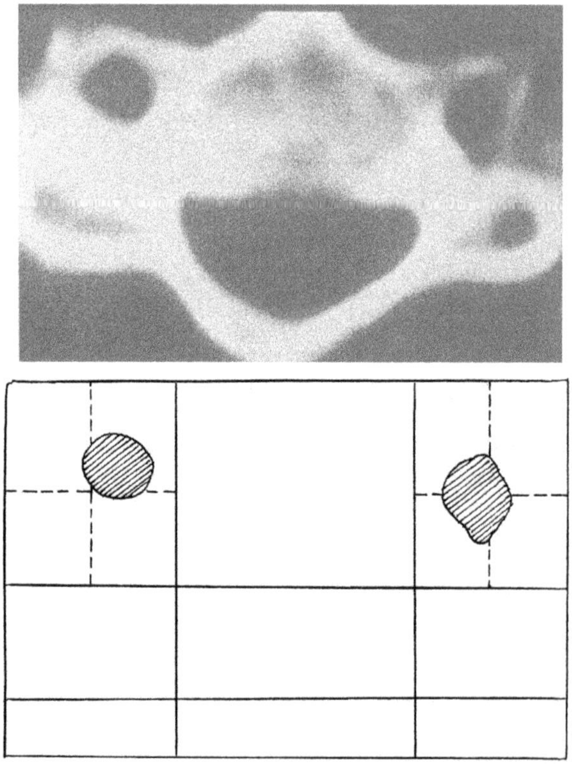

Fig. 11. The foramen transversarium is located in the anterior part of sector 1 and 3 in this case of canal stenosis due to achondroplasia

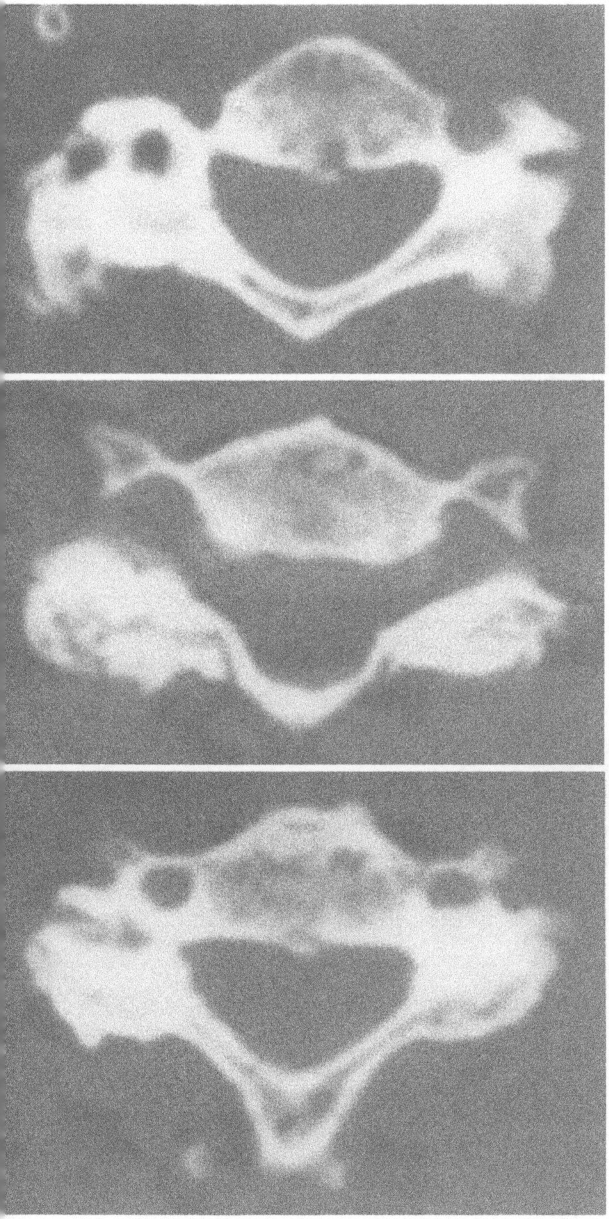

12

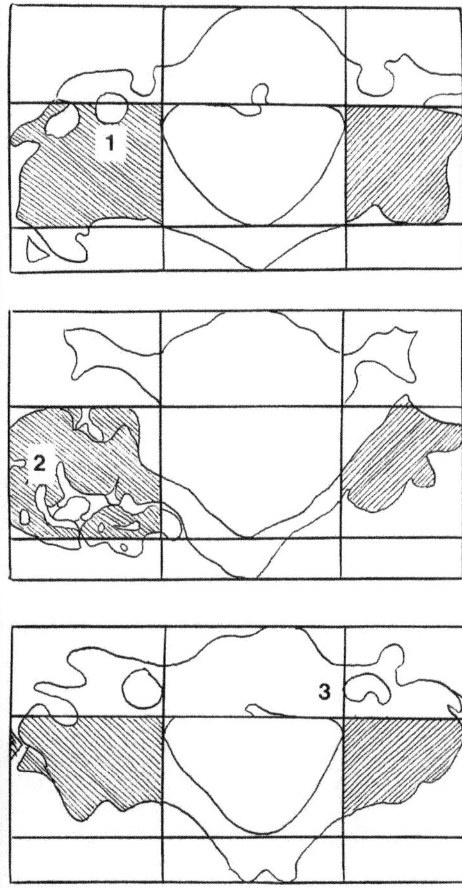

13

Figs. 12 and 13. Axial views of three vertebrae: C_3 (*above*), C_4 (*middle*), and C_5 (*below*). Notice the false foramen at the level of C_3 on the right side (*1*), the marked hypertrophy in the posterior parts of the articular pillar of C_4 (*2*) and finally the stenosis of the left foramen transversarium at the level of C_5 (*3*)

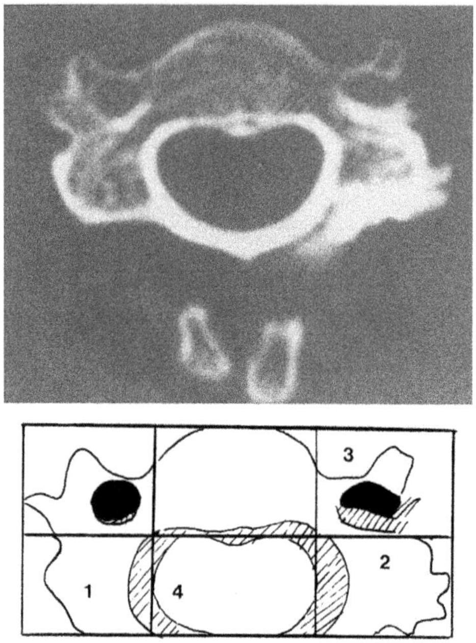

Fig. 14. The automatic analysis of this axial view has to find out that the articular pillars are hypertrophied posteriorly on the right (*1*), posteriorly and anteriorly on the left (*2*), that the foramen transversarium is altered on the left (*3*) and that the corticalis of the vertebral canal is hypertrophied (*4*)

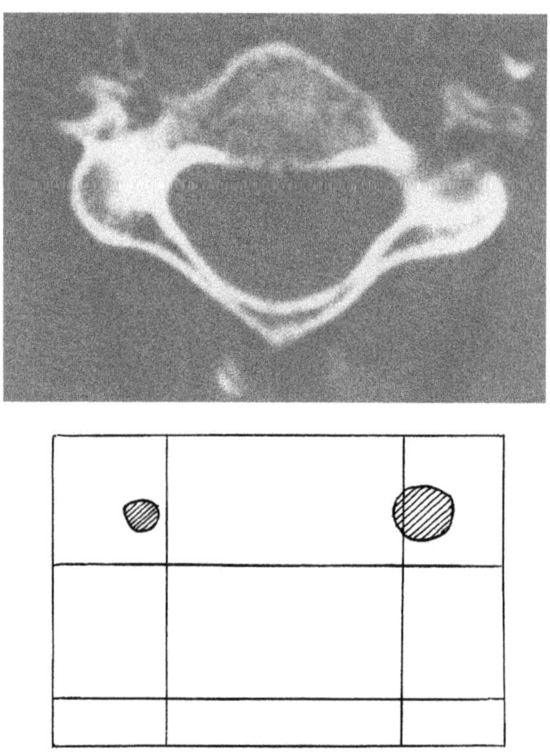

Fig. 15. Asymmetry of the foramen transversarium which is small on the right side (see Fig. 16)

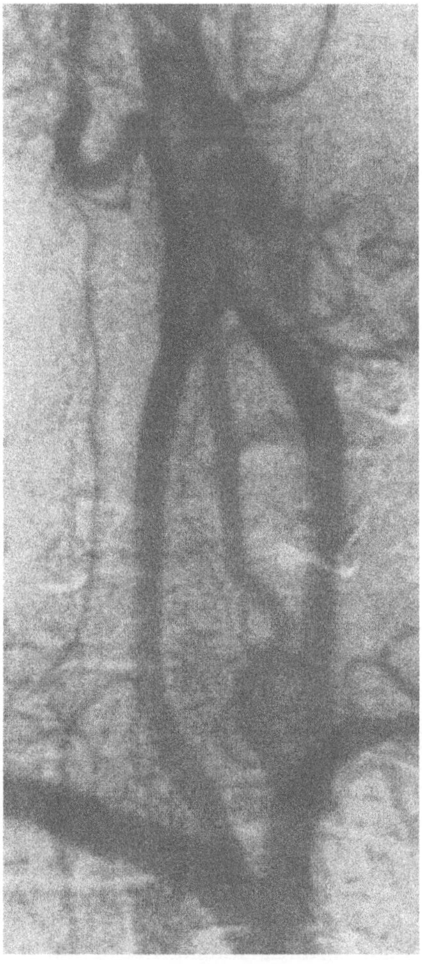

Fig. 16. Hypoplasia of the right vertebral artery in its cervical segment. This angiography corresponds to the patient illustrated in Fig. 15

4. The Diagnosis of the Variety of Spondylolisthesis

With the help of the lines and sectors illustrated in Fig. 3, the program has to distinguish the three varieties of spondylolisthesis schematized in Fig. 17.

Discussion

In this paper we tried to demonstrate the very first steps we adopted to create an expert system in reading and interpreting radiologic images. The reader certainly understands that thousands of programs have to be available for a first model of A. I. The heuristic rules have a considerable importance and they have to be written down by a team in which one medical and one surgical specialist of the matter have to participate.

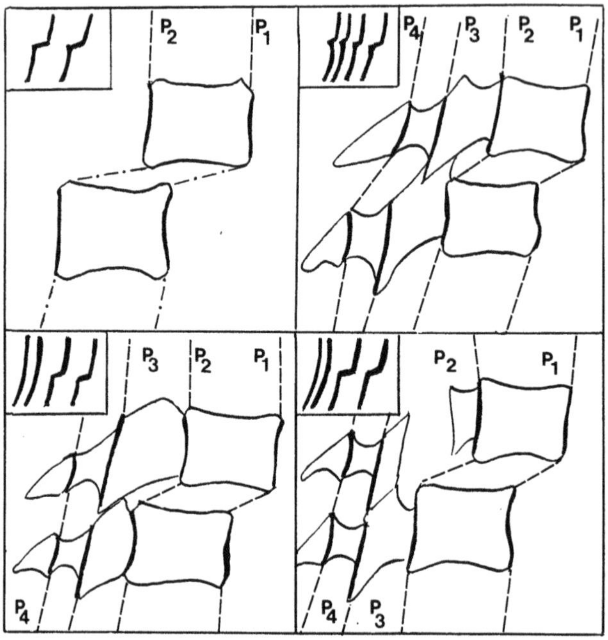

Fig. 17a–d. Three varieties of spondylolisthesis are very easy to recognize: **a** the deviation of the P_1, P_2 lines characterizes the spondylolisthesis, **b** the variety due to sagittalization of the articular interspaces is characterized by the deviation of P_1, P_2, P_3 and P_4, **c** and **d** the deviation of P_1 and P_2 without deviation of P_3 and P_4 characterizes the spondylolisthesis type Junghanns and type spondylolysis

Summary

The author describes the first steps of a program for artificial intelligence in radiology of the cervical spine. He limited his demonstration to the so-called "cervical triplet", made of three vertebrae: C_3–C_4–C_5.

Key-words: cervical triplet – vertebra – expert system – artificial intelligence.

References

1. Wackenheim A (1984) La ségrégation d'unités figurales par la proximité et la ressemblance de leurs composants. J Radiol 65:6–7, 437–441
2. Wackenheim A (1984) La lecture structuraliste de l'image radiologique. J Radiol 65:61–69
3. Wackenheim A (1984) Analyse structuraliste de l'image radiologique. Radiologie J CEPUR 4:289–290

Brain Stem and Tentorial Notch

M. Nadjmi, Würzburg/FRG

Tentorium cerebelli is one of the most significant and clinically important anatomic structures of the brain. Tentorial roof corresponds to the great vein of Galen. This is where the tentorial notch begins, subsequently ending on the level of the posterior clinoid process. In the computed tomogram the two lateral tentorial walls are usually cut axially. On the roof level they have the shape of "V" or "Y", whereas the basal cuts diverge. The intersection of two walls is always the Sinus rectus. The region between these two lines is infratentorial, laterally it is supratentorial, and ventrally there is the tentorial notch.

Only with coronal cuts the supratentorial region is above this line and vice versa (Fig. 1).

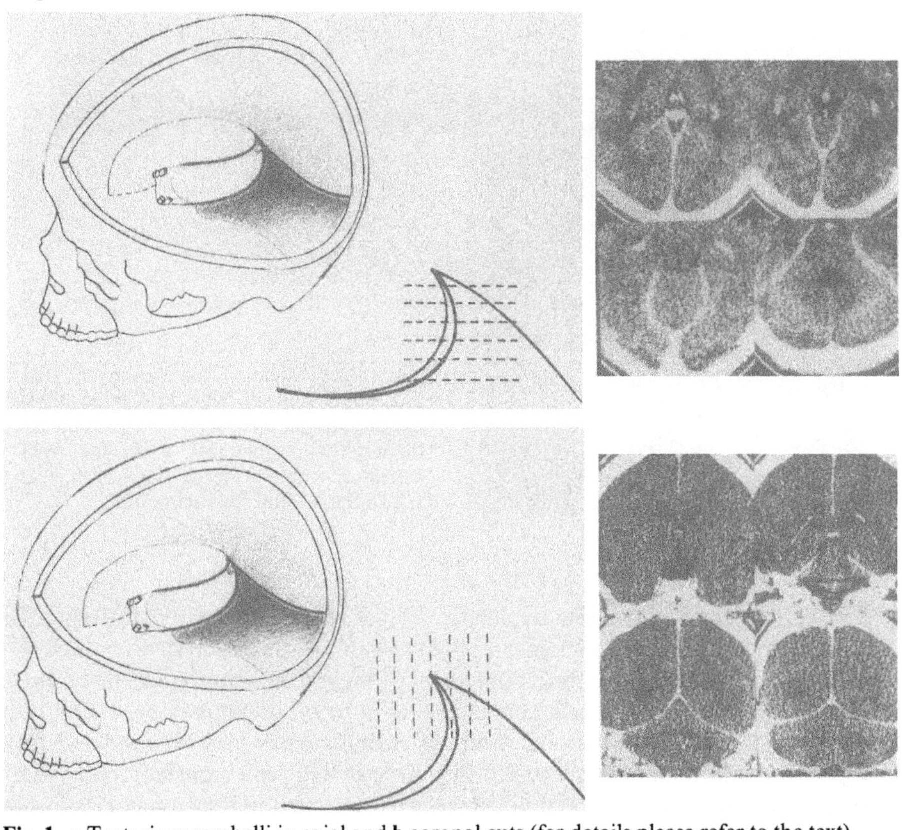

a

b

Fig. 1. **a** Tentorium cerebelli in axial and **b** coronal cuts (for details please refer to the text)

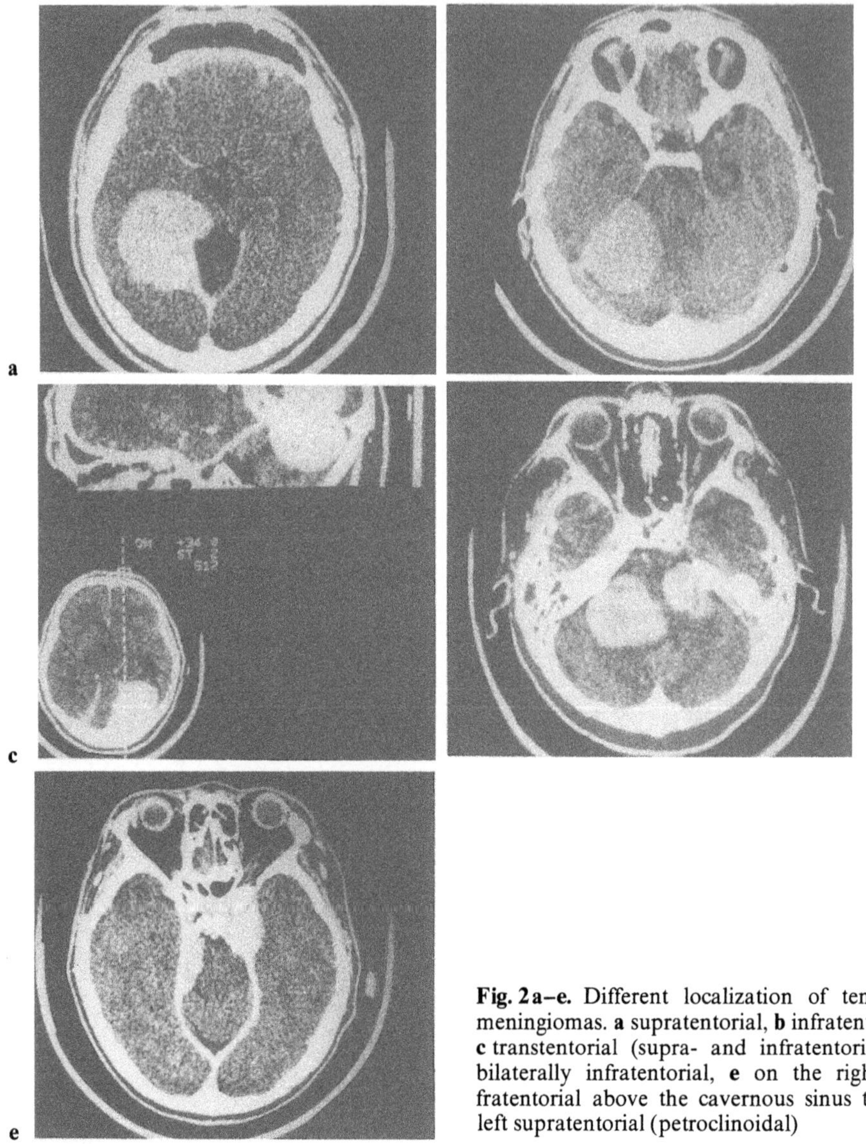

Fig. 2a–e. Different localization of tentorial meningiomas. **a** supratentorial, **b** infratentorial, **c** transtentorial (supra- and infratentorial), **d** bilaterally infratentorial, **e** on the right infratentorial above the cavernous sinus to the left supratentorial (petroclinoidal)

The most important primary tumors of the tentorium are meningiomas. This term summarizes all meningiomas of the median and posterior fossa with close relation to the tentorium cerebelli. Only part of these meningiomas originate directly from the tentorium, whereas meningiomas of different origin may penetrate during their growth into the tentorium. Tentorial meningiomas may be restricted to the supra- and infratentorial region. But they may as well grow transtentorially with or without relation to the tentorial notch. In rare cases, tentorial meningiomas may extend from one side to the other (Fig. 2).

Another rare localization of meningiomas with close relationship to the tentorial notch is the free falx margin of the inferior sagittal sinus of the great vein of Galen, i.e. the highest point of the tentorial roof (Fig. 3).

Modern high resolution computed tomography with the possibility of sagittal and coronal reformations allow for exact definition of site and extent of tentorium-connected meningiomas; thus, constituting a prerequisite of the correct decision on what therapeutic measures to take. Angiography is especially important in evaluating the origin of meningiomas of this region.

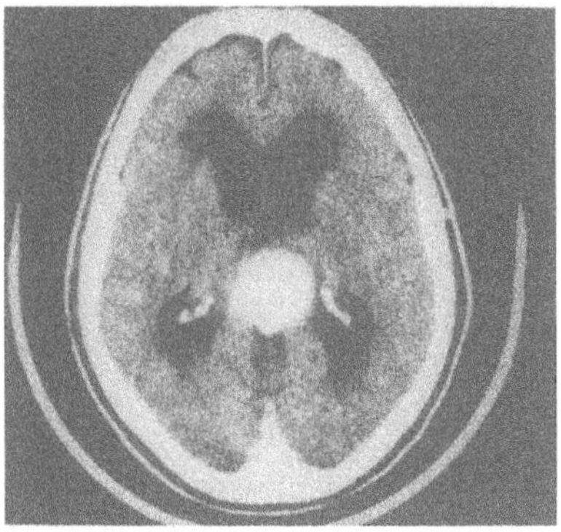

Fig. 3. Supratentorial meningioma at the tentorial roof parting from the inferior margin of the falx cerebri with close relationship to the tentorial notch

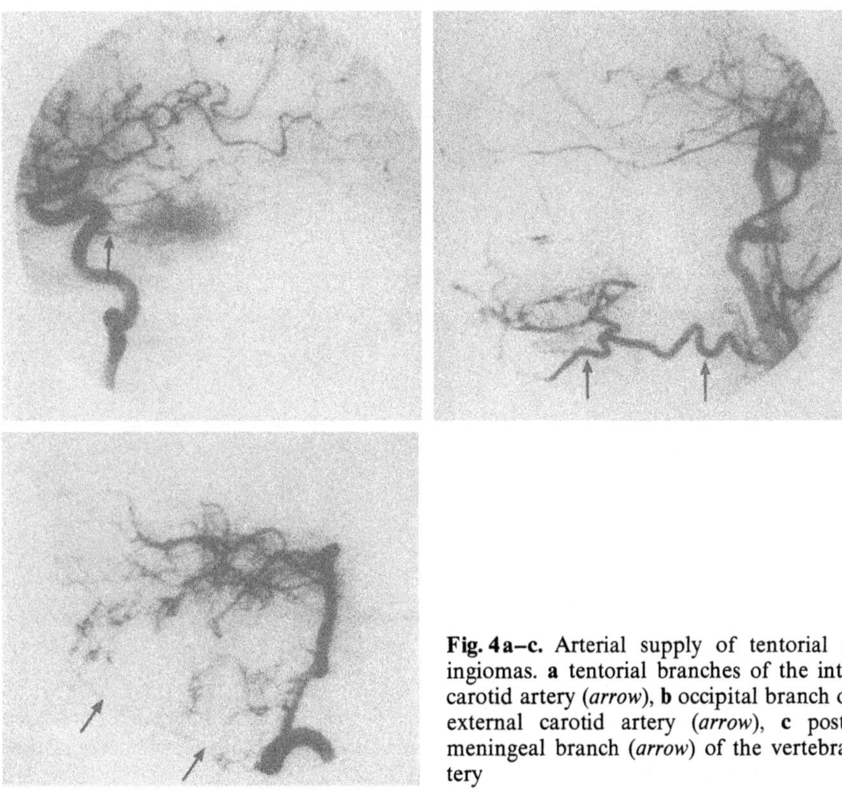

a b c

Fig. 4 a–c. Arterial supply of tentorial meningiomas. **a** tentorial branches of the internal carotid artery (*arrow*), **b** occipital branch of the external carotid artery (*arrow*), **c** posterior meningeal branch (*arrow*) of the vertebral artery

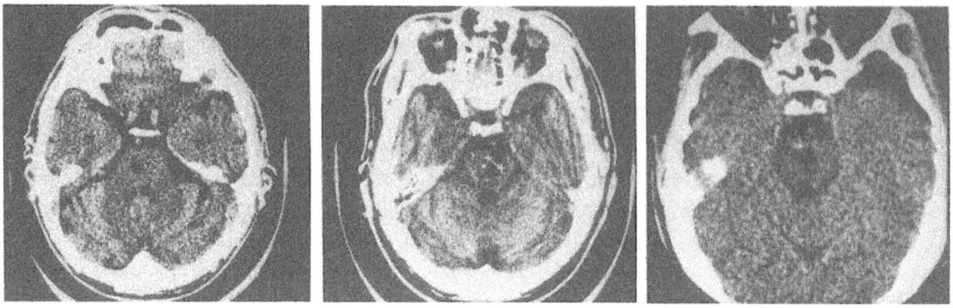

a b c

Fig. 5a–c. Brain stem infarction of different sizes: **a** paramedian pons lesion with a diameter of more than 10 mm, **b** considerably large infarction defect nearly half as large as the pons, **c** fresh hemorrhage pons infarction

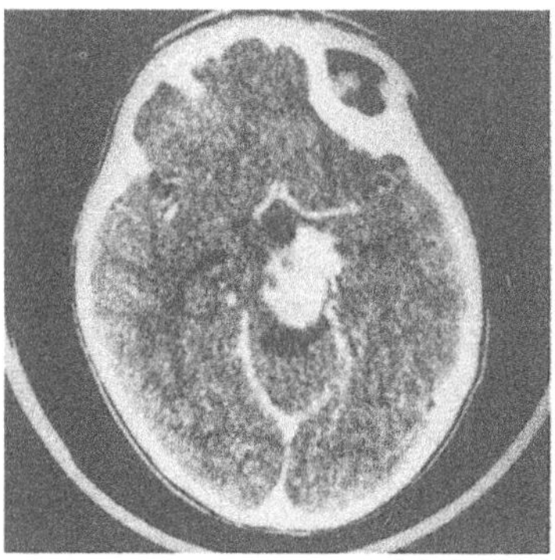

Fig. 6. Polycystic astrocytoma of a three-year-old child. The tumor has grown through the tentorial notch

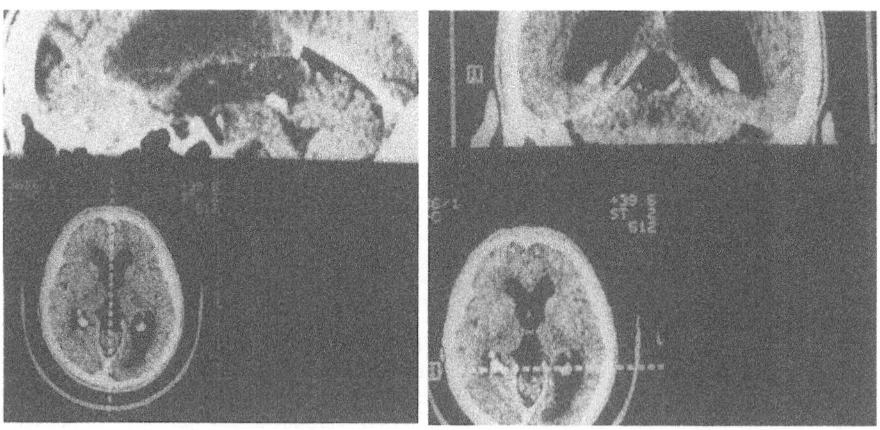

Fig. 7. Cystic supra- and infratentorial tumors of the quadrigeminal region with close relationship to the tentorial notch

Today it is absolutely necessary to investigate the vascular supply of each meningioma by means of selective and superselective angiography, last but not least, to decide on possible interventional proceedings before operation.

DSA renders a relatively quick and precise angiographic demonstration of tentorial meningiomas.

The most important arterial branches feeding meningiomas of the posterior fossa are the tentorial branches of the internal carotid artery and the branches of the external carotid artery, especially the occipital artery, whereas vertebral angiography of both sides can nearly always be negative (Fig. 4).

The second part of my presentation deals with some aspects of primary brain stem lesions. Today, high-resolution tomography is able to demonstrate lesions with a diameter of less than a few millimeters. Part of these lesions are ischemic brain stem lesions. It is often difficult to find a corresponding angiographic correlate, thus, differential diagnosis may also suggest a brain stem tumor.

The next patients show brain stem infarctions of different sizes (Fig. 5).

Large lesions with clinical progress can be reliably diagnosed by means of biopsy. The following brain stem tumor of a 3-year-old child is a polycystic astrocytoma (Fig. 6). The tumor has grown through the tentorial notch. The angiogram only demonstrated signs of displacement, but no tumor-specific vascularisation.

We still have another group of disease to be described: Here you will see a cystic tumor above the quadrigeminal region closely related to tentorial roof. Galenic vein, tentorial sinus and pineal body. Aqueduct is narrow. This process, as well, is growing through the tentorial notch. Coronal reconstructions demonstrate the supratentorial and infratentorial sections (Fig. 7).

When summarizing these points we have come to the conclusion that high-resolution computed tomography still remains an especially sensitive method of diagnosing brain stem tumors as long as we perform this examination more patiently and continue with this method until we have gained more experience with MRI.

Local Cerebral Blood Flow Measurements in the Deep Seated Brain Structures

K.-D. Lerch, N. Nemati, E. Kohmura, K. Holl, and M. Samii, Hannover/FRG

With the recent advancements of computed tomography (CT) and Magnetic Resonance Imaging System (MRI), it is now possible to have a precise anatomical information in and around the brain stem. In cases of ischemic processes involving the brain stem, information about the anatomical changes are not sufficient in the management of patients, but also information about the hemodynamics – cerebral blood flow (CBF) – is inevitable as in surface region cases. It had been impossible to measure CBF in the deep seated brain structures by the conventional stationary head detector system using ^{133}Xe, which cannot provide tomographic information.

The newly developed Single-Photon-Emission-Computed Tomography (SPECT) can give us tomographic CBF information, but its spatial resolution is not sufficient to measure CBF in the deep seated structures. Although Positron-Emission Tomography (PET) can provide us not only with information about CBF but also about metabolism, which is highly important and interesting, its clinical utility is still rather limited because of the high costs and the need of a cyclotron.

Since 1978, another tomographic CBF method, which uses computed tomography with stable Xenon-enhancement, has been developed (Xenon-CT) [2, 4, 6]. Recent advancements of computed tomography and the software systems have now made it possible to measure CBF with a high spatial resolution and to reduce the Xe-concentration to 33%, which is below the anesthetic concentration.

Method

The system is composed of a GE 9800 CT, a Xenon supplying and monitoring machine and a special software package to calculate CBF. The precise theoretical statements can be seen from the literature [3, 8, 9].

During the study the patient lays on the CT-table with a closely fitted mask. Using a scout view we choose a slice on which the brain stem is well to be seen and the artefacts are minimal (Fig. 1). Three parallel slices can be examined maximally in one study, using an incremental table moving system. Afterwards two baseline scans (80 kV, 240 mA, 4 sec) are performed in each chosen slice, while the patient still breathes room air. Then a 33% Xenon-oxygen mixture is inhalated through the mask. During the xenon inhalation six dynamic enhanced scans are performed in each slice, according to the predetermined time schedule. The xenon inhalation lasts only about five minutes. Endtidal xenon and CO_2 concentrations are continuously monitored. Blood pressure is also registrated manually before and after the xenon inhalation. Both CBF and partition coefficient are calculated in each CT voxel

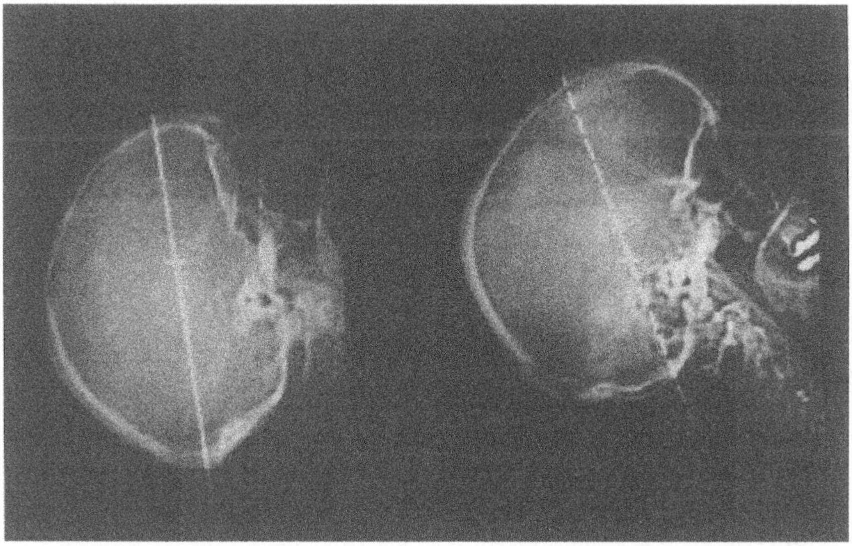

Fig. 1. Typical scout views of a usual slice (*left*) and a special slice (*right*) to evaluate CBF in the deep seated brain structures

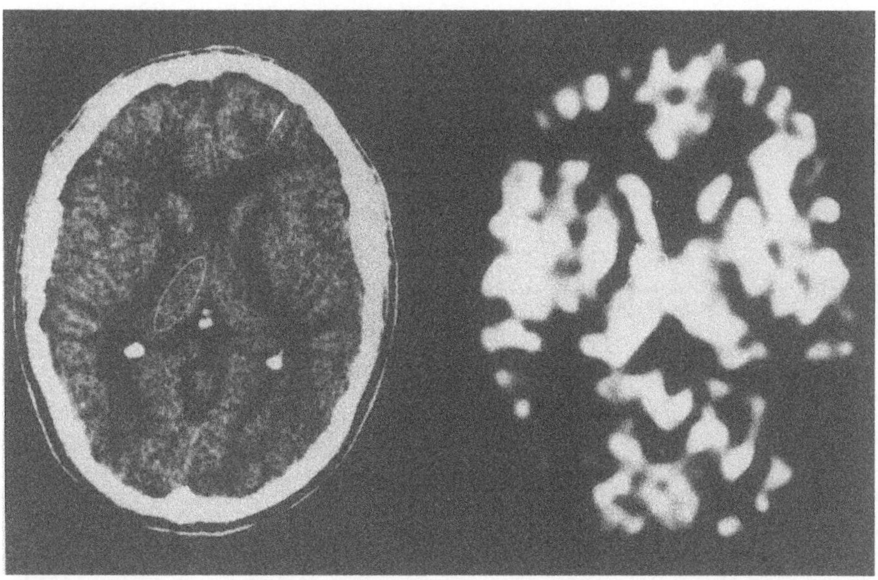

Fig. 2. A measurement of CBF in a R.O.I. in the right thalamus. As the R.O.I. in the CT picture (*left*) is transferred into the corresponding area in the flow map (*right*), absolute CBF data can be obtained with an exact anatomy. (In this case local CBF in the right thalamus is 110 ml/100 g/min)

(0,78 × 0,78 × 5 mm), solving a mono-compartimental Kety equation by using a weighted least square fit routine. The flow data are displayed as a flow map after smoothing the data to reduce the pixel-to-pixel variation. The spatial resolution is 4 × 4 × 5 mm. The flow map is evaluated not only by the optical impression, but also by the absolute flow data that can be obtained in a region of interest (ROI) (Fig. 2). The Xenon-CT-method is a significant help in evaluating CBF in the deep seated brain structures because of

1. high spatial resolution
2. possibility to measure CBF with precise anatomical correlation.

Results

The following three studies demonstrate examples of CBF measurements in the deep seated brain structures using Xenon-CT. One patient (Case I) had lacunar infarction, one (Case II) ischemia after subarachnoidal hemorrhage due to aneurysmal rupture, and the third (Case III) was in a vegetative state.

Case I: This 63-year-old female presented with right hemiparesis two years ago. She had recovered almost completely. A doppler ultrasound examination suggested a stenosis of the left internal carotid artery. CT-scan could reveal only mild brain atrophy. A Xenon-CT study was performed (Fig. 3). The flow map showed that she

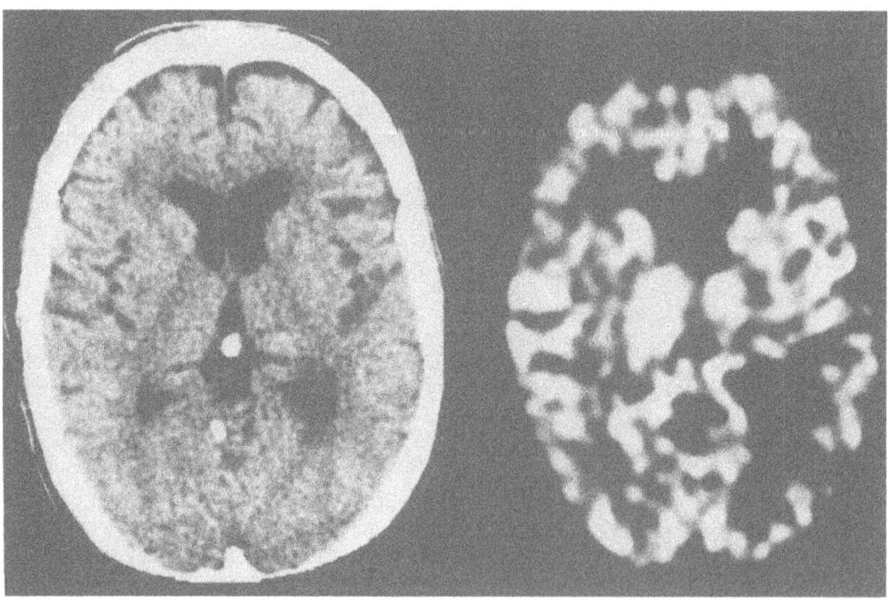

Fig. 3. Xenon-CT study in case I. The baseline CT-scan (*left*) shows only mild brain atrophy. The flow map (*right*) shows almost good flow except small areas in the left posterior thalamus and in the left internal capsule

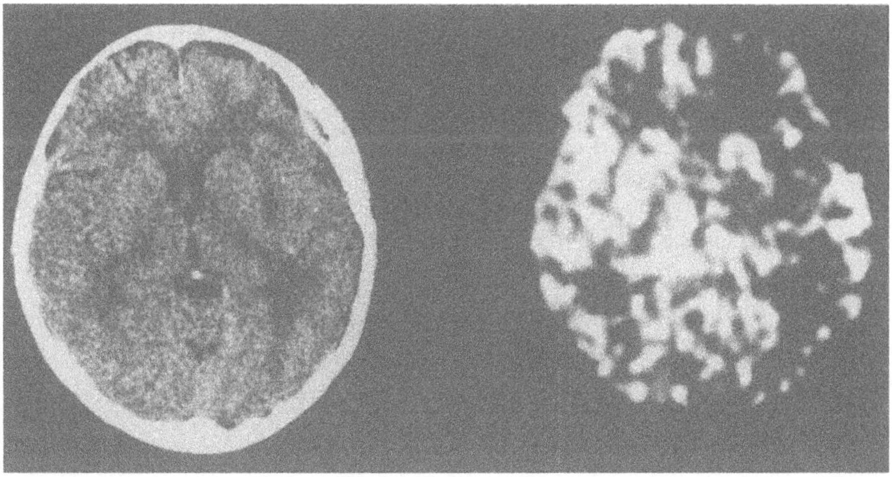

Fig. 4. Xenon-CT study in case II. The baseline CT-scan (*left*) shows only a small low density area in the left external capsule. The flow map (*right*) does not only show the zeroflow area in that region but also a decreased flow in the entire left hemisphere (34 ml/100 g/min). Furthermore it reveals decreased flow (26 ml/100 g/min) in the left internal capsule

has almost good flow except in the regions of the left internal capsule and the left posterior thalamus. This fact correlates well with her clinical history. It was diagnosed as lacunar infarction.

Case II: This 40-year-old female was admitted to our department on the same day of her subarachnoidal hemorrhage (SAH), due to rupture of a left internal carotid artery aneurysm. She was operated on the following day. Eight days after the operation she presented with a right hemiparesis, that deteriorated to a hemiplegia three days later. Figure 4 depicts the Xenon-CT study on the 11th postoperative day. The CT-scan showed only a small low density area in the left external capsule, that could not explain her clinical findings. On the contrary, the flow map demonstrated reduced CBF in the entire left hemisphere. The left external capsule had almost zero flow, which corresponded well to the CT. Moreover, it revealed a reduced flow area in the left internal capsule. The clinical course thereafter improved and she had only minimal weakness of the right hand at discharge. Follow-up Xenon-CT studies showed also normalisation of CBF except in the region of the left external capsule.

Case III: This 58-year-old female had been in a vegetative state for 10 months. The CT-scan showed severe brain atrophy and a hypodensity area in the left cerebellar hemisphere. The flow map (Fig. 5) proved diffusely reduced flow throughout the cerebral cortex. Figure 6 shows the same slice of a volunteer with normal clinical findings. In comparison with Figs. 5 and 6, the CBF at the floor of the 4th ventricle is reduced in case III. As CBF is usually coupled with metabolism, we can correlate reduced CBF with reduced activity in that area.

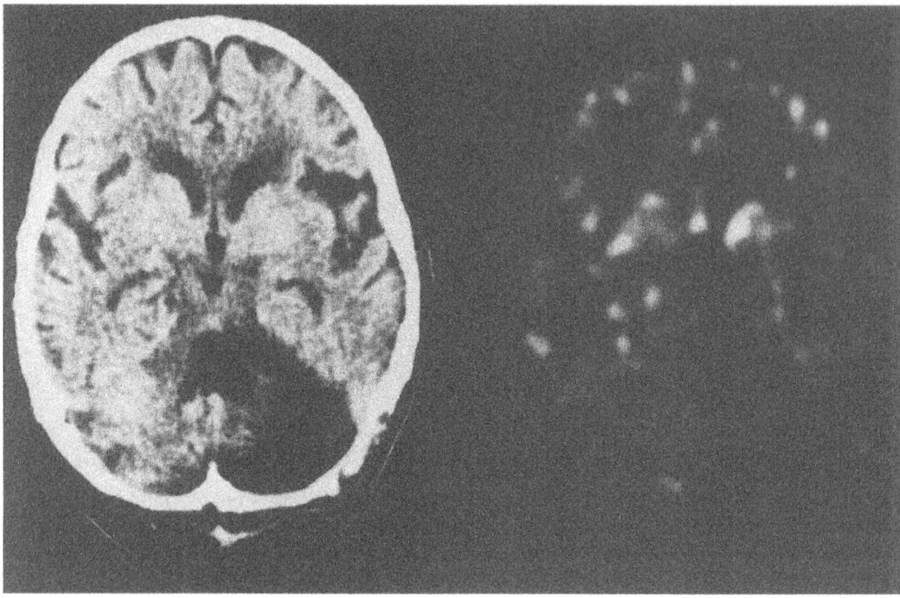

Fig. 5. Xenon-CT study in case III

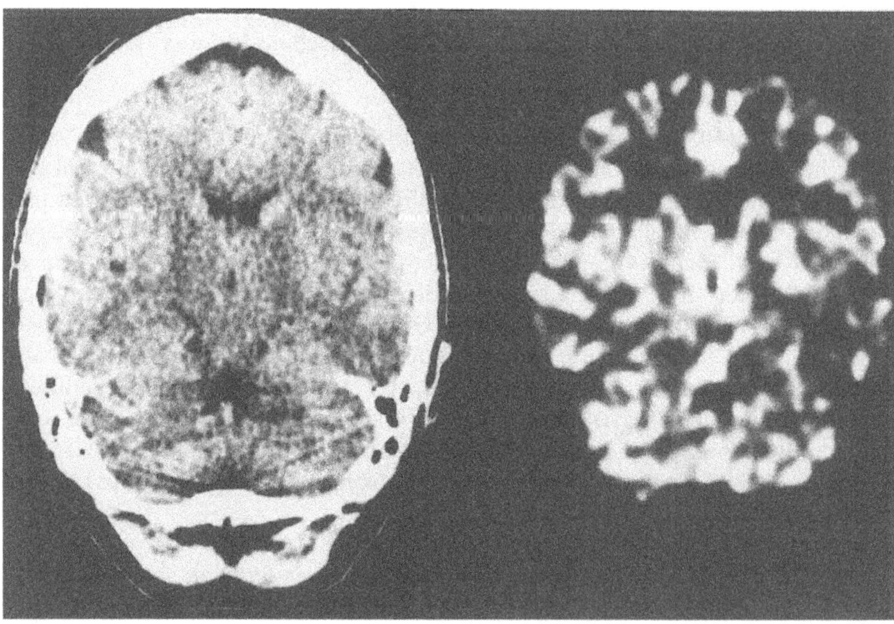

Fig. 6. Xenon-CT study of a volunteer with normal clinical findings, using the same slice as in case III

Discussion

Xenon-CT enables us to measure CBF routinely in the deep seated brain structures, but the problems of this method have also to be mentioned:

1. Relatively high radiation dose (15–20 rads/slice) [8]
2. Need for precise head positioning
3. Side effects of Xenon inhalation
4. Possibility of data errors

To examine CBF, especially in and around the brain stem, it is sometimes very difficult to select the concerned slice. Artefacts due to the petrous bone are the most limiting factors. It is also very important to keep the head position during the study, thus uncomfortable positions must be avoided. The xenon gas has an anesthetic effect in a high concentration [1, 3, 5]. In case of inhalation of 33% xenon for five minutes, there have been no serious side effects [7, 9]. The commonest reactions to xenon inhalations are euphoria and paresthesia, which disappear briefly after the cessation of xenon inhalation. The overall error to calculate CBF using this system is estimated to be about 11% in 0,5 cm × 0,5 cm R.O.I. [9]. By improving the signal-to-noise ratio it could be reduced.

Conclusion

Using the Xenon-CT method we can now measure CBF changes in the deep seated brain structures. The information can be very useful in the management of patients because it provides more pathophysiologic data.

Acknowledgement: We are very thankful to the radiologic technicians for their cooperative work and to Mrs. R. Nitsche and Miss H. Töllner for their secretarial efforts relating to this manuscript.

References

1. Cullen SC, Gross EG (1951) The anesthetic properties of xenon in animals and human beings with additional observations of krypton. Science 113:580–582
2. Drayer BP, Wolfson SK Jr, Reinmuth OM, Dujovny M, Boehnke M, Cook EE (1978) Xenon enhanced CT for analysis of cerebral integrity, perfusion and blood flow. Stroke 9:123–130
3. Gur D, Wolfson SK Jr, Yonas H, Good WF, Shabason L, Latchow RE, Miller DM, Cook EE (1982) Progress in cerebrovascular disease: Local cerebral blood flow by xenon enhanced CT. Stroke 13:750–758
4. Kelcz F, Hilal SK, Hartwell P, Soseph PM (1978) Computed tomographic measurement of the xenon brain-blood partition coefficient and implication for regional cerebral blood flow: a preliminary report. Radiology 127:385–392
5. Lawrence JH, Loomis WF, Tobias CA, Turpin FH (1946) Preliminary observations on the narcotic effect of xenon with a review of values for solubilities of gases in water and oils. Physiol 105:197–204

6. Meyer JS, Hayman LA, Sakai F, Yamamoto M, Nakajima S, Armstrong D (1979) High resolution three dimensional measurement of localized cerebral blood flow by CT scanning and stable xenon clearance. Trans Am Neurol Assoc 104:85–89
7. Yonas H, Grundy B, Gur D, Shabason L, Wolfson SK Jr, Cook E (1981) Side effects of xenon inhalation. J Comput Assist Tomogr 5:591–592
8. Yonas H, Good WF, Gur D, Wolfson SK Jr, Latchaw RE, Good BC, Leanza R, Miller SL (1984) Mapping cerebral blood flow by xenon-enhanced computed tomography: clinical experience. Radiology 152:435–442
9. Yonas H, Wolfson SK Jr, Gur D, Latchaw RE, Good WF, Leanza R, Jackson DL, Jannetta PJ, Reinmuth OM (1984) Clinical experience with the use of xenon-enhanced CT blood flow mapping in cerebral vascular disease. Stroke 15:443–450

Remote Metabolic Disturbances in Lesions of Brain Stem and Diencephalon – A PET-Study

W.-D. Heiss, G. Pawlik, K. Herholz, B. Szelies, C. Beil, R. Wagner, and K. Wienhard, Köln/FRG

Functional hypometabolism in morphologically intact projection areas distant from the site of a typical cerebral infarct is a common finding in positron emission tomography (PET) of ischemic stroke (Kuhl et al. 1980; Baron et al. 1981; Heiss et al. 1983; Martin and Raichle 1983; Kushner et al. 1984). The extent of remote metabolic deactivation is dependent mainly on the location of an infarct, but also the size and the severity of the ischemic damage modulates the degree of hypometabolism in areas of the central nervous system connected to the affected structure. The thalamus as the most important relay station in the brain modulates and coordinates almost all other cerebral functions; its projections reach nearly all areas of the telencephalon sparing only a few. From previous experience with lesions in other brain centers it might be expected that rather small destructions in the diencephalon and in the nearby brain stem depress function and consequently metabolism in various distant related areas. The present study was designed to investigate the pattern of metabolic depression consequent to thalamic infarction.

Methods

The study of glucose metabolism with PET of FDG (Reivich et al. 1979) was performed on eighteen patients with thalamic infarction (6 bilateral, 2 unilateral) all verified by X-ray computed tomography. For the PET the patients were placed on a reclining chair in a room with low ambient light and noise, eyes closed and ears emplugged. Approximately 15 min before starting the examination short catheters were inserted into one cubital vein for injection and into a vein of the contralateral hand that was subsequently kept in a thermostat-controlled water bath at 44° C for blood sampling as described by Phelps et al. (1979). Plasma glucose levels remained stable around 5.4 mmol/l throughout the examination.

(^{18}F)-2-fluoro-2-deoxyglucose (FDG) was synthetized according to a modification of the method of Ido et al. (1978) using a remote-controlled injection of approximately 5 mCi FDG in sterile pyrogen-free normal saline solution (specific activity 10–20 mCi/mg). Seven equally spaced parallel planes, from the canthomeatal line (CML) up to 81 mm above it, were simultaneously scanned with a four-ring positron camera (Scanditronix PC 384) at a spatial resolution of approximately 8 mm FWHM in 11 mm slices (Eriksson et al. 1982). Recordings were taken at consecutive intervals increasing from 1 to 5 min during a period of 40 min, starting at FDG injection. Subsequently, another set of 7 images was obtained with the lowest section positioned at 7 or 20 mm above CML. From these data and the plasma FDG activites from time of injection to end of measurement a VAX 11/780 (DEC) computer calculated metabolic maps (for details of data handling and calculations see Heiss et al. 1984; Wienhard et al. 1985) giving regional cerebral metabolic rates for glucose consumption (rCMRGl) in µmol/100 g/min. On these images an average of 210 standardized regions of interest per case defining infarcted and normal brain structures were outlined employing a user-written interactive program (Herholz et al. 1985).

Results

As observed in ischemic infarction in the territory of the middle cerebral artery (Heiss et al. 1983) metabolic changes were most severe in the infarct proper, also in thalamic lesions. Glucose consumption also was significantly decreased in various remote cortical, subcortical and posterior fossa structures but usually those effects were less localized in thalamic than in extrathalamic infarction. The pattern of distant metabolic depression was dependent on location and extent of bi- or unilateral infarction of thalamic structures.

Bithalamic Infarction

The bilateral ischemic lesions of 6 patients ranged from bilateral lesions afflicting the anterior parts of the medial nuclei and the anterior nuclei to large lesions comprising the mesencephalic tegmentum as well as the anterior and medial thalamic nuclei (Fig. 1). According to the extent of the infarction the neurologic syndrome varied between dementia with marked impairment of short time memory, disorientation, aspontaneity and affective unresponsiveness and a hypersomnic state with bilateral oculomotor paresis. In all the 6 FDG-studies the lowest rCMRGl values were found in the infarcted thalamus (rCMRGl in both thalami between 16 and 28.5 µmol/100 g/min). While in the cases with smaller bilateral lesions the remote glucose hypometabolism was confined to a few brain structures – usually the precentral cortex, the hypocampal structures, cerebellum and to a lower extent the basal ganglia – in the patient with the large mesencephalic and diencephalic lesion (Fig. 1) glucose metabolism was severely depressed in most cortical areas, in the basal ganglia and in the cerebellum.

Unilateral Infarction

Again, the neurologic syndrome and the pattern of hypometabolism were dependent on location and extent of the lesion in the thalamus. The lesions usually reduced glucose metabolism specifically in the ipsilateral parietal and prefrontal cortex, the upper brain stem and the contralateral cerebellum. In other regions observed reductions of glucose consumption were bilateral and related to a more global effect on brain function. In the most often occurring ischemic lesion in the posterior capsula and the nuclei ventralis intermedius and ventroposterior – a lesion which causes a typical Déjerine-Roussy syndrome combined to amnestic disturbances and reduction of intellectual capability – deactivated glucose metabolism was found in

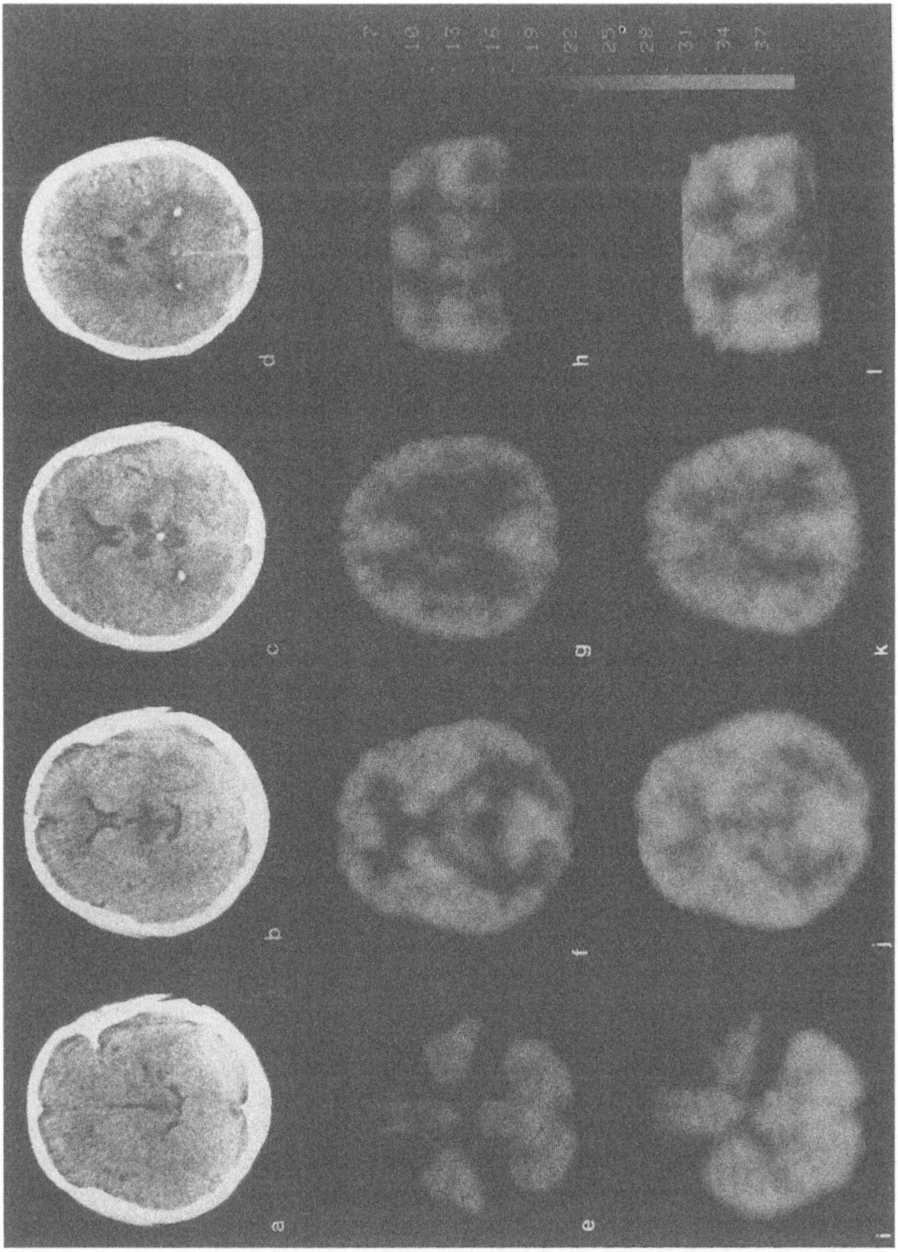

Fig. 1. CT and FDG-PET in a 39-year-old female patient with bilateral thalamic and mesencephalic infarction. **a–d** CT shows bilateral, right larger than left, low-density areas in the paramedian thalami and midbrain, involving the medial nuclei, partially the anterior nuclei, quadrigeminate plate, pretectal area, and the posterior commissura. **e–h** FDG-PET 0, 40 and 60 mm above canthomeatal line and reconstructed in frontal slice through the thalamus 18 days after onset of symptoms shows generalized depression of glucose metabolism (μmol/100 g/min) according to scale on the right by approximately 40% of normal. Within the thalamus reduction by more than 50% (right: 18, left: 20 μmol/100 g/min). **i–l** FDG-PET 10 weeks after onset of symptoms shows increase of glucose metabolism in most brain structures; basal ganglia, temporo-parietooccipital cortex 20%, frontal cortex 30% below normal

many ipsilateral cortical regions and the contralateral cerebellum in addition to the metabolic disturbance in the infarcted thalamus. In smaller lesions, e.g. in the anterior thalamus, the deactivation only affected small areas in the frontal lobe.

Changes of Glucose Metabolism Related to the Course of the Clinical Syndrome

Glucose metabolism in areas remote from the ischemic lesion was in some instances related to the clinical syndrome. This was especially the case in the patient with a large bilateral mesencephalic and diencephalic infarction (Fig. 1): a repeat FDG study two months after the first examination in an improved clinical condition – patient was awake, but drowsy, with severe amnestic disturbance, dysarthria, polyphagia, and bilateral oculomotor paresis – showed a better demarcated decrease of rCMRGl in the thalamus and the midbrain (25 μmol/100 g/min) with specific deactivation of frontal cortical areas. In the other cortical regions and the basal ganglia glucose consumption was improved as was global brain function, especially consciousness and vigilance.

Effect of Thalamic Stimulation on Glucose Metabolism

In one case with a Déjerine-Roussy syndrome severe thalamic pain was treated by implantation of a stimulating electrode. When this patient was studied the first time during pain the lowest metabolic rate was in the infarcted thalamus, some areas showed decreased glucose consumptions in the otherwise normal ipsilateral cortex. A second PET-study under permanent stimulation with short impulse trains relieving the pain revealed markedly decreased glucose metabolism in most brain regions. This result might indicate that thalamic stimulation inhibits transmission through the thalamus by electrophysiological or humoral mechanisms; thereby transmission of pain sensation to the cortex is blocked and metabolism in the cortex is depressed.

Discussion

In addition to the decrease in glucose metabolism in the infarct proper – an information corresponding to the hypodense lesion in CT or the prolonged T_2 values in MRI – FDG-PET yields information on distant brain structures influenced by a localized lesion. In thalamic infarction two types of deactivation might be differentiated: a specific deactivation due to the interruption of projecting fiber systems, and an unspecific, more global glucose hypometabolism caused by impairment of global brain function. As in lesions of other location the specific deactivation is permanent because the input to the dependent region is irreversibly damaged. The unspecific hypometabolism corresponds to the impairment of consciousness or vigilance and to disturbances of integrative brain function; with the improvement of these functional disorders glucose metabolism is globally improved leaving only those areas hypometabolic whose input fibers are morphologically destroyed. This unspecific influence of the thalamus on the brain can also be deducted from the effect of thalamic stimulation on brain metabolism. The results demonstrate that thalamic infarction deactivates specifically function and metabolism in the ipsilateral parietal and prefrontal cortex, the upper brain stem and the contralateral cerebellum; in other cortical regions and the basal ganglia the accompanying glucose hypometabolism is due to a global, unspecific influence on cerebral activity. It is of importance for our understanding of unlocalized neurologic symptoms accompanying focal ischemic lesions to compare these remote effects of thalamic infarcts to those of lesions at other locations (Pawlik et al. 1985): lesions in the frontal cortex have a specific effect on temporopolar and temporooccipital cortex, and the contralateral cerebellum and unspecific influences on various other structures. Temporal and parietal infarcts affect specifically the thalamus and the posterior temporal region; their influence on other regions is less localized and more connected to a bilateral global effect. Striatal lesions exert also unspecific deactivation in many brain structures, but usually do not affect considerably the thalamus: Isolated lesions in the internal capsule deactivate the contralateral cerebellum – as do lesions in the cerebral peduncles – and at higher locations also the thalamus. Lesions in the upper brain stem only cause hypometabolism in the contralateral cerebellum when the corticopontine fibers are disrupted. In some instances of brain stem and cerebellar infarctions a retrograde deactivation in higher centers, e.g. in the thalamus, can be observed, but additional lesions in these structures could not be ruled out.

All these results emphasize once more the highly interactive nature of brain function, where a small localized lesion in a critical region can affect function and metabolism in many distant structures. The observations of the widespread metabolic deactivation help to explain why perceptive, cognitive, emotional and expressive disorders are so common in ischemic stroke, particularly in thalamic infarction.

References

Baron JC, Bousser MG, Comar D, Castaigne P (1981) "Crossed cerebellar diaschisis" in human supratentorial brain infarction. Trans Am Neurol Ass 105:459–461

Eriksson L, Bohm C, Kesselberg M, Blomqvist G, Litton J, Widén L, Bergström M, Ericson K, Greitz T (1982) A four ring camera system for emission tomography of the brain. IEEE Trans Nucl Sci 29:539–543

Heiss WD, Ilsen HW, Wagner R, Pawlik G, Wienhard K (1983) Remote functional depression of glucose metabolism in stroke and its alteration by activating drugs. In: Heiss WD, Phelps ME (eds) Positron emission tomography of the brain. Springer, Berlin Heidelberg New York, pp 162–168

Heiss WD, Pawlik G, Herholz K, Wagner R, Göldner H, Wienhard K (1984) Regional kinetic constants and cerebral metabolic rate for glucose in normal human volunteers determined by dynamic positron emission tomography of (^{18}F)-2-fluoro-2-deoxy-D-glucose. J Cereb Blood Flow Metab 4:212–223

Herholz K, Pawlik G, Wienhard K, Heiss WD (1985) Computer assisted mapping in quantitative analysis of cerebral positron emission tomograms. J Comput Assist Tomogr (in press)

Ido T, Wan CN, Casella V, Fowler JS, Wolf AP, Reivich M, Kuhl DE (1978) Labelled 2-deoxy-D-glucose analogs. ^{18}F-labelled 2-FDG, 2-FDM and ^{14}C-2-FDG. J Label Comp Radiopharm 14:175–183

Kuhl DE, Phelps ME, Howell AP, Metter EJ, Selin C, Winter J (1980) Effects of stroke on local cerebral metabolism and perfusion: Mapping by emission computed tomography of ^{18}FDG and $^{13}NH_3$. Ann Neurol 8:47–60

Kushner M, Alavi A, Reivich M, Dann R, Burke A, Robinson G (1984) Contralateral cerebellar hypometabolism following cerebral insult: A positron emission tomographic study. Ann Neurol 15:425–434

Martin WRW, Raichle ME (1983) Cerebellar blood flow and metabolism in cerebral hemisphere infarction. Ann Neurol 14:168–176

Pawlik G, Heiss WD, Herholz K, Beil C, Szelies B, Wienhard K, Grünewald G (1985) Positron emission tomographic study of variations in brain glucose metabolism related to spontaneous speech. In: Heiss WD (ed) Functional mapping of the brain in vascular disorders. XIII World Congress of Neurology, Hamburg, September 1985. Springer, Berlin Heidelberg New York (in press)

Phelps ME, Huang SC, Hoffman EJ, Selin C, Sokoloff L, Kuhl DE (1979) Tomographic measurement of local cerebral glucose metabolic rate in humans with (F-18)2-fluoro-2-deoxy-D-glucose: validation of method. Ann Neurol 6:371–388

Reivich M, Kuhl D, Wolf A, Greenberg J, Phelps M, Ido T, Casella V, Fowler J, Hoffman E, Alavi A, Som P, Sokoloff L (1979) The (^{18}F)fluorodeoxyglucose method for the measurement of local cerebral glucose utilization in man. Circ Res 44:127–137

Wienhard K, Pawlik G, Herholz K, Wagner R, Heiss WD (1985) Estimation of local cerebral glucose utilization by positron emission tomography of (^{18}F)2-fluoro-2-deoxy-D-glucose: A critical appraisal of optimization procedures. J Cereb Blood Flow Metab 5:115–125

Vascular Malformations Involving the Mesencephalic Region (Review of 26 Personal Cases)

P. Lasjaunias, C. Manelfe, L. Lopez Ibor, K. Ter Brugge, and M. Chiu,
Kremlin Bicêtre/France

Introduction

The diagnosis and treatment involving the mesencephalic region are particularly challenging. Deeply located, and containing vital functions, the mesencephalic region regroups most of the problems that can be encountered in CNS vascular malformations (Smith and Holla 1982):

- "cortical" lesions (temporal lobe–cerebellum)
- "deep" lesions (diencephalon–brain stem)
- dural structures (tentorium–falx) involvement
- cranial nerves (IIIrd, IVth and Vth) involvement.

In addition, every type of neurological disorders can be found as a presenting symptom, or as a complication of the treatment: high cortical functions (speech–memory), endocrine dysfunction, sensorimotor or sensorial deficits, peripheral nervous system impairment.

The vascular malformations involving this area can be discovered either in young patient ("vein of Galen aneurysms"), or in adults (cerebral AVM, tentorial dural AVM). Obviously each type mentioned can be described in every population group, however, each one of them is usually considered as representative of a specific type of problems and solutions. One can easily understand that too sharp a delineation between these types of lesions would be artificial, since multiple overlapping situations can occur, and passage forms be recognized.

General Considerations

Regardless of their locations, cerebral AVMs can produce different types of symptoms: hemorrhages, deficits (transient or permanent), seizures or mass effects.

Vein of Galen aneurysms and mesencephalic AVMs are known to give cardiac failure, epilepsy, neurological deficits, bleeding, hydrocephalus (Hoffman et al. 1982).

Furthermore it is of importance to point out that dural AVMs draining into the cerebral venous system can have *the same* symptomatology. The only, but paramount difference is absence of parenchymatous nidus in dural AVM. On the other hand, the only common feature is the venous outlet of the AVM (dural or parenchymatous).

The clinical analysis of any type of AVM can therefore be related to its venous characteristics (Lasjaunias et al. 1986). The arterial feeders and nidus disposition will be secondarily analyzed to predict the functional risks of the different type of interventions to be discussed (surgical or endovascular since they both act on the arterial side of the lesion); assessment of a symptomatic arterial steal is very difficult, however, it was thought to be absent in our series of patient with CBF studies.

If our observation is coherent, the clinical goal to assign to any treatment can be directed primarily to the venous hemodynamic effects of the AVM:

- *flow through the shunt:* cardiac failure, intrasinusal hyperpressure with CSF malabsorption producing communicating hydrocephalus, papilledema and visual atrophy.
- *retrograde congestion into the cerebral vein:* CNS deficits, thrombosis, and bleeding.
- *pressure and venous ectasias induced:* creating by mass effect communicating hydrocephalus, venous aneurysms and bleeding.

Following this schematic presentation, two remarks should be made:

1. The arterial steal of adjacent cerebral supply may create additional symptoms, that can theoretically be corrected with the shunt treatment. However, partial correction of the shunt may correct as well the retrograde venous congestion in healthy territory. Therefore, reversal of symptoms does not necessarily mean arterial steal. The same dramatic clinical improvement is observed in dural AVM draining into the cerebral veins, in which the regression of the symptoms (purely venous) can be obtained after treatment of the dural shunt.
2. The topographic significance of symptoms is exceptionally correlated with the location of the nidus. The retrograde hyperpressure within the draining veins of the AVM may produce symptoms far from the shunt area. The venous dilatation may even absorb the increase of the venous flow and pressure from the AV shunt leading to an absence of symptoms. Simultaneously, the healthy territories drain through collateral pathways with almost no hemodynamic constraints.

However, one type of mechanism will desequilibrate this durable situation and induce complications, the venous occlusion, or insufficiency with or without an increase of the arteriovenous shunt (Laine et al. 1981; Nombela et al. 1984).

This mechanism can be due to:

- anatomical (mechanic) obstacle to dilatation (junction vein of Galen–straight sinus),
- secondary stenosis (Kinking of a dolicho-mega draining vein),
- venous thrombosis (mechanical, hormonal, iatrogenic or idiopathic).

These hemodynamic changes will produce an upstream hyperpressure leading to further ectasia (vein of Galen) or venous rupture with intradural hemorrhage.

In the specific area of the mesencephalon the converging character of the venous system (deep cerebral vein and basal vein) into the vein of Galen is relatively unfavorable for alternate venous route to absorb or bypass an increase flow coming from a deep AVM (Fig. 1). The normal venous outlet is the straight sinus.

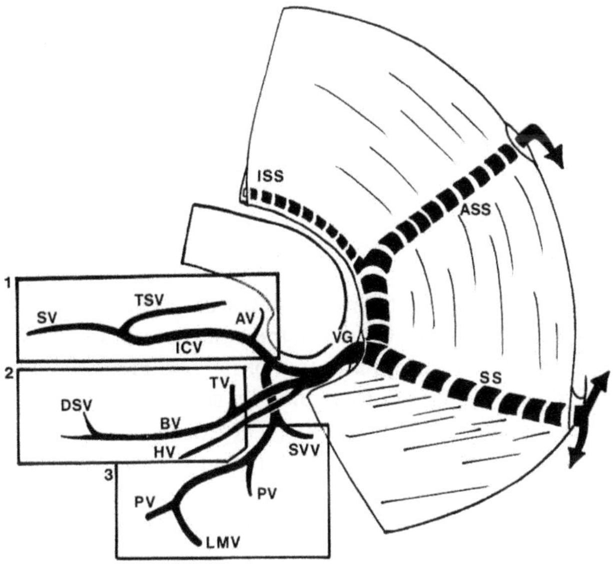

Fig. 1. Schematic representation of the mesencephalic confluence and its changes when draining AVM

		Venous channels	Remarks in cases of AVM
	ISS	Inferior sagittal sinus	Rarely involved
	SS	Straight sinus	Atresic or thrombosed in "VofG aneuryms"
	ASS	Accessory straight sinus	Persistent in case of V of G aneurysms
	VG	Vein of Galen	Constant venous channel
1	ICV	Internal cerebral vein	Drainage of telencephalic AVMs extending at least to the corpus callosum
	AV	Atrial vein	
	TSV	Thalamostriate vein	
	SV	Septal vein	
2	BV	Basal vein	Drainage of diencephalic lesions, deep temporal (T5-T4-Hyppocampus) and some fronto orbital AVMs
	TV	Thalamic vein	
	DSV	Deep sylvian vein	
	HV	Hippocampal vein	
3	SVV	Superior vermian vein	Drainage of brain stem, cerebellum and tentorial AVMs
	PV	Precentral vein	
	LMV	Latero mesencephalic vein	
	PV	Petrous vein	

When there is a thrombosed straight sinus, two systems can be recruited:

- *infratentorially:* the latero mesencephalic and superior vermian veins opening either into the petrous vein or the torcular, or caudally into the spinal cord venous system;
- *supratentorially:* the deep sylvian vein and the cavernous sinus via the basal vein of Rosenthal.

In rare anatomic situations, the mesencephalic venous system uses the persistent embryonic accessory straight sinus; it courses within the falx, opens into the longitudinal sinus close to the occipital fontanelle and corresponds to the most commonly observed venous drainage of the vein of Galen malformations (Dobbelaere et al. 1979).

Material and Method

Since the last 5 years one of us (P. L.) has been involved in the diagnostic and treatment planning of 80 intracranial AVMs. 50% were dural, the others cerebral.

26 AVM cases were located in the mesencephalic area or in its immediate vicinity. Cortical AVMs extending deeply to the ventricle margin, corpus callosum and even temporal lobe have been excluded from this series. They rise different therapeutic problems or challenges, although they partially drain into the deep venous system.

Table 1 summarizes the types of lesion we have reviewed. Few comments must complete this presentation of our material.

9 of the 26 cases of our series have not received any treatment, although almost all of them presented with major symptoms (Table 2):

Table 1. Location and treatment chosen

	Number	Radiation therapy	Surgery	Embolization	No treatment
Posterior fossa AVM (brain stem and cerebellum)	8	–	2	3 (10 procedures)	3
Diencephalic AVM (hypothalamus, thalamus ...)	8	1	1	3 (6 procedures)	3
Tentorial AVM with mesencephalic venous drainage	5	–	–	4 (8 procedures)	1
Vein of Galen ectasia	5	–	2	1 (1 procedure)	2
Total	26	1	5	11 (25 procedures)	9

Table 2. Dominant symptoms

	Posterior fossa (8 cases)	Diencephalic (8 cases)	Tentorial (5 cases)	Vein of Galen (5 cases)	Total (26 cases)
Hemorrhages	5	6	3	1	15 (58%)
CNS deficit	3	7	3	1	14 (54%)
PNS deficit	2	–	1	–	3 (11%)

- In 3 of them venous abnormalities were demonstrated (Valavanis et al. 1983): two were diencephalic and one was a complete thrombosis (or absence) of the venous sinuses of the middle cranial fossa leading to an exclusive venous drainage via the vein of Galen and its ectasia.
- 2 others were incidental discoveries during the pretherapeutic angiographic protocol of maxillofacial AVMs.
- The remaining 4 cases were thought to be resistant to any treatment: they were seen at the beginning of this series, and they would be considered for embolization today. They are followed by the neurologic department.

Among our 26 cases, only three were asymptomatic, two already mentioned, the third was associated with ruptured aneurysms located far from the AVM. In the 23 remaining cases more than half of them had bleedings (some twice), or presented a neurologic deficit.

The embolization performed (25 procedures in 11 patients) have been indicated and performed mainly in Bicêtre (with L. L.) or in Toulouse (with C. M.) or in Toronto (with K. T. and M. C.).

Results and Discussion

The technique of embolization has always been the same for the same type of patients or location using different type of materials (PVA in two cases, IBCA in the others). The results are indicated in Table 3.

2 deaths are reported in this series: a 35-year-old male with a cerebellar and mesencephalic AVM which had bled twice, during the second session of embolization by rupture of the malformation and fatal hemorrhage. This case had been previously considered as non-surgical.

The second case was a 3-day-old baby (2.3 kg) presenting with a vein of Galen malformation with major cardiac failure, multiple cardiac arrests occurred during surgery leading to myocardic infarction and death. This case was considered as non-embolizable due to the multiple small feeders.

Concerning the other patients which received some types of treatments a few further comments should be made. Following 4 surgical attempts, 3 cures were ob-

Table 3. Results of treatment (6 months to 5 years follow-up)

Results / Treatment	N°	In process	"Anatomic" cure	Significantly improved	Mild improvement or no change	Impaired complication	Recurrent bleeding
Embolization	11	–	3	5	2	1 death	–
Surgery	5	–	3	–	1	1 death	–
Radiation	1	1	–	–	–	–	–
No treatment	9	–	–	–	9	–	–
Total	26	1	6	5	12	2	0

tained, whereas the same result could be noticed after 11 embolizations. None – but one – of the cases embolized was considered as surgical. In fact the embolization goal to reach was not the complete eradication of the AVM, particularly in the cases with no previous bleeding, but a venous drainage effect. Since we do not know whether a post embolization residue carries the same risks as a post operative one (should a residual corresponding to 25% of the pretherapeutic lesion with 20% or less flow remaining, be treated?) Therein it has to be emphasized that the surgical extirpability of an AVM or its accessibility to embolization depends on the surgeon and the angiographer.

Besides, for the same reason it is difficult to choose which approach should be preferred if a given AVM is both embolizable and surgical.

The angiographic analysis of the lesions involving the mesencephalic area must provide answers to the questions of the clinicians, as well as the informations required by every therapeutic team (surgical, endovascular if they are available) for the technical decisions.

As mentioned above, the feeders and the nidus may be far from the symptomatic area since the venous drainage is most likely responsible for the clinical signs.

The adjacent territories and their venous drainage, the dural surrounding, the circle of Willis have to be studied carefully. The dominant vertebral, both internal carotid arteries, both middle meningeal, ascending pharyngeal and occipital arteries (depending on the variant) should be studied selectively.

From our experience there is *no indication of an intravenous injection,* which *never* gives the necessary informations that both a neurosurgeon and a therapeutic angiographer require for therapeutic strategy.

The femoral approach, selective injections, magnification, subtraction (digital or conventional) associated with functional tests (transient occlusions, compressions, drug injections), represent the best present modality of the pretherapeutic evaluation.

The pediatric population requires the use of small catheters (3; 3.7; or 4 F) which usually give enough flow to allow a satisfactory study of the AVM. In our experience high rate injections are not necessary to properly image an AVM; 3.5 or 4 cc/per second for the total of 10 cc is enough in these pediatric cases (5 cc for a total of 12 in adults).

The filming program that we use is also very simple: 1 film per second during 5 seconds, then 1 film in the 7th, 9th and 12th second. We never had to use 2 films per second in any of our AVM studies. The future developments of digital imaging will even solve this type of problem when the matrix (1024 × 1024) will have routinely a similar definition as conventional films.

Besides the angiographic study our feeling is that some other studies should be carried out to appreciate the precise location of the AVM with regard to the eloquent areas of the brain and the effects of the AVM on the surrounding structures: CT, MRI, flow study with speech stimulation, neuropsychological tests for hemispheric dominance.

Even with these examinations multiple morphological insufficiency can be already found. As pointed out by G. Yaşargil (personal comments) even if an angiographic procedure is of best possible quality the feeders imaged may still be different (usually inferior) from those found at surgery. Three reasons related to the vascular architecture of the AVM may explain this problem:

a) intralesional steal phenomenon, a compartment will never be seen entirely,
b) one compartment is of a cavernous type and its flow is so slow compared to the adjacent one that neither it nor its feeder will be seen,
c) previous hemorrhage transiently compromises the visibility of part of the lesion, by modifying its hemodynamics.

Nevertheless several technical achievements have made intracerebral navigation safer (Kerber 1976; Pevsner 1977; Berenstein 1981; Debrun et al. 1982; Vinuela et al. 1984; Picard et al. 1984). In 1984, we have developed* a calibrated leak balloon device through a 4 F introducer sheath to be used in the pediatric population, particularly in vein of Galen malformations therefore allowing preservation of the femoral artery in newborn or infants (Fig. 2).

All these cases need further follow-up, but there is evidence from experiences of similar treatment of AVM in other locations that proper delivery *within* the nidus gives a stable occlusion. Some lesions remain that could not have been seen entirely at the time of embolization (quiescent) and may secondarily reveal and develop. Only late angiographic control can confirm the consistency of the result obtained. However, we should emphasize that so far none of the cases of the present series has rebled.

Conclusion

Our feeling is that more attention should be paid to the anatomic variation and hemodynamics of the veins draining both the lesion, and the normal brain.

Accurate pretherapeutic evaluation should be done to allow every therapeutic team to answer its specific technical questions.

The decision for treatment should be multidisciplinary (with each time every fully trained team available).

Endovascular procedures do represent a serious therapeutic chance, particularly in the AVM in general and that location in particular. Actually our results are still below their real possibilities and need follow-up. But the low rate of morbidity and mortality and the recent technical improvements are very encouraging.

---

* This research program was realized (P. L.; K. T. and M. C.) in the Playfair Institute (B. Tatton director), Toronto, Western Hospital, Canada

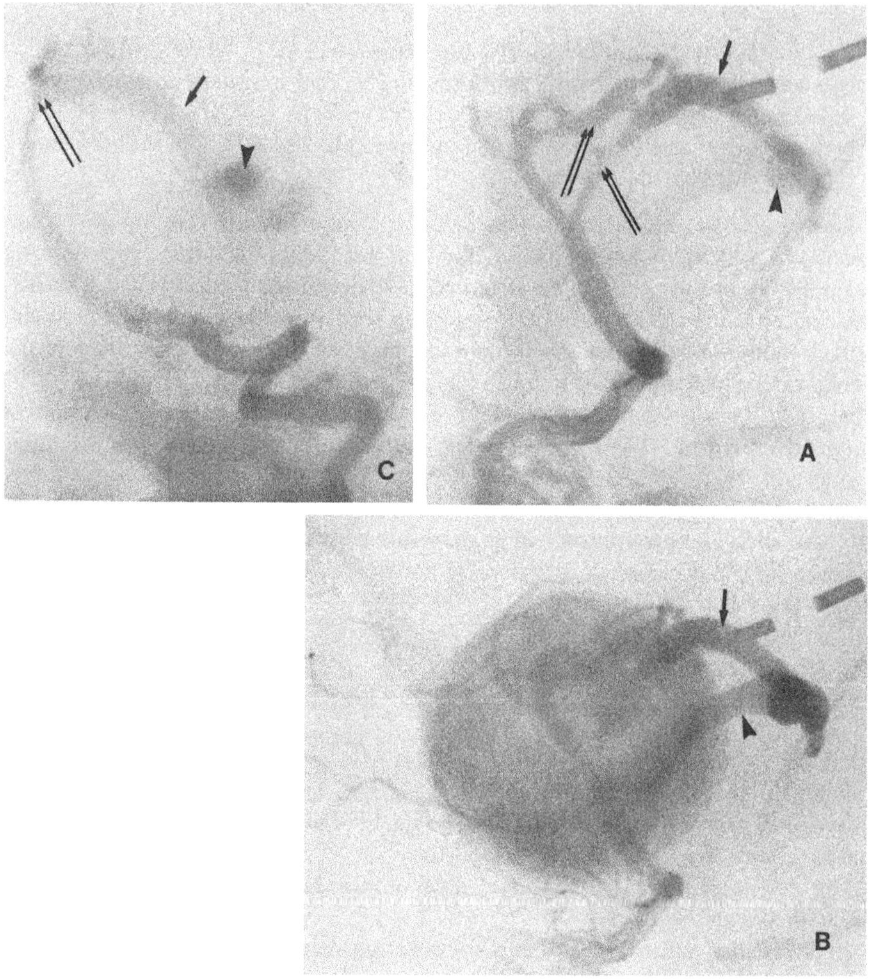

Fig. 2 A–G. *Vein of Galen Aneurysm:* A 6-month-old (6 kg) male infant with hydrocephalia but satisfactory development and normal cardiac function presented with a high flow AVM of the choroïd plexus of the right lateral ventricle, draining via the thalamostriate vein (*arrow*) and the medial cerebral vein (*arrow-head*) into a dilated vein of Galen. A ventriculo peritoneal shunt had already been performed to stabilize the hydrocephalia. At the time of admission the right femoral artery pulse could not be felt following previous arteriographies done somewhere else.

The lesion was considered non-surgical (Dr. Hoffman – Sick Children Hospital – Toronto). The therapeutic angiography thought to be technically feasible was chosen and achieved via the

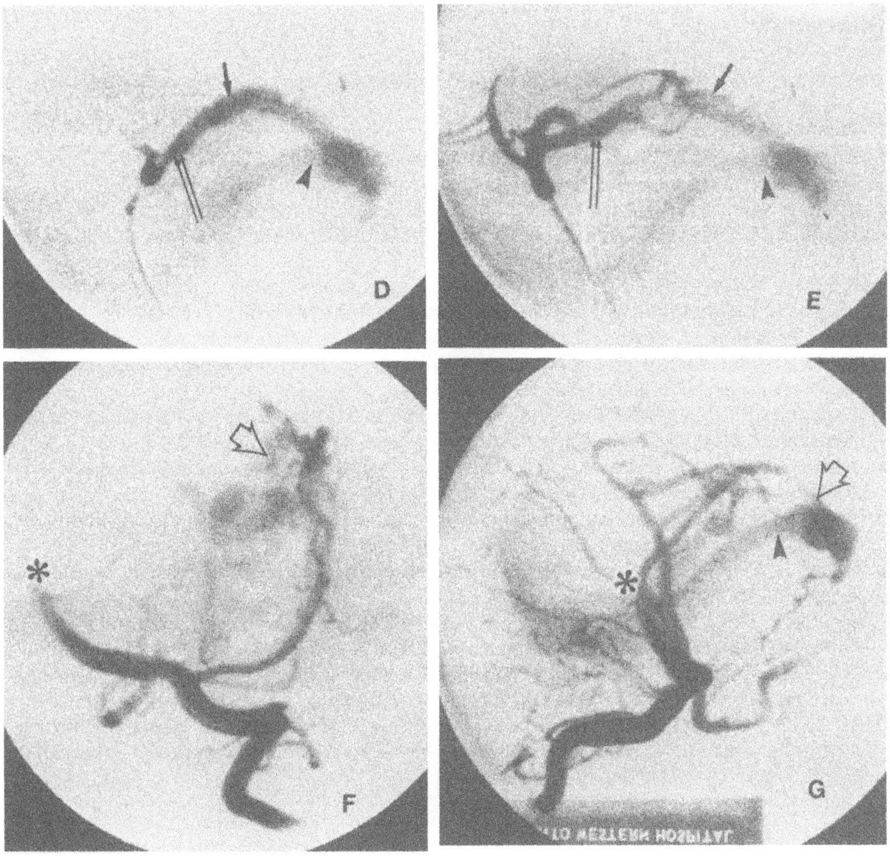

left side with the 4 F sheath. 1 h 20 after the arterial puncture, the two feeders of the right AVM (*double arrows*) identified on the previous angiogram were, selectively, catheterized and embolized with IBCA. On the control angiogram, another small AVM was found at the level of the left foramen of Monro (*open arrow*), however, the flow was so reduced in the vein of Galen that it was decided to stop the procedure. The left femoral pulse was present at the end of the procedure; systematic heparin therapy was used for 24 h to ensure the distal pulses to be satisfactorily palpated. Five days following the embolization the baby was discharged from the hospital. The intracranial bruit could not be perceived any more.
In this particular case the follow-up is still too short, although the technical and immediate clinical results achieved are extremely encouraging; the left femoral approach is still usable for complementary embolization if needed. Vertebral angiogram before embolization **A** and **B** early and later phase in lateral projection. **C** Frontal projection. **D, E** Selective catheterization of the arterial feeders. **F, G** Vertebral control after embolization

References

1. Berenstein A (1981) Technique of catheterization and embolization of lenticulostriate arteries. J Neurosurg 54:783–789
2. Debrun G, Vinuela F, Fox AJ, Kan S (1982) Two different calibrated leak balloons: experimental work and application in humans. AJNR 3:407–414
3. Dobbelaere P, Jomin M, Clarisse J, Laine E (1979) Interêt pronostique de l'étude du drainage veineux des anévrysmes arterioveineux cerebraux. Neurochirurgie 25:178–184
4. Hoffman H, Chuang S, Hendrick B, Humphreys R (1982) Aneurysms of the vein of Galen. J Neurosurg 57:316–322
5. Kerber CW (1976) Catheter with a calibrated leak: A new system for super selective angiography and occlusive catheter therapy. Radiology 120:547–550
6. Laine E, Jomin M, Clarisse J (1981) Les malformations arterioveineuses cérébrales profondes: classification topographique, possibilités et résultats thérapeutiques à propos de 46 observations. Neurochirurgie 27:147–160
7. Lasjaunias P, Chiu M, Ter Brugge K, Tolia A, Hurth M, Berenstein M (1986) Spontaneous intracranial dural AVM: neurological manifestations. J Neurosurg 64, 724–730
8. Nombela L, Vinuela F, Fox AJ, Pelz DM (1984) Occlusion of the venous drainage of deep AVMs of the brain. AJNR 5:670
9. Pevsner PH (1977) Micro balloon catheter for superselective angiography and therapeutic occlusion. Am J Roentgenol 128:225–230
10. Picard L, Moret J, Lepoire J (1984) Traitement endovasculaire des angiomes arterio-veineux intracérébraux. J Neuroradiol 11:9–28
11. Smith RR, Holla PS (1982) Arteriovenous malformations of the posterior cranial fossa. In: Smith RR, Haerer A, Russell WF (eds) Raven Press, New York, pp 65–76
12. Valavanis A, Wellaver J, Yaşargil MG (1983) The radiological diagnosis of cerebral venous angioma: cerebral angiography and computed tomography. Neuroradiology 24:193–199
13. Vinuela F, Fox AJ, Debrun G, Pelz DM (1984) Pre embolization superselective angiography: role in the treatment of brain AVM with isobutyl 2 cyanoacrylate. AJNR 5:765–770

New Embolization Method for Inoperable AVMs and Vascular Rich Tumors – Chemical Embolization Using Conjugated Estrogen

J. SUZUKI, Y. NAGAMINE, and A. TAKAHASHI, Sendai/Japan

A chemical embolization method using conjugated estrogen has been introduced as a new method for the treatment of inoperable arteriovenous malformations (including dural AVMs, and AVMs in central nervous system) and vascular rich tumors such as meningiomas. Forty-seven cases were treated, good results were achieved, and no remarkable complications were encountered.

Materials and Methods

According to the location of lesions, the cases can be divided into two groups, the external carotid lesions and the lesions of the central nervous system. Forty cases of external carotid lesions (including 11 cases of dural AVMs in the area of the cavernous sinus and/or in the posterior fossa, 20 cases of meningiomas and 9 cases of other diseases such as venous angioma of the scalp) were treated, as well as 7 cases of AVMs in the central nervous system (including 6 cases of intracranial AVMs and one case of spinal AVM).

To treat the external carotid lesions, a Teflon or polyethylene cannula (0.5 mm inner diameter, 1.0 mm outer diameter) was inserted through the common carotid artery, and the tip of the cannula was positioned in the main feeder or just proximal to it. The tube was connected to an infusion pump, and conjugated estrogen (Premarin) dissolved in normal saline was administered continuously. The concentration was varied from 5 to 20 mg/ml, and the dose of estrogen was varied from 30 to 120 mg a day. The duration of infusion ranged from 2 to 24 days (10 days on the average). Only in cases of venous angioma of the scalp was conjugated estrogen injected directly into the cavity by the one shot-injection-method.

For AVMs in the central nervous system, a calibrated leak balloon catheter (Dow-Corning) was introduced into the feeder or the parent artery of the feeder via the transaxillary or transfemoral route, and conjugated estrogen was continuously infused by a pump (100 mg a day) under careful monitoring of neurological signs and angiography.

Results

Forty cases with external carotid lesions are summarized in Table 1. In 11 cases with dural AVM, angiograms showed complete disappearance of the nidus of AVM in 3 cases (cases 3, 4 and 5). Case 5 is shown in Fig. 1. In 6 cases, reduction of the nidus

Table 1. Summary of cases with external carotid lesions

Case	Age	Sex	Location	Dose/duration (mg) (days)	Effect CT-scan	Effect Angiogram	Result
Dural AVM							
1	46	F	Cavernous sinus temporal	480/6		+	Improved
2	34	F	Cavernous sinus posterior fossa temporal	500/5, 400/8		+	Improved
3	43	M	Cavernous sinus	L 1000/12, 740/12, 1070/11 R 960/8		++	Improved
4	10	M	Cavernous sinus	440/15		++	Cured
5	57	M	Cavernous sinus	960/12		++	Cured
6	48	M	Cavernous sinus	1100/11		+	Improved
7	64	F	Cavernous sinus fronto-temporal	L 790/10 R 130/2		+	Improved
8	50	M	Cavernous sinus posterior fossa	900/9, 420/7		±	Improved
9	59	M	Posterior fossa	1025/18		–	Unchanged
10	39	M	Posterior fossa	L 490/7 R 450/5		+	Improved
11	70	M	Posterior fossa	700/10, 1000/12		+	Improved
Meningioma							
12	46	M	Sphenoidal ridge	745/15	–	+	Subtotal resection
13	70	F	Sphenoidal ridge	360/12	+	++	Not operated
14	24	F	Sphenoidal ridge	850/10	+	++	Total resection
15	58	F	Sphenoidal ridge	550/8	++	++	Total resection
16	52	F	Sphenoidal ridge	250/2	–	+	Total resection
17	31	M	Sphenoidal ridge	1100/12	++	++	Total resection
18	50	M	Sphenoidal ridge	650/12	–	–	Partial resection
19	42	M	Middle fossa	700/12	+	+	Not operated
20	31	M	Middle fossa	660/12	++	++	Total resection
21	47	F	Middle fossa	650/12	+	++	Total resection
22	46	M	Convexity	640/24	–	+	Total resection
23	41	M	Convexity	420/6	–	±	Total resection
24	62	F	Convexity	405/6	+	++	Total resection
25	45	F	Convexity	750/7	–	++	Total resection
26	57	M	Convexity	2000/16	±	++	Total resection
27	45	F	Falx	970/10	–	++	Total resection
28	68	F	Falx	L 400/4 R 500/5	–	+	Total resection
29	64	M	Falx	L 1200/12 R 400/4	–	+	Total resection
30	63	M	Tentorial	300/5	–	–	Total resection
31	53	M	Posterior fossa	850/14	–	+	Total resection
Other diseases (Diagnosis)							
32	77	F	Skull metastasis of thyroid cancer	400/10	–	+	Total resection
33	23	F	Angiosarcoma (skull)	L 720/10 R 700/6	+	++	Total resection

Table 1. (continued)

Case	Age	Sex	Location	Dose/duration (mg) (days)	Effect		Result
					CT-scan	Angio-gram	
34	48	F	Aneurysmal bone cyst	900/10	+	+ +	Cured
35	14	M	Nasopharyngeal tumor	1370/22	+	+	Total resection
36	33	M	Traumatic dural AV fistula	500/5		+ +	Cured
37	31	M	Scalp AVM	880/11		+	Improved
38	15	F	Venous angioma (scalp)	500/4	+	+ +	Cured
39	13	M	Venous angioma (scalp)	1100/11	+	+	Cured
40	4	F	Venous angioma (scalp)	200/2	+	+	Improved

L: left, R: right, + +: very effective, +: effective, ±: slightly effective, –: not effective

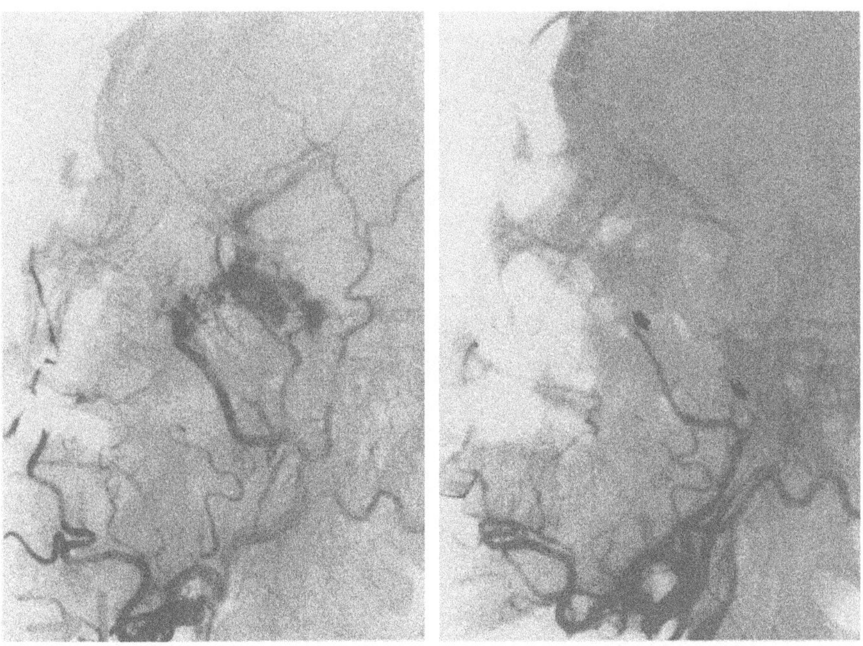

Fig. 1. A 57-year-old man with a dural AVM in the region of the cavernous sinus. Note the dural AVM before chemical embolization (*left*), and its disappearance after treatment (*right*)

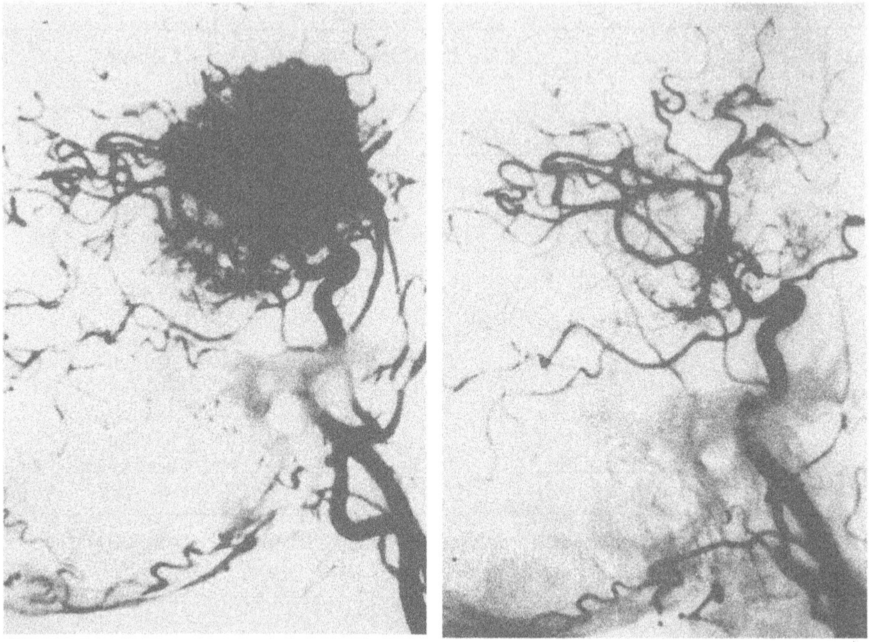

Fig. 2. A 58-year-old woman with meningioma of the right sphenoidal ridge. Before chemical embolization (*left*), a marked tumor stain mainly supplied by the middle meningeal artery was observed. After embolization (*right*), note the disappearance of the tumor stain and the feeders

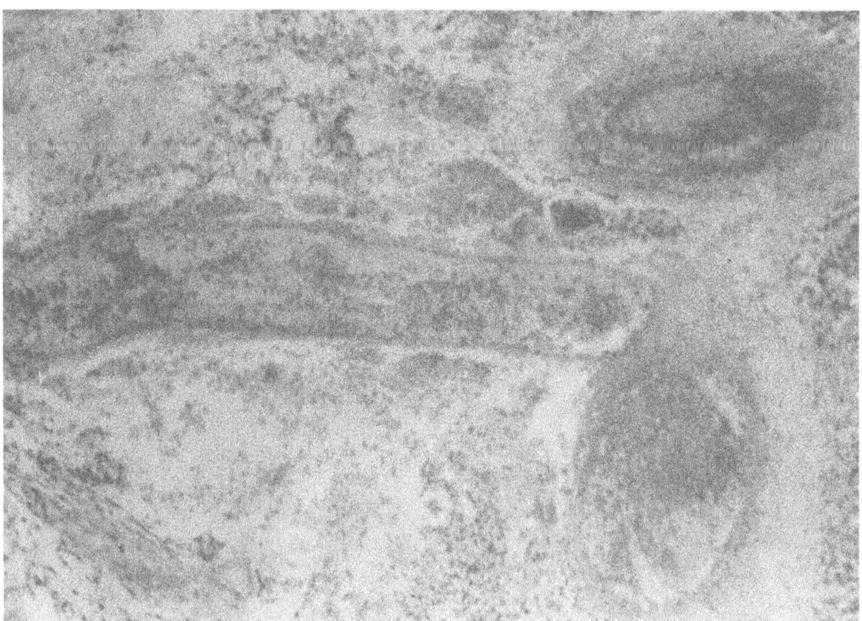

Fig. 3. Histological findings on a meningioma obtained at operation. Note the thrombosis of the tumor vessels. HE stain ×30

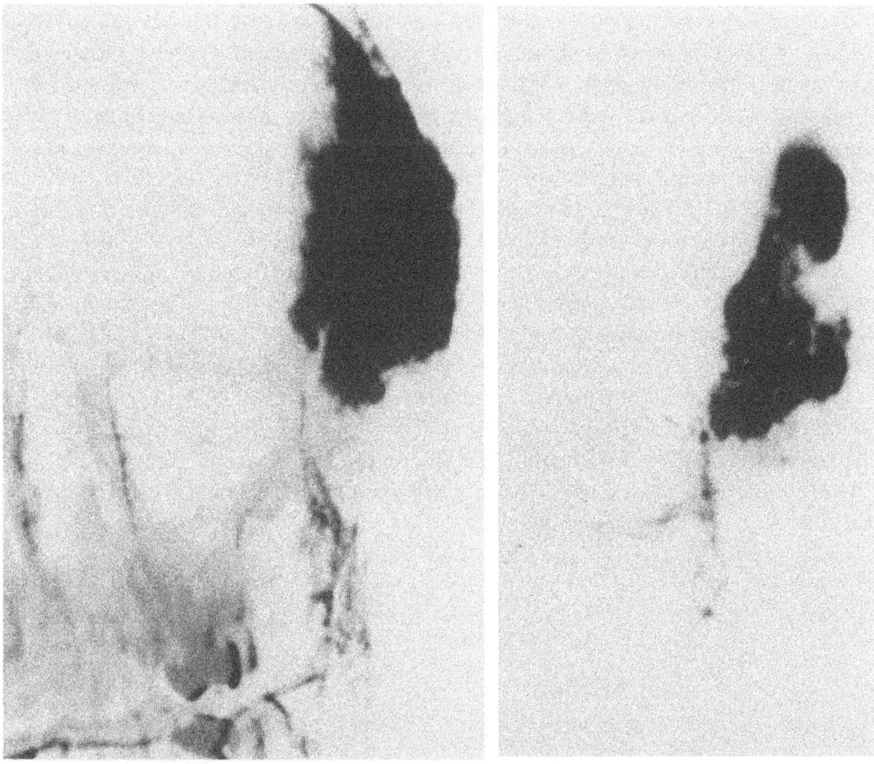

Fig. 4. A 15-year-old girl with a venous angioma of the scalp in the left temporal region. A direct puncture venogram before chemical embolization (*left*) shows a large pooling of venous blood. After embolization (*right*), a marked decrease in the size of the cavity is seen. This cavity disappeared after one month

and/or occlusion of the feeders were noticed with the improvement of symptoms (cases 1, 2, 6, 7, 10 and 11). In 2 cases in the posterior fossa, no good result could be achieved because of too many feeders and collateral circulation (cases 8 and 9). Of the 9 cases out of 11 (81.9%), in which embolization was effective, there was no recurrence of symptoms during follow-up, the longest period of observation being 9 years.

In 20 cases with meningioma, decrease in the enhancement of the computed tomograms (CT) of 8 cases (40%) was observed and disappearance or reduction of the tumor stain on angiograms was obtained in 17 cases (85%). A representative case (case 15) is shown in Fig. 2. Of eighteen cases of meningioma operated upon, 16 cases were totally resected. Surgical treatment of these cases was carried out easily and without blood transfusion as a result of decreased bleeding. Histological examination of the specimen obtained from the operations revealed the thrombosis of the vessels (extending even into the arterioles and venules) (Fig. 3).

In 9 cases of other diseases, reduced enhancement of CT was encountered in 6 cases out of 7 (85.7%), and effective findings on angiograms or venograms were obtained in all cases. A representative case (case 38) is shown in Fig. 4.

Complications in the 40 cases mentioned above were as follows; 17 cases of parotitis, 3 cases of liver dysfunction, and one case each of gynecomastia, facial palsy, trismus and convulsion. Convulsion was induced by accidental injection into the internal carotid artery, after which the procedure was interrupted. Each of these complications cleared up or disappeared following interruption of the procedure. No remarkable complications were observed.

Seven cases with AVM in the central nervous system are summarized in Table 2. Conjugated estrogen (40–850 mg) was infused for 5 hours to 13 days. The nidus of the AVM was totally obliterated in one case (case 42), subtotally obliterated in 3 cases (cases 41, 44 and 47), partially obliterated in one case (case 46), while the procedure was discontinued in 2 cases for some reasons (accidental severance of the catheter and anemia). Cases 42 and 47 are shown in Fig. 5 and Fig. 6, respectively. During embolization all patients sometimes complained of anorexia, nausea or vomiting. Other complications were as follows; 2 cases of transient neurological deficits, 2 cases of liver dysfunction, and one case each of anemia, convulsion and extravasation of estrogen. Each of these complications disappeared with cessation of the infusion.

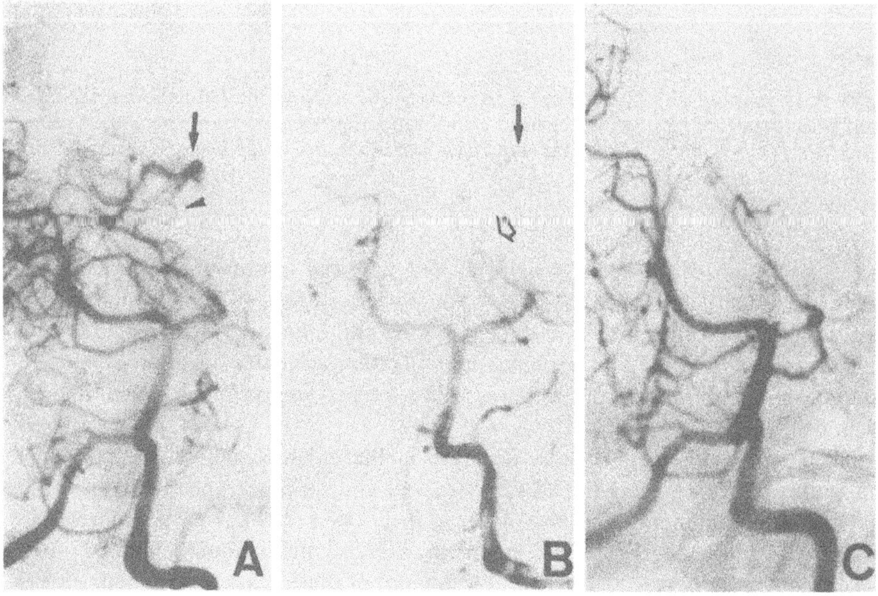

Fig. 5A–C. A 19-year-old male with thalamic AVM. **A** Before chemical embolization (left VAG). Note the small thalamic AVM (*black arrow*) fed by medial and lateral posterior choroidal arteries (*arrow head*). **B** Continuous infusion of estrogen into the left posterior cerebral artery for 5 days resulted in the disappearance of one feeder and diminished size of the nidus (*black arrow*). The *open arrow* indicates the other main feeder. **C** After embolization, note the disappearance of the nidus. In this case, the region of the left posterior cerebral artery was perfused by collateral circulation

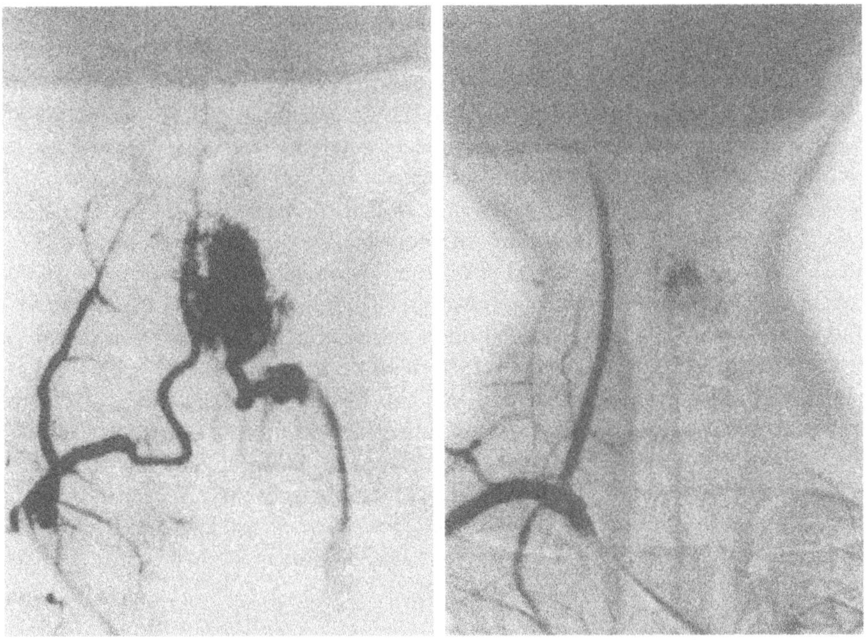

Fig. 6. An 11-year-old boy suffering from severe subarachnoid hemorrhage, in which an angiogram revealed no intracranial lesion. Before embolization (*left*), the nidus of the AVM was situated on the ventral surface of the cervical spinal cord (C_4–C_6) and was fed by the right ascending cervical artery. After 2 unsuccessful attempts at transcatheter embolization (Spongel), chemical embolization was carried out and almost all of the nidus was embolized (*right*)

Table 2. Summary of cases with AVMs in the central nervous system

Case No.	Age	Sex	Location of nidus	No.	Procedure of embolization		Results
					Site of infusion	Dose/duration (mg) (days)	
41	10	F	Rt. cerebellum	1	Rt. PICA	220/ 3	Subtotal obliteration
				2	Rt. SCA	120/ 2	
				3	Rt. AICA	60/ 1	
42	19	M	Rt. thalamus	1	Rt. P_3, P_2, P_1	850/10	Total obliteration
43	19	M	Lt. frontal	1	Lt. M_1	280/ 4	Discontinued[a]
44	30	F	Rt. thalamus	1	Rt. P_3	310/ 3	Subtotal obliteration
				2	Rt. P_1	520/ 6	
45	45	F	Rt. occipital	1	Lt. P_2	560/ 4	Discontinued[a]
46	50	F	Rt. frontal	1	Rt. M_2	20/ 5 hours	Partial obliteration
				2	Rt. M_2	770/ 8	
47	11	M	Spinal cord C_4–C_6	1	ascending cervical a.	440/13	Subtotal obliteration

[a] Total resection

Discussion

For the treatment of AVMs and vascular rich tumors, transcatheter embolization methods using various emboli, such as muscle fragments, Gelfoams, polyvinyl alcohols (Ivalon), silastic spheres and cyanoacrylates have recently been employed. However, some disadvantages such as a tendency towards early recanalization, high risk of embolism of the unwanted lesion and difficulties in occlusion of the nidus itself exist. The chemical embolization method that we recently developed [4], originated from animal experiments made to study the relationship between the etiology of chronic subdural hematoma and estrogen [1, 3]. In those studies, estrogen was found to cause disturbance in circulation of the dura mater. Further study showed that conjugated estrogen induced microcirculatory disturbances [2]. In this report, we presented cases treated successfully with this new embolization method. The results were good and there were no remarkable complications. As opposed to embolization with other emboli, this method appeared to be safer and has many advantages. Since obliteration of the AVM or vascular beds of the tumor may occur at the capillary level, obliteration is more radical and recurrence is reduced. With regard to cases of AVM in the central nervous system, ours is the first report of treatment with chemical embolization.

References

1. Komatsu S (1975) Estrogen as a cause of chronic subdural hematoma. Brain Nerve (Tokyo) 27:645–656
2. Nagamine Y, Komatsu S, Suzuki J (1983) New embolization method using estrogen: effect of estrogen on microcirculation. Surg Neurol 20:269–275
3. Suzuki J, Komatsu S (1977) Estrogen in patients with chronic subdural hematoma. Surg Neurol 8:243–247
4. Suzuki J, Komatsu S (1981) New embolization method using estrogen for dural arteriovenous malformation and meningioma. Surg Neurol 16:438–442

Surgical Management of Specific Lesions: Vascular Lesions, Trauma

Cavernous Angioma in the Brain Stem
Report of Successfully Operated Cases

T. YOSHIMOTO and J. SUZUKI, Sendai/Japan

Although there have been several autopsy studies on cavernous angioma developing at the brain stem, there have been few reports of direct neurosurgical intervention in such cases. None the less, with the widespread use of CT scanning and the advent of NMR-CT in clinical use, it has become possible to make accurate diagnosis of lesions of the brain stem. As a consequence, the possibility of surgical intervention in cases with lesions at this region of the brain – which has previously been thought unsuitable for surgical repair – must be reconsidered. In the present study, we report on our experiences with three cases of cavernous angioma developing in the brain stem, which could be totally and successfully removed.

Case 1

The patient was a 35-year-old man who six months previously had had a transient gait disturbance and sense of bodily instability diagnosed as vertebro-basilar insufficiency at another clinic. In January 1979, however, he experienced nausea, vomiting and numbness of the left side of the tongue. In CT scan on February 1, a high density area and mild contrast enhancement effects indicating a mass lesion were found at the base of the fourth ventricle and slightly left to the midline at the pons. A diagnosis of pontine bleeding was made but the symptoms were mild and his condition was followed as an outpatient. In 1980, he became aware of loss of sensation of the left side of his face, left auditory deficits and slight dysphagia. On March 13, he was admitted to our clinic for detailed examination.

On admission, deficits of cranial nerves 5, 7, 8, 9, 10 and 12 and mild left cerebellar signs were noted. In the subsequent CT scan (Fig. 1), the high density area was seen to have enlarged. No notable findings were obtained from vertebral angiograms.

Operative Findings: Radical surgery was performed on March 18, 1980 under the diagnosis of pontine bleeding. After cauterising the lower ⅔ of a vermis incision, the 4th ventricle was inspected. A protruding 0.7 × 0.7 cm sized process of brownish stain was found on the dorsal pons laterally from the left eminentia medialis (Fig. 2). The border between this tissue and the surrounding healthy tissue was relatively distinct. A small mass with fine blood vessels and including a dark red hematoma, thought to be due to a relatively recent hemorrhage, and containing a small, old and dirty hematoma and a cyst of xanthochromic fluid was removed. Most of the excised tissue was scar tissue, but a 3 × 3 mm abnormal vascular system was discovered in the cyst wall. Histologically, it contained abnormal blood vessels

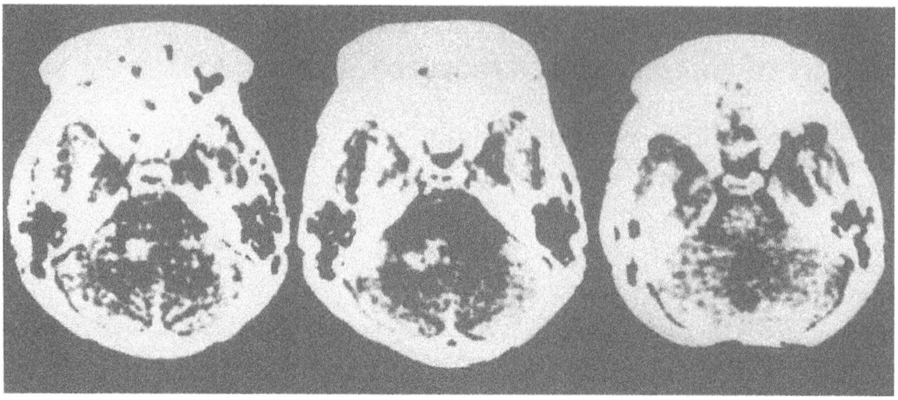

Fig. 1. CT scans of case 1. *Left:* Preoperative CT (February 1, 1979), *Middle:* Preoperative CT (March 3, 1980), *Right:* Postoperative CT (May 16, 1980)

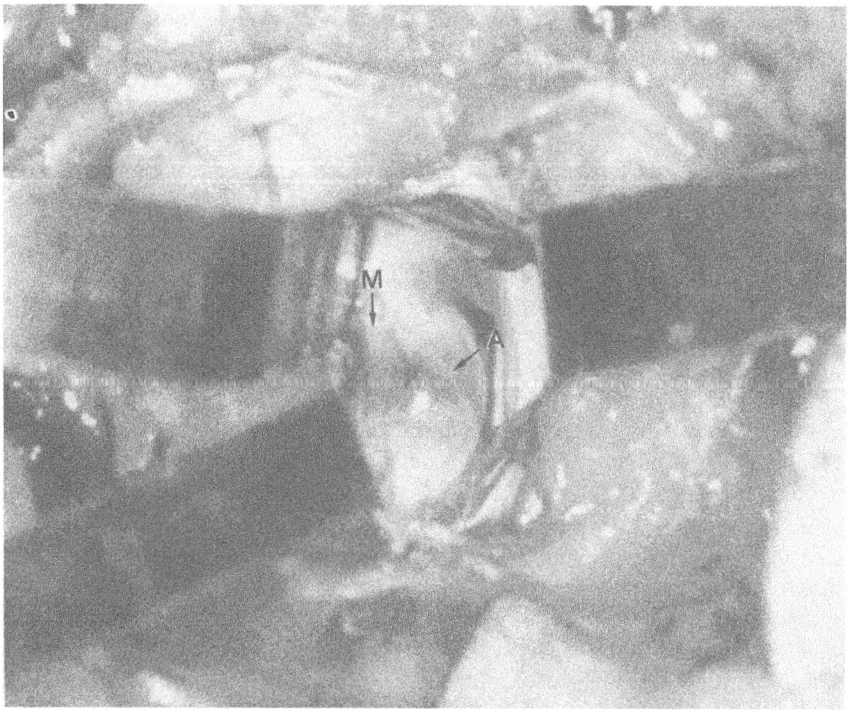

Fig. 2. Operative view of case 1. *A* = Cavernous Angioma, *M* = Midline of the floor of 4th ventricle

with hypertrophied walls, including dilated veins and organized thrombi. These findings are compatible with cavernous angioma.

Postoperative Course: He was discharged one month after surgery. In CT scan taken on May 16, no high density areas were seen and there were no positive enhancement effects. Neurologically, mild deficits of cranial nerves 5, 7, 8 and 9 on the left and mild left-side cerebellar signs have remained, but he has been able to return to a normal life.

Case 2

The patient was a 40-year-old man who had been to our clinic six months earlier complaining of polydipsia, polyuria, genital hypofunction and headache. On admission in April 1980, he was neurologically normal, but sero-biochemical tests showed diabetes insipidus. In craniograms and carotid angiograms, no abnormalities were found, but CT scans revealed an irregular high density area extending from the anterior portion of the third ventricle to the left hypothalamus. Surrounding a portion of the high density area, there was positive contrast enhancement. Under the diagnosis of ectopic pinealoma, he was administered 5000 rads of ^{60}Co and chemotherapy. Two months later the diabetes insipidus had disappeared and he was discharged in good condition. CT scans at that time showed that the high density area had contracted considerably but the enhancement effect was still evident.

Six months later, on January 7, 1982, he experienced a sudden headache and on January 29, he was re-admitted to our hospital without alleviation of the headache. Neurologically, right homonymous hemianopsia, which had not been present previously, was found. CT scans revealed that the high density area had enlarged posteriorly (Fig. 3).

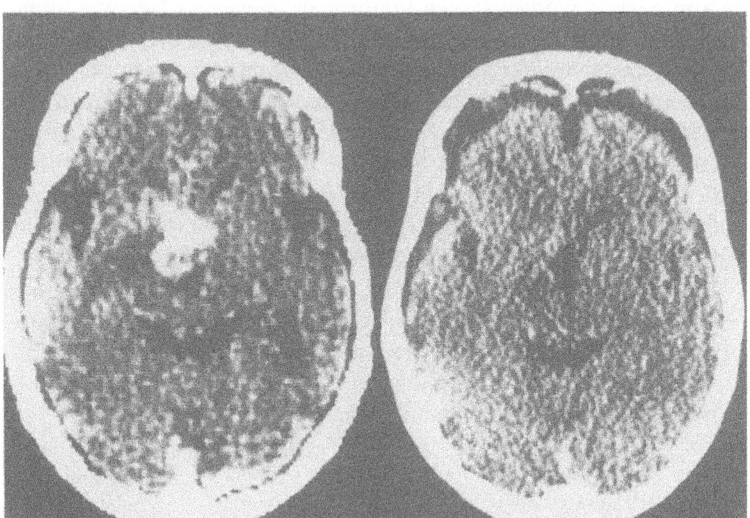

Fig. 3. Enhancment CT scans of case 2. *Left:* Preoperative CT (January 29, 1982), *Right:* Postoperative CT (March 2, 1982)

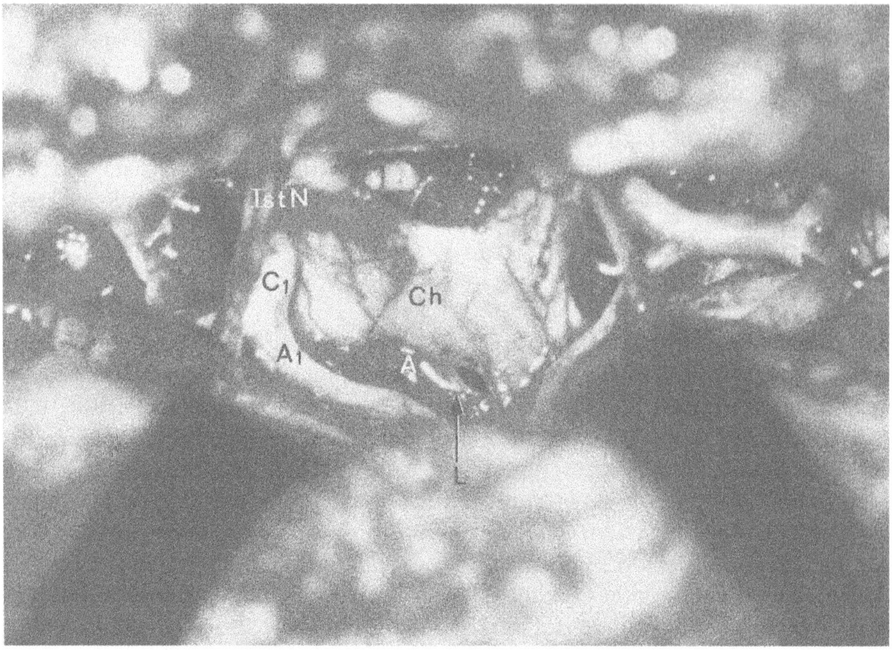

Fig. 4. Operative view of case 2. *A* = Cavernous Angioma, *L* = Lamina Terminalis, *Ch* = Optic Chiasma, C_1 = Carotid Artery, A_1 = Anterior Cerebral Artery, *IstN* = Olfactory Nerve

Operative Findings: Under a diagnosis of tumor of the left wall of the third ventricle, surgery was undertaken on February 2. After bifrontal craniotomy, using an interhemispheric approach, a reddish-brown tumor with uneven surface was found to the left and posterior to the optic chiasma and extending inferiorly (Fig. 4). By dissecting the tumor from surrounding tissue and entering the third ventricle from the lamina terminalis, it was possible to excise the tumor piece by piece which was present from the left of the optic chiasma to the lateral and anterior walls of the third ventricle. The volume of the excised tissue was 2 × 3 × 3 cm and contained various old and new blood clots. Histologically, many blood vessels ranging from large vessels to small capillaries were found. The interstice had scanty neural tissue, with hyalinisation and surrounding, adherent hemosiderin.

Postoperative Course: Diabetes insipidus appeared transiently and the homonymous hemianopsia remained, but otherwise the patient was neurologically well. CT scans obtained one month postoperatively showed disappearance of the high density area and there were no positive enhancement effects.

Case 3

The patient was a 16-year-old boy, who during fencing practice on May 9, 1984, became aware of the instability to place the saber as intended. On the following day, he experienced numbness of the right arm and leg and went to a hospital for exami-

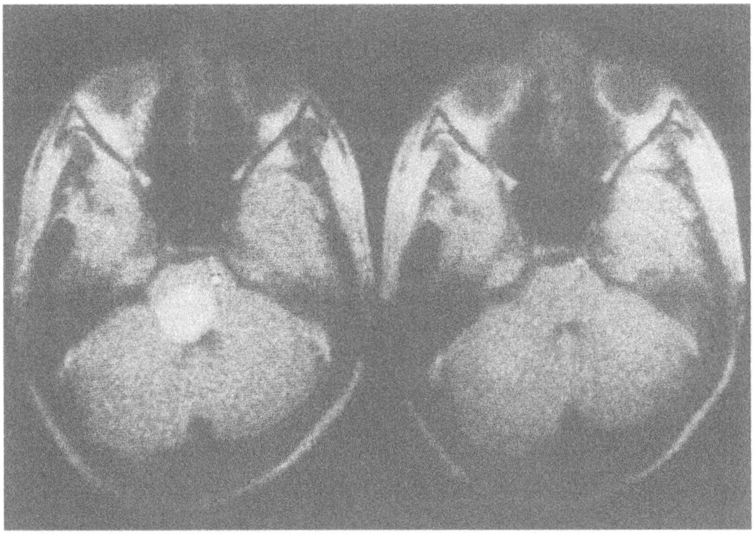

Fig. 5. NMR-CT of case 3. *Left:* Preoperative, *Right:* Postoperative

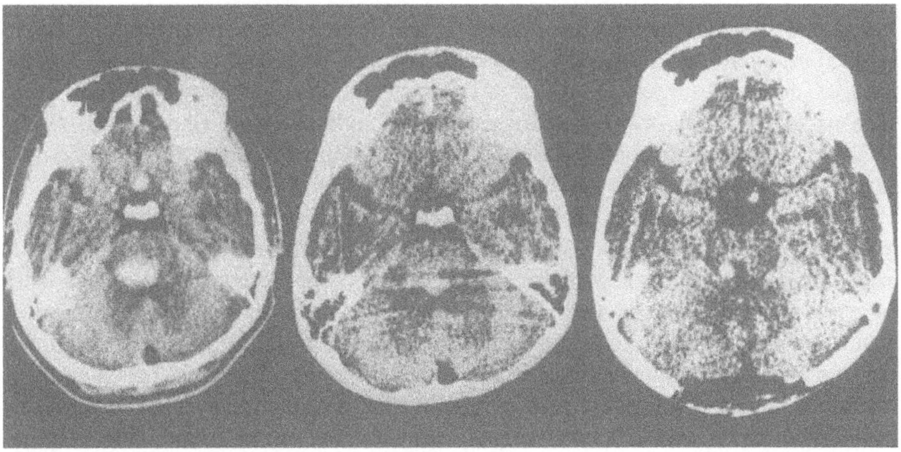

Fig. 6. CT scans of case 3. *Left:* Preoperative CT (May 15, 1984), *Middle:* Preoperative CT (June 7, 1984), *Right:* Postoperative CT (June 30, 1984)

nation. CT scans suggested pontine mass with a high density area at the dorsal pons. On May 22, he was admitted to our clinic. His consciousness was normal but mild sensory and motor deficits of the body including the face, were found. These symptoms gradually improved. NMR-CT, done on May 23, showed a distinct high signal intensity lesion confined to the posterior pons (Fig. 5). It had the appearance of a relatively recent hematoma, rather than that of a tumor or ischemic lesion. Although slight contrast enhancement was evident in CT scans on June 7, the high density area had become smaller (Fig. 6) and no abnormality was evident in angiogram.

Operative Findings: Surgery was undertaken on June 10 under the diagnosis of cavernous angioma of the posterior pons with a portion facing the floor of the 4th ventricle. After making a vermis splitting incision, a 1 × 1 cm yellowish process was seen on the floor of the 4th ventricle slightly left of the midline of the striae medullares. A vertical incision at the site revealed a mass of abnormal blood vessels, and a hematoma of both new and old composition. Peripherally, there was granulation and scar tissue with hemosiderin deposits. The borders of the lesion were relatively distinct and its complete removal together with a vascular mass in the dorsal pons (1 × 1 × 1.5 cm) was successfully achieved. Histologically, most of the tissue was scar tissue, and a portion was abnormal blood vessels containing thrombi. Normal tissue was not evident.

Postoperative Course: Motor and sensory functions did not deteriorate, but an ocular movement deficit similar to one-and-a-half syndrome appeared and slowly disappeared. On the 40th postoperative day, he was discharged and postoperative NMR-CT showed disappearance of the high signal intensity region.

Discussion

Based upon the anatomical knowledge, it has been thought impossible to allow surgical intervention in this region up until recently. Although there have been reports of successful surgery of lesions of the posterior fossa including the brain stem, such as hemangioblastoma and arteriovenous malformation (Chou et al. 1975; Drake 1975), reports of complete excision and histological examination of lesions located within the pons are extremely rare (Terao et al. 1979).

In our first case, over a year of observation elapsed from the identification of the lesion at the pons until radical surgery. This lengthy delay was not only due to the mild nature of the clinical symptoms, but also due to our reluctance to proceed with surgery on the brain stem. In the light of the experience, radical surgery was performed on case 2 and 3, at the time of the identification of the cavernous angioma. Our results suggest that even in cases of brain stem lesions, the tissue surrounding a cavernous angioma will often already have formed reactive scar tissue, so that it is possible for an experienced neurosurgeon to excise the entire lesion while keeping damage to surrounding normal tissue to a minimum.

With regard to diagnosis, in the present series of patients, the most characteristic findings were dynamic changes in the high density areas in follow-up CT scans, findings which were in relatively close agreement with changes in clinical symptoms. NMR-CT was carried out in case 3 only, but was useful in making the diagnosis. In comparison with X-ray CT, it is possible with NMR-CT to make diagnosis of tumor or hematoma, and to obtain an accurate understanding of the anatomic relationships of the cavernous angioma with the brain stem.

Conclusion

Although surgical intervention at the brain stem has previously been considered impossible, among the operative findings of three cases we have found that the lesions were delimited by reactive scar tissue, so that by means of a careful surgical technique severe associated disorders need not appear postoperatively.

It is thought likely that, henceforth, surgical indication in cases with brain stem lesions will greatly increase.

References

1. Chou SN, Erickson DL, Oritz-Suarez HJ (1975) Surgical treatment of vascular lesions in the brain stem. J Neurosurg 42:23–31
2. Drake CG (1975) Surgical removal of arteriovenous malformation from the brain stem and cerebello pontine angle. J Neurosurg 43:661–670
3. Terao H, Hori T, Matsutani M et al (1979) Detection of cryptic vascular malformation by computerized tomography. J Neurosurg 51:546–551

Surgical Management of Deep Seated Angiomas

M. Samii and R. Ramina, Hannover/FRG

Introduction

The surgical treatment of deep seated angiomas, as well as of extensive cortical AVMs remains a challenge [5, 7–9, 17, 20, 22, 23, 26, 29, 37]. Because of the location and size of these lesions, alternative methods of treatment have been proposed [7, 14, 15, 21, 24, 31, 32, 34–36]. In this paper we report on our experience in the treatment of 15 patients presenting deep seated angiomas who were admitted to our clinic between January 1978 and April 1985. All these angiomas were approached directly using microsurgical techniques and bipolar coagulation. In this report we discuss the indications for the operation of these cases and compare the results obtained with the surgical treatment and the alternative methods.

Clinical Material

From January 1978 to April 1985, 15 patients harboring deep seated angiomas were operated on in our clinic. A summary of the clinical presentation and clinical features is presented in Table 1. Twelve patients presented with intracranial bleeding. Ten patients showed in the CT-scan examination an intraventricular bleeding.

Hemiparesis and psychosyndrome were the most frequent neurologic symptoms observed preoperatively. One patient, a 10-year-old boy, was operated on because of intractable headaches. This was the reason why he had not been able to attend school. Another patient, who had an extensive AVM at the brain stem, was operated because of a progressive hemiparesis and cranial nerves palsies. The localization of the lesions and the age of the patients are presented in Table 2.

Table 1. Deep seated AVMs (15 cases)

Clinical presentation		*Clinical symptoms*	
Intracranial bleeding	12	Hemiparesis	9
First bleeding	8	Psychosyndrome	5
Repeated bleeding	4	Steal phenomenon	4
Intractable headaches	1	Headaches	3
Progressive intractable neurological		Cranial nerve palsy	3
disability	2	Seizures	2
		Aphasia	1
		Decreased visual acuity	1

Case Reports

Case 1: Three months before admission to our clinic this 16-year-old girl had one episode of intracerebral bleeding. She remained unconscious for three days. At examination she presented an aphasia and a right-sided hemiparesis. The CT-scan

Table 2. Deep seated AVMs (15 cases)

Localization		*Age*	
Corpus callosum	1	10 to 30 years	8
Thalamus	2	30 to 50 years	6
Lateral ventricle	2	Over 50 years	1
Pineal region	2		
Brain stem	6		
C.P.A.	1		
IV ventricle	1		

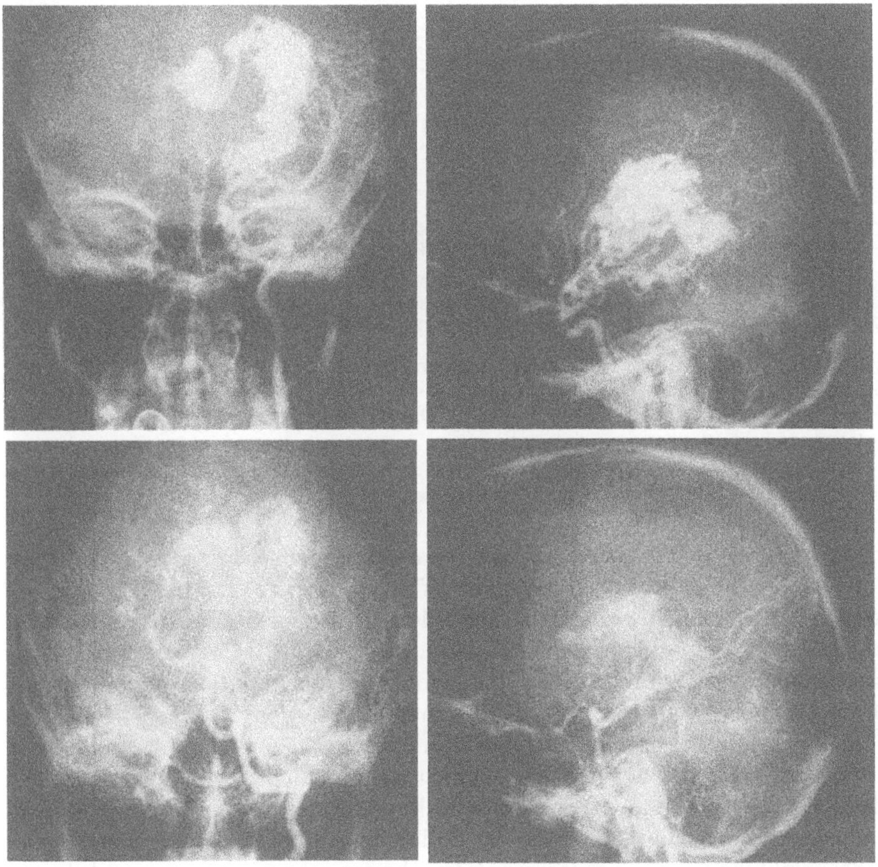

Fig. 1. *Above.* Left carotid angiography showing a large AVM in the deep temporal and basal ganglia region.
Below. Left vertebral angiography. The lesion is supplied by perforating branches from the basilar and posterior cerebral arteries

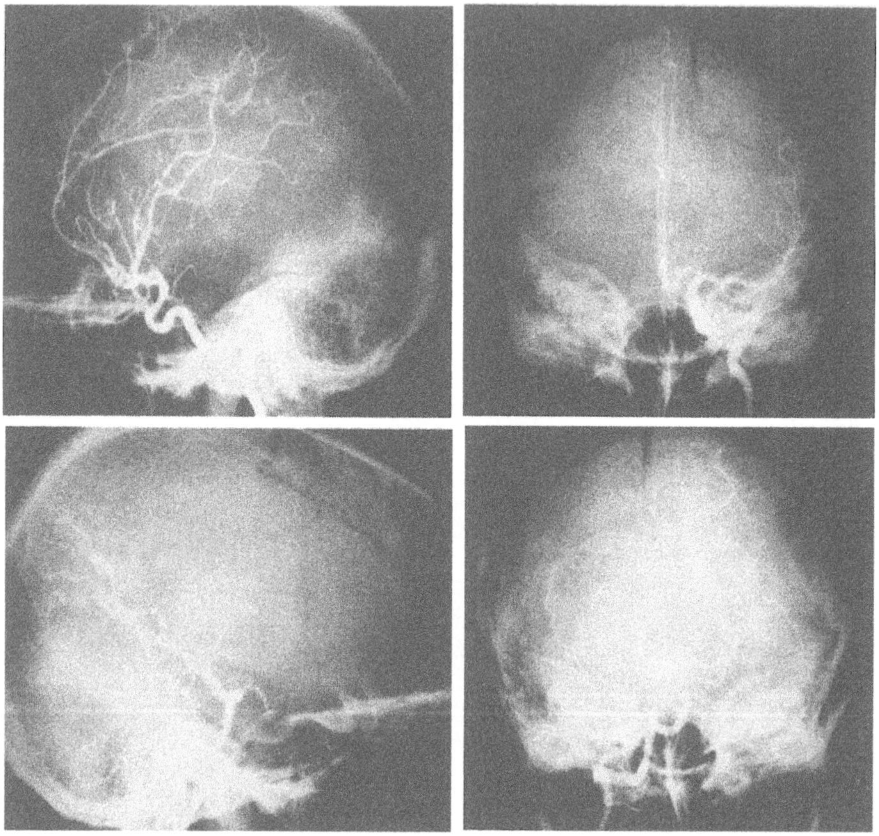

Fig. 2. *Above.* Postoperative left carotid angiography demonstrating total removal of the angioma.
Below. Postoperative left vertebral angiography. The perforating branches from the basilar and posterior cerebral arteries were preserved

examination revealed intracerebral and intraventricular bleeding. An angiography showed a very large AVM occupying the left deep temporal and basal ganglia region (Fig. 1). The lesion was mainly supplied by the lenticulo-striatae artery and by branches from the posterior communicating artery. The AVM drained into the internal cerebral vein. On June 7, 1983 the lesion was exposed through a left pre-frontal, transventricular approach. The intraventricular portion of the AVM and the choroid plexus, which had changed into arteriovenous malformation, were removed at first. With controlled hypotension and high magnification the lesion was removed totally. Postoperatively the patient initially showed a complete aphasia and a right hemiplegia. The hemiplegia improved gradually, but the aphasia remained unchanged until the discharge four weeks later. The control angiography revealed a total removal of the lesion (Fig. 2). In the control examination one year after the operation the patient presented only a mild hemiparesis and an improvement of the aphasia.

Case 2: This 27-year-old man suffered an intracerebral hemorrhage in November 1983. He was admitted to another clinic presenting a right abducent palsy, neck stiffness and nystagmus. The CT-scan revealed an intrapontine bleeding. The angiography (Fig. 3) showed an AVM in the brain stem, fed by branches of the right cerebellar superior artery, right AICA and right PICA. The lesion drained into the rectus sinus. Using a middle-line posterior fossa approach, the fourth ventricle was exposed. The angioma was found in the floor of the IV ventricle. The angioma bleeding created a sheet between the lesion and the brain stem, as a pseudo-capsule. Under high magnification the lesion was extirpated totally. The postoperative course was uneventful, the patient recovered without neurologic deficits. The control angiography (Fig. 4) confirmed the total removal of the AVM.

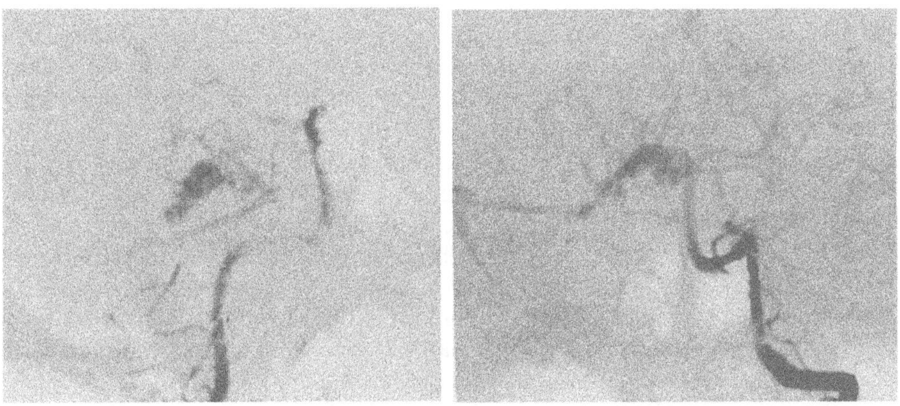

Fig. 3. Preoperative right vertebral angiography showing an angioma in the brain stem, supplied by branches of the superior cerebellar artery, anterior inferior cerebellar artery and by the posterior inferior cerebellar artery

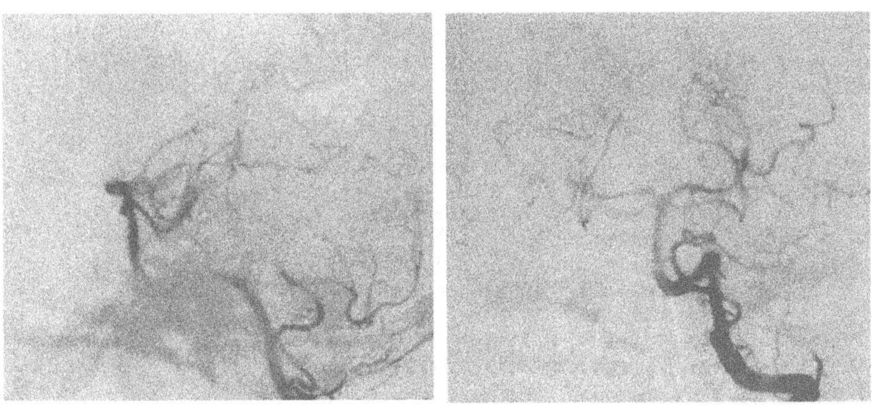

Fig. 4. Postoperative vertebral angiography demonstrating a total removal of the AVM

Discussion

The indications for surgical treatment of large cortical and deep seated AVMs remain controversial, because the natural history of these lesions is not well known [2, 3, 8, 10, 12, 18, 19, 22, 27]. According to the literature angiomas in general present a risk of bleeding of about 47% in 20 years, if they bled before, and of 39% in 20 years without previous bleeding [11]. The mortality rate increases with the recurrence of the hemorrhage. So it is about 10% after the first bleeding, 13% after the second and 20% after the third bleeding [25]. The morbidity caused by bleeding from these deep seated lesions remains unknown. Size and location are important factors related to the neurological deficits caused by these malformations [1, 4, 30]. Bleeding from deep seated AVMs often causes an intraventricular hemorrhage, which can occlude the ventricular system completely [13]. Some authors report a mortality of 100% in these cases [28]. These factors should be considered when determining whether or not to operate [30]. Fourteen of our 15 cases presented intracranial bleeding or clinical symptoms related to the angioma before the 50th year of life. Eight of these patients were even under 30 years of age. This suggests that about half of our patients could die or be severely disabled within twenty years.

All cases were operated on with the surgical microscope. Angiomas which bled before often created a sheet between the brain tissue and the lesion, like a pseudocapsule, which permits the removal of the AVM without damaging the surrounding brain. We try to remove these angiomas like a "tumor", i.e. bipolar coagulation of the angiomatous vessels and step by step resection of it. The major draining veins are preserved until the end of the procedure. In contrast to other authors we did not observe in any case the so-called "Normal Perfusion Pressure Breakthrough Syndrome" [6, 33, 37]. In many cases we observed a bleeding from the "angioma bed" after the removal of the main angioma mass. This bleeding is produced by small angiomatous vessels surrounding the major portion of the lesion. These vessels can usually not be seen on the angiography because they are compressed by the main portion of the angioma or by a hematoma, or because of the high flow-shunt inside the malformation.

Alternative methods for treatment of these lesions have been used (Table 3). However, in most cases these methods fail to completely obliterate the lesion. Of all these alternative methods, the embolization with bucrylate, and the high focused energy irradiation seem to be the methods which can achieve the best results [7, 8,

Table 3. Deep seated AVMs. Alternative therapy

1. Flow-directed percarotid embolization (Luessenhop 1975; Drake 1979)
2. Direct selective feeder embolization (Drake 1979)
3. Embolization with bucrylate (Drake 1979; Debrun et al. 1982)
4. Occlusion of the feeders by detachable balloon (Serbinenko 1979)
5. Radiotherapy (Johnson 1975)
6. High focused energy. Proton beam (Kjellberg et al. 1978); (Stereotactic gama radiation – Steiner et al. 1974)
7. Cryo-coagulation (Walder 1978)
8. Combined open-stereotactic operation (Riechert + Mundinger 1964)

Table 4. Deep seated AVMs (15 cases)

Results		*Complications*	
Good	12	Transient aphasia	2
Fair	2	Hemiparesis	4
Death	1	Seizures	1
		Hemianopsia	1
Control Angiography		Cranial nerve palsy	1
Total removal	12	Death (pulm. embolism)	1
Partial removal	3	No complications	10
		Recurrent bleeding	0

35]. Size, number of feeders and the location of the AVM are usually the limiting factors of these alternative methods. A longer follow-up of the patients treated with this therapy is, however, required.

In our series we achieved good results in twelve cases (80% of the cases) (Table 4). These patients returned after the operation to a normal social life. Two patients became disabled and needed help in their daily lives, and one patient died 3 weeks after an uneventful removal of a large angioma in the brain stem, due to a fulminating pulmonary embolism.

A total removal of the lesion could be achieved in 12 cases. In two cases a total removal was not attempted because those patients had had no intracranial bleeding and the lesions were very large and located inside the brain stem. In the last case the postoperative angiography disclosed a small portion of the angioma within the lateral ventricle, probably angiomatous choroid plexus.

The operative results of this series with complete extirpation of the lesions in 80% of the cases speak in favor of the surgical management of these malformations.

References

1. Amacher AL, Allcock JM, Drake C (1972) Cerebral angiomas: The sequelae of surgical treatment. J Neurosurg 37:571–575
2. Bonnal J, Serratrice G, Winninger J (1960) Angiome arterio-veineux (A.A.V.). Des territoires choroideus anterieur et posterieur juxta thalamique avec hematoma dans le pulvinar. Ablation partielle etude des sequeles. Neurochirurgie 6: 173–185
3. Bonnal J, Petrou U, Gillet J (1978) Aneurysmes arterioveineux interessant la toile choroidienne du IIIe ventricule. Neurochirurgie 24: 15–21
4. Bushe KA, Bockhorn J, Schäfer ER (1975) Macro- and microsurgery of central angiomas. In: Pia HW, Glaeve J, Grote E, Zierski J (eds) Cerebral angiomas, advances in diagnosis and therapy. Springer, Berlin Heidelberg New York, pp 123–128
5. Da Pian R, Pasqualin A, Scienza R (1982) Microsurgical treatment of juxta-peduncular angiomas. Surg Neurol 17: 16–29
6. Day AL, Friedman WA, Sypert GW et al. (1982) Successful treatment of the normal perfusion pressure breakthrough-syndrome. Neurosurgery 5:625–630
7. Debrun G, Vinuela F, Fox A, Drake CG (1982) Embolization of cerebral arteriovenous malformations with bucrylate. J Neurosurg 56:615–627
8. Drake CG (1979) Cerebral arteriovenous malformations: Considerations and experience with surgical treatment in 166 cases. Clin Neurosurg 26: 145–208
9. French LA, Chou SN, Story JL (1964) Cerebrovascular malformations in "Clinical Neurosurgery". In: Shillito J (ed) Williams & Wilkens Co., Baltimore, pp 171–182

10. French LA (1977) Surgical treatment of arteriovenous malformations: A history. Clin Neurosurg 4:22–33
11. Graf CJ, Perret GE, Torner JC (1983) Bleeding from cerebral arteriovenous malformations as part of their natural history. J Neurosurg 58:331–337
12. Hodge CJ jr, King BB (1975) Arteriovenous malformation of choroid plexus – case report. J Neurosurg 42:457–461
13. Jellinger K (1980) Pathology and etiology of ICM. In: Pia HW, Langmaid C, Zierski J (eds) Spontaneous intracerebral haematomas. Diagnosis and therapy. Springer, Berlin Heidelberg New York, pp 13–29
14. Johnson RT (1975) Radiotherapy of cerebral angiomas with a note on some problems in diagnosis. In: Pia HW, Glaeve JRW, Grote E, Zierski J (eds) Cerebral angiomas: Advances in diagnosis and therapy. Springer, Berlin Heidelberg New York, pp 256–266
15. Kandel EL, Peresedov UU (1977) Stereotactic clipping of arterial aneurysm and arteriovenous malformations. J Neurosurg 46:12–24
16. Kjellberg RN, Poletti CE, Robertson GH, Adams DA (1978) Bragg peak proton beam treatment of arteriovenous malformations of the brain. In: Carrea R (ed) Neurological surgery. Proceedings of the 6th international congress of neurological surgery, Sao Paulo, June 19–25, 1977. Excerpta Medica, Amsterdam, pp 181–187
17. Kunc Z (1972) Surgery of arteriovenous malformations in the speech and motor-sensory regions. J Neurosurg 103:107–111
18. Laine E, Jomin M, Clarisse J, Combelles O (1981) Les malformations arterio-veineuses cerebrales profundes. Neurochirurgie 27:147–160
19. Lapras C (1975) Angiomas of cerebellum and brain stem in cerebral angiomas: Advances in diagnosis and therapy. Springer, Berlin Heidelberg New York, pp 136–141
20. Logue U, Mockton G (1954) Posterior fossa angiomas. A clinical presentation of nine cases. Brain 77:252–273
21. Luessenhop AJ (1975) Artificial embolization of inoperable arteriovenous malformations. In: Pia HW, Glaeve JRW, Grote G, Zierski J (eds) Cerebral angiomas. Advances in diagnosis and therapy. Springer, Berlin Heidelberg New York, pp 198–205
22. Natsumura M, Hakita Y, Someda K, Kondo A (1977) Arteriovenous malformations in the posterior fossa. J Neurosurg 47:50–56
23. McCormick WF, Hardman JM, Boulter TH (1968) Vascular malformations ("angiomas") with special reference to those occurring in the posterior fossa. J Neurosurg 28:241–251
24. Mullan S, Kawanaga H, Patronas NJ (1979) Microvascular embolisation of cerebral arteriovenous malformations. J Neurosurg 51:621–627
25. Nibbelink DW (1975) Cooperative aneurysm study in cerebral vascular disease. Ninth conference. In: Whisnant JP, Sandok BA (eds) Grune & Stratton, New York, pp 155–165
26. Patul AA (1980) Surgical excision of arteriovenous malformations of the cerebellum and brain stem. A case presentation. Acta Neurochir (Wien) 54:117–125
27. Perret C, Nishicka H (1966) Report on the cooperative study of intracranial aneurysms and subarachnoid hemorrhage. Arteriovenous malformations in analysis of 545 cases of cranio-cerebral arteriovenous malformations and fistulae reported to the cooperative study. J Neurosurg 25:467–490
28. Pia HW (1980) Location, indications and prognosis. In: Pia HW, Langmaid C, Zierski J (eds) Spontaneous intracerebral haematomas. Advances in diagnosis and therapy. Springer, Berlin Heidelberg New York, pp 329–330
29. Pool JL (1962) Treatment of arteriovenous malformations of the cerebral hemispheres. J Neurosurg 19:136–141
30. Ramina R, Samii M (1983) Operative Behandlung von tiefliegenden Angiomen mit Eindringen in das Ventrikelsystem. Paper presented at the "Arbeitstagung Mikroneurochirurgie" Hamburg, 8–10 Dec., 1983
31. Riechert T, Mundinger F (1964) Combined stereotaxic operation for treatment of deep seated angiomas and aneurysms. J Neurosurg 21:358–363
32. Serbinenko FA (1979) Balloon catheterization and occlusion of major cerebral vessels. J Neurosurg 41:125–145
33. Spetzler RF, Wilson CB, Weinstein P et al. (1978) Normal perfusion pressure breakthrough theory. Clin Neurosurg 25:651–672

34. Stein BM, Wolpert SM (1977) Surgical and embolic treatment of cerebral arteriovenous malformations. Surg Neurol 7:359–369
35. Steiner L, Leksell L, Forster DMC et al (1974) Stereotactic radiosurgery in intracranial arteriovenous malformations. Acta Neurochir [Suppl] (Wien) 21:196–209
36. Walder HAD (1978) Freezing arteriovenous anomalics in the brain. In: Pia HW, Glaeve JRW, Grote E, Zierski J (eds) Cerebral angiomas. Advances in diagnosis and therapy. Springer, Berlin Heidelberg New York, pp 183–193
37. Wilson CB, Domingue J (1979) Microsurgical treatment of intracranial vascular malformations. J Neurosurg 51:446–454

Surgical Treatment of Para- and Intraventricular Vascular Lesions Complicated by Intraventricular and Periventricular Hemorrhage

M. MIRCEVSKI, A. POPOVSKI, R. BASEVSKA, P. RUŠKOV and I. DZONOV,
Skopje/Yugoslavia

Key Words: Intraventricular Hemorrhage, Cryptic A-V malformation, Ruptured aneurysm, Surgical treatment.

Abstract: During the last 10 years (1975–1984), 31 patients with clinical manifestations of compressive bleeding in brain ventricles and caused by A-V malformations, atypical location of aneurysms, and hemangioblastic tumors with bleeding in brain ventricles, were surgically treated.

The main characteristic of our patients is that all of them are young children and adults up to 25 years of age.

The hospital admission of all patients was accompanied by severe .disorder of brain functions, unconsciousness with palsy and fast evolution.

The diagnosis of the pathologic process and the compressive bleeding had to be performed as soon as possible after the hospital admission, because of the compressive bleeding.

The analysis of the surgically treated 31 patients indicates that the patients had vascular benign pseudotumorous or tumorous processes without any symptoms in the preclinical phase or the symptoms were almost unnoticed (compensated hydrocephalus, arterial hypertension, epilepsy and etc.).

The surgical treatment is indispensable, the results especially those in benign intravascular processes complicated with bleeding and compressive, are not always encouraging but we are obliged to continue with surgical activity based on our experience and modern equipment.

Introduction

Spontaneous intracranial hemorrhages with or without initial symptoms are characteristic for cerebral lesion, rapid evolution and functional change of the central nervous system manifested with disturbances of consciousness, neurological deficits and worsening of the general status of the patient.

Localization of the cause for the hemorrhage and spatial elements of the spilled blood in the brain tissue and cavities are key elements for the clinical evaluation and manifestation of this vascular syndrome [3–5, 8, 9, 11, 13, 14].

Evolution of the manifestation and the localization of the pathological process are especially due to spontaneous acute compressive hemorrhages detected in the brain ventricles and concerning the lesions A-V malformation, ruptured aneurysm and not exceptionally hemoblastic tumor or metastasis.

It is well acknowledged that most of these patients die immediately after the initial hemorrhage and do not reach hospital treatment. It is most commonly: *first:* A-V malformation spotted paraventricularly or near this zone, the hemorrhage being intracerebral with secondary penetration in the ventricles; *secondly:* tiny A-V malformations spotted paraventricularly or ventricularly in relation with chorioid plexus; and *thirdly:* quite tiny angiomas with ventricular localization as big as a small knot and even smaller than that. The aneurysms belong frequently to anterior cerebral artery with most common localization on the floor of the third ventricle, very big and with initial hemorrhage [3–5, 8, 12–14].

In 1956, Crawford and Russell, used the term 'cryptic' to define some small vascular malformations that had certain clinical features in common; they occurred in the younger age groups, and the bleeding source often remained obscure on clinical and complete investigation. Gerlach [5] prefers to call them microangiomas defining them as masses of vessels with an arbitrary maximal diameter of 2 cm. Finally, some other authors, such as Krayenbühl and Siebenmann [8], call them small vascular malformations.

In this report we describe our experience of operated cases with compressive bleeding in the brain ventricles caused by small vascular malformations with either ventricular or paraventricular localization with direct rupture in the ventricle or paraventricular hematoma with secondary penetration in the ventricle. Similar mechanism or evolution is a property of aneurysm or bleeding tumor.

Clinical Material and Methods

During the last 10 years (1975–1984), we have surgically treated 31 patients with intraventricular hemorrhage with ventricular or paraventricular localization of A-V malformation, aneurysm or hemoblastic tumor (Table 1–3).

The main characteristic of our patients is that all of them are young:
In the history of the disease in our material we noticed that two thirds of the operated cases had no symptoms, while in one third of adults over 20 years of age there were transient headaches, prostration, blood pressure changes and the patients had been treated as cardiac patients.

On the contrary the vascular affliction was with a sudden onset of loss of consciousness with rapid or gradual worsening of the state and rapid admission to the hospital.

Table 1. Age distribution of the cases

Age	Number of cases
0 to 1 year	3
1 to 2 years	1
2 to 8 years	1
8 to 15 years	2
15 to 35 years	24
Total	31

Table 2. Manifestional forms of the pathologic process

Pathologic manifestation	Number of cases
A-V malformation	21
Aneurysm of the ACA	3
Aneurysm of the PCA	4
Hemoblastic ventricular tumor	3
Total	31

Table 3. Localization of the compressive hemorrhage

Lateral ventricles	Right ventricle	3
	Left ventricle	2
Third ventricle		1
Fourth ventricle		4
All the ventricles/intracer. and ventr./		21
Total		31

Diagnosis

Because of the rapid evolution of the compressive syndrome and worsening of the patient's general status the diagnosis has been immediately established on admission of the patient to hospital.

We commonly used the history, neurological finding, evolution of the consciousness, EEG, fundus, the dilatation of the pupils, carotid or vertebral arteriography and since 1978 CT-scan (78% of the patients).

Surgical Treatment

The operative technique that we used consisted of osteoplastic opening of the head, corticotomy and entrance in the engaged ventricle at frontal, occipital and temporal aspect or the posterior fossa for fourth ventricle, consequently extirpation of the blood clots, step by step and definitively coagulation of the blood pathological vessels which were aspirated and sucked into the aspirator. After the definitive hemostasis we terminated the operation without drainage.

Results

All 31 patients that were operated survived operation. Everyone of them was observed and reanimated in acute care unit, after the operation. In the course of the first six hours 14 patients (45%) were extubated while the rest, 17 patients, were still on assisted ventilation.

In the next 18 hours extubation was performed in further 7 patients, which gives a total of 21 patients or 68%, with spontaneous respiration, normal vital functions, normal reactions, capable of awakening themselves and with full consciousness and nutrition by tube or per os. In the next 24 hours, further 2 patients were extubated while the rest were still on assisted ventilation.

9 patients died: 3 in the first 4 days after the operation, 4 in the next 14 days, one from pulmonal infection and one as a cause of a cerebrospinal meningitis.

The total mortality rate in our series is 27% (5 patients died (or 24%) with A-V malformation, 3 (or 47%) with aneurysm and ventricular bleeding, one patient with

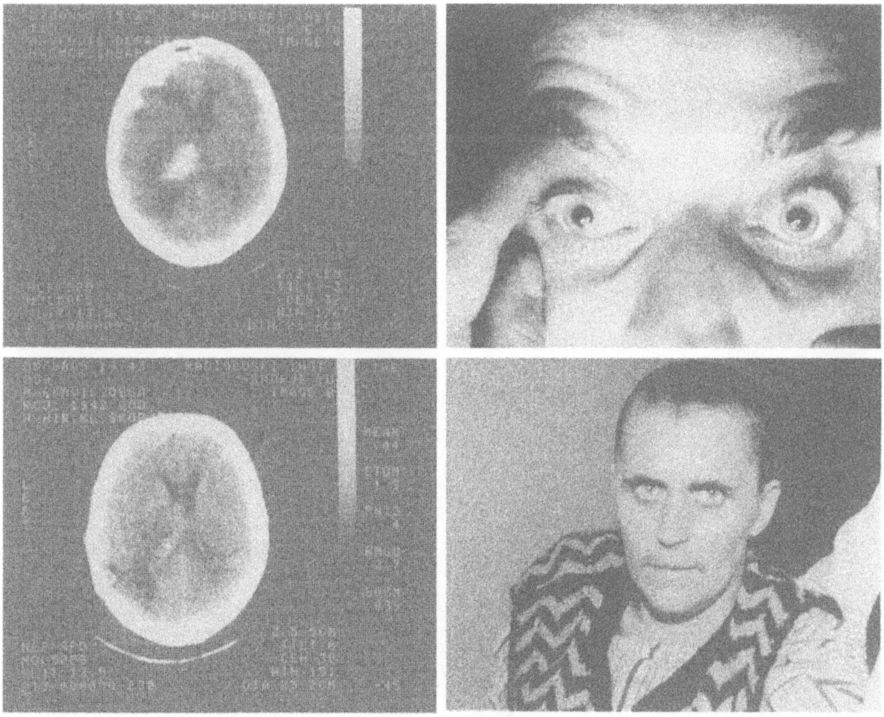

Fig. 1. A woman, aged 42: CT-scan of the brain before and after the operation; A-V malformation of the plexus chorioides; Operated in coma condition with dilated pupils and spontaneous breathing. After the operation completely reconvalescenced

metastatic hypernephroma, while the rest, two patients with hemoblastic tumor, survived).

22 survivors recovered in this order: 15 in the first 3–6 months, the rest in the next 9–12 months.

All 22 survived without marked sequellae which recupirated by means of light sedatives like valium and vitamins (Figs. 1, 2a and b).

Discussion

Spontaneous intraventricular and paraventricular bleeding with direct flooding either in the ventricle or the brain and afterwards in the ventricle, are acute intracranial processes whose onset, manifestation and evolution are atypical with rapid neurologic worsening and, simultaneously, of the general status.

The key problems are the diagnosis and localization which are supposed to be performed any time during day and night, which is difficult to do especially in the pre-CT-scan era. Since 1978, we use CT-scan and we had the diagnosis and localization in 11 cases (36%), which guided our planning for arteriography and surgical treatment.

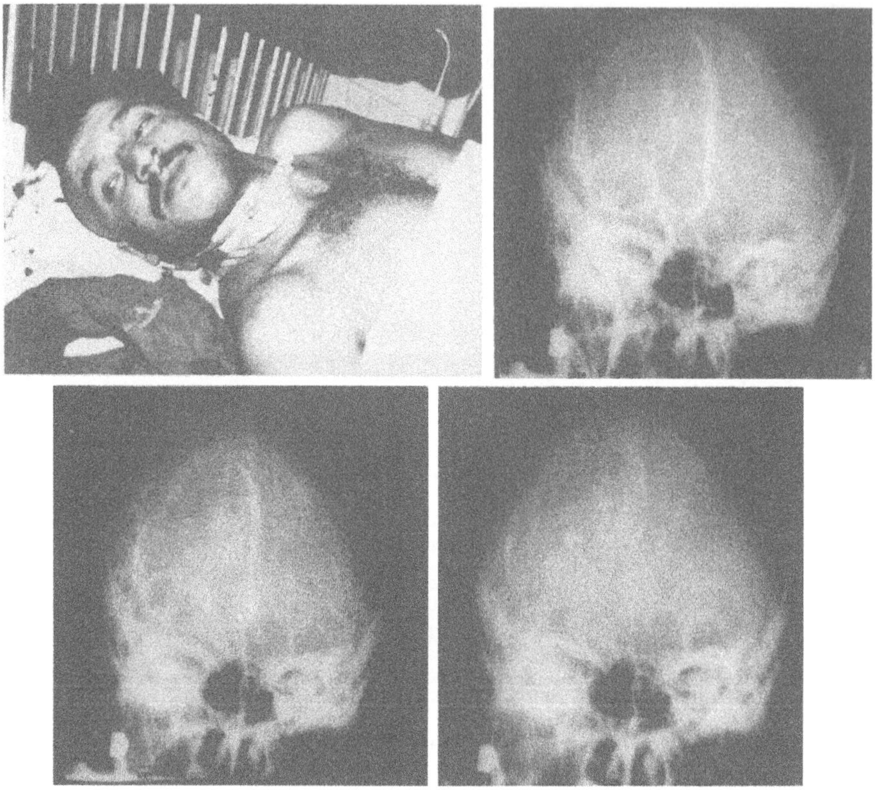

Fig. 2. a A patient, aged 22, student of medicine, in coma condition with ventricular hemorrhage; Cryptic A-V malformation; Right carotic angiography; Operated and completely reconvalescenced

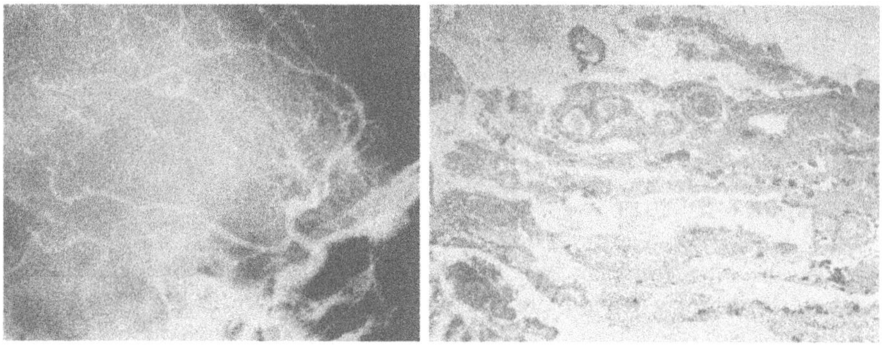

Fig. 2. b Right carotic angiography profile and hystologic finding of the patient in Fig. 2a

Arteriography is inevitable and must be performed in excellent condition, its diagnosis being the localization and the distribution of the normal vessels. But we must stress that the importance of the arteriography for ventricular and paraventricular bleeding is not in the same rate as in other brain regions. Especially in case of an aneurysm the localization is given by CT-scan and not by arteriography although it helps [6–8, 14].

Localization of the A-V malformation is even harder and in some forms it is impossible, such as cryptic malformations [6–8, 14] and it is due to local brain destruction, darkening of the spot, small caliber of the vessels, slugging, internal circulation and spasm of the feeding vessels after the hemorrhage. The majority of cryptic vascular malformations has not been detected by angiography, but in the last two decades advances in neuroradiological techniques have made it possible to demonstrate some of them, especially with the use of the so-called selective angiography [6–8, 14].

Based on all these facts and especially on CT-scan, we do not approve of the general opinion that the cryptic bleeding is a rarity since we have met them during the last 7 years in an increasing number, although we know that some of them die before admission to hospital or in the course of the diagnosing process [1–5, 8].

Histology, above all other means, establishes the diagnosis of the bleeding source although in some cases it is impossible due to brain destruction, clots, and ruptured vessels [2, 3, 8, 10]. Arteriographic findings, histology and other means give rise to this diagnosing process since the operation gives benign evolution. Sometimes, even post mortem examinations are necessary [3, 8, 13]. Only in a small number of intraventricular hemorrhage the outcome is gloomy. The compression of the bleeding gives us the right to operate and we are supposed to extirpate not only the hematoma but the cause at the same time: A-V malformation or clipped aneurysm. There are authors who place ventriculo-external drainage in cases of intraventricular hemorrhage and then as circumstances require they continue with operative treatment [2, 5].

Our experiences show that this treatment is completely unsuccessful because of blocking the drainage and possible infection. Finally, we are posing our question: Is it necessary to operate patients with intraventricular lesions complicated by intraventricular and periventricular hemorrhage?

Our answer is: Rapid admission of the patient into hospital, observation and fast diagnostic procedures and indication for operative treatment.

The indication for operative treatment depends on the pathologic process, hemorrhage compression and consciousness of the patients. The key role in treating the hemorrhage of compressive character plays the team work of neurosurgeons, neurologists, anesthesiologists and other specialists.

This team work enables synthesis of the past attitudes and knowledge thus solving the problem of the compressive hemorrhage according to its localization and evolution.

References

1. Britt RH, Slivebreg GD, Enzmann DR, Hanbery JW (1980) Third ventricular choroid plexus arteriovenous malformation simulating a colloid cyst. J Neurosurg 52:246–250
2. Butler AB, Partain RA, Netsky MG (1972) Primary intraventricular hemorrhage. Neurology (NY) 22:675–687
3. Crawford JV, Russell DS (1956) Cryptic arteriovenous hematomas of the brain. J Neurol Neurosurg Psychiatry 19:1–11
4. Doe FD, Shuangshoti S, Netsky MG (1972) Cryptic hemangioma of the choroid plexus. Neurology (NY) 22:1232–1239
5. Gerlach J (1969) Intracerebral hemorrhage caused by microangiomas. Prog Neurol Surg 3:362–396
6. Golden JB, Kramer RA (1978) The angiographically occult cerebral vascular malformation. J Neurosurg 48:292–296
7. Kramer RA, Wing SD (1977) Computed tomography of angiographically occult cerebral vascular malformation. Radiology 123:649–652
8. Krayenbühl H, Siebenmann R (1965) Small vascular malformations as a cause of primary intracerebral hemorrhage. J Neurosurg 22:7–20
9. Malik GM, Horoupian DS, Boulos RS (1980) Hemorrhagic/colloid/cyst of the third ventricle and episodic neurologic deficits. Surg Neurol 13:73–77
10. McCormick WF, Nofzinger JD (1966) "Cryptic" vascular malformations of the central nervous system. J Neurosurg 24:865–875
11. Pozzati E, Padovani R, Morrone B, Finicio F, Gaist G (1963) Cerebral cavernous angiomas in children. J Neurosurg 53:826–832
12. Roda MJ, Monso HJ, Vilarejo JF, Morales C, Blazquez GM (1981) Cryptic arteriovenous malformation of the choroid plexus of the third ventricle. Surg Neurol 16:353–357
13. Russell DS (1954) The pathology of spontaneous intracranial haemorrhage. Proc R Soc Med 47:689–693
14. Voigt K, Yaşargil MG (1976) Cerebral cavernous haemangiomas or cavernomas. Incidence, pathology, localization, diagnosis, clinical features and treatment. Review of the literature and report of an unusual case. Neurochirurgia (Stuttg) 19:59–68

Surgical Management of Deep-Seated Cerebrovascular Lesions by Means of Temporary Vascular Occlusion Using Sendai Cocktail

J. SUZUKI, T. KAYAMA, and T. YOSHIMOTO, Sendai/Japan

Introduction

In surgery of deep-seated arterio-venous malformation or basilar giant aneurysm, the surgeon should be fully aware of the fact that the bleeding of inaccessible vessels or aneurysms is sometimes inevitable. Consequently, prior to dissection of the arterio-venous malformation and aneurysm, at least feeding arteries must be occluded.

In order to prolong the period of temporary occlusion of cerebral vessels, 20% mannitol was used as we reported previously [3]. After a dose of 2 mg/kg of 20% mannitol is given intravenously over 30 min, vascular occlusion is undertaken. With this method, occlusion of any of the intracranial vessels can be performed safely for up to 40 min within 100 minutes from the time of the administration of mannitol [7].

In all our cases of radical surgery on cerebrovascular lesions, we used temporary vascular occlusion method with mannitol and obtained good surgical results [6, 7].

Furthermore, we newly developed the cerebral protective agents (Sendai Cocktail) which increases prevention of ischemic insults [2, 5, 8].

This time, surgical management of deep-seated cerebrovascular lesions such as large basilar aneurysm, cerebellar and deep-seated arterio-venous malformation by means of temporary vascular occlusion method using our newly developed brain protective agent (Sendai Cocktail: 20% mannitol 500 ml, Vitamin E 300 mg, steroid 50 mg) is reported. Also mentioned are the advantages of balloon catheter which is applied to the temporary occlusion method.

Case Reports

Case 1: A 59-year-old housewife was admitted to our hospital suffering from sudden onset of severe headache, nausea and vomiting. On admission, the symptoms of the patient were headache, slight IIIrd and IVth cranial nerve dysfunction, with clear consciousness. CT scan revealed a round shaped, high density area (diameter 25 mm) existing at the right portion of the basal cistern (Fig. 1). Cerebral angiography showed a large basilar artery aneurysm with thrombosed cavity (Fig. 2). Surgery was performed with keel form skin incision and subtemporal approach. Before surgery, vascular balloon catheter was inserted through femoral artery to basilar artery in order to temporarily occlude the basilar artery during surgery (Fig. 3). After administration of Sendai Cocktail, the balloon was inflated to the basilar artery, consequently the tip of balloon catheter was flown into the aneurysm down

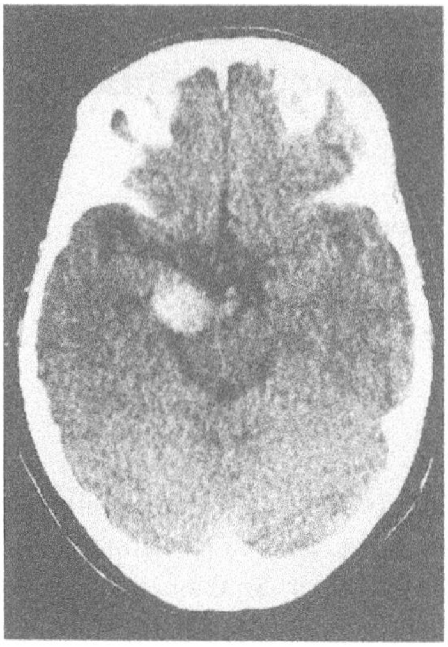

Fig. 1. CT scan of case 1 shows mass lesion at left interpeduncular cistern

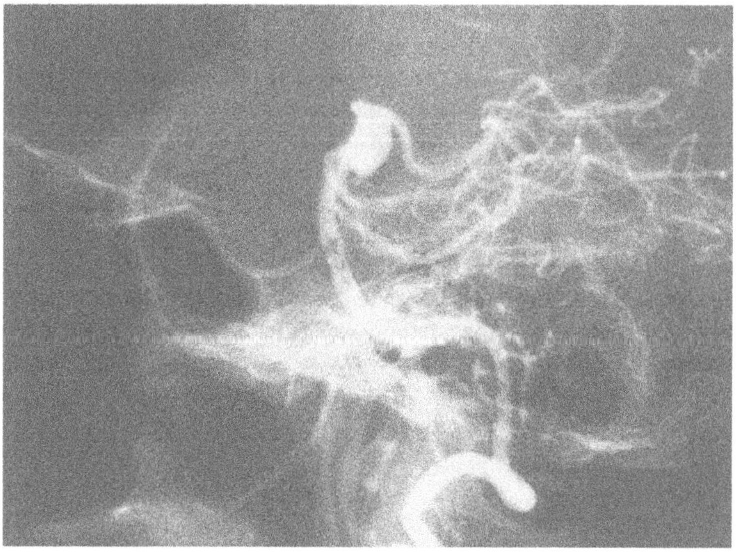

Fig. 2. Left VAG of case 1 shows giant aneurysm, between left PCA and SCA

where the orifice between basilar artery and aneursym was. Because of occlusion of the orifice of the basilar artery aneurysm, dissection of aneurysm was performed safely and resection of aneurysm was also undertaken with little bleeding. After the aneurysm was reduced, temporary vascular clips were used on the basilar, bilateral posterior cerebral artery and then the neck of the aneurysm was permanently clipped. During surgery, temporary occlusion time was 34 min 28 sec. The postoperative course was eventless, she was discharged and was clinically the same as before with slight left IIIrd cranial nerve dysfunction (Fig. 4).

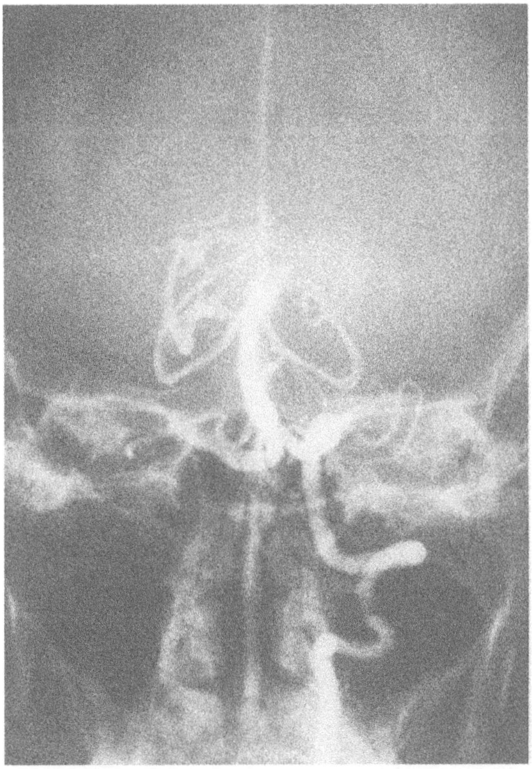

Fig. 3. Intraoperative left VAG shows that the orifice of aneurysm was occluded by a balloon catheter

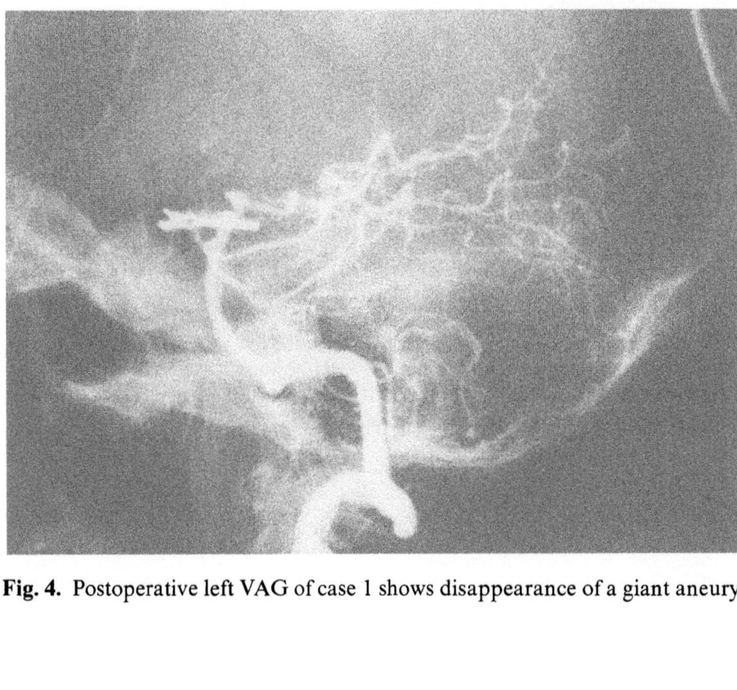

Fig. 4. Postoperative left VAG of case 1 shows disappearance of a giant aneurysm

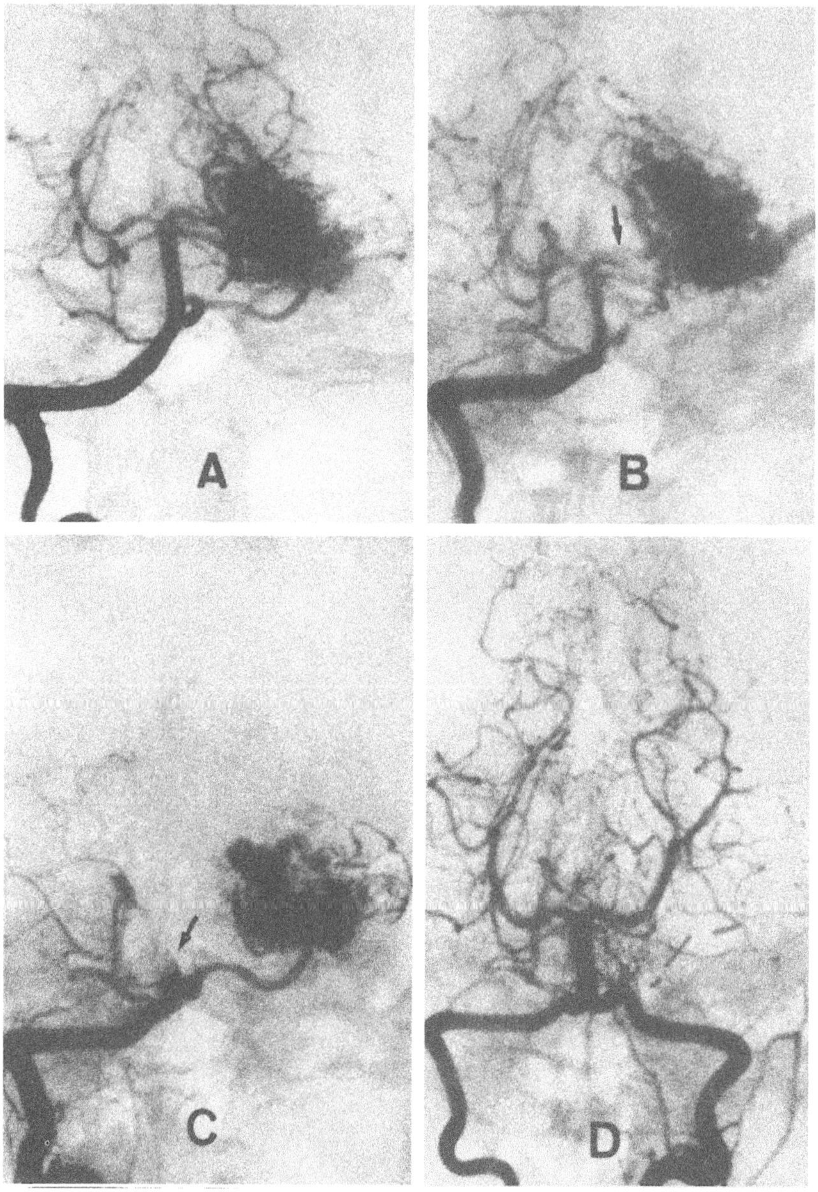

Fig. 5 A. Right VAG of case 2 shows deep-seated cerebellar AVM fed by double left SCA and left AICA. **B.** Intraoperative angiogram reveals that left P_1 is occluded by a balloon catheter. **C.** shows that the basilar artery just distal to the left AICA is occluded by a balloon catheter. **D.** Postoperative angiogram. The AVM is completely resected

Case 2: A 14-year-old female was admitted to our clinic suffering from sudden onset of a headache, vertigo and tinnitus. CT scan showed subarachnoid hemorrhage with ventricular rupture and left cerebellar hemorrhage. Cerebral angiography revealed a large left cerebellopontine angle arteriovenous malformation fed by double left superior cerebellar arteries and a left anterior inferior cerebellar artery (Fig. 5). The superior anterior part of the nidus was mainly fed by the double left superior cerebellar arteries and the inferior posterior part by the left anterior inferior cerebellar artery. Before the operation, the tolerance test for balloon occlusion of the basilar artery for 15 min by means of administration of Sendai Cocktail was performed. Auditory brain stem response showed that no change and no neurologic deficits had occurred during temporary occlusion of the basilar artery.

Operation was performed by the unilateral suboccipital approach. Before surgery, two balloon catheters were introduced via femoral artery into the left anterior inferior cerebellar artery and the basilar artery where the double left superior cerebellar arteries originated. The ABR was monitored continuously and intraoperative angiography was also performed. Before the temporary occlusion, Sendai Cocktail was administered and then temporary occlusion was performed. Arterio-venous malformation was removed totally without massive bleeding during operation. During surgical procedures, the anterior inferior cerebellar artery was occluded for 26 min and the basilar artery for 46 min.

The postoperative course was uneventful, and the postoperative angiography revealed the disappearance of the arteriovenous malformation. The patient was discharged and is now rehabilitated.

Discussion

Over 20 years ago, I found out that mannitol protects ischemic brain by an experience in a case of middle cerebral artery aneurysm where temporary vascular occlusion was performed for 50 min and in which postoperative course was uneventful. Thereafter, many kinds of animal experiments were conducted for extending the knowledge of the mechanism of the effectiveness of mannitol against ischemic brain [1, 2, 4, 8, 9]. Now, the scavenge reaction might be thought as the main mechanism of the effectiveness of mannitol. Nowadays, if the ischemic insults break out in the brain, it is well known that free radicals ($'O_2$ $O_2^{-}\cdot$, H_2O_2, $OH\cdot$), arise immediately after ischemic insults. By our experimental data, mannitol suppresses the increase in the counts of chemiluminescence which occurs as the results of singlet oxygen ($'O_2$) in hypoxic and ischemic rat brain. So that the effectiveness of mannitol might be thought as free radical scavenger [9].

At the same time, we newly developed cerebral protective agents among free radical scavengers. Using a canine model of completely ischemic brain regulated by infusion method, in which cerebral blood flow is freely controlled [1], a model of 10% cerebral blood flow as the normal one was produced. Many kinds of free radical scavengers were analysed. It was evaluated the recovery of the activity of EEG after 1 hour ischemia and 3 hours recirculation to know the effectiveness of each drug [8]. As a result, mannitol, Vitamin E and steroids were indicated as the protective agents, and furthermore the mixture of these 3 drugs, which we named Sen-

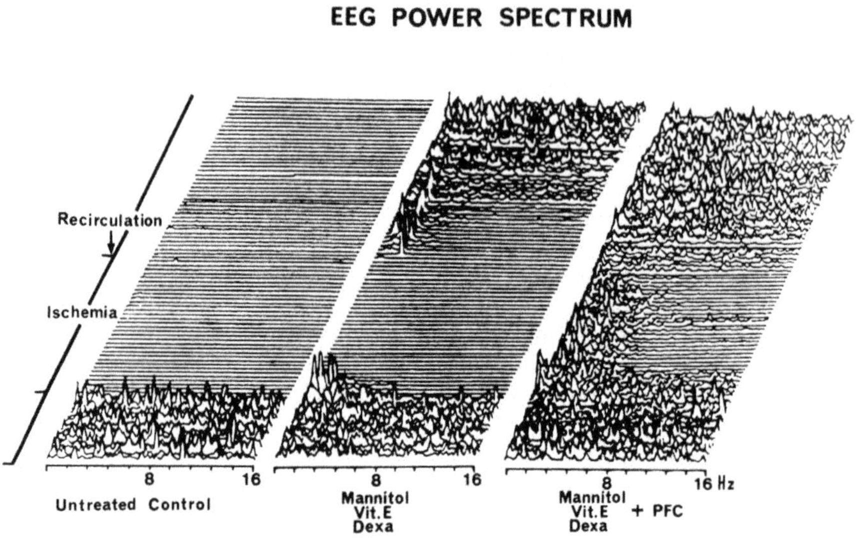

Fig. 6. The result of animal experiment; evaluation of the recovery of EEG activity after 1 hour ischemia (10% CBF), 3 hours recirculation indicates that Sendai Cocktail protects the brain against ischemia

dai Cocktail (20% mannitol 500 ml, Vitamin E 300 mg, Steroid 50 mg) has more protective effect against ischemia (Fig. 6).

It is sometimes difficult to control the accidental massive bleeding in surgery such as deep-seated AVM and giant basilar aneurysm. Previously our reports overstated that the method of temporary cerebrovascular occlusion using mannitol is useful to make the surgery of cerebrovascular lesions safe, radical and obtain good results [3, 7]. It is, however, possible that the temporary vascular occlusion could be performed for 40 min or more if Sendai Cocktail was administered prior vascular occlusion, without cerebral ischemic insults.

However, in these kinds of surgery to inaccessible feeding and draining vessels of cerebrovascular lesions, it is impossible to put temporary clips. For this reason, a balloon catheter technique was applied instead of temporary clips. By using balloon catheter method it is possible to occlude an inaccessible vessel such as in cases of giant basilar aneurysm and deep-seated AVMs.

Also now, new cerebral protective agents are being developed by animal experiments. Sendai Cocktail was also applied to the surgical treatment of acute stage of cerebral infarction, because it is able not only to protect ischemic insults but also to prevent hemorrhagic infarction and cerebral edema due to surgical revascularization [4]. Over 40 cases of acute stage of cerebral infarction were treated by this procedure [5].

References

1. Kayama T, Mizoi K, Suzuki J (1981) A canine model of a completely ischemic brain regulated with perfusion method. Surg Neurol 16: 167–172
2. Mizoi K, Yoshimoto T, Suzuki J (1981) Experimental study of new protective substances – Functional recovery of severe incomplete ischemic brain lesions, pretreated with mannitol and perfluorochemicals. Acta Neurochir (Wien) 56: 157–166
3. Suzuki J, Yoshimoto T (1979) The effect of mannitol in prolongation of permissible occlusion time of cerebral artery – clinical data of aneurysm surgery. Neurosurg Rev 1: 13–19
4. Suzuki J, Tanaka S, Yoshimoto T (1981) Suppression of brain swelling with mannitol and perfluorochemicals. An experimental study. Acta Neurochir (Wien) 58: 149–160
5. Suzuki J, Yoshimoto T, Kodama N et al. (1982) Development of a new therapeutic method for the acute period of brain infarction. Revascularization following administration of mannitol and perfluorochemicals. Preliminary report. Surg Neurol 17:332–352
6. Suzuki J, Onuma T, Kayama T (1982) Surgical treatment of intracranial arteriovenous malformation. Neurol Res 4: 191–207
7. Suzuki J, Yoshimoto T, Kayama T (1984) Surgical treatment of middle cerebral artery aneurysms. J Neurosurg 61: 17–23
8. Suzuki J, Fujimoto S, Mizoi K et al. (1984) The protective effect of combined administration of anti-oxidants and perfluorochemicals on cerebral ischemia. Stroke 15:672–679
9. Suzuki J, Imaizumi S, Kayama T (1985) Chemiluminescence of hypoxic Brain – The 2nd report: Cerebral protective effect of mannitol, Vitamin E and betamethasone. Stroke 16:695–700

Revascularization of the Brain Stem and Posterior Fossa

R. F. SPETZLER and M. N. HADLEY, Phoenix AZ/USA

Refined microneurosurgical techniques, sophisticated neurophysiologic monitoring and contemporary neuroanesthetic practices have greatly contributed to the advancement of neurovascular surgery. Revascularization of the cerebral hemispheres with extracranial to intracranial (EC-IC) bypass has long been possible. The concept of surgically treatable brain stem ischemia has gained increased attention in recent years; and technically more difficult posterior fossa EC-IC microvascular anastomoses have become feasible [1–3, 10, 13, 18].

We present our experience with 51 patients with debilitating symptoms of brain stem ischemia from both intracranial and extracranial vertebrobasilar disease and describe their surgical management.

Methods

All 51 patients underwent extensive neurologic and neuroradiologic evaluations including computerized cranial tomography and 4-vessel head and neck angiography with views of the aortic arch. Twenty-four patients were found to have extracranial vertebral artery compromise. Twenty-seven patients had intracranial vertebrobasilar pathology.

The same neurosurgeon (RFS) performed each of the 51 surgical procedures. Intraoperative neurophysiologic monitoring was utilized in each of the last 35 cases and included brain stem auditory and somatosensory cortical evoked potential recording. Barbiturate protection and blood pressure reduction therapy were administered by the neuroanesthetist in all 27 cases of EC-IC bypass and in the 3 cases of extracranial occipital to vertebral artery (VA) bypass.

All patients were followed postoperatively for a mean of 16 months. All but two patients underwent postoperative angiography or digital venous subtraction angiography.

Results

All 51 patients experienced recurrent episodes of transient brain stem ischemia despite antiplatelet or anticoagulation therapy. All had symptoms referable to the vertebrobasilar vascular tree and had correlative lesions on angiography (Table 1). These patients reported marked disability and compromise of their quality of life but were either without permanent brain stem or cerebellar deficits or had only mild dysfunction between ischemic events.

Table 1. Twenty-four patients were found to have extracranial pathology while twenty-seven patients had intracranial lesions as depicted above

	Angiographic findings	*Cases*
Extra-cranial	Proximal innominate or subclavian artery disease with steal	8
	Proximal band occlusion of vertebral artery (VA)	1
	Spondylitic compression, stenosis of VA	3
	Proximal VA occlusion	4
	Proximal VA stenosis with contralateral VA compromise	5
	Distal extracranial VA stenosis or pseudoaneurysm with contralateral VA compromise	3=24
Intra-cranial	Distal VA stenosis	3
	Distal VA occlusion	2
	Bilateral VA stenosis	1
	Bilateral VA occlusion	5
	VA occlusion with contralateral VA stenosis	8
	Proximal basilar artery (BA) occlusion	1
	Distal BA stenosis	2
	Distal BA occlusion	2
	Branch occlusions BA	1
	BA stenosis with unilateral VA occlusion	2=27
Total		=51

Table 2. Classification of procedures performed for vertebro-basilar insufficiency

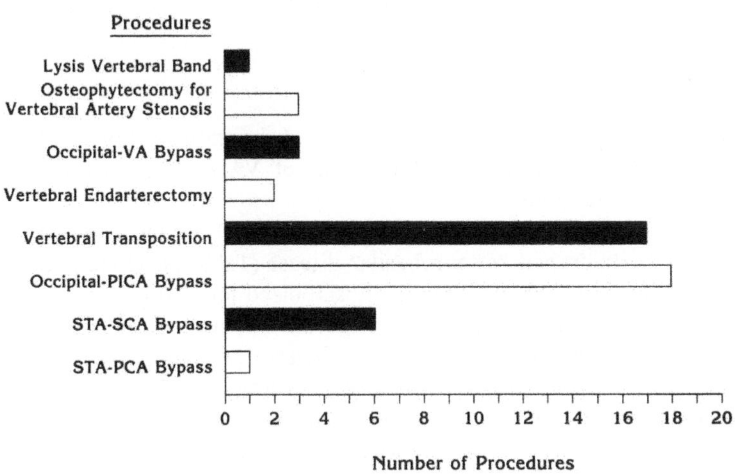

Extracranial

We performed 17 vertebral artery transpositions for proximal VA stenosis (16 of 17 cases had contralateral VA compromise), (Figs. 1, 2), one lysis of fascial bands for intermittent proximal VA occlusion [14], three cervical osteophytectomies for mid-portion VA spondolytic compromise and 3 extracranial-extradural occipital artery to distal VA anastomoses [11], (two for distal VA stenosis, one for a traumatic C-1–C-2 level pseudoaneurysm with dissection) (Table 2).

1 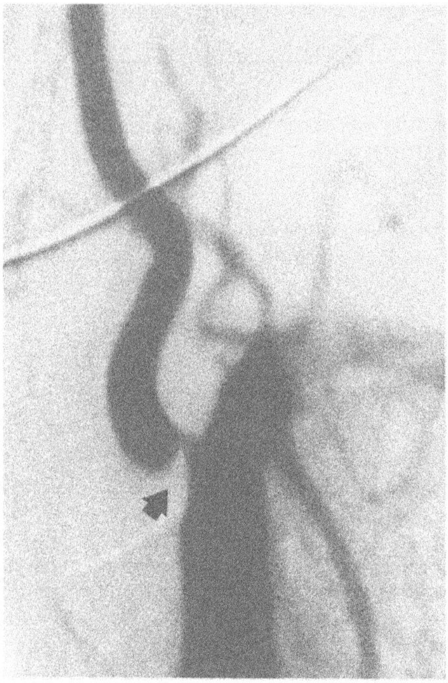

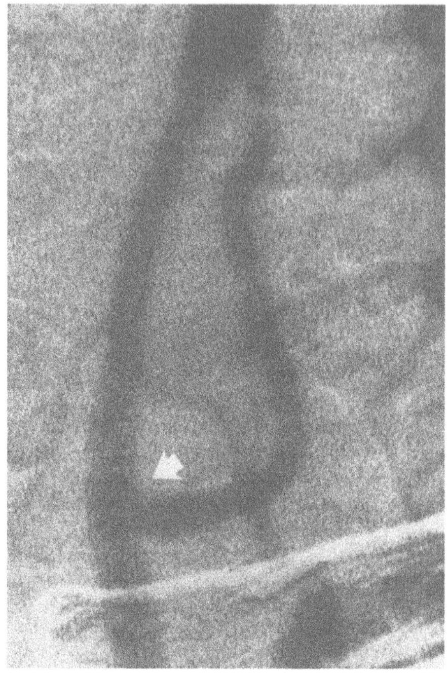 2

Fig. 1. Severe proximal VA stenosis (*arrow*)

Fig. 2. Digital subtraction study demonstrating end-to-side VA to common carotid artery transposition (*arrow*)

Postoperative angiography revealed 100% patency of the transpositions and bypasses (occipital to VA), and complete elimination of VA compromise due to spondylitic disease or fascial bands.

There were no significant postoperative complications (early or late) among the 24 patients treated for extracranial vertebrobasilar disease (Table 3). Three patients with fluctuating neurologic deficits preoperatively stabilized following vertebral artery transposition. Two subsequently improved; the third continued to have "vertebrobasilar symptoms". He was the only patient in the transposition group who did not have contralateral vertebral artery hypoplasia, agenesis or occlusion. He remains a diagnostic enigma. All of the other patients showed progressive neurologic recovery and have had no evidence of further ischemic symptoms. A few patients on whom we performed vertebral artery transposition developed a transient postoperative Horner's syndrome. They all cleared within a period of two weeks. These minor postoperative complications were due to the surgical manipulation of the cervical sympathetic chain during dissection of the proximal vertebral artery.

Intracranial

Eighteen of the 27 procedures performed in the treatment of intracranial vertebrobasilar insufficiency were occipital artery to posterior inferior cerebellar artery

Table 3. An analysis of early post-operative complications (0 to 30 days) in fifty-one procedures for vertebro-basilar insufficiency. There were no late complications or deaths

Complications	Comp/Cases	Description
Extracranial		
VA transposition	5/17	(1)–(5) Transient Horner's syndrome
Osteophytectomy	0/3	
VA band lysis	0/1	
Occipital-VA	0/3	
	5/24	
Intracranial		
Occipital-PICA	4/18	(1) Hydrocephalus (2) Aseptic meningitis (3) + (4) Respiratory insufficiency
STA-SCA	4/6	(1) Temporary worsening of deficits (2) Confusion, agitation, disorientation (3) Aseptic meningitis (4) Seizure, cardiac dysrhythmias
STA-PCA	1/1	(1) Seizure, post-op hematoma
VA endarterectomy	2/2	(1) Marked confusion/hydrocephalus (2) Marked confusion, disorientation, transient hydrocephalus
	11/27	

anastomoses. There were six STA-SCA and one STA-PCA anastomoses and two intracranial distal vertebral artery endarterectomies (Table 2).

These patients, like those with extracranial vertebrobasilar disease, were severely disabled from hemodynamic compromise of brain stem blood flow. In each case there was either a tandem lesion in the contralateral vertebral artery – or the opposite vertebral was absent, hypoplastic or terminated in the posterior inferior cerebellar artery. Eight patients had stenotic lesions or occlusion of the basilar artery with incomplete collateral blood supply to cerebellar or brain stem structures.

Only one of the 25 bypasses was not patent on postoperative examination (STA-SCA). Both of the intracranial vertebral artery endarterectomies were widely patent on follow-up angiography (total intracranial patency rate was 96%). There were no new strokes noted on postoperative computerized cranial tomography. Of the eight patients with preoperative stroke, seven have shown improvement following posterior fossa revascularization with time and rehabilitative therapy. One patient with significant right facial paresis, slurred speech and right body ataxia remains unchanged (Occip-PICA).

We had eleven transient postoperative complications in this group (Table 3). Four of the eighteen patients with an occipital to PICA bypass (Figs. 3, 4), developed either aseptic meningitis, respiratory insufficiency or hydrocephalus. These patients were treated with steroids, supportive therapy, and a lumboperitoneal shunt respectively. All improved to their preoperative baseline. An additional four complications occurred among the six patients who had a STA-SCA anastomosis (Figs. 5 and 6). One patient had temporary worsening of his severe cerebellar defi-

3 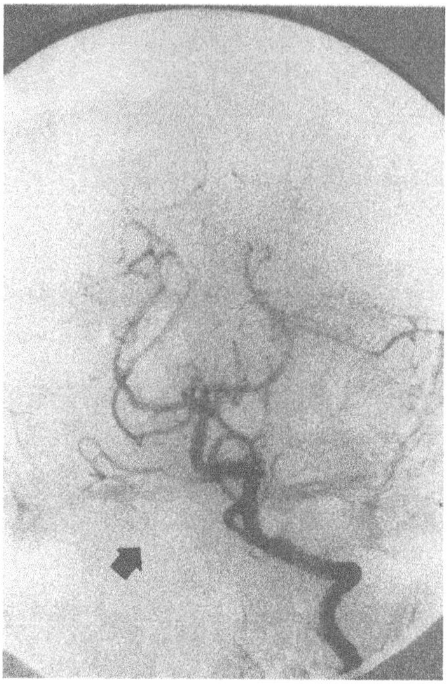 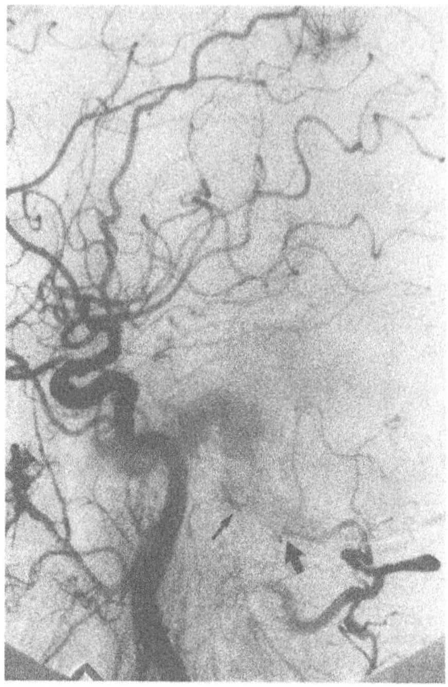 4

Fig. 3. Anteroposterior view of vertebrobasilar circulation. Note absence of PICA territory blood supply due to proximal PICA occlusion (*arrow*)

Fig. 4. Lateral view, common carotid injection demonstrating occipital to PICA anastomosis (*large arrow*) and flow into PICA distribution and vertebral artery (*small arrow*)

cits. Postoperative angiography demonstrated occlusion of the bypass graft. He improved with supportive therapy but not beyond his preoperative condition. One patient had multiple cardiac dysrhythmias and a single generalized seizure on the seventh postoperative day. Both conditions were effectively treated with appropriate medication. Two patients developed confusion and irritability and were found to have aseptic meningitis. Both responded well to steroid and supportive therapy. Our only patient with a STA-PCA bypass developed generalized seizures on the third postoperative day with worsening of his preoperative hemiparesis. The bypass was patent on angiography but a CT scan revealed a small hematoma with mass effect at the operative site. The patient's seizures and hemiparesis resolved correlating with resolution of the hematoma on serial CT studies. Both patients who underwent vertebral artery endarterectomy developed postoperative aseptic meningitis. One also manifested persistent ventriculomegally (communicating hydrocephalus) which resolved with placement of a lumboperitoneal shunt. Both patients were back to full activities and employment on last examination.

5 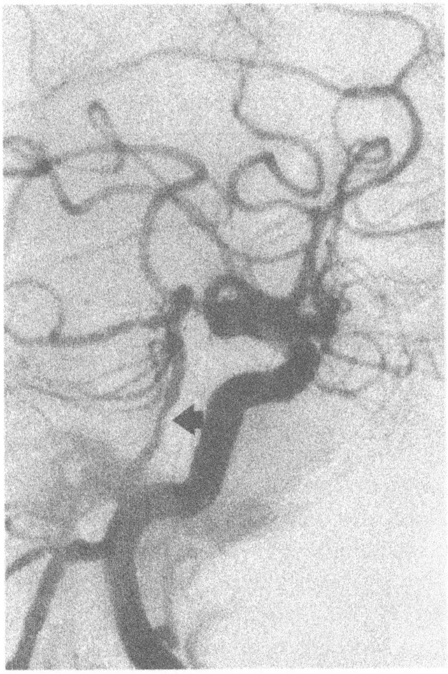 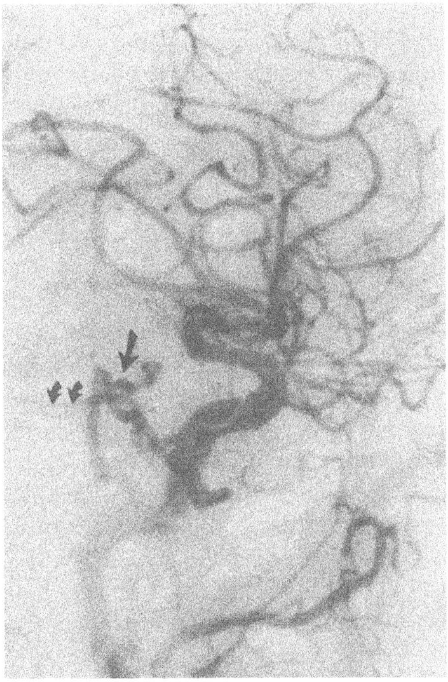 6

Fig. 5. Lateral view depicting mid-basilar stenosis (*arrow*)

Fig. 6. Postoperative common carotid angiogram demonstrating STA-SCA anastomosis (*large arrow*) and SCA flow (*small arrows*)

Discussion

Symptoms of vertebrobasilar insufficiency (i.e. cerebellar and brain stem ischemia) are often poorly characterized and are usually less concrete than symptoms of TIA or stroke in the anterior circulation. Accordingly, symptoms of vertebrobasilar insufficiency may be recognized less frequently than symptoms of anterior circulation ischemia, further confusing the issue of the natural history of the disease. It is well known that patients with transient ischemic events in the vertebrobasilar distribution can progress to frank infarction. While vertebrobasilar TIAs were only half as common as anterior circulation TIAs in the series reported by Cartlidge and associates, they were not less ominous [6, 20]. The risk of stroke following a TIA in either vascular distribution appears to be equal, roughly 7% per year.

Patient selection is important when considering the efficacy of posterior fossa revascularization. Only those patients with severe symptoms referable to cerebellar or brain stem ischemia, with correlative angiographic evidence of hemodynamic compromise should be considered as surgical candidates [5, 10, 12, 18]. Castaigne and colleagues discovered that most brain stem infarctions were the result of thrombosis or branch occlusion of a preexisting stenotic lesion [7]. It is those stenotic or preocclusive lesions in the vertebral or basilar arteries, symptomatic despite antiplatelet or anticoagulation therapy, which we feel are most amenable to surgical intervention. However, not all patients with vertebral artery stenosis or occlusion should be considered for decompression or transposition. While thromboembolic TIAs do occur in the vertebrobasilar distribution, the great majority of TIAs are due to transient hemodynamic insufficiency [5, 8, 16]. In all but one case in our series, patients had significant compromise of posterior fossa collateral blood flow from either contralateral vertebral artery compromise (disease, hypoplasia, agenesis, PICA termination), or significant basilar artery stenosis, or both. The diverse and often multiple pathologic causes of vertebrobasilar ischemia may be treated by a number of bypass alternatives. New, refined microsurgical techniques allow revascularization to be directed to the area(s) of greatest need [1–4, 9–13, 15, 18].

Anastomotic revascularization procedures, particularly those for intracranial disease, require considerable skill, patience and microvascular surgical experience. Neurophysiologic monitoring and contemporary neuroanesthetic practices are important surgical adjuncts. We employ continuous intraoperative EEG and spectral array analysis in conjunction with somatosensory cortical and brain stem evoked potential recording. Analysis of our results indicates that this sensitive combination of intraoperative patient evaluation is of considerable value for determining the depth and effect of barbiturate anesthesia and provides a sensitive warning system for potential ischemic or retraction injury [17]. Our experience with barbiturate anesthesia, with and without systemic hypotension, has been positive [19, 21]. We have had no major operative morbidity and zero operative mortality utilizing these microneurosurgical techniques and intraoperative adjuncts.

The intracranial revascularization procedures are the most difficult to perform as evidenced by our significant occurrence of postoperative complications (11 of 27 procedures). Fortunately, these were transient complications and did not contribute to long-term patient morbidity or mortality. Based on this experience involving 51 patients, we feel that brain stem and posterior fossa revascularization benefits selected patients and in most cases improves their quality of life.

References

1. Allen GS, Cohen RJ, Preziosi TJ (1981) Microsurgical endarterectomy of the intracranial vertebral artery for vertebrobasilar transient ischemic attacks. Neurosurgery 8:56–59
2. Ausman JI, Diaz FG, de los Reyes RA, Pak H, Patel S, Boulos R (1981) Anastomosis of occipital artery to anterior inferior cerebellar artery for vertebrobasilar junction stenosis. Surg Neurol 16:99–102
3. Ausman JI, Diaz FG, de los Reyes RA, Pak H, Patel S, Mehta B, Boulos R (1982) Posterior circulation revascularization. J Neurosurg 56:766–776
4. Camp PE (1984) Carotid to distal vertebral artery bypass for vertebrobasilar ischemia. J Neurosurg 60:187–189
5. Caplan LR (1981) Current concepts of cerebrovascular disease – stroke. Vertebrobasilar disease – time for a new strategy. Stroke 12:111–114
6. Cartlidge NEF, Whisnant JP, Elveback LR (1977) Carotid and vertebral-basilar transient cerebral ischemic attacks. A community study, Rochester Minnesota. Mayo Clin Proc 52:117–120
7. Castaigne P, Lhermitte F, Gautier JC, Escourolle R, Derouesne C, Der Agopian P, Popa C (1973) Arterial occlusions in the vertebro-basilar system: A study of 44 patients with post-mortem data. Brain 96:133–154

8. Fisher CM (1977) Occlusion of the vertebral arteries. Arch Neurol 22:13–19
9. George B, Laurian C (1980) Surgical approach to the whole length of the vertebral artery with special reference to the third portion. Acta Neurochir (Wien) 51:259–272
10. Hadley MN, Masferrer R, Zabramski JM, Spetzler RF (1985) Management of vertebrobasilar insufficiency. In: Spetzler RF, Selman WR, Carter LP, Martin NA (eds) Cerebral Revascularization for Stroke. Thieme-Stratton, New York, pp 475–482
11. Hadley MN, Spetzler RF, Masferrer R, Martin NA, Carter LP (1985) Occipital artery to extradural vertebral artery bypass: A case report. J Neurosurg (in press)
12. Hopkins LN, Budny JL (1985) A rational surgical approach to vertebrobasilar ischemia. In: Spetzler RF, Selman R, Carter LP, Martin NA (eds) Cerebral Revascularization for Stroke. Thieme-Stratton, New York, pp 490–504
13. Hopkins LN, Budny JL, Spetzler RF (1982) Revascularization of the rostral brain stem. Neurosurgery 10:364–369
14. Mapstone T, Spetzler RF (1982) Vertebrobasilar insufficiency secondary to vertebral artery occlusion from a fibrous band. J Neurosurg 56:581–583
15. Nagashima C (1970) Surgical treatment of vertebral artery insufficiency caused by cervical spondylosis. J Neurosurg 32:512–521
16. Naritomi H, Sakai F, Meyer JS (1979) Pathogenesis of transient ischemic attacks within the vertebrobasilar arterial system. Arch Neurol 36:121–128
17. Raudzens PA, Spetzler RF, Carter LP, Wilkinson E (1985) Cerebral electrical activity during low flow states. In: Spetzler RF, Selman WR, Carter LP, Martin NA (eds) Cerebral Revascularization for Stroke. Thieme-Stratton, New York, pp 189–196
18. Roski RA, Spetzler RF, Hopkins LN (1982) Occipital artery to posterior inferior cerebellar artery bypass for vertebrobasilar ischemia. Neurosurgery 10:44–49
19. Spetzler RF, Selman WR, Roski RA, Bonstelle C (1982) Cerebral revascularization during barbiturate coma in primates and man. Surg Neurol 17:111–115
20. Whisnant JP, Cartlidge NEF, Elveback LR (1978) Carotid and vertebral-basilar transient ischemic attacks: Effect of anticoagulants, hypertension, and cardiac disorders on survival and stroke occurrence – a population study. Ann Neurol 3:107–115
21. Wilkinson E, Spetzler RF, Carter LP, Raudzens PA (1985) Intraoperative barbiturate therapy during temporary vessel occlusion in man. In: Spetzler RF, Selman WR, Carter LP, Martin NA (eds) Cerebral Revascularization for Stroke. Thieme-Stratton, New York, pp 397–402

Revascularization of the Brain Stem: Anatomical Basis, Clinical Results and Long-Term Angiographic Follow-Up – Ten Years Experience

J. I. Ausman, F. G. Diaz, M. Dujovny, C. Shrontz, J. Pearce, R. A. De Los Reyes, S. Patel, B. Mehta and R. Boulos, Detroit MI/USA

The first report of vertebral basilar bypass surgery appeared in 1975 with an occipital artery (OA) to posterior inferior cerebellar artery (PICA) bypass procedure (Ausman et al. 1976). Then the OA to anterior inferior cerebellar artery (AICA) (Ausman et al. 1981) and superficial temporal artery (STA) to superior cerebellar artery (SCA) bypass (Ausman et al. 1979) were introduced to provide additional blood flow to presumed hemodynamically compromised areas of the brain stem. The principle followed was to allow the revascularization of the vertebral basilar arterial system distal to a stenotic or an occlusive lesion. Thus, the OA-PICA bypass was used for stenosis or occlusions in the vertebral artery (VA) proximal to PICA. The OA-AICA bypass was utilized for stenotic or occlusive lesions proximal to AICA and the STA-SCA anastomosis for lesions proximal to SCA. We are reporting the results of 10 years of experience with vertebral basilar revascularization in 50 patients.

Methods

The methods for the anatomical studies of the resin injected vessels of fresh autopsied brains have been previously written and reviewed (Gomes et al. 1984).

The operative approaches for the OI-PICA, OA-PICA, and STA-SCA bypasses have been described and summarized in other articles and will not be reviewed here (Ausman et al. 1985).

Cerebral angiography is performed by neuroradiologists, usually through the transfemoral route. The origins, extra- and intracranial courses of each of the carotid and vertebral arteries are selectively studied preoperatively. In some patients who are clinically unstable, angiography was performed after low molecular weight dextran was given to prevent rouleaux formation and after volume loading of the patients. In those unstable patients who were referred with adequate angiographic studies, a repeat preoperative angiogram was not performed.

An *unstable* patient is defined as one who has frequent symptoms of vertebral basilar insufficiency (VBI) requiring intravenous anticoagulation, a *stable* patient as one who has episodic VBI not requiring intravenous anticoagulant therapy.

Vertebral basilar insufficiency has been defined for our patients previously. Patients must have two or more symptoms or signs indicating involvement of brain stem structures or occipital lobes. Dizziness alone is not a sufficient symptom for VBI. Our patients had four or five symptoms or signs consistent with the clinical diagnosis VBI.

Results

Anatomical

Superior Cerebellar Artery

The best site for anastomosis was in the lateral midbrain segment of the superior cerebellar artery. This segment is seen underneath the arachnoid at the edge of the tentorium usually before the 4th nerve enters the dura. It has less branches to the brain stem in this segment. It is single or paired and has a diameter in this location of 1.1 to 1.4 mm. If it is the major source of collateral to the distal basilar artery, the anastomosis and temporary clipping should be done on the vessel after it branches to allow uninterrupted flow in the vessel during the anastomosis.

Anterior Inferior Cerebellar Artery

First, the vessel is confirmed as being the AICA by following it towards the basilar artery. The optimum site of the anastomosis is in the region after the vessel leaves the area of the 7th and 8th nerves in the cistern before it reaches the cerebellum. Its size in this location is 1.0 to 1.1 mm. There are the least branches to the brain stem in this segment.

Posterior Inferior Cerebellar Artery

As PICA exits from the vertebral artery, it travels between the 9th and 10th cranial nerves in its course along the lateral medulla. In this area the artery is 1.7 to 1.8 mm in diameter and has few small perforating branches which make it optimal for anastomosis with the occipital artery. The site has less perforating branches and is of larger caliber than the tonsillar segment or the hemispheral branch of PICA.

Clinical

The clinical results are divided between those patients who present with unstable VBI and those with stable VBI.

Table 1.

		Mortality	Morbidity	Asymptomatic improved
STA-SCA	Unstable (15)	(4) 27%	(5) 33%	(6) 40%
	Stable (14)	(1) 7%	(2) 14%	(11) 79%
OA-AICA	Unstable (2)	0%	0%	(2) 100%
	Stable (7)	0%	0%	(7) 100%
OA-PICA	Unstable (2)	(1) 50%	0%	(1) 100%
	Stable (10)	(1) 10%	(1) 10%	(8) 80%
Total		(7) 14%	(8) 16%	(35) 70%

Table 1 depicts the results of three different vertebral basilar revascularization operations in stable and unstable patients with VBI. In the STA-SCA bypass where there are sufficient numbers to establish a trend, it appears as though those who are unstable have a lower chance of improvement than those who are stable. Overall 35 of 50 patients have been helped (70%) with posterior circulation revascularization operations. Forty-seven percent (9 of 19) unstable patients were helped and 83% (26 of 31) stable patients can benefit from surgical revascularization.

Angiography

As in the anterior circulation bypass, the size of the STA and the number of vessels filled in the vertebral basilar revascularization operation increase with time.

Discussion

Our anatomical studies have revealed the most optimum sites for the anastomosis in the SCA, AICA, and PICA vessels. These sites, at the lateral midbrain, beyond the 7th and 8th nerve segments, and at the lateral medulla near the 9th and 10th nerves respectively, have the fewest perforators to the brain stem and have an adequate diameter.

Clinically the operation is based on a hypothesis that a flow deficiency is the cause of symptoms and if corrected, the patients will improve. The data supports this hypothesis that the bypass actually is correcting a blood flow related to symptomatology.

Obviously those unstable VBI patients in our series are medical treatment failures. They have continued to be symptomatic even on intravenous anticoagulants. It is probable that a high percentage of these patients would succumb to their disease. The fact that 40% of the unstable patients can be helped with surgical bypass, while 60% have mortality or morbidity must be viewed in the perspective of patients who have no other alternative treatment.

It can be stated that to continue to treat patients until they are medically unstable also will compromise the surgical alternative.

Only long term follow-up of medically and surgically treated series of patients can prove the ultimate benefit of either therapy.

References

Ausman JI, Lee MC, Klassen AC, Seljeskog EL, Chou SN (1976) Stroke: Whats new? Cerebral revascularization. Minn Med 59:223–227

Ausman JI, Lee MC, Chater N, Latchaw RE (1979) Superficial temporal artery to superior cerebellar artery anastomosis for distal basilar artery stenosis. Surg Neurol 12:277–282

Ausman JI, Diaz FG, de los Reyes RA, Pak N, Patel S, Boulos R (1981) Anastomosis of occipital artery to anterior inferior cerebellar artery for vertebrobasilar junction stenosis. Surg Neurol 16:199–202

Ausman JI, Diaz FG, de los Reyes RA, Pearce JR, Shrontz C, Pak H (1985) Microsurgery for arteriosclerosis in the distal vertebral and basilar arteries. In: Rand R (ed) Microneurosurgery. CV Mosby, St. Louis, pp 497–512

Gomes FB, Dujovny M, Umansky F, Ausman JI, Diaz FG, Ray WJ, Mirchandani NG (1984) The recurrent artery of Huebner. J Neurosurg 60:130–139

Prognostic Factors Implicated in the Microsurgical Treatment of Trigeminal Neuralgia

M. SINDOU and J. SZAPIRO, Lyon/France

An ever growing number of publications concerning the results of Micro-Vascular Decompression (MVD) in cases of Neuro-Vascular Conflict (NVC) has appeared during the last years, and a motivated optimism as to its further perspectives has been expressed. However, the very fact that the patient has to face an open intracranial operation versus percutaneous procedures (RF-thermocoagulation and glycerol injection) remains incontestable (Apfelbaum 1984; Burchiel et al. 1981; Penzholz and Kühner 1981).

This study analyzes a series of 100 patients referred with the diagnosis of idiopathic Trigeminal Neuralgia (TN) and operated on through a direct microsurgical approach, with the aim of getting insight into the influence of some clinical, angiographic, anatomical and operative factors on the results of MVD.

Material and Method

In the last 6 years, 100 TN have been operated upon at the cerebellopontine angle, i.e. 20% of the total series of 513 patients with tic douloureux, 413 of them having been submitted to percutaneous RF-thermocoagulation.

In 10 of the above patients, 8 tumors and 2 angiomas have been found and removed. In all but 3 of the other 90 patients, a NVC has been revealed (Table 1). In 17 of them a selective section of the trigeminal root had to be performed, as its

Table 1. Etiologies of trigeminal neuralgia in 100 cases treated with direct CPA approach

Symptomatic neuralgias (10 cases)

Total removal	Meningioma	3	Arach. cyst.	1	VIIIth neurinoma	1
	Cholesteatoma	2	Vth neurinoma	1	Angioma	2

Neuro-vascular conflicts (87 out of 100 cases)

	Vert-bas.	SCA	AICA	SCA+ AICA	SCA+ Vein	Vein	Art.+ Pre[a]	None
Part rhiz (20 cases)	9	0	1	1	2	0	4	3
MVD (70 cases)	0	48	4	7	7	4	0	0
Total	9	48	5	8	9	4	4	3

[a] Pre: predominant petrous ridge elevation

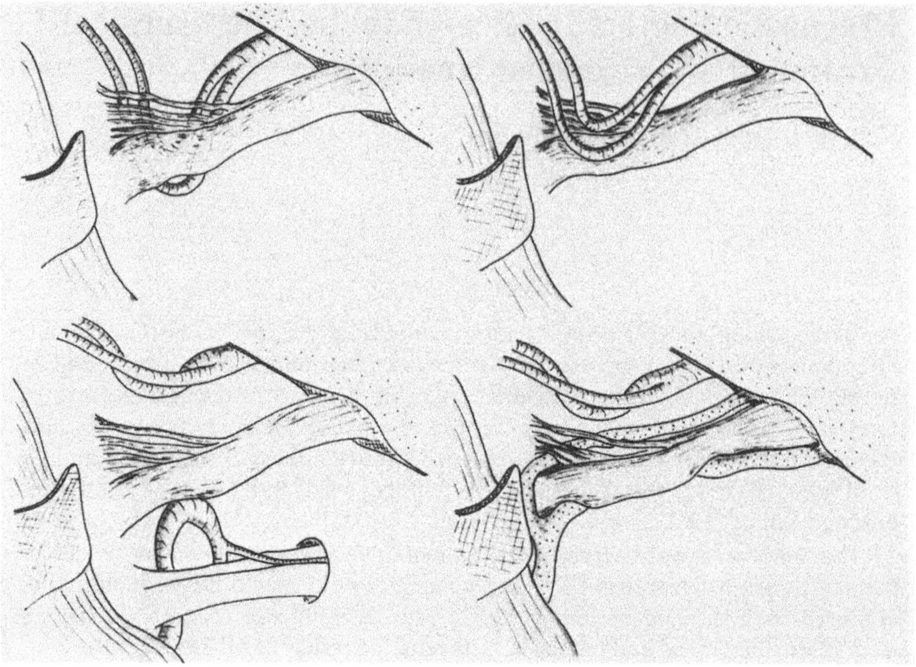

Fig. 1. Various types of Neuro-Vascular Conflicts: SCA in antero-superior (*upper left*) or postero-superior (*upper right*) position. AICA inferiorly cross-compressing the Vth REZ (*lower left*). Satellite trigeminal veins embedded in nerve tissue (*lower right*)

cross-compression could not be completely eliminated. *In 70 patients, a MVD was performed* according to Jannetta's microsurgical technique (1976, 1981) (Fig. 1).

In most cases, the conflicting agent was *a vascular loop of a cerebellar megadolicho-artery,* usually compressing the root entry zone (REZ) into the pons. The superior cerebellar artery (SCA) was the most frequent compressive agent either isolated in 48 cases, or associated with another factor in 14 cases. It compressed the REZ, antero-superiorly (AS) in 43.3% and postero-superiorly (PS) in 56.7% of the cases. When the antero-inferior cerebellar artery (AICA) was responsible (4 cases), the cross-compression was always located inferiorly to the nerve. The treatment consisted of detaching and transposing the arterial loop away from the nerve. Then the conflicting vessel was maintained apart in the most normal situation as possible, i.e. upwards for the SCA and downwards for the AICA. This was achieved by interposing a small piece of periosteum in the 29 first cases of the series or a square of Dacron stretch N° 09114 (Meadox Medicals Inc., Oakland N.J.) – 1 mm thick and 5 to 10 mm in size – in association with the periosteum in the 36 following cases.

When NVC was *a satellite trigeminal vein* coursing alongside the nerve (4 times isolately, 7 in association), it was suppressed by coagulating and resecting the venous compressing segment.

Overall Results

The results of this series of 100 patients have been analysed after a one year to five years follow-up.

The neurological complications related to the CPA approach were the following: 2 transient and 1 permanent occipital neuralgias; 2 transient diplopias after manipulation of the IVth nerve; 1 severe and 1 mild decrease of hearing, 1 transient tinnitus and 1 facial nerve paresis. The 3 latter complications occurred in the early cases of the series, and have not been observed since pre-operative monitoring of the Auditory Evoked Potentials had shown us that the stretching of acoustic-facial nerves could be avoided in approaching the trigeminal root via the supra-cerebellar rather than the latero-cerebellar route (Grundy et al. 1982; Fischer et al. 1985). Except for the cases with partial juxta-pontine rhizotomy, impairment of trigeminal functions was scarce and, when present, always transient. One death out of two was related to surgery; it was due to a large hemorrhagic cerebellar infarct secondary to extensive coagulations of the cerebellopontine angle (CPA) veins and a prolonged spasm of the SCA.

As regards to *the results on pain,* we must mention that a total relief was obtained in all of the 10 symptomatic neuralgias, after total removal of the causal lesions; as well as in 17 of the 20 cases treated with partial rhizotomy.

The next part deals with the results obtained in the 68 MVD group: A complete and hopefully permanent cure has been obtained in 82.36% of these patients. The word "hopefully" has been used, because out of 56 patients with excellent results, 11 have been followed for 12 months only, further 16 for 1 year–2 years, while the remaining 29 for 2–5 years. A rubric of a dissociated cure concerns 2 patients (2.94%) in whom a total relief of paroxysmal pain has been obtained, but still a background of a permanent pain at least partially persisted. This result has been evaluated as fairly good. The same estimation concerned 2 further patients (2.94%) who had a satisfactory improvement, which means that intensity and frequency of pain has been remarkably diminished so that it could be controlled with very low doses and/or episodic medical therapy. So the rate of *excellent and good results amounts to 88.23%.*

In turn, 3 patients (4.41%) have been placed in the rubric of unsatisfactory improvement. The intensity and/or frequency of their pain has also been diminished, but to a lesser degree, and they need an every day pharmacological treatment. There were, finally, 3 cases of failure (4.41%) and 2 cases of recurrence (2.94%), after respectively 8 and 12 months of follow-up. These 8 cases can be evidently grouped as *bad results (11.77%).*

Clinical Prognostic Factors

The mode of painful manifestations and the territorial extent of the neuralgia significantly influenced the quality of MVD results, whereas age, duration of symptoms, pain intensity and frequency did not.

Out of the 44 patients with paroxysmal pain only, in 42 a complete cure has been obtained (95.45%). Conversely, out of 24 patients with paroxysmal pain occurring

Table 2. Correlation of mode of pain manifestation and pain area with cure/total ratio

	Cure/total (%)		
Mode of pain manifestation \ Pain area	One branch	2–3 branches	Total
Paroxysmal pain only	20/20 (100.0)	22/24 (91.6)	42/44 (95.5)
Paroxysmal and permanent pain	7/ 8 (87.5)	7/16 (43.8)	14/24 (58.3)
Total	27/28 (96.4)	29/40 (72.5)	56/68 (82.4)

on the background of a permanent pain, 14 only have had a total relief of their pain (58.3%). This negative influence of *permanent pain* on postoperative results was found to be highly significant ($p < 0.001$).

The extent of pain also influenced the prognosis. Out of 28 patients whose pain involved only one branch of the Vth nerve, 27 were completely cured (96.4%). In turn, out of 40 patients with pain extending to 2–3 branches, 29 were cured (72.5%). This difference proved to be significant ($p < 0.05$).

Although the distribution of the two above cited factors were not correlated in our series, they were found to combine for prognosis evaluation (Table 2). Indeed out of 20 patients with paroxysmal pain only and its extent to one branch, all were cured, whereas out of 16 patients with paroxysmal and permanent pain extending to 2–3 branches, 7 only obtained a total relief (43.8%). It is interesting to note that both these factors, mode of painful manifestations ($P < 0.01$) and extent of pain ($P < 0.05$), have been derived from anamnestic data only.

Angiographic Studies

A vertebral angiogram on the TN side has been done in all the cases of MVD, in order to predict the agent of the NVC. Only the course of SCA – the most frequent cause (77.5%) – could be correctly analysed, in the AP Towne semi-axial view.

The course of the *SCA circumpontic loop,* at the level of the trigeminal REZ, was evaluated by measuring the distance of its infero-lateral extreme point (P), 1) from the horizontal line corresponding to the basilar bifurcation, and 2) from the median vertical axis. Then P co-ordinates on the TN side were compared to the contralateral ones.

This study which has been done in 57 interpretative angiograms, has led to the following conclusions (Fig. 2):

1) When P on TN side was both more inferior and more lateral in comparison with contralateral P, SCA was the only NVC agent in all the 18 patients of this group (100%)

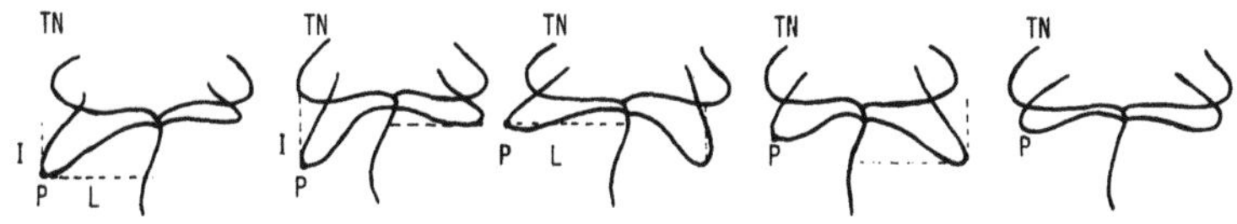

TOTAL	I+, L+ = 18 CASES	I+, L- = 14 CASES	I-, L+ = 18 CASES	I-, L- = 4 CASES	NORMAL = 3 CASES
SCA	18 AS = 15 , PS = 3	10 AS = 7 , PS = 3	13 AS = 4 , PS = 9		
AICA		1		2	2
SCA + AICA		2 AS = 0 , PS = 2	2 AS = 0 , PS = 2	2 AS = 0 , PS = 2	
VEIN		1	1		1
SCA + VEIN			2 AS = 1 , PS = 1		

Fig. 2. Vertebral angiographic studies: correlations between SCA position and operative findings
P = extreme infero-lateral point of the SCA circum pontic loop

2) When P was either more inferior or more lateral on TN side (32 cases), SCA was the only cause in 23 cases (71.8%) or one of the conflicting vessels in 6 other cases (18.7%)
3) When SCA on TN side was in a normal position (3 cases), i.e. strictly parallel to the posterior cerebral artery course, or making a loop, but with a less inferior and lateral P than on the unaffected side (4 cases), NVC resulted from an SCA, in association with another factor, in only two cases.

Anatomical Findings and Operative Modalities Implicated in MVD Prognosis

The *anatomical data* concerning the various agents of NVC, as well as those related to the site and degree of nerve compression, have been detailed in Table 1 and Fig. 2. A correlative study of these findings with the results did not show any statistically significant influence of these factors on MVD prognosis.

In turn, some *operative modalities* have been revealed to play a significant role. They concern this part of the procedure with aims to maintain the artery apart from the root and to prevent the possibility of recurrence of NVC. In 29 cases, a piece of periosteum was interposed between the root and the conflicting artery, and in 36 cases a piece of Dacron has been added to ascertain the protection of the root. The results proved to be excellent in almost all the cases of paroxysmal pain only, independently of the material used, respectively in 20 out of 21 (95.2%) and in 21 out of 22 (95.4%). But among 22 cases with a permanent pain component, 11 patients were cured out of 14 in whom pieces of periosteum and Dacron have been applied (78.6%), while 2 only have been relieved out of 8 patients in whom a piece of periosteum alone has been interposed (25%). This difference proved to be significant ($p < 0.02$) (Table 3).

The favorable effect of Dacron interposition seems to be related to the fact that this non-absorbable prosthesis, thanks to its semi-rigidity, reduces nerve compression by the transposed artery, the arterial pulsations being damped down by the soft piece of periosteum. With Dacron it was easier to restitute a normal course of the nerve, in suppressing its angulation when crossing the petrous ridge (Fig. 3). This technical point might contribute to the cure of the permanent pain component, that could be at least partly related to the nerve angulation, as previously mentioned by Gardner et al. 1956, Gardner 1958 and Malis 1967.

Table 3. Correlation of operative procedure with cure/total ratio

	Cure/total (%)		
Mode of pain manifestation \ Operative procedure	Periosteum only	Periosteum and dacron	Total
Paroxysmal pain only	20/21 (95.2)	21/22 (95.4)	41/43 (95.3)
Paroxysmal and permanent pain	2/ 8 (25)	11/14 (78.6)	13/22 (59)
Total	22/29 (75.8)	32/36 (88.8)	54/65 (83.1)

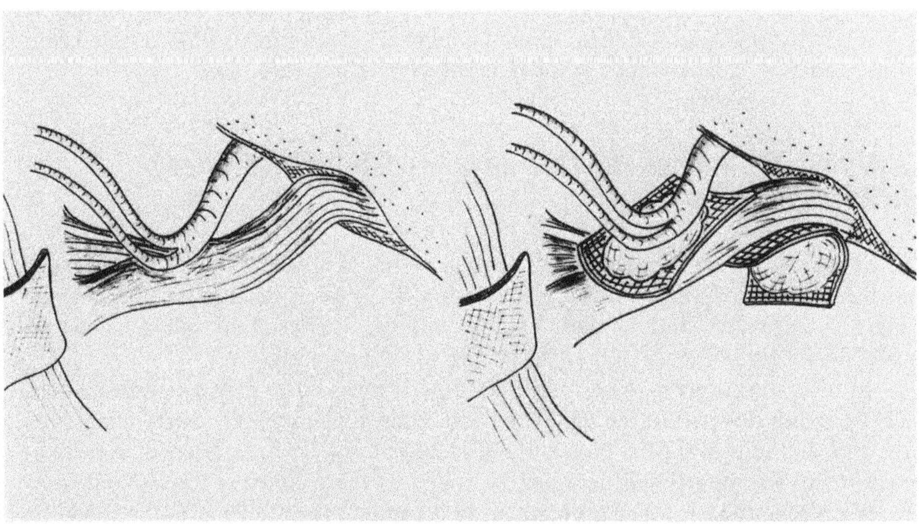

Fig. 3. Neuro-Vascular Conflict depressing the Vth REZ by SCA, associated with nerve angulation when crossing the petrous ridge (*left*). Micro-Vascular Decompression and restitution of the normal course of the nerve, using Dacron and periosteum (*right*)

Conclusions

This critical study (Szapiro 1985) has been made in search for the causes of unsatisfactory results and for the possibilities of making MVD efficacy ascertained in a higher percentage of patients.

Some *clinical factors* proved to be of paramount importance for the prognosis. The most evident has been a highly significant difference in the rate of a total cure in patients with attacks of tic douloureux only (94.5%) and in those with associated permanent pain (58.3%).

The analysis of the *operative findings* and of the details of the *surgical procedures* indicated to a necessity of restitution of the normal course and shape of the trigeminal root from the petrous ridge up to the entry-zone and completed by an adequate root protection (for instance with Dacron), after the Vth nerve had been detached from the conflicting vessel.

A correlation of the above findings with *the angiographic studies* has been made. Although the presence of cerebellar megadolicho-arteries is far from being specific, a careful study of their course – mainly of SCA, which was the most frequent NVC cause (77.5%) – may be of some help in predicting the conflicting agent. The absence of a significant displacement of SCA must incite the surgeon to search for another factor or several associated factors.

Acknowledgement: The authors thank Professor Jerzy Szapiro from Warsaw (Poland) for his participation in this study.

References

Apfelbaum RI (1984) Surgery for tic douloureux. Clin Neurosurg 31:351–368

Burchiel KJ, Steege TD, Howe JF, Loeser JD (1981) Comparison of percutaneous radiofrequency gangliolysis and microvascular decompression for the surgical management of tic douloureux. Neurosurgery 9:111–119

Fischer C, Ibanez V, Mauguiere F (1985) Evalution of BAEP changes in intra-operative monitoring. XIth Int. Congress of E.E.G., London (to be published)

Gardner WJ, Todd EM, Pinto JP (1956) Roentgenographic findings in trigeminal neuralgia. Am J Roentgenol 76:346–350

Gardner WJ (1958) Trigeminal neuralgia. Clin Neurosurg 15:1–56

Grundy BL, Jannetta PJ, Procopio PI, Ling A, Boston R, Doyle E (1982) Intraoperative monitoring of Brainstem Auditory Evoked Potentials. J Neurosurg 57:674–681

Jannetta PJ (1976) Microsurgical approach to the trigeminal nerve for tic douloureux. In: Krayenbühl H, Maspes PE, Sweet WH (eds) Progress in Neurosurgery, vol 7. Karger, Basel, pp 180–200

Jannetta PJ (1981) Vascular decompression in trigeminal neuralgia. In: Samii M, Jannetta PJ (eds) The cranial nerves. Springer, Berlin Heidelberg New York, pp 331–340

Malis LI (1967) Petrous ridge compression and its surgical correction. J Neurosurg 26:163–167

Penzholz H, Kühner A (1981) Critical remarks on different surgical methods in trigeminal neuralgia. In: Samii M, Jannetta PJ (eds) The cranial nerves. Springer, Berlin Heidelberg New York, pp 341–346

Szapiro J, Jr (1985) Prognostic factors for microvascular decompression in trigeminal neuralgia. Med. Thesis, Lyon

Ectatic Basilar Artery: An Unusual Cause of Trigeminal Neuralgia

R.H. Lye, Manchester/England

Elongation and tortuosity of the basilar artery is variously referred to as ectasia (Yu et al. 1982), arteriectasis (Stebhens 1972) or cirsoid ('S' shaped) aneurysm of the basilar artery. The last term was used to denote "an 'S' shaped elongation of the basilar and/or vertebral arteries with consequent lateral bulging that compresses either the fifth or eighth nerve or both". The lateral bulging of the basilar artery is more often to the left than to the right (Dandy 1945). Basilar artery ectasia is an unusual cause of trigeminal neuralgia (Campbell and Keedy 1947; Gardner 1962) secondary to vascular compression. The case history of a patient suffering from this vascular anomaly is reviewed and the management discussed. Comparison is made with the case histories of three similarly afflicted patients.

Case Report

A 59-year-old Caucasian female presented with a five year history of intractable trigeminal neuralgia affecting the second and third divisions of the right trigeminal territory. Her pain was associated with an occasional tremor of her left arm. Tegretol failed to afford relief. The patient was otherwise well apart from being mildly hypertensive (BP 170/100). Computerised axial tomography (CT scan) revealed an ectatic basilar artery (Fig. 1) with evidence of lacunar infarcts in both internal capsules. An intravenous digital subtraction angiogram[1] (Fig. 2) confirmed the presence of an ectatic basilar artery extending into the right cerebellopontine angle and crossing the midline to extend superiorly to the left.

Posterior fossa exploration revealed a complex anatomical arrangement (Fig. 3). The anterior inferior cerebellar artery passed between the facial and auditory nerves before sending a labyrinthine branch to the internal auditory meatus. It is interesting that this patient had no evidence of hemifacial spasm, presumably because the artery was not in contact with the root entry zone of the facial nerve (Jannetta 1981). The dilated atheromatous basilar artery passed deep to the facial and auditory nerves and deep to the anterior inferior cerebellar artery. The latter vessel was compressed against the root entry zone of the trigeminal nerve, indenting the nerve and elevating it. The petrosal vein ran below the trigeminal nerve proximal to the site at which the nerve penetrated the dura and it appeared to hitch the nerve to the under-side of the tentorium. Decompression of the trigeminal nerve involved three

[1] Manufacturer: IGE, LVA isocentric orbiting angiographic unit with DF 3000 digital system

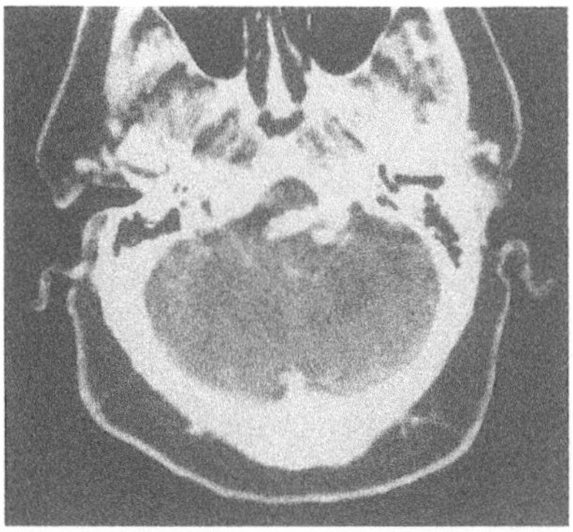

Fig. 1. CT scan after enhancement with intravenous contrast, demonstrating ectatic basilar artery

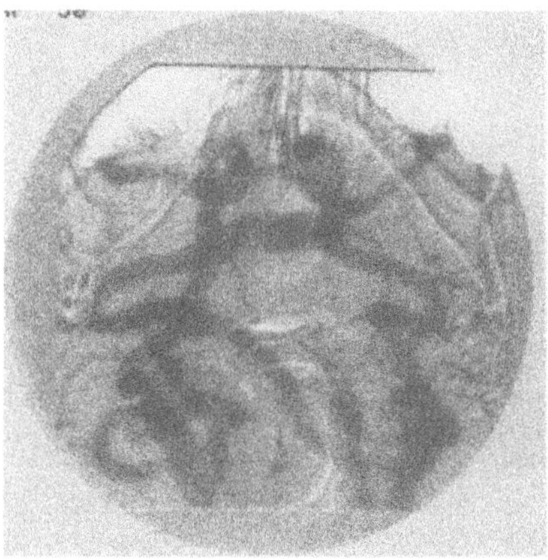

Fig. 2. Intravenous digital subtraction angiogram demonstrating ectatic basilar artery – frontal view

manoeuvres. Firstly, the anterior inferior cerebellar artery was mobilised and delivered from under the trigeminal nerve whilst preserving the labyrinthine artery. Secondly, a muscle graft was placed between the inferior surface of the nerve and the anterior inferior cerebellar artery and the basilar artery which was now in contact with the nerve. Thirdly, the petrosal vein was divided, so releasing the nerve from any tendency to be hitched up to the under-side of the tentorium (Fig. 4).

Postoperatively, the patient had no neurological deficit and was relieved of her pain. She had an episode of cerebrospinal rhinorrhoea, the source of which was an incompletely occluded mastoid air cell. A minor repair to seal the mastoid air cells cured this problem and she was soon discharged home. She has remained free from her trigeminal neuralgia until the present (30 months).

Review of our records revealed three further examples of trigeminal neuralgia associated with basilar artery ectasia (Table 1). The first, a 67-year-old female, had a 3 year history of right trigeminal neuralgia which had failed to respond to carbamazepine. On examination, she had minimal hypalgesia and hypaesthesia in the ophthalmic division of the right trigeminal territory and mild nystagmus on looking right. A CT scan demonstrated an ectatic basilar artery curving into the right cerebellopontine angle. Angiography was not performed. Initial relief following per-

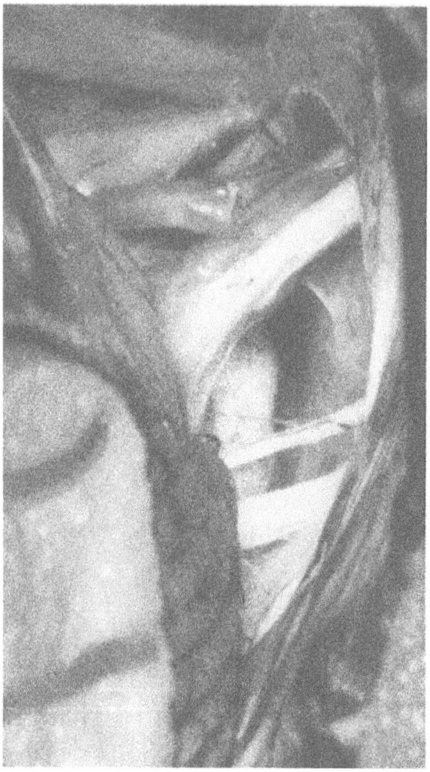
3

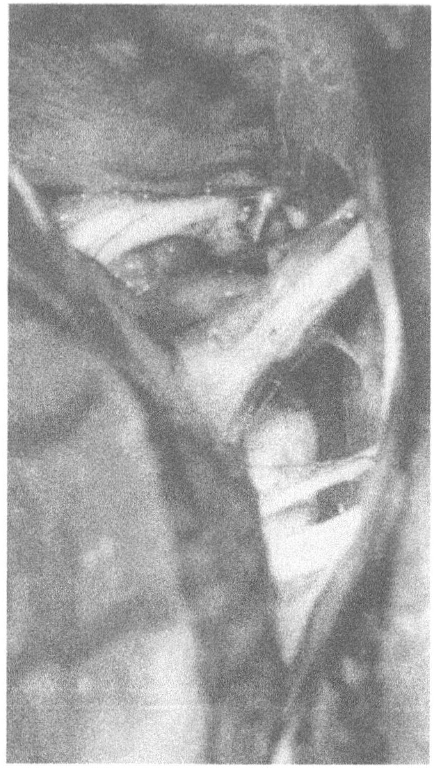
4

Fig. 3. Operative findings. An ectatic basilar artery can be seen compressing a loop of the anterior inferior cerebellar artery against the inferior and posterior aspect of the trigeminal nerve. Note the distortion of this nerve

Fig. 4. A muscle patch has been inserted between the trigeminal nerve and the anterior inferior cerebellar artery. The labyrinthine artery can be seen running from the anterior inferior cerebellar artery towards the internal auditory meatus

Table 1.

	No.	Incidence of basilar ectasia
Dandy (1945)	108 peri-operative findings	11 (10.2%)
Sunderland (1948)	210 autopsies	2 (0.95%)
Present series (CT diagnosis)		
(a) Patients with trigeminal neuralgia	92	4 (4.3%)
(b) Patients with atypical facial pain	17	0
(c) Patients with symptoms/signs suggestive of a posterior fossa lesion (excluding trigeminal neuralgia)	100	0
(d) Patients undergoing CT scan with no symptoms/signs referable to posterior fossa	100	0

cutaneous thermocoagulation was followed by recurrence of her pain one year later. She refused further treatment and her pain persists 23 months after the recurrence.

The second patient, an 82-year-old female, had a 9 month history of left sided trigeminal neuralgia affecting the second and third trigeminal divisions. Previous treatment with carbamazepine and alcohol injections had failed. A CT scan confirmed an ectatic basilar artery occupying the left cerebellopontine angle. Angiography was not performed. Percutaneous thermocoagulation gave initial relief but her pain returned after one year. A second thermocoagulation procedure gave temporary relief but was soon followed by relapse. Her pain persists 26 months later.

Finally, a 71-year-old mildly hypertensive male presented with an 8 year history of left trigeminal neuralgia affecting the first and second divisions. He could not tolerate carbamazepine. A CT scan revealed an ectatic basilar artery extending to the apex of the left petrous bone and this was confirmed by digital subtraction angiography examination. Posterior fossa exploration and microvascular decompression of his left trigeminal nerve relieved his pain but he suffered a myocardial infarction in the postoperative period and died one month later.

Discussion

Basilar artery ectasia is associated with hypertension and atherosclerosis (Ekbom et al. 1969; Greitz and Löfstedt 1954) as was the case with two of the four patients here reported. There is a high incidence of generalised vascular disease in patients with trigeminal neuralgia (Lew and Grant 1938) although this may be a reflection of the age group so afflicted with this complaint.

The incidence of basilar artery ectasia amongst patients with trigeminal neuralgia is difficult to assess. It will depend on the frequency with which such patients are investigated by angiography or posterior fossa exploration. The advent of CT scanning and more recently of intravenous digital subtraction angiography might be expected to increase the rate of detection since these investigations are less invasive and therefore more likely to be performed. Table 1 summarizes our experience and compares it with that of others.

Basilar artery ectasia has been described in association with trigeminal neuralgia (Dandy 1945) and trigeminal neuralgia combined with hemifacial spasm (Campbell and Keedy 1947; Gardner 1962). As the above case histories demonstrate, trigeminal neuralgia caused by basilar ectasia is refractory to a variety of therapies including partial section of the trigeminal nerve, nerve avulsion and foramen ovale injection, although successful thermocoagulation has been reported (Yu et al. 1982). Posterior fossa exploration and vascular decompression, however, has proved effective (Campbell and Keedy 1947).

The operative findings described above emphasize the complex anatomical neuro-vascular relations which may occur in the posterior fossa. The possibility of vascular cross-compression as a cause of trigeminal neuralgia (Jannetta 1981) is clearly demonstrated by the first patient, where the anterior inferior cerebellar artery, basilar artery and petrosal vein all appeared to contribute to compression of the trigeminal nerve. The value of the operating microscope in providing good illumination and magnification, thus facilitating preservation of fine but important vessels such as the labyrinthine artery, is obvious.

Clearly, caution must be exercised when recommending microvascular decompression as treatment since thermocoagulation is safer, although the latter procedure is not without risk (Penzholz and Kühner 1981). It should be remembered that patients with this type of vascular anomaly are likely to have generalised arterial disease and this may adversely affect the outcome of surgery. However, vascular decompression of the trigeminal nerve appears to be a logical and effective operation for the alleviation of trigeminal neuralgia caused by an ectatic basilar artery, especially in the younger and otherwise fit patient.

Acknowledgements: The author wishes to thank Miss Pamela Brown for typing the manuscript and the Department of Medical Illustration, Manchester Royal Infirmary for help in preparing the illustrations.

References

Campbell E, Keedy C (1947) Hemifacial spasm: a note on etiology in two cases. J Neurosurg 4:342–347

Dandy WE (1945) Intracranial arterial aneurysms. Comstock Publishign Co. Inc, Ithaca, pp 64–66

Ekbom K, Greitz T, Kugelberg E (1969) Hydrocephalus due to ectasia of the basilar artery. J Neurol Sci 8:465–477

Gardner WJ (1962) Concerning the mechanism of trigeminal neuralgia and hemifacial spasm. J Neurosurg 19:947–958

Greitz T, Löfstedt S (1954) The relationship between the third ventricle and the basilar artery. Acta Radiol 42:85–100

Jannetta PJ (1981) Vascular decompression in trigeminal neuralgia. In: Samii M, Jannetta PJ (eds) The cranial nerves. Springer, Berlin Heidelberg New York, pp 331–340

Jannetta PJ (1981) Hemifacial spasm. In: Samii M, Jannetta PJ (eds) The cranial nerves. Springer, Berlin Heidelberg New York, pp 484–493

Lew FH, Grant FC (1938) Physiopathologic and pathoanatomic aspects of major trigeminal neuralgia. Arch Neurol Psychiatr 40:1126–1134

Penzholz H, Kühner A (1981) Critical remarks on different surgical methods in trigeminal neuralgia. In: Samii M, Jannetta PJ (eds) The Cranial Nerves. Springer, Berlin Heidelberg New York, pp 341–346

Stebhens WE (1972) Pathology of the cerebral blood vessels. CV Mosby, Saint Louis, p 82

Sunderland S (1948) Neurovascular relations and anomalies at the base of the brain. J Neurol Neurosurg Psychiatry 11:243–257

Yu YL, Moseley IF, Pullicino P, McDonald WI (1982) The clinical picture of ectasia of the intracerebral arteries. J Neurol Neurosurg Psychiatry 45:29–36

Microneurosurgical Findings of Glossopharyngeal Neuralgia

J. HAMER, Heidelberg/FRG

Introduction

The term glossopharyngeal neuralgia was first used by Harris in 1921, and the similarities with tic douloureux of the 5th cranial nerve were soon noticed by others. As Dandy stated as early as 1927: "The term 'tic douloureux' is no longer synonymous with trigeminal neuralgia, but must now include glossopharyngeal neuralgia. The characteristic sudden ticlike paroxysms of excruciating pain and the induction of pain by external stimuli are common to each." The pain is located in the back of the tongue and the tonsillar part of the pharynx. Swallowing, yawning, coughing or even talking triggers off the painful attacks. Via the tympanic branch of the glossopharyngeal nerve (so-called Jacobson's nerve), the pain is also felt deep in the ear. Occasionally, the auricular branch of the vagal nerve seems to be involved and the projection of the pains extends to the external ear. This is why some authors speak of "vagoglossopharyngeal" neuralgia (Chawla and Falconer 1967; White and Sweet 1969; Rushton et al. 1981). In later years Dandy proposed cutting the upper branch of the intracisternal vagus nerve in addition to the resection of the 9th cranial nerve. Other surgeons such as Bohm and Strang (1962) recommend this procedure only in cases where the glossopharyngeal nerve is remarkably thin. To establish the differential diagnosis between pure glossopharyngeal neuralgia and vagoglossopharyngeal neuralgia the application of cocain solution to the throat for relief of pain has been used (Robson and Bonica 1950).

When the more comprehensive case reports in the pertinent literature since Harris and Dandy are studied, it becomes obvious that vagoglossopharyngeal neuralgia is rather the exception and pure glosso-pharyngeal neuralgia more common. In comparison with the incidence of tic douloureux of the 5th cranial nerve, glossopharyngeal neuralgia is very rare, the ratio being 100 : 1 (Bohm and Strang 1962). Considering the microneurosurgical findings in the cerebellopontine angle in cases with trigeminal neuralgia and in view of the very good prognosis after neurovascular decompression, it was tempting to assume that offending vessels and neurovascular contact also play an important pathogenetic role in glossopharyngeal neuralgia. Arterial compression of the glossopharyngeal nerve has been noticed on occasion in earlier case reports (Brihaye et al. 1956; Kempe and Smith 1969; Rushton et al. 1981). In the large clinical series of the Mayo-Clinic covering the years 1922 to 1977 there were 19 cases among 129 patients treated by Dandy's operation where an arterial compression was expressly stated by the surgeon (Rushton et al. 1981). But here as in other similar case reports definite therapeutic conclusions were not drawn from these observations. But the first case reports of Laha and Jannetta

(1977) and Jannetta (1981) who explored the cerebellopontine angle and the root entry zone in glossopharyngeal neuralgia, gave strong evidence that arterial compression of the 9th cranial nerve is the major cause of this type of neuralgia. Another case was published in 1977 by Morales et al. However, with regard to the very few cases hitherto documented, more extensive observations on this subject are extremely desirable.

Case Report and Discussion

A 74-year-old male patient is presented who has suffered for 16 years from glossopharyngeal neuralgia on the right side. For many years he had to take between 8 and 10 tablets of Tegretal per day to relieve his pain adequately. A few weeks before emergency admission to our department glossopharyngeal neuralgia became so severe that in spite of an increase in the dosage of Tegretal pain attacks were no longer controlled. Even frequent application of cocain to the throat did not lead to temporary relief to enable the patient to eat and drink, and artificial intravenous nutrition became necessary. There was no neurologic deficit. Cranial CT-scan and vertebral angiograms were normal. There was no enlarged styloid process visible on plain X-rays of the skull.

In spite of the age and the reduced general condition of the patient the decision was taken to explore the right cerebellopontine angle and to look for neurovascular compression, and to decompress if necessary, or otherwise to perform Dandy's operation. Figure 1 shows the intraoperative finding at the root entry zone of the glossopharyngeal nerve: We found a dorsal compression of the cranial nerve caused by a loop of the PICA which crossed the nerve shortly after its origin from the vertebral artery. This course of the PICA in front and above the glossopharyngeal nerve is not common and occurs in only 14% of the cases according to the investigations of

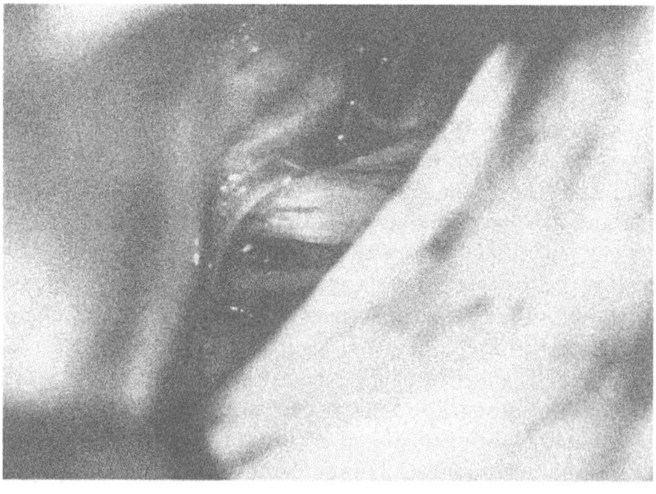

Fig. 1. Compression of the glossopharyngeal nerve caused by a loop of the PICA

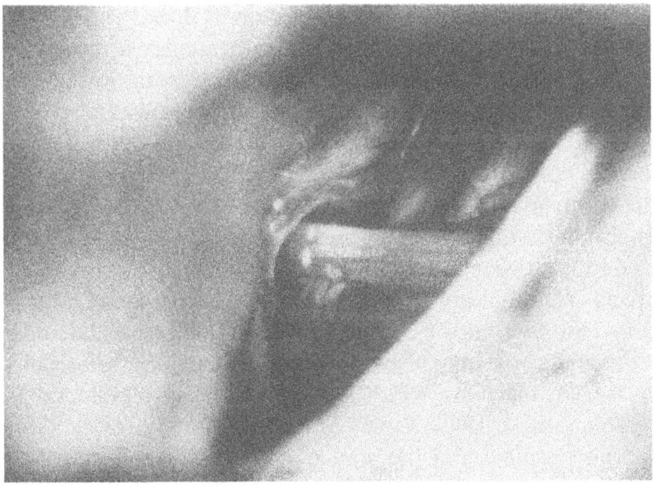

Fig. 2. Mobilization of the arterial loop from the cranial nerve

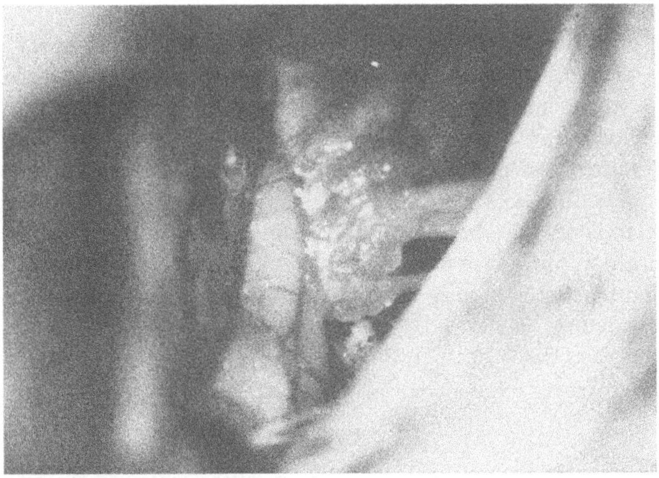

Fig. 3. Definite neurovascular decompression achieved by plugging a piece of muscle between glossopharyngeal nerve and artery

Lang (1981). Figure 2 demonstrates the mobilization of the arterial loop, and Fig. 3 shows the definite neurovascular decompression achieved by plugging a piece of muscle between the nerve and the arterial vessel. The postoperative course was uncomplicated and no neurologic deficit was observed. The patient was immediately painfree without any more Tegretal medication. He could drink and eat normally the day after the operation. He has now remained without tic douloureux attacks for 6 months.

According to the 17 published cases by Jannetta (1981), the initial dorsal and medullary segment of the PICA is most commonly the compressing vessel.

The compression may be located beneath the nerve or on its dorsal surface. It is less common that the vertebral artery is the origin of neurovascular compression, and the AICA seems to be a very rare cause of neurovascular contact to the glossopharyngeal nerve. In view of the scanty case reports on neurovascular glossopharyngeal decompression we are not yet able to answer the question whether true venous compression can play a decisive role.

The advantage of the neurovascular decompression procedure over Dandy's section of the glossopharyngeal nerve and the upper two filaments of the vagal nerve is obvious: Neurovascular decompression is non-destructive and lowers the risk of unforeseen neurologic sequela. We should bear in mind that – although many patients were definitely cured from pain by Dandy's operation – section of the cranial nerves IX and X may be accompanied by immediate severe and sustained arterial hypertension and cardiovascular reactions which can jeopardize cerebellopontine angle exploration (Nagashima et al. 1976; Ripley et al. 1977; Alonso et al. 1981). The same is true for thermocoagulation of the jugular foramen where – in spite of refined techniques and careful monitoring – dangerous risks remain prevalent (Ori et al. 1983). According to Tew (1977) and Lazorthes and Verdie (1979) this last procedure should be reserved for patients with cancer-induced glossopharyngeal neuralgia.

The exploration of the cerebellopontine angle offers the possibility to detect a curable vascular lesion and still leaves the option for nerve section if no persuasive vascular compression is seen. Finally, however, it should be stressed that during exploration of the cerebellopontine angle it is not sufficient to visualize the cranial nerve at the jugular foramen and in the lateral half of the basal cistern alone as Dandy's operation requires, but to follow the nerve more medially to the brain stem. The neurovascular contact is here and not distal at the skull base. The neurovascular decompression procedure is necessarily more delicate and technically more difficult than simple nerve section at the jugular foramen. Microsurgical experience is therefore mandatory.

References

Alonso T, Pujol J, Aynso AL (1981) Sustained hypertension after section of the glossopharyngeal nerve. J Neurol Neurosurg Psychiatry 44:369
Bohm E, Strang RR (1962) Glossopharyngeal Neuralgia. Brain 85:371–388
Brihaye J, Périer O, Smulders J, Franken L (1956) Glossopharyngeal neuralgia caused by compression of the nerve by an atheromatous vertebral artery. J Neurosurg 13:299–302
Chawla JC, Falconer MA (1967) Glossopharyngeal and vagal neuralgia. Br Med J 3:529–531
Dandy WE (1927) Glossopharyngeal Neuralgia (Tic Douloureux). Its Diagnosis and Treatment. Arch Surg 15:198–214
Harris W (1921) Persistent pain in lesions of the peripheral and central nervous system. Brain 44:557–571
Jannetta PJ (1981) Cranial Nerve Vascular Compression Syndromes (Other than Tic douloureux and Hemifacial Spasm). In: Clinical Neurosurgery, vol 28. Williams and Wilkins, Baltimore/London, pp 445–456
Kempe LG, Smith DR (1969) Trigeminal Neuralgia, Facial Spasm. Intermedius and Glossopharyngeal Neuralgia with Persistent Carotid-Basilar Anastomosis. J Neurosurg 31:445–451
Laha RK, Jannetta PJ (1977) Glossopharyngeal Neuralgia. J Neurosurg 47:316–320

Lang J (1981) Klinische Anatomie des Kopfes. Springer, Berlin Heidelberg New York, pp 364–365
Lazorthes Y, Verdie JC (1979) Radiofrequency coagulation of the petrous ganglion in glossopharyngeal neuralgia. Neurosurgery 4:512–516
Morales F, Alberca P, de Valle B, Narros A (1977) Glossopharyngeal and vagal neuralgia secondary to vascular compression of the nerves. Surg Neurol 8:431–433
Nagashima CH, Sakaguchi A, Kamisasa A, Kawanuma S (1976) Cardiovascular complications on upper vagal rootlet section for glossopharyngeal neuralgia. J Neurosurg 44:248–253
Ori C, Salar G, Giron G (1983) Percutaneous glossopharyngeal thermo-coagulation complicated by syncope and seizures. Neurosurgery 13:427–429
Ripley RC, Hollifield JW, Nies AS (1977) Sustained hypertension after section of the glossopharyngeal nerve. Am J Med 62:297–302
Robson JT, Bonica J (1950) The vagus nerve in surgical consideration of glossopharyngeal neuralgia. J Neurosurg 7:482–484
Rushton JG, Stevens JC, Miller RH (1981) Glossopharyngeal (Vagoglossopharyngeal) Neuralgia. A Study of 217 cases. Arch Neurol 38:201–205
Tew JM (1977) Percutaneous rhizotomy in the treatment of intractable facial pain (trigeminal, glossopharyngeal and vagus nerves). In: Schmideck HH, Sweet WH (eds) Current techniques in operative neurosurgery. Grune and Stratton, New York, pp 409–426
White JC, Sweet WH (1969) Pain and the Neurosurgeon: A 40-Year Experience. Charles C. Thomas, Springfield, Ill, pp 265–283

Traumatic Intraventricular, Basal Ganglia, and Brain Stem Haematomas

G. TEASDALE, E. TEASDALE and P. MACPHERSON, Glasgow, Scotland/Great Britain

Introduction

It was realised rapidly that one of the main benefits of CT scanning was in the early detection of acute extradural, subdural, and other space-occupying traumatic intracranial bleeds and that its use could lead to improved outcome in operated cases (Teasdale et al. 1984). Further experience with CT then led to the recognition of certain less dramatic, less common deep traumatic haemorrhagic lesions, which previously had been seen only at post mortem. This paper reviews knowledge of these lesions; perhaps unusually in a symposium focussed upon surgery, it sounds a cautionary note about the place of operation in their management.

Lesions Considered

Radiologically it is appropriate to recognise three main varieties of haemorrhage:

1. Intraventricular haemorrhage – which may involve one, or more often two or more ventricles.
2. Haematomas in the vicinity of the third ventricle, in particular in the basal ganglia.
3. Primary brain stem haematomas.

No single study so far has considered all of these kinds of lesions and the present analysis has been derived from several previous reports (Tsai et. al. 1980; Zuccarello et al. 1981; Oliff et al. 1978; Kim et al. 1981; Cordobes et al. 1983) and from a review of more than 2000 head injured patients in Glasgow (Macpherson et al. 1985).

Radiological Features

Intraventricular bleeding (Fig. 1) varies in extent from a small precipitation, recognised only when the occipital horns are carefully inspected, to extensive collections occupying the lateral, third, and fourth ventricles. Commonly the CT scan also shows intracerebral bleeding, sometimes in direct contact with the ventricular surface, suggesting that bleeding in the latter was secondary to a primary parenchymal lesion. *Basal Ganglia haematomas* (Fig. 1) likewise vary greatly in size and in a third of cases are associated with a space-occupying surface clot or with major lacerations and contusions of the frontal and temporal poles (Macpherson et al. 1985). *Hae-*

matomas in the brain stem occur as a component of primary impact damage but also may be secondary to tentorial herniation and mid brain infarction due to compression. *Primary brain stem haematomas* (Fig. 2) characteristically are placed laterally in the rostral brain stem. Although intracranial pressure may be raised diffusely, so that the basal cisterns may be obliterated (Teasdale et al. 1982), major intracranial shifts are absent. By contrast, secondary haematomas are usually central and either associated with or follow major intercompartmental shifts.

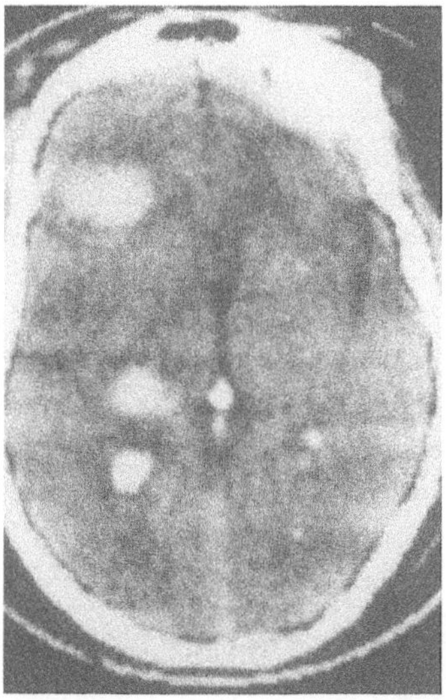

Fig. 1. CT scan of 21-year-old man, two hours after a road traffic accident, since when he had been in coma (Glasgow Coma Score 4). There is blood in the occipital horn, a haematoma in the basal ganglia and a frontal intracerebral clot

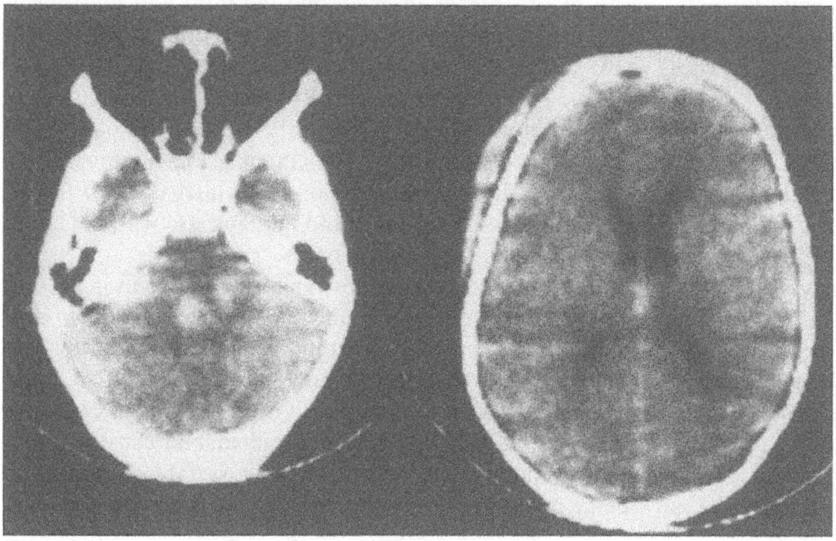

Fig. 2. CT scan of a 20-year-old girl in deep coma since a road traffic accident. There is evidence of haemorrhage in the dorsolateral part of the rostral brain stem and in the corpus callosum

Table 1.

Site of bleed	Frequency in CT scans of head injuries (%)	Unconscious from time of injury (%)	Other lesions on CT (%)	Mortality (%)
Intraventricular	1 – 6	95	90	75
Basal ganglia	3	98	55	55
Brain stem	≪1	100	100	>99

Other intracranial lesions are commonly seen in association with deep traumatic haematoma (Table 1). These other lesions include surface clots, and contusions, but a striking feature is the frequency with which haemorrhages are observed in the corpus callosum. Such small haemorragic lesions in the corpus callosum are the computer tomographic hallmark of diffuse primary shearing injury to white matter (diffuse axonal injury) (Zimmerman et al. 1978).

A corpus callosum (Fig. 3) haematoma is seen in the majority of patients with either intraventricular haemorrhage (Cordobes et al. 1983) and/or primary brain stem lesions. Among patients with basal ganglia bleeding who do not have a major surface collection, a third of cases have a corpus callosum lesion (Macpherson et al. 1985).

Frequency and Clinical Features

Although criteria for the selection of head injured patients for CT scanning vary from centre to centre, in all reports bleeds in or around the third and fourth ventricles have occurred in only a very small proportion of cases (Table 1). When only those patients in coma at the time of the scan are considered the incidence is higher. This is because an overwhelming majority of patients with deep haematomas are in deep coma from the time of the injury (Table 1). Nevertheless, even amongst head injured patients in coma it is in only a minority (< 10%) that deep haematomas have been detected. However, the recognition of these lesions may increase with the increasing availability of high definition CT scanning and perhaps also with the use of magnetic resonance imaging in head injured patients.

Patients with a deep traumatic haematoma are typically young, usually < 40 years old, more than ¾ have been injured in a road traffic accident or other high velocity injury, but less than half have a skull fracture. In these respects they resemble patients with diffuse primary shearing (axonal) injury more than those whose depression of consciousness is due to a surgically significant surface lesion. The latter patients are older, have often fallen or been assaulted, and usually have a skull fracture. The majority of patients with space-occupying surface clots, even in the posterior fossa, now make a good recovery. By contrast the outcome in patient

Fig. 3 a, b. Brain sections at post mortem corresponding to CT scan in Fig. 2. **a** The primary haemorrhages in the brain stem are shown, and **b** a tear of the corpus callosum

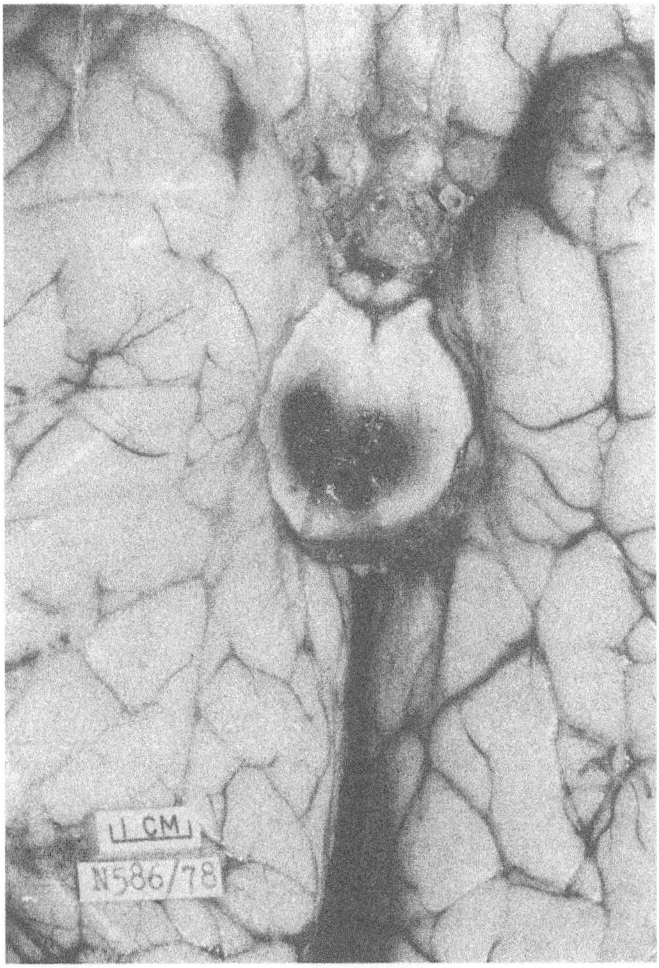

a

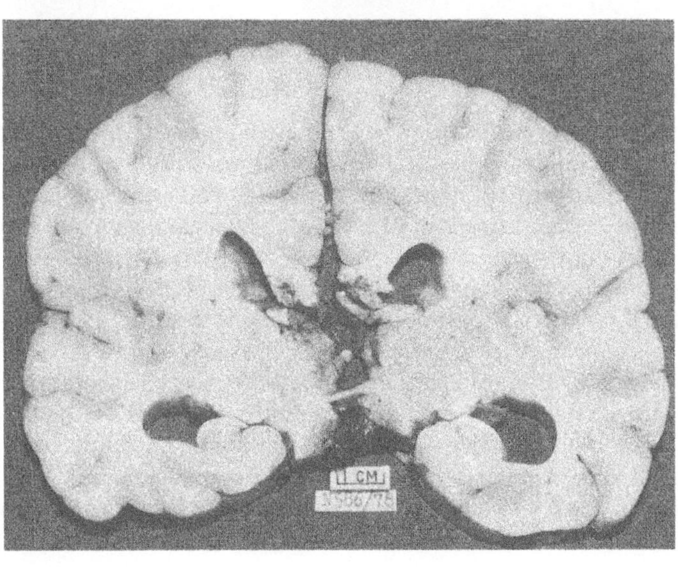

b

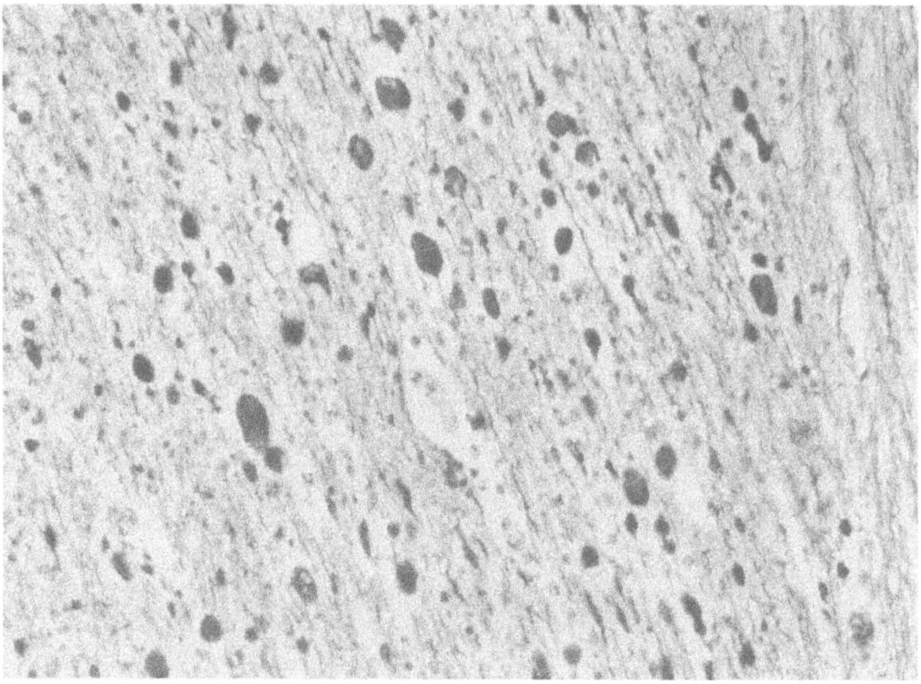

Fig. 4. Section from the white matter of the brain shown in Fig. 3, stained to show nerve fibres, and also showing numerous 'retraction balls' at the site of damaged axons

with a deep haematoma is poor. More than half of the patients with a basal ganglia haematoma die as do more than three out of four of those with intraventricular bleeding. Convincing evidence of recovery after primary brain stem bleeding is lacking.

Pathology

Comprehensive studies in all types of lesion have not been reported. However, when full neuropathological examination has been carried out on patients with intraventricular or brain stem haemorrhage almost invariably the finding at post mortem has been the pattern of damage associated with shearing forces at the time of impact and now referred to as diffuse axonal injury (Adams et al. 1977). Macroscopical inspection of the cut surface of the brain shows small haemorrhagic tears in the corpus callosum and in the dorsolateral aspect of the rostral brain stem (Fig. 4), and these correspond to the haemorrhagic lesions seen on the CT scan. Thus, in a series of 12 patients in Glasgow whose CT scans had shown intraventricular haemorrhage, corpus callosum lesions were found in each case at post mortem and in each case axonal injury was confirmed histologically by the finding of retraction balls, of microglial stars, or of long tract degeneration depending upon the duration of survival. Diffuse axonal injury is also found in many patients with basal ganglia bleeding, but is not invariable.

Discussion

This review makes it clear that operation is not appropriate in most of these patients. The radiological association with corpus callosum lesions, the clinical features of severe primary brain damage, and the post mortem findings provide convincing evidence that the demonstration on CT of intraventricular, basal ganglia or primary brain stem haemorrhages signifies a severe primary diffuse shearing injury in almost all cases.

This pattern of brain damage seems to result from shearing forces, brought about by inertial acceleration or deceleration forces, applied for a specific duration. It appears that in most instances the axons of the tracts in the white matter are preferentially vulnerable to these forces and that when discrete haemorrhage develops, axonal lesions are already severe. It may be that in some rare circumstances blood vessels may be more susceptible, as in certain patients with basal ganglia bleeding. However, in most patients the CT scan finding of a deep central traumatic bleed represents merely the visible tip of the iceberg of severe diffuse shearing injury, the full extent of which becomes apparent only after detailed neuropathological and histological examination.

Intraventricular haemorrhage appears to be associated with and perhaps is usually derived from primary white matter lesions. Alternative sources that are suggested include a tear of the choroid plexus, rupture of a subependymal vein or even spontaneous rupture of a vascular malformation at the time of injury. One or other of these mechanisms may account for the very rare instances in which extensive intraventricular bleeding and hydrocephalus are found in association with a delayed deterioration of consciousness. This has occurred in patients who were lucid initially and who therefore could not have had severe primary brain damage; such patients may be helped by ventricular drainage (Kim et al. 1981).

The treatment of spontaneous intraventricular, basal ganglia and brain stem haematomas by either microsurgical or stereotactic evacuation is sometimes followed by success. By contrast, it is important to realize that these techniques are not going to benefit a patient with a deep traumatic haematoma who has been in coma from the time of the injury. In such cases it is the accompanying severe diffuse axonal injury that determines the patient's fate.

References

Adams JH, Mitchell DE, Graham DI, Doyle D (1977) Diffuse brain damage of immediate impact type: its relationship to primary brain stem damage in head injury. Brain 100:489–502

Cordobes F, de la Fuente M, Lobato RD, Roger R, Perez C, Miltan JM, Barcena A, Lamas E (1983) Intraventricular haemorrhage in severe head injury. J Neurosurg 58:217–222

Kim CH, Tanaka R, Kawakami K, Ito J (1981) Traumatic Primary Intraventricular Haemorrhage. Surg Neurol 16:415–417

Macpherson P, Teasdale E, Dharker S, Allerdyce G, Galbraith S (1985) The significance of traumatic haematoma in the region of the basal ganglia. Submitted to J Neurol Neurosurg Psychiatry

Oliff M, Fried AM, Young AB (1978) Intraventricular haemorrhage in blunt head trauma. J Comput Assist Tomogr 2:625–629

Teasdale E, Cardoso E, Galbraith S, Teasdale G (1984) CT scan in severe diffuse head injury: physiological and clinical correlations. J Neurol Neurosurg Psychiatry 47:600–603
Teasdale G, Galbraith S, Murray L, Ward P, Gentleman D, McKean M (1982) Management of Traumatic Intracranial Haematoma. Br Med J 285:1695–1697
Tsai FY, Teal JS, Quinn MF, Itabashi HH, Huprich JE, Ahmadi J, Segall HD (1980) CT of Brain Stem Injury. Am J Radiol 134:717–723
Zimmerman RA, Bilaniuk LT, Gennarelli T (1978) Computer Tomography of Shearing Injuries of the Cerebral White Matter. Radiology 127:393–396
Zuccarello M, Ivacoli A, Pardatscher L, Cervellini P, Fiore D, Mingrino S, Gerosa M (1981) Post traumatic intraventricular Haemorrhages. Acta Neurochir (Wien) 55:283–293

Neurosurgical Advances Relating to Pontine Hemorrhage

W. J. BOCK and C. SPRICK, Düsseldorf/FRG

The treatment of pontine hemorrhage still presents a major problem. Any concept of therapy will have to take into account both the initial neurologic deficit, the clinical course, and the size and position of the hemorrhage.

Reviewing both, the literature and our own cases, we try to set up a concept of treatment and to present for discussion the operative possibilites and the approaches to the lesion favoring our own access via the cerebellopontine angle.

Spontaneous brain stem hemorrhages are rare compared to those of the supratentorial white matter and basal ganglia. Because of the numerous vital functions represented within a very limited area they are carrying a poor prognosis and frequently a lethal outcome. Major problems are encountered both by getting access to the lesion and avoiding additional damage to surrounding structures.

Early descriptions of an operative approach can be found in Fedor Krause's 1914 textbook "General Surgery of the Diseases of the Brain". He is commenting both, on a transclival approach, which he rejects, and on a dorso-lateral way, on which, however, he failed to succeed. The approach via the cerebellopontine angle is also mentioned in Hoff and Schönbauer's 1933 textbook "Brain Surgery", where it is suggested to remove parts of the petrous bone to get a better lateral view. In 1948, Tönnis in his book "Surgery of the Head, Spine and Nerves" mentions the subtemporal access providing better visualization of the lateral pons.

We may now present a case report from our own patients: A 15-year-old boy developed ataxia and weakness of his right hand 4 weeks prior to admission. 3 days before admission he also showed right hemisensory defect and weakness of the lower right extremity. In another hospital symptoms were thought to be due to a poliomyelitis revaccination 4 weeks before the onset of the disease. There were increased deep tendon reflexes and plantar response was extensor on the right. There was slight supranuclear facial nerve palsy on the right but no more nuclear cranial nerve dysfunction. Initial CT scans performed in another department revealed a hypodense area in the left brain stem next to the IVth ventricle. Initially inflammatory disease was suspected but with negative result. Clinically, left cerebellar ataxia, dysmetria, impairment of rapid alternating movements, left nuclear facial nerve palsy and paresis of left horizontal gaze developed. The level of consciousness became fluctuating, the patient being mostly somnolent. A repeated scan confirmed the hypodense lateralized left pontine lesion. Progression of symptoms led us to operative intervention via the left cerebellopontine angle. The pons was prominent and dark stained. On incision we found a brownish-black old liquefied clot of blood followed by prompt diminution of the size of the pons. A small biopsy was taken which showed an older tissue necrosis. In the months to follow the boy recovered completely and is free of symptoms to the present day.

Discussion

Brain stem hemorrhages can occur spontaneously or as a result of trauma (Table 1). In head injuries they are either primary lesions mainly to be found in the dorsolateral quadrants of the brain stem or else secondary hemorrhages of the central or the entire pons following supratentorial masses. In both cases the hemorrhages represent symptoms of a mainly supratentorial lesion and are never the only cause of clinical symptoms, mainly coma III° and IV°. There is no operative indication in these cases.

In opposition spontaneous brain stem hemorrhages are the primary and circumscribed infratentorial cause of the clinical situation. There are hemorrhages into tumors as well as bleedings from dysplastic vessels which cannot always be demonstrated angiographically. Of main interest to us in this context are those hemorrhages without other identifiable causes. In these, two clinical entities can be distinguished (Arseni and Stanciu 1973; Wong and Duffy 1982); (Table 2).

The rather more frequent type I hemorrhage of Arseni represents 6–10% of intracerebral hematomas (Dinsdale 1964; Zimmermann 1949). Mainly older patients are affected (5th and 6th decades) (Dinsdale 1964; Okudera et al. 1978). Hyperten-

Table 1. Classification of pontine hemorrhage

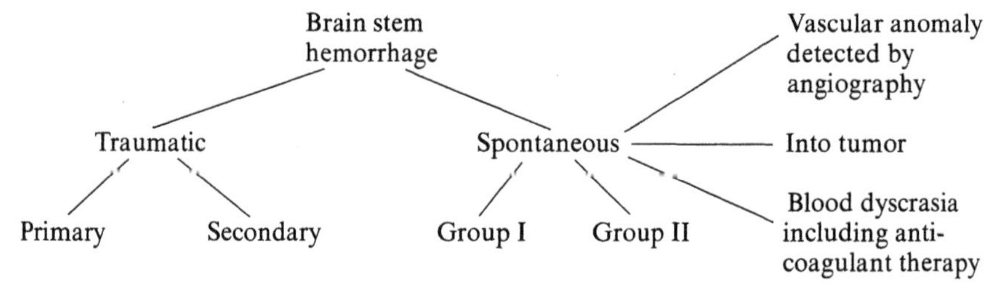

Table 2. Primary pontine hemorrhage

	Group I	Group II
Incidence	6–10% of ICH	Rare
Age	5th and 6th decade	Younger patients
Etiology	Hypertension/atherosclerosis	No risk factors "cryptic microangioma"
Localization	Central pons diffuse laceration	Lateralized circumscribed space occupying haematoma
Onset and course	Ictal	Progressive in several stages
Symptoms	Cf. Table 3	Cf. Table 3
Treatment	Conservative	Operative
Prognosis	Poor	Good

sion and atherosclerosis are frequent underlying diseases (Arseni and Stanciu 1973; Dinsdale 1964; Goto et al. 1980; Okudera et al. 1978; Russell 1954). In these cases there is a major tissue laceration compromising the mid-pons. The onset of symptoms is ictal, they are headed by deep coma (III° or IV°). Therapy has uniquely been conservative and the outcome invariably fatal.

Typ II hematomas of Arseni are definitely rarer. There are less than 30 well documented cases to which we contribute another two, one more was recently added by Bosch and Beute in the Journal of Neurosurgery, Jan. 1985. Reviews of operated cases were compiled by Vaquero et al. 1980 and Wong and Duffy 1982. Patients tend to be younger than in Type I. Usually there are no risk factors. In a few cases trivial trauma in the previous history is mentioned, the etiological value of which, however, is rather doubtful. "Cryptic microangiomas" appear to be of major etiological relevance (McCormick and Nofzinger 1966; Margolis et al. 1961; Scott et al. 1973); they usually escape angiographic detection, and pathological evidence within or close to a hematoma is often lacking. Hematomas tend to be lateralized and circumscribed space-occupying lesions. Sparing or rather compressing midpontine structures they are associated with lesser degrees of impairment of consciousness. Extra-axial localization has given rise to the differential diagnosis of cerebellopontine angle tumor as both in our case and in the literature (Pouyanne et al. 1967; Vaquero 1980).

Onset and clinical course of symptoms are often pseudotumoral or progressive in several stages and can extend over a period of weeks or months. This has even suggested multiple sclerosis as the most likely diagnosis (Abroms et al. 1971). Differential diagnosis can also be brain stem tumor (Scoville and Poppen 1949; Myers et al. 1961; Scott 1973), cerebellopontine angle tumor (Gros et al. 1948; Pouyanne et al. 1967; Vaquero et al. 1980), vertebrobasilar vascular insufficiency (Kempe 1964) and meningo-encephalitis (Koos et al. 1969). Symptoms of type I and type II hematomas are compiled in Table 3. In type II cases there is an operative indication. The few results in the literature are encouraging (Abroms et al. 1971; Arseni and Stanciu 1973; Dandy 1932; Doczi and Thomas 1979; Gros et al. 1948; Kempe 1964; Koos et al. 1969; Kowada et al. 1971; Matson 1969; Myers et al. 1961; Obrador et al. 1970; Papo et al. 1976; Pouyanne et al. 1967; Scoville and Poppen 1949; Vaquero

Table 3. Symptoms of pontine hemorrhage

Group I	Group II
Coma III–IV	Lesser, often fluctuating impairment of consciousness
Tetraplegia or decerebrate posturing	Hemiplegia, alternating brain stem syndromes
(Covered by coma)	Ataxia, Nystagmus
Vegetative dysfunction esp. of respiration and body temperature regulation	Lesser dysfunction
Miotic pupils	No miosis, double vision, paresis of horizontal gaze
(Covered by coma)	Nuclear dysfunction of cranial nerves, esp. CN V and VII

et al. 1980; Wong and Duffy 1982). Our own cases are two operated patients of type II with excellent results.

Since the first description of a successfully removed brain stem hematoma by Dandy (1932) diagnostic techniques have been considerably improved. Whereas in the past pneumencephalography and ventriculography including tomography (Kowada et al. 1971) were required and showed dorso-convex bulging of the floor of the IVth ventricle or aqueductal occlusion (Abroms et al. 1971; Kempe 1964; Koos et al. 1969; Obrador et al. 1970; Pouyanne et al. 1967; Scott et al. 1973; Scoville and Poppen 1949), computerized tomography has taken over and permits to assess localization and extent of the hematoma with sufficient exactness to suggest the operative approach. In addition NMR imaging allows hematomas to be visualized as areas of increased proton density on cross sections of the pons in axial views and their rostro-caudal area in the sagittal plane. This new technique is even superior to CT since tissue structures around the hematoma can be outlined far better.

In addition to clinical symptoms functional impairment can be demonstrated by evoked potential studies. Vertebrobasilar angiography should always be performed to exclude major vascular anomalies. Most cases of type II hematomas, however, show normal angiograms.

For operative treatment both timing and approach to the lesion have to be discussed. In our own two cases as well as in the literature surgery was not performed until 10–15 days after the insult provided vital functions were absolutely stable (Kowada et al. 1971; Pouyanne et al. 1967). Since a demarcation of the hematoma from the functionally vital surroundings is desirable to avoid additional damage, surgery should rather be delayed.

Several operative approaches to type II pontine hematomas have been advanced by various authors. Frequently a midline posterior fossa craniectomy via the cerebellar vermis and floor or the IVth ventricle was selected (Abroms et al. 1971; Arseni and Stanciu 1973; Gros et al. 1948; Kempe 1964; Koos et al. 1969; Kowada et al. 1971; Obrador et al. 1970; Scott et al. 1973). These reports comprise 9 patients. Both midline incisions of the rhomboid fossa and directly via a bulging dome created by the lesion were described. The lateral approach via the cerebellopontine angle was chosen in 6 patients (Doczi and Thomas 1979; Pouyanne et al. 1967; Wong and Duffy 1982). Scoville's access to a mesencephalic hematoma of the crus cerebri via the tentorium following left occipital lobectomy should be considered an exceptional case and not a routine approach.

A stereotactic puncture of a pontine hematoma has recently been presented in the Journal of Neurosurgery (Bosch and Beute 1985). The main argument advanced for the procedure was rapid deterioration of the patient's condition so that there remained no time for formal posterior fossa craniectomy. In our opinion fixing a Leksell stereotactic frame, calculating the position of the hematoma and advancing the probe should take up at least the time necessary to proceed with the craniectomy.

There appears to be a relation of extra-axial hematoma position in the pons and clinical state. Almost all operatively treated hematomas tended to be lateralized towards the cerebellopontine angle. For this reason the danger involved in proceeding through the floor of the rhomboid fossa is avoided and the lateral access favored. In addition to the self-evident use of the operating microscope the sitting position is suggested in younger patients.

With correct operative indication the results of surgery are encouraging. The number of published cases, however, is too small for a definitive answer to the problem. Further literature will remain to be limited to case reports.

References

Abroms IF et al. (1971) Spontaneous intracerebral haemorrhage in patients suspected of multiple sclerosis. J Neurol Neurosurg Psychiatry 34: 157–162

Arseni C, Stanciu M (1973) Primary haematomas of the brain stem. Acta Neurochir (Wien) 28:323–330

Bosch DA, Beute GN (1985) Successful stereotaxic evacuation of an acute pontomedullary hematoma. J Neurosurg 62: 153–156

Dandy W (1932) In: Lewis D, Prior Hagerstown W (ed) Practice of Surgery, vol 12

Dinsdale HB (1964) Spontaneous hemorrhage in the posterior fossa. Arch Neurol 10:200–217

Doczi T, Thomas GT (1979) Successful removal of an intrapontine haematoma. J Neurol Neurosurg Psychiatry 42: 1058–1061

Goto N et al (1980) Primary Pontine Hemorrhage: Clinicopathological Correlations. Stroke 11:84–90

Gros C, Giraud G, Latour H (1948) Hématome spontané de la calotte protubérantielle. Presse Med 56:890

Kempe LG (1964) Surgical removal of an intramedullary haematoma simulating Wallenberg's syndrome. J Neurol Neurosurg Psychiatry 27: 78–80

Koos WT, Sunder-Plassmann M, Salah S (1969) Successful removal of a large intrapontine hematoma. J Neurosurg 31:690–694

Kowada M et al. (1971) Primary pontine haemorrhage revealed by pneumoencephalo-roulette tomography, and a report on surgically treated cases. Acta Neurosurg 25:269–276

Krause F (1914) Die Allgemeine Chirurgie der Gehirnkrankheiten. Enke, Leipzig

Margolis G, Odom GI, Woodhall B (1961) Further experiences with small vascular malformations as a cause of massive intracerebral bleeding. J Neuropathol Exp Neurol 20:161

Matson DD (1969) Neurosurgery of Infancy and Childhood, 2nd ed. Thomas, Illinois, pp 749–772

McCormick WF, Nofzinger JD (1966) "Cryptic" vascular malformations of the central nervous system. J Neurosurg 24: 865–875

Myers J, Scott M, Silverstein A (1961) Cystic hemangioblastoma of pons. J Neurosurg 18:694–697

Obrador S, Dierssen G, Odoritz BJ (1970) Surgical evacuation of a pontine-medullary hematoma. J Neurosurg 33: 82–84

Okudera T et al. (1978) Primary pontine hemorrhage: Correlations of pathologic features with postmortem microangiography, and vertebral angiographic studies. M Sinai J Med (NY) 45:305–321

Papo I, Pasquini U, Salvolini I (1976) Subependymal brain stem hematomas. A report of two cases. Neuroradiology 11:279

Pouyanne MMH et al. (1967) Deux cas d'hématomes intraprotubérantiels opérés. Etude critique. Neurochirurgie 13:738–742

Russell DS (1954) Spontaneous Intracranial Haemorrhage. Proc R Soc Med 47:689–693

Scott BB, Seeger JF, Schneider RC (1973) Successful evacuation of a pontine hematoma secondary to rupture of a pathologically diagnosed "cryptic" vascular malformation. J Neurosurg 39: 104–108

Scoville WB, Poppen JL (1949) Intrapeduncular hemorrhage of the brain. Arch Neurol Psychiatr 61:688–694

Vaquero J et al. (1980) Hematomas of the Pons. Surg Neurol 14: 115–118

Wong SKK, Duffy GP (1982) Surgical treatment of spontaneous pontine haematoma. J Royal Soc Med 75:206–208

Zimmermann HM (1949) Cerebral apoplexy: mechanism and differential diagnosis. NY State J Med 49:2153–2157

Surgical Removal of an Intrapontine Hematoma. Case Report

M. SCHÄFER (†), H.-P. RICHTER and H.J. KLEIN, Günzburg and Fulda/FRG

Introduction

The majority of brain stem hematomas is located within the pons [5]. Nowadays, these hematomas most often are clearly diagnosed by CT scan. Patients suffering from brain stem hematoma rarely show an acute onset of symptoms [1, 2, 8–11, 18]. They tend to have a history of progressive or alternating neurological deficits. In most patients reported in the literature, surgical evacuation of the hematoma led to rapid clinical improvement [1, 2, 4, 6–11, 13, 14, 16–18, 20].

The following case report deals with our experience in one patient with a pontine hematoma whose postoperative course differed from those reported by most other authors.

Case Report

The 43-year-old male patient complained of dysarthria for several weeks before he sustained a sudden left-sided hemiparesis without impairment of consciousness on April 12, 1983. When admitted to a neurologic clinic one month later, he showed a flaccid left-sided hemiparesis and hemihypesthesia including the face, together with increased tendon reflexes and extensor plantar response on that side. In addition, vertical nystagmus was present. Appreciation of vibration sense was decreased on both legs.

On admission, there was no arterial hypertension. But the family doctor reported later on that in the past he sometimes had measured diastolic blood pressure values up to 105 mmHg, the systolic value never exceeding 145 mmHg. Blood tests were normal except for an increased gamma-GT (42 mU). CSF was not examined.

The first CT scan also performed one month after the acute onset of hemiparesis revealed an area of increased density of about two cm diameter within the right pontine brain stem (Fig. 1). Both temporal horns appeared somewhat dilated suggestive of a narrowing of the CSF pathways caudally. The fourth ventricle was displaced. There was no enhancement after i.v. injection of iodinated contrast material. Right-sided brachial angiography was found to be normal.

Because either a pontine hematoma or a tumor adjacent to the pons was suspected, surgical exploration was performed on June 23, 1983 (71 days after the acute onset of symptoms) by a right suboccipital approach. The cerebellopontine angle was found to be normal, but the right pontine brain stem appeared swollen.

Its surface around and rostral to the entry zone of the trigeminal root presented a yellowish discoloration.

The brain stem was incised two mm rostral to the entry zone of this nerve over a length of three mm. After penetrating its wall lying close to the surface, the hematoma discharged its liquid contents immediately followed by a collapse of the brain stem in this region. Microscopic examination of this material which also included small blood clots revealed no abnormality.

The postoperative course was uneventful, but neurologic signs have not changed dramatically since then. When seen the last time 1½ years after surgery, he was able to walk – which was impossible before – but still presented left-sided motor and sensory deficits, dysarthria and gait ataxia. In addition, he showed trigeminal hypesthesia and hearing deficit on the right side.

The bulk of the hematoma had diminished on the CT scan done four months following surgery (Fig. 2). The fourth ventricle was in normal position again. However, in later controls one year and 1½ years after the operation, a high attenuation area

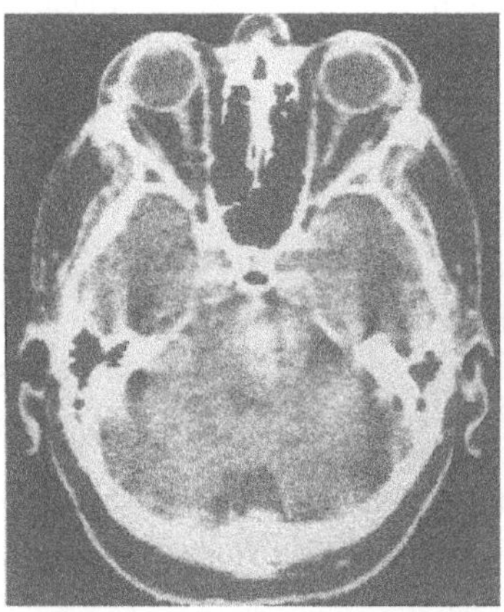

1

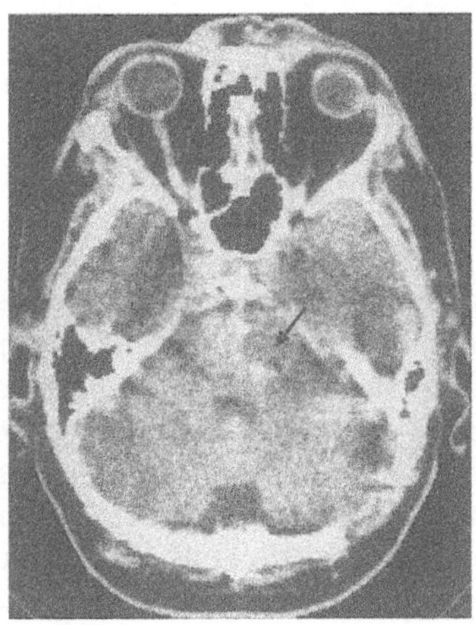

2

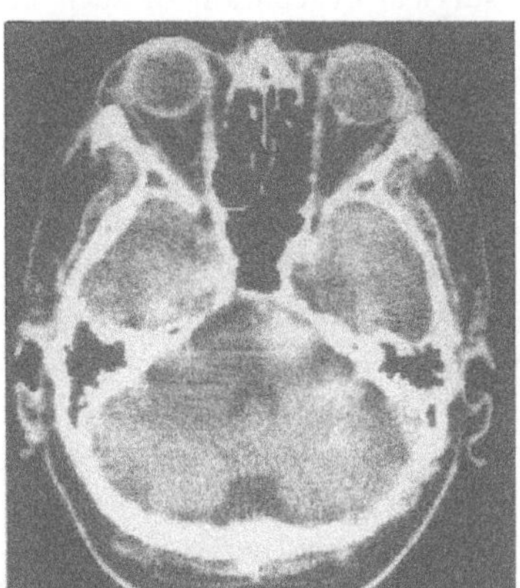

3

Fig. 1. Contrast enhanced CT scan showing a right intrapontine hematoma. Fourth ventricle displaced

Fig. 2. Plain CT scan four months after evacuation of a right-sided intrapontine hematoma shows the hematoma's cavity (*arrow*). Fourth ventricle in normal position

Fig. 3. Plain CT scan one year after evacuation of a right-sided intrapontine hematoma. Note area of increased density (60 HE) within the right pons. Fourth ventricle not displaced

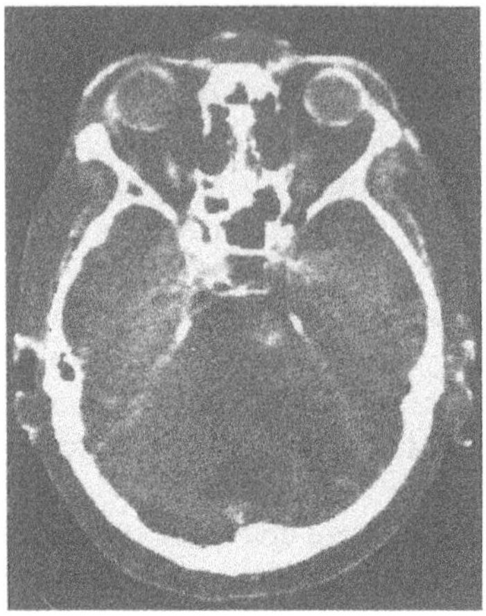

Fig. 4. Plain CT scan 1½ years after evacuation of a right-sided intrapontine hematoma resembling the CT scan done six months previously (Fig. 3)

reappeared but did not attain the same dimension as prior to surgery (Figs. 3, 4) and did not displace the fourth ventricle. Interestingly, there was no concomitant clinical impairment but rather a slow and steady improvement, as mentioned above.

Discussion

Most brain stem hematomas reported in the literature were found in the pontine or medullary areas [5, 23]. Only few were located in the midbrain [4, 7, 9, 21]. The clear prevalence of hemorrhages into the pontine area is related to the greater incidence in this region of "cryptic" vascular malformations [15]. Their rupture most often is considered the basic pathology in brain stem hematomas [15].

If not operated on, brain stem hematomas most often are fatal. Among the seven patients described by Kowada et al. [12], five untreated patients died. The two remaining were operated on after a six weeks period of coma and did not improve following surgery.

On the other hand, reports dealing with the surgical evacuation of such hematomas, first performed by Dandy in 1932, are encouraging. The majority of patients showed a rapid improvement, often towards complete recovery.

Most of the patients reported in the literature were young, normotensive and did not show vascular abnormalities on cerebral angiography, although "cryptic" vascular malformations were considered by the majority of authors who reported their surgically treated cases to be the cause of the hematoma [1, 6, 8–14, 16, 20]. Among these patients in whom a biopsy was taken from the hematoma's wall, fragments of abnormal vessels have so far been reported only once [20]. In the case described by Pak et al. [19] a venous angioma in the floor of the fourth ventricle was seen during postoperative angiography. However, microscopic examination of the biopsy taken in the course of surgery had been normal.

Our patient was also young, normotensive on admission and had a normal angiogram. A CT scan done three years previously following a traffic accident had been normal. He never had suffered of impaired consciousness. Symptoms and signs appeared in two stages, which is considered typical for a hematoma rather than a hemorrhage [2, 24]. He therefore was amenable to surgical therapy. This should be undertaken as soon as the diagnosis is established [2]. However, diagnosis of a brain stem hematoma may be delayed because typical clinical signs are failing [2, 18], and such a hematoma may be misinterpreted as multiple sclerosis, e.g. [1, 22].

The cause of the hematoma in our patient remained unclear. Like most authors we did not biopsy the wall of the hematoma because biopsy in that region carries a certain risk and often does not provide the desired histopathologic information to explain the patient's lesion [8, 10, 11, 16, 19].

Several surgical approaches have been practiced since Dandy performed the first successful evacuation of a brain stem hematoma in 1932: The suboccipital approach through the floor of the fourth ventricle [1, 2, 4, 8, 10–12, 16, 18, 20], cerebellopontine angle [6, 18], subtemporal [7, 9] and suboccipital transtentorial [21] approach. The decision depends on the location of the hematoma. Contrary to many authors, we did not evacuate the hematoma by needle aspiration [4, 18] but incised the brainstem under microscopic control over the hematoma. This might have been the cause for the postoperative trigeminal hypesthesia on one side of the operation although most hematomas reported in the literature had been evacuated by incision of the overlying parenchyma, obviously without causing additional harm to the patient's neurological state.

Whereas most patients reported by other authors improved very well and rapidly after evacuation of the hematoma, our patient showed only a slow and gradual improvement of symptoms and signs, being able to walk on his own 1½ years after surgery which was impossible before the operation. Lack of dramatic improvement following surgery might be explained by the long time which had elapsed between onset of symptoms and surgery. Some authors, however, reported an important clinical improvement even after longer intervals [2, 6, 21], although the majority of patients was operated on more rapidly than our patient [1, 3, 8–11, 13, 16, 18–20].

CT scans performed during the postoperative period showed a decrease of the hematoma four months after surgery. At that time, there was still a ring of increased density in the region of the hematoma, and one year and 1½ years following surgery a homogenous hyperdense area was seen, being smaller than before the surgical evacuation. The explanation of this phenomenon is unclear, particularly since there was no clinical impairment but rather a steady although weak improvement of symptoms and signs. Maybe a cryptic vascular malformation had rebled without causing additional deficits.

Summary

A case of a spontaneous pontine hematoma is reported. Clinical and CT presentation was suggestive of either a hematoma or a tumor. Operative evacuation by a cerebellopontine angle approach led to slow improvement of symptoms and signs over a follow-up period of 1½ years. The presentation of brain stem hematomas, their cause and their treatment are discussed.

References

1. Abroms IF et al. (1971) Spontaneous intracerebral haemorrhage in patients suspected of multiple sclerosis. J Neurol Neurosurg Psychiatry 34:157–162
2. Arseni C, Stanciu M (1973) Primary haematomas of the brain stem. Acta Neurochir (Wien) 28:323–330
3. Beatty RM, Zervas NT (1983) Stereotactic aspiration of a brain stem hematoma. Neurosurgery 13:204–207
4. Burns J et al. (1980) Recovery following brainstem hemorrhage. Ann Neurol 7:183–184
5. Dinsdale HB (1969) Spontaneous hemorrhage in the posterior fossa. Arch Neurol 10:200–217
6. Doczi T, Thomas DGT (1979) Successful removal of an intrapontine haematoma. J Neurol Neurosurg Psychiatry 42:1058–1061
7. Durward GJ et al. (1982) Presentation and management of mesencephalic hematoma. Report of two cases. J Neurosurg 56:123–127
8. Gros C et al. (1948) Hématome spontané de la calotte protubérantielle opéré et guéri. Presse Med 56:890
9. Humphreys RP (1978) Computerized tomographic definition of mesencephalic hematoma with evacuation through pedunculotomy. J Neurosurg 49:749–752
10. Kempe LG (1964) Surgical removal of an intramedullary haematoma simulating Wallenberg's syndrome. J Neurol Neurosurg Psychiatry 27:78–80
11. Koos WT et al. (1969) Successful removal of a large intrapontine hematoma. Case report. J Neurosurg 31:690–694
12. Kowada M et al (1971) Primary pontine haemorrhage revealed by pneumoencephalo-Roulette Tomography, and a report on surgically treated cases. Acta Neurochir (Wien) 25:269–276
13. La Torre E et al. (1978) Hematoma of the quadrigeminal plate. Case report. J Neurosurg 49:610–613
14. Matson DD (1968) Surgery of posterior fossa tumors in children. Clin Neurosurg 15:247–264
15. McCormick WF, Nofziger JD (1966) "Cryptic" vascular malformations of the central nervous system. J Neurosurg 24:865–875
16. Murphy MG (1972) Successful evacuation of acute pontine hematoma. Case report. J Neurosurg 37:224–225
17. Obrador S et al. (1970) Surgical evacuation of a pontine-medullary hematoma. J Neurosurg 33:82–84
18. O'Laoire SA et al. (1982) Brain-stem hematoma. A report of six surgically treated cases. J Neurosurg 56:222–227
19. Pak H et al. (1981) Successful evacuation of a pontine hematoma secondary to rupture of a venous angioma. Surg Neurol 15:164–167
20. Scott BB et al. (1973) Successful evacuation of a pontine hematoma secondary to rupture of a pathologically diagnosed "cryptic" vascular malformation. J Neurosurg 39:104–108
21. Scoville WB, Poppen JL (1949) Intrapeduncular hemorrhage of the brain. Arch Neurol Psychiatr 61:688–694
22. Stahl SM et al. (1980) The clinical and pathological spectrum of brain-stem vascular malformations. Arch Neurol 37:25–29
23. White RJ et al. (1958) A study of fifty intracranial vascular tumors found incidentally at necropsy. J Neuropathol Exp Neurol 17:392–398
24. Zuccarello M et al. (1980) Primary brain stem hematomas: Diagnosis and treatment. Acta Neurochir (Wien) 54:45–52

Surgical Management of Lesions in Specific Locations: Pineal Region, Anterior Third Ventricle

Treatment of Tumors in the Pineal and Posterior Third Ventricular Region

K. SANO, Tokyo/Japan

René Descartes (1596–1650), the greatest philosopher of 17th century in France, thought that the pineal body might act as a valve or sphincter to regulate the passage of spirits between the ventricular chambers, and this tiny organ thus gained supreme importance as "the seat of the soul". What we have to deal with today is that the pineal body or gland can often be the seat of various kinds of tumors.

Tumors in the pineal region occupy 4% of all intracranial primary neoplasms in Japan (583/14672 cases) (Sano 1983). This high incidence mostly comprises the so-called germinoma, or pinealoma, of the two-cell-pattern type (PTC), which forms 2.6% of all intracranial primary neoplasms according to the most recent Japanese statistics. In these same statistics, pineocytoma occupies 0.2%, pineoblastoma 0.1%, and teratoma including malignant teratoma 0.7%.

Table 1 shows 133 cases of tumors in the pineal region and the posterior third ventricle (excluding falco-tentorial meningiomas) experienced in the author's clinic and its affiliated hospitals (cases treated by radiotherapy only were excluded). The pineal tumor of the two-cell-pattern type, which has been called pinealoma or germinoma, is described in this Table as PTC. Pineoblastoma corresponds to medulloblastoma of the pineal of Zülch. Mixed germ cell tumors are composed of two or three types of tumors such as germinoma (seminoma), teratoma, teratoma with

Table 1. Tumors in the pineal region (133 cases) histologically verified

	Age: below 20 years	Age: 20 years and older
PTC	44 (41 M+3 F) (incl. pineal+suprasellar 1)	18 (17 M+1 F) (incl. pineal+suprasellar 1)
Pineoblastoma	1 (1 M)	4 (3 M+1 F)
Teratoma	15 (15 M)	2 (2 M)
Teratoma with malignant transformation	4 (4 M)	1 (1 M)
Mixed germ cell tumors	13 (13 M)	2 (2 M)
Unclassified germ cell tumor	1 (1 M)	0
Epidermoid	1 (1 M)	2 (2 F)
Ependymoma	3 (3 M)	5 (1 M+4 F)
Other gliomas	4 (2 M+2 F)	13 (11 M+2 F)
Total	86 (81 M+5 F)	47 (37 M+10 F)

M: male, F: female, PTC: pinealoma of two-cell-pattern type or germinoma malignant transformation, embryonal carcinoma, choriocarcinoma, and endodermal sinus tumor. According to the studies of the author's group (Sano 1983), PTC can be divided into germinoma (seminoma) of germ cell origin and pinealoma of pineal parenchyma origin. If we admit, though there is no convincing evidence, the germ cell theory that teratoma, teratoma with malignant transformation, germinoma (seminoma), embryonal carcinoma, endodermal sinus tumor, choriocarcinoma, and mixed germ cell tumors all arise from the imaginary germ cell (Friedman 1947, 1951; Teilum 1965), they can be grouped under the term "germ cell tumors". Then, tumors in the pineal region and the posterior third ventricle are classified as follows:

A. Germ cell tumors
   - Germinoma (seminoma) (one of PTC here described)
   - Teratoma (and epidermoid or dermoid)
   - Teratoma with malignant transformation
   - Embryonal carcinoma
   - Endodermal sinus tumor
   - Choriocarcinoma
   - Mixed germ cell tumors

B. Tumors of pineal parenchyma origin
   - Pinealoma (one of PTC here described)
   - Pineocytoma
   - Pineoblastoma

C. Gliomas

D. Tumors of the velum interpositum
   - Meningioma
   - Hemangiopericytoma
   - Angiomas
   - Cysts

In this paper, the author will deal mainly with groups A and B.

Based on the criterion that in a true tumor of pineal origin, tumor cells should be, as in any endocrine neoplasm, in close proximity to the capillaries (sinusoids) without intervening mesenchymal tissues, PTC can be divided into two groups: one group corresponds to a true tumor of pineal origin, which may be called *pinealoma,* and the other to seminoma, which, according to Friedman, may be called *germinoma* (Sano 1983). Of PTC involving the pineal region, pinealoma accounted for two-thirds of the cases examined; in contrast, 80% of suprasellar-hypothalamic PTC cases were germinoma. In both, pinealoma and germinoma, males were predominant (83–88%). However, in pinealoma and germinoma in the suprasellar region, the male predominance was not marked.

Therapeutic Principles

Examination of levels of alpha-fetoprotein (AFP), human chorionic gonadotrophins (HCG), and carcinoembryonic antigen (CEA) in the serum or in the cerebrospinal fluid should be done in all cases. The first two tumor markers (AFP and HCG) are especially informative as to the nature of tumors in this region.

If HCG is positive, the tumor must be choriocarcinoma or a mixed germ cell tumor with choriocarcinomatous elements. If AFP is positive, the tumor must be an endodermal sinus tumor or a mixed germ cell tumor with endodermal sinus elements. In both cases, prognosis is rather poor even after surgical removal of the tumor and postoperative radiotherapy of the whole neuraxis. Recently, chemotherapeutic agents such as actinomycin D, cis-platinum, vinblastine, bleomycin, etc., or their combinations are reported to be worthy of use.

If AFP and HCG are negative, the tumor may be either pinealoma, germinoma, embryonal carcinoma, teratoma with malignant transformation, or mature teratoma. If 2000 rad of local radiation effectively abolishes the tumor on CT (computed tomography), it may be pinealoma or germinoma, and radiotherapy should be continued with or without shunting procedure. However, if the size of the tumor is more than 2 cm (or sometimes more than 1.5 cm) in diameter, direct surgery and removal of the tumor followed by radiation (for pinealoma and germinoma, local radiation is usually sufficient) should be recommended. Mature teratoma can be cured only by removal of the tumor, and its prognosis is good. Embryonal carcinoma and teratoma with malignant transformation usually show poor prognosis even after surgical removal and postoperative radiotherapy of the whole neuraxis. The above mentioned chemotherapeutic agents are also recommended as being worthwhile. These principles are shown in Table 2.

Stereotaxic biopsy of tumors of this region has recently been gaining in popularity. The author, however, is not particularly enthusiastic about this procedure, because different parts of the same tumor of this region may show different histology so that biopsy of a small piece of the tumor may be misleading as to the true nature of the tumor. Therefore, the author prefers exploration and debulking (unless removal is possible) of the tumor.

Among various operative approaches to tumors in this region, the author prefers (i) the *occipital transtentorial approach* (Poppen and Marino 1968; Jamieson 1971), or (ii) the *infratentorial supracerebellar approach* (Oppenheim and Krause 1913; Krause 1926; Zapletal 1956; Stein 1971), if the tumor is medium-sized or small. If, however, the tumor is large enough to reach anterior to the abhesio interthalamica, (iii) the *anterior transcallosal transventricular trans-velum interpositum approach* (originally described as the frontal transcallosal approach by Sano in 1983) may be recommended.

Anterior Transcallosal Transventricular Trans-Velum Interpositum Approach

The patient is positioned supine. A coronal or horseshoe-shaped skin incision is made on the right (non-dominant) side, in the frontal region. A quadrangular bone flap extending to the midline and anterior to the coronal suture is elevated. The dura is hinged toward the midline. The right frontal lobe is retracted away from the falx to expose the corpus callosum and the anterior cerebral arteries. The anterior part of the corpus callosum is split between these arteries, 3 to 4 cm in length, proceeding posteriorly to open the pars centralis of the right lateral ventricle (Figs. 1, 2). The velum interpositum is cut just lateral to the tenia fornicis and medial to the cho-

Table 2. Principles of treatment of germ cell tumors and pinealoma. Modified from Sano (1983)

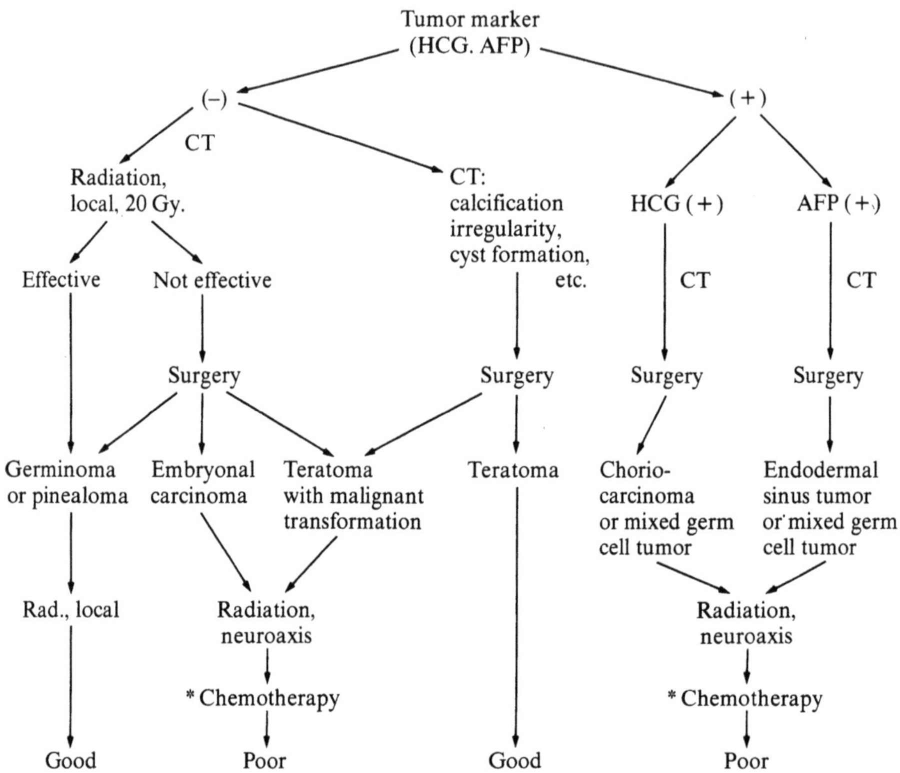

* Chemotherapy: Actinomycin D, cis-Platinum, Vinblastine, Bleomycin, etc.
= When Tumor Size is more than 1.5–2 cm in diameter,
Surgical Removal is recommended as an initial treatment in most cases.

roid plexus (Figs. 2, 3) under the microscope. The bilateral fornices and the internal cerebral veins are retracted to the medial side to explore the tumor between these structures and the right thalamus (Fig. 3). Section of the choroid plexus or the thalamostriate vein is not necessary. Thus the tumor and the surrounding structures are viewed from above and before. Microsurgical manipulation of the tumor is easy because of the ample space. So far, 4 cases of large tumors in the pineal region were operated on by this approach, i.e., 2 cases of huge AFP positive tumors (reported, Sano 1983), one case of anaplastic astrocytoma, and one case of mature teratoma. The last case is a 21-year-old man whose computed tomography (CT) scan is shown in Fig. 4. The tumor was removed en bloc (Fig. 5). The postoperative CT (Fig. 6) reveals no tumor.

The author has experienced no operative mortality either by the occipital or by the infrantentorial or by this transcallosal approach. Steroid is administered before, during, and after the operation.

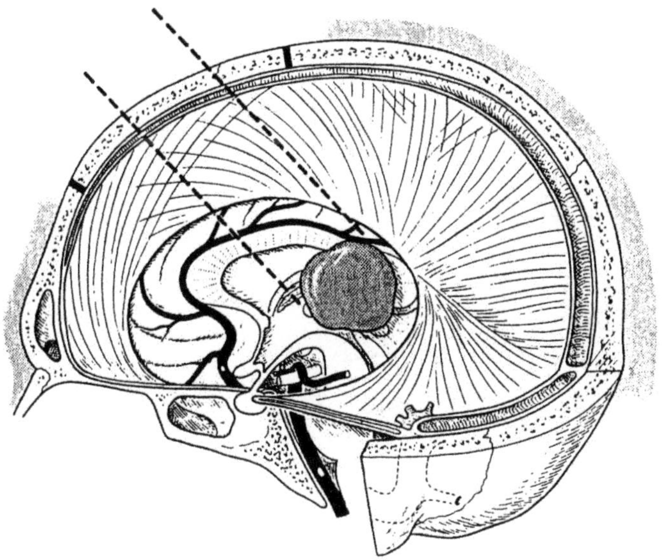

Fig. 1. Anterior transcallosal transventricular trans-velum interpositum approach to a huge pineal tumor. Taken from Sano (1983)

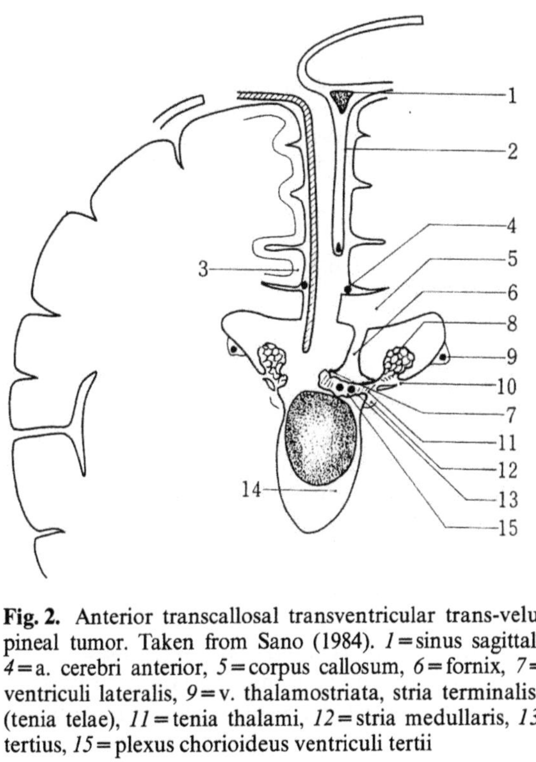

Fig. 2. Anterior transcallosal transventricular trans-velum interpositum approach to a huge pineal tumor. Taken from Sano (1984). *1* = sinus sagittalis superior, *2* = falx, *3* = gyrus cinguli, *4* = a. cerebri anterior, *5* = corpus callosum, *6* = fornix, *7* = tenia fornicis, *8* = plexus chorioideus ventriculi lateralis, *9* = v. thalamostriata, stria terminalis, lamina affixa, *10* = tenia chorioidea (tenia telae), *11* = tenia thalami, *12* = stria medullaris, *13* = v. cerebri interna, *14* = ventriculus tertius, *15* = plexus chorioideus ventriculi tertii

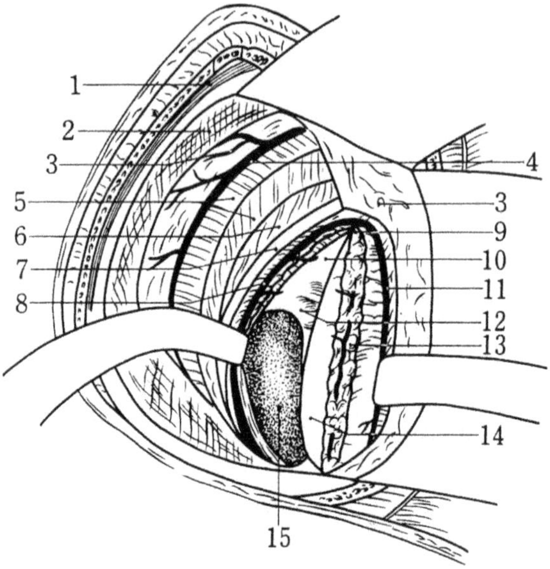

Fig. 3. Anterior transcallosal transventricular trans-velum interposium approach to a huge pineal tumor. Taken from Sano (1984). *1* = sinus sagittalis superior, *2* = falx, *3* = gyrus cinguli, *4* = a. cerebri anterior sinistra, *5* = corpus callosum, *6* = septum pellucidum, *7* = fornix, *8* = v. cerebri interna dextra, *9* = foramen interventriculare, *10* = ventriculus tertius, *11* = v. thalamostriata dextra, lamina affixa, *12* = adhesio interthalamica, *13* = plexus chorioideus ventriculi lateralis dexter, *14* = thalamus dexter, *15* = tumor

Table 3. Follow-up results of tumors in the pineal region submitted to surgery

	Cases	One-year survival (%)	3-year-survival (%)	5-year-survival (%)	10-year-survival (%)
Teratoma (mature)	16	93.7	87.1	78.3	78.3
Epidermoid	2	100.0	100.0	100.0	100.0
PTC (pinealoma and germinoma)	32	96.9	83.3	79.6	74.9
{ PTC ≧ 20 years	14	92.9	78.6	71.4	71.4
{ PTC < 20 years	18	100.0	87.1	87.1	78.3

Postoperative irradiation for pinealoma or germinoma was done with Co-60 or LINAC, the total dose being 5000–6000 rad (the daily dose, 100–200 rad). The field of irradiation was 6×6 cm to 8×8 cm, centering on the pineal region. In cases of malignant tumors, whole brain irradiation and spinal cord irradiation were added, but even in these cases the total dose did not exceed 5000–6000 rad.

Table 3 shows the survival rates calculated by Kaplan-Meier method (1958) of teratoma, epidermoid, and PTC cases. The 10-year-survival rates were 78.3%, 100.0%, and 74.9% respectively. PTC cases were divided into the group 20 years or older and the group younger than 20 years, the latter showing better results (78.3%) than the former (71.4%).

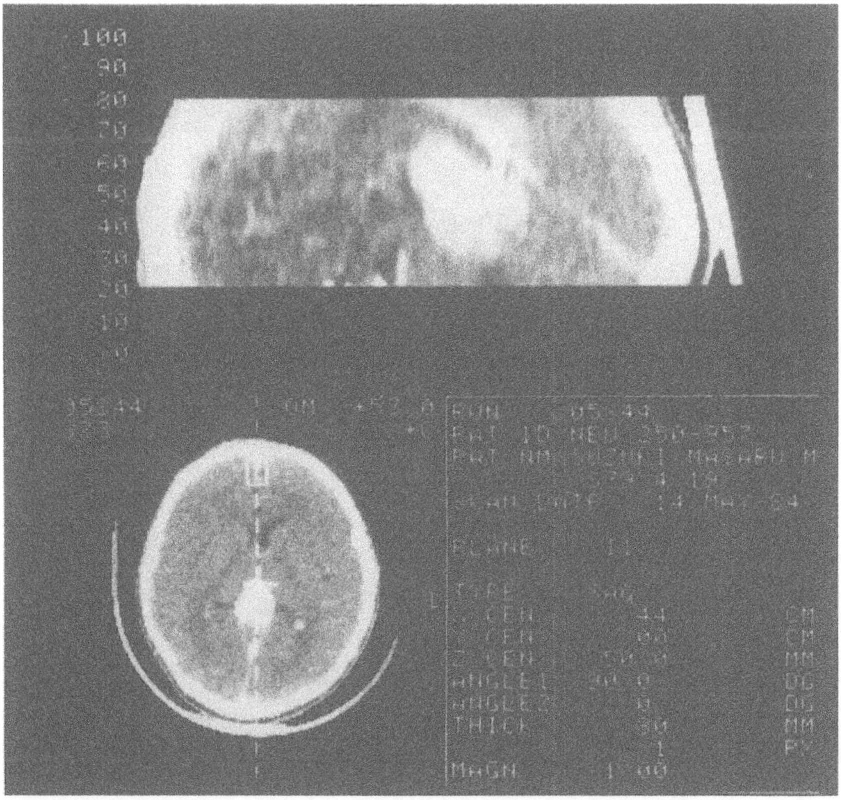

Fig. 4. A 21-year-old man. Contrast-enhanced CT. Horizontal and sagittal sections. A huge tumor in the pineal region

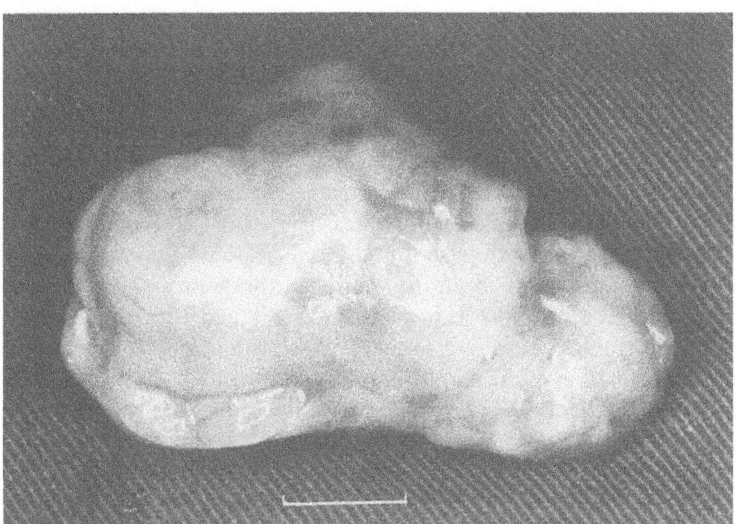

Fig. 5. Extirpated tumor of the case in Fig. 4. Teratoma

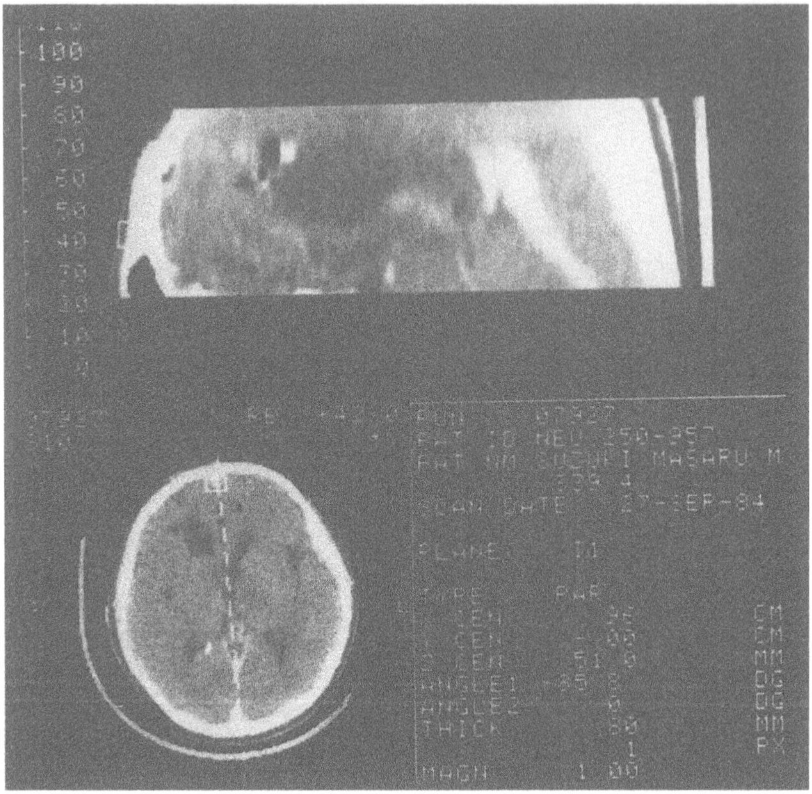

Fig. 6. The same case as in Fig. 4. Postoperative CT (contrast-enhanced). No tumor is seen

Summary and Conclusion

There are various kinds of tumors in the pineal-posterior third ventricular region. Among them, the so-called two-cell pattern tumor (PTC) is most frequent. These tumors can be divided into tumors of pineal parencyma origin (pinealoma) and tumors of germ cell origin (germinoma or seminoma). These two-cell pattern tumors and the so-called germ cell tumors are also found in other areas of the brain, most frequently, however, in the area of the third ventricle. The germ cell tumors are grossly divided into two groups by the tumor markers (AFP and HCG), with those being either positive or negative. However, exact diagnosis can be made only by surgery and histologic examination of the surgical specimens.

As for treatment, mature teratoma and epidermoid should be surgically removed because it is not radiosensitive. Pinealoma and germinoma (seminoma) are radiosensitive; if they are of a considerable size, however, surgical removal and postoperative radiotherapy should be recommended (for these tumors, local radiation may be sufficient in usual cases, since dissemination metastases are not frequent). Embryonal carcinoma, teratoma with malignant transformation, choriocarcinoma, endodermal sinus tumor, or their combinations (mixed germ cell tumors) should be submitted to surgery and postoperative radiation (whole neuraxis) combined with chemotherapy.

Among the various surgical approaches to tumors in the pineal-posterior third ventricular region, the infratentorial supracerebellar approach and the occipital transtentorial approach may be the methods of choice if the tumor is confined posterior to the adhesio interthalamica. If the tumor is large and reaches anterior to the adhesio interthalamica, the anterior transcallosal transventricular trans-velum interpositum approach may be preferable.

References

Friedman NB (1947) Germinoma of the pineal. Its identity with germinoma ("seminoma") of the testis. Cancer Res 7:363–368

Friedman NB (1951) The comparative morphogenesis of extragenital and gonadal teratoid tumors. Cancer 4:265–276

Jamieson KG (1971) Excision of pineal tumors. J Neurosurg 35:550–553

Kaplan EL, Meier P (1958) Non-parametric estimation for incomplete observations. J Am Stat Assoc 53:457–481

Krause F (1926) Operative Freilegung der Vierhügel nebst Beobachtungen über Hirndruck und Dekompression. Zentralbl Chir 53:2812–2819

Oppenheim H, Krause F (1913) Operative Erfolge bei Geschwülsten der Sehhügel- und Vierhügelgegend. Berl Klin Wochenschr 50:2316–2322

Poppen JL, Marino R Jr (1968) Pinealomas and tumors of the posterior portion of the third ventricle. J Neurosurg 28:357–364

Sano K (1983) Pineal region tumors: problems in pathology and treatment. Clin Neurosurg 30:59–91

Sano K (1984) Surgery of pineal tumors – anatomical consideration of various approaches. Neurol Surg 12:1119–1129 (Japanese)

Stein BM (1971) The infratentorial supracerebellar approach to pineal lesions. J Neurosurg 35:197–202

Teilum G (1965) Classification of endodermal sinus tumor (mesoblastoma vitellinum) and so-called embryonal carcinoma of the ovary. Acta Pathol Microbiol Immunol Scand 64:407–429

Zapletal B (1956) Ein neuer operativer Zugang zum Gebiet der Incisura Tentorii. Zentralbl Neurochir 16:64–69

Tumor Markers: Their Role and Limit for Management of Pineal Tumor

N. Arita, Y. Ushio, T. Hayakawa, S. Bitoh, M. Kano, Y. Oku, S. Mori, H. Hasegawa, Y. Maeda, and H. Mogami, Osaka/Japan

Introduction

The 5 year survival rate of patients with pineal tumor has been reported to be between 25 and 79% in the literature (Abay et al. 1981). One of the reasons for this wide variation may be the different therapeutic regimens chosen by each neurosurgeon. The most important reason, however, might be the fact that the treated tumors in each series consisted of histologically different types. Pineal tumors include germ cell tumors, pineoblastomas, pineocytomas, gliomas, and other cystic tumors, and they show different responses to treatments. Recently, specific tumor markers such as alphafetoprotein (AFP) and human chorionic gonadotropin (HCG) were reported to be useful indicators for the management of intracranial germ cell tumors (Allen et al. 1979; Arita et al. 1980; Arita 1985). In this report, we discuss the rational treatment of tumors in the pineal region, especially the surgical indications and the role of tumor markers in the management of germ cell tumors.

Clinical Materials

During the 15 years from June 1970 through December 1984, we encountered 78 pineal and posterior third ventricular tumors. Sixty-three tumors (81%) were diagnosed as primary germ cell tumors, while 15 tumors (19%) were non-germ cell tumors. Germ cell tumors originating in the suprasellar region or basal ganglia are included since the tumor is not necessarily localized in the pineal region and disseminated and multiple tumors are not infrequent upon diagnosis.

Therapeutic Regimens and Results

Germ Cell Tumor

Conservative treatment, consisting of irradiation of the whole neuro-axis and, if necessary, shunt procedures to alleviate the accompanying hydrocephalus, has been our standard treatment of choice for the germ cell tumor. In 40 of 63 patients with germ cell tumors, the serum and/or CSF levels of both AFP and HCG were determined before the initial treatment. Based on the results of these data, the patients were divided into 2 groups. In 18 patients, both markers were negative (Group A), and in 22, one or both markers were positive (Group B). In Group A, 2 patients

(11%) died: one who had not received irradiation to the spine died of wide-spread dissemination of the tumor in the subarachnoid space, and the other died of an unknown cause not directly related to the tumor. The other 17 patients (89%) have now survived for 8 months to 13 years since the diagnosis. In Group B, 12 patients (55%) died, and the remaining 10 (45%) have now survived for 8 months to 10 years since the diagnosis. Figure 1 shows the correlation between the level of tumor markers and the outcome for the patients in group B. Most of the patients with high levels of the tumor markers died, while the survivors are in the subgroup of patients with relatively lower marker levels. And all the patients positive for HCG only in the CSF are alive. The survival curves (Kaplan-Meier) of the patients in Groups A and B are shown in Fig. 2. The difference in the survival times of the groups is statistically significant ($p < 0.05$, generalized Wilcoxon test). Even if the statistical evaluation is made only of the patients with a tumor localized in the pineal region, the difference is still significant ($p < 0.05$).

Non-Germ Cell Tumor

In these cases, different therapeutic approaches were used depending upon the clinical situation. Seven of 15 tumors were histologically verified; they consisted of 3 ependymomas, 2 glioblastomas, one pineocytoma, and one pineoblastoma. All except for the patient with a pineocytoma died one month to 2 years and 2 months after diagnosis. No histological examinations were made of the 8 remaining patients. Three of these 8 patients died, and the remaining 5 are alive.

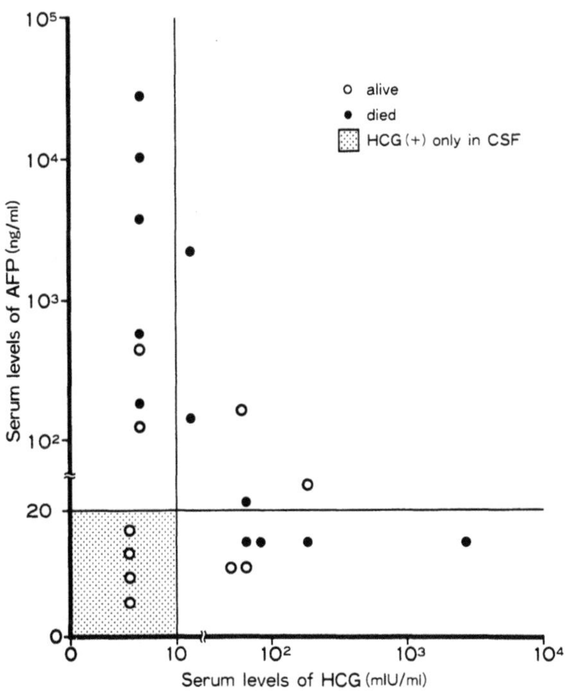

Fig. 1. Correlation of outcome of the patients with serum and cerebrospinal fluid levels of the tumor marker

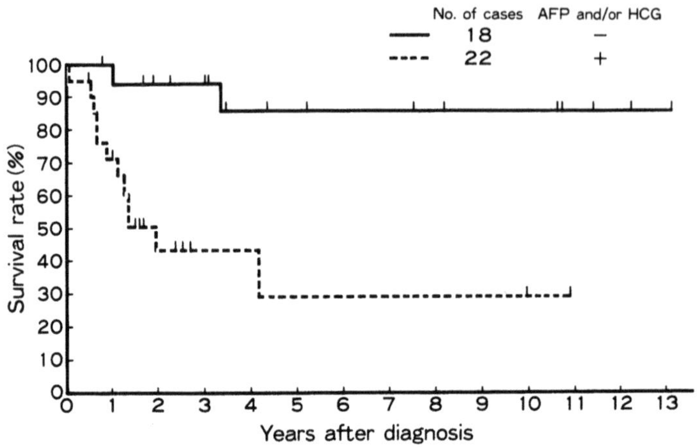

Fig. 2. Survival curves (Kaplan-Meier) of patients with germ cell tumor, in whom serum and/or cerebrospinal fluid levels of AFP and HCG were determined before treatment

Table 1. Treatment of germ cell tumor with AFP and HCG (–) (pre.: before radiotherapy, post.: after radiotherapy, Ara-C: cytosine arabinoside, MTX: methotrexate, PVB: combination chemotherapy with cisplatinum, vinblastine and bleomycin, RT: radiotherapy)

		CT	CSF cytology		Treatment
			Pre.	Post.	
Stage I		Localized	(–)	(–)	Local or whole neuro-axis RT
Stage II	A	Localized	(+)	(–)	Whole neuro-axis RT
	B	Multi-focal or disseminated	–		Whole neuro-axis RT
	C	–	(+)	(+)	Chemotherapy (Ara-C, MTX)
Stage III		Extra-CNS metastasis	–		Systemic chemotherapy (PVB)

Table 2. Treatment of germ cell tumor with AFP and/or HCG (+) (PVB: combination chemotherapy with cisplatinum, vinblastine and bleomycin, RT: radiotherapy)

	Marker	Treatment
Stage I	HCG (+) only in CSF	Same as for germinoma
Stage II	Moderate elevation of AFP and/or HCG	RT, Surgery
Stage III	Marked elevation of AFP and/or HCG	Surgery, RT Chemotherapy (PVB)

Surgery

Seventeen patients underwent surgical removal of the tumor. In the earlier part of this series, a parietal transventricular approach was used in 8 patients. No more than partial resection of the tumor could be achieved in these cases. We experienced one operative death. Recently, we used an infratentorial supracerebellar approach in 5 patients and an occipital transtentorial approach in 4 patients. The surgical approach was determined by each surgeon on the basis of experience. In 8 of these 9 cases, subtotal or total resection of the tumor was attained. We have not experienced any operative death or major postoperative morbidity. Some representative cases are described below.

Case 1 (Figs. 3, 4): A 33-year-old female was admitted because of headaches. The CT appearance, absence of tumor markers and negative CSF cytology were suggestive of a non-germ cell tumor, and a posterior fossa craniectomy was performed. A well demarcated tumor with a cyst was removed in total via an infratentorial supracerebellar approach with the patient in the Concorde position (Kobayashi et al. 1983). The tumor was histologically a pineocytoma. The postoperative course was uneventful except for a transient upward gaze palsy of 3 weeks' duration.

Case 2 (Fig. 5): An 8-year-old boy developed headaches and vomiting. The serum levels of AFP and HCG were 240 ng/ml and 71 mIU/ml, respectively. Radiation therapy was started. However, the tumor was not reduced in size after irradiation with 2000 cGy. Therefore, the patient underwent direct surgical intervention. Total resection of a well-circumscribed tumor was performed by an infratentorial supracerebellar approach with the patient in the sitting position. The tumor was histologically an embryonal carcinoma.

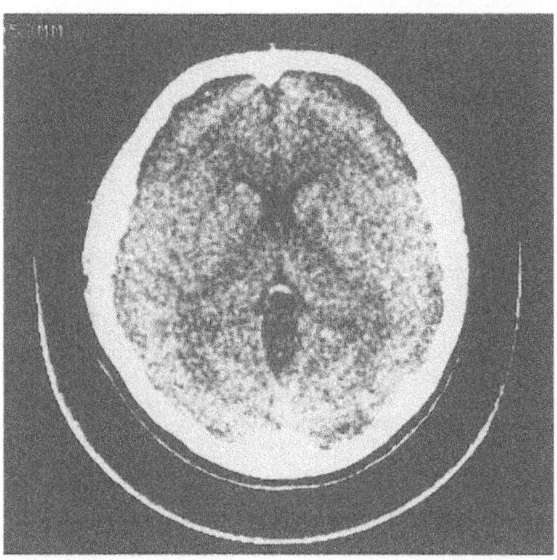

Fig. 3. Plain CT scan obtained on admission showing an isodense tumor with calcification in the pineal region in Case 1

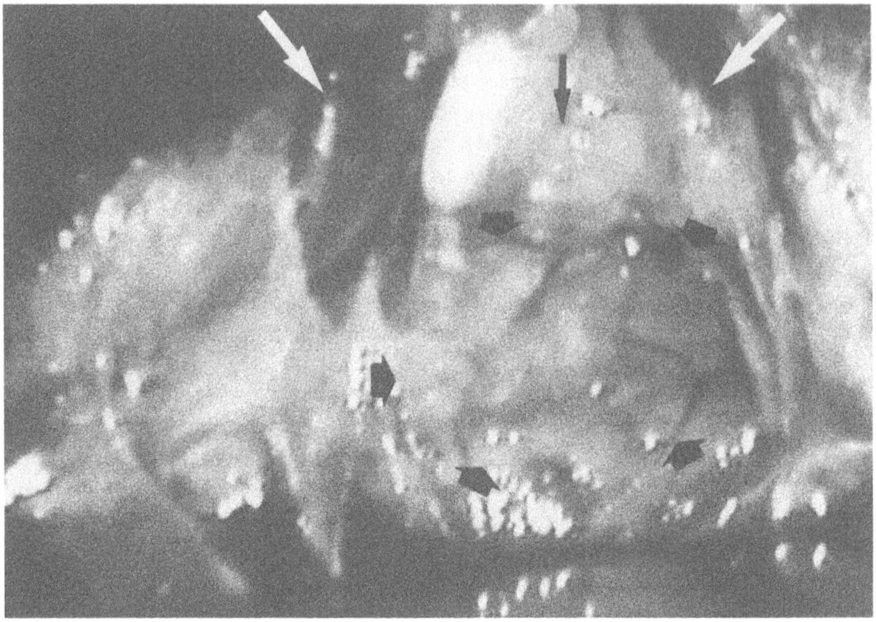

Fig. 4. Operative microphotograph of infratentorial supracerebellar approach in Case 1 demonstrating a tumor (*large arrows*), basal veins of Rosenthal (*white arrows*) and suprapineal resessus of third ventricle (*small arrow*)

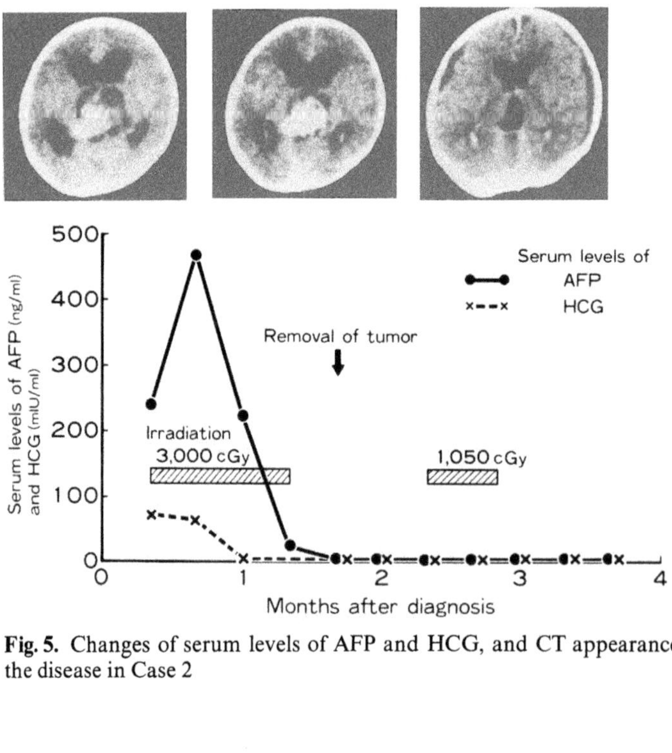

Fig. 5. Changes of serum levels of AFP and HCG, and CT appearances during the course of the disease in Case 2

a 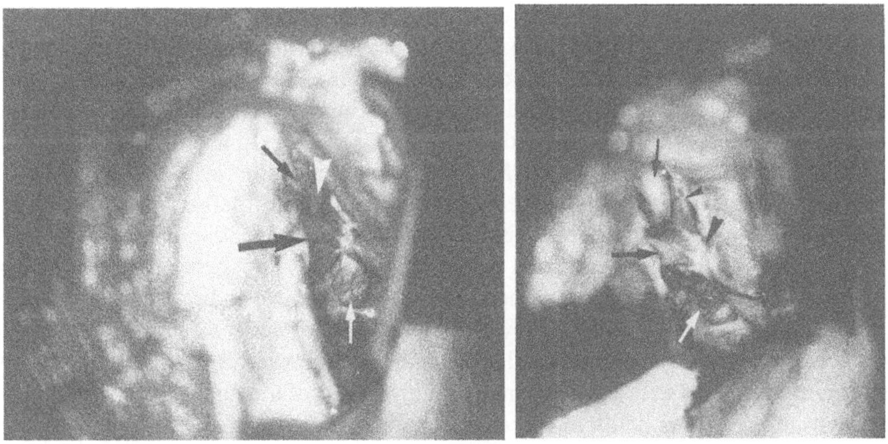 b

Fig. 6 a. Operative microphotograph of right occipital transtentorial approach in Case 3 demonstrating a tumor (*small arrow*), quadrigeminal plate (*white arrow*), vein of Galen (*large arrow*) and right internal cerebral vein (*white arrow-head*). **b** After removal of the tumor, third ventricle (*small arrow*), quadrigeminal plate (*white arrow*), vein of Galen (*large arrow*), right basal vein of Rosenthal (*large arrow-head*) and right internal cerebral vein (*small arrow-heads*)

Case 3 (Figs. 6a, b): A 17-year-old male was admitted because of headache and vomiting. First, 2200 cGy was irradiated, but the tumor increased somewhat in size. Therefore, an occipital transtentorial exposure of the tumor was made, and it was removed in total. The histological diagnosis was ependymoma.

Discussion

During the past decade, encouraging results with direct surgical approaches to pineal tumors have been described (Jamieson 1971; Stein 1971; Lazar and Clark 1974; Sano 1983), and some neurosurgeons believe that surgical exploration should be performed initially in all cases of pineal tumor. In our recent series using the occipital transtentorial and infratentorial supracerebellar approaches, no operative death or major complication occurred. However, this therapeutic modality should be further evaluated by a long-term follow-up study (Jooma and Kendall 1983). Accordingly, at present, surgery should be determined not on the basis of the operative risk, but by benefit to the patient. Our results suggest that irradiation is preferable for germinomas, while multidisciplinary treatment is required for marker-positive germ cell tumors. Tables 1 and 2 show our present treatment schedule of the germ cell tumor based on the provisional staging of the patients, derived from the results concerning about the tumor marker.

In the case of pineal tumors, direct surgical intervention is attempted (1) to remove the tumor in total for permanent cure by surgery alone, (2) to reduce the tumor burden for the postoperative adjuvant therapies and (3) to obtain a firm histological diagnosis of the tumor to determine the most beneficial schedule of treatment. Benign cystic lesions clearly demonstrated by CT can be cured by surgical resection. In patients in whom a non-cystic tumor other than a germ cell tumor is suspected by both the CT appearance and the absence of tumor markers, histological confirmation of the tumor is considered to be mandatory. Although surgical cure cannot be expected in malignant gliomas such as in Case 3, other less malignant tumors like pineocytoma or low-grade astrocytoma may be resectable as in Case 1, and long survival can be expected. Most patients in our series, who had a high level of a tumor marker and were treated conservatively, died. Malignant germ cell tumors like embryonal carcinomas are often well demarcated despite their histologically malignant features, and total removal was achieved. Therefore, we consider that the tumor bulk should be reduced as much as possible to be followed by combined irradiation and chemotherapy. In patients with a moderate level of a marker, the level often declines upon irradiation, but the tumor hardly changes in size, as shown in Case 2. In such cases, the major components of the tumor have been transformed into a mature teratoma, necrosis or fibrosis, and permanent cure could be expected by surgical removal.

The occipital transtentorial (Lazar and Clark 1974) and infratentorial supracerebellar approaches (Stein 1971) have been most commonly used for pineal tumors in the last decade. We have used both approaches, and in all cases satisfactory exposure of the tumor has been anatomically attained. As described previously, there are two disadvantages in the infratentorial supracerebellar approach with the patient in the sitting position: first there is danger of an air embolism and second, the surgeon tires easily (Reid and Clark 1978). However, we feel that both can be avoided by placing the patient in the Concorde position. We consider that each neurosurgeon can determine the surgical approach on the basis of his experience.

Acknowledgment: The authors are grateful to all the staff of the Department of Neurosurgery, Osaka University Medical School in the management of these patients, and thank Miss Reiko Fujita for her help in this investigation.

This investigation was supported by Grant-in-Aid from the Ministry of Welfare (NO. 59-22) and the Ministry of Education (No. 58480304) in Japan

References

Abay EO, Laws ER Jr, Grado Gl, Bruckman JE, Forbes GS, Gomez MR, Scott M (1981) Pineal tumors in children and adolescents. Treatment by CSF shunting and radiotherapy. J Neurosurg 55:889–895

Allen JC, Nisselbaum J, Epstein F, Rosen G, Schwartz MK (1979) Alphafetoprotein and human chorionic gonadotropin determination in cerebrospinal fluid. An aid to the diagnosis and management of intracranial germ-cell tumors. J Neurosurg 51:368–374

Arita N, Ushio Y, Hayakawa T, Watanabe M, Mori T, Mogami H (1980) Serum levels of alphafetoprotein, human chorionic gonadotropin and carcinoembryonic antigen in patients with primary intracranial germ cell tumor. Oncodev Biol Med 1:235–240

Arita N (1985) The role of tumor markers in the management of primary intracranial germ cell tumors. Neurosurgeons 4:101–113 (in Japanese)

Jamieson KG (1971) Excision of pineal tumors. J Neurosurg 35:550–553

Jooma R, Kendall BE (1983) Diagnosis and management of pineal tumors. J Neurosurg 58:654–665

Kobayashi S, Sugita K, Tanaka Y, Kyoshima K (1983) Infratentorial approach to the pineal region in the prone position: Concorde position. J Neurosurg 58:141–143

Lazar ML, Clark K (1974) Direct surgical management of masses in the region of the vein of Galen. Surg Neurol 2:17–21
Reid WS, Clark WK (1978) Comparison of the infratentorial and transtentorial approaches to the pineal region. Neurosurgery 3:1–8
Sano K (1983) Pineal region tumors: Problems in pathology and treatment. Clin Neurosurg 30:59–91
Stein BM (1971) The infratentorial supracerebellar approach to pineal lesions. J Neurosurg 35:197–202

A New Operative Approach to the Pineal Region

J. I. Ausman, G. M. Malik, J. Pearce, and J. S. Rogers, Detroit, MI/USA

A variety of approaches to the pineal region has been advocated, however, all have some significant disadvantages. A new operative approach to the pineal tentorial region is introduced to eliminate these disadvantages: the three-quarter prone operated side down occipital parietal transtentorial approach.

Methods

After the patient is intubated while supine on the operating table, the patient is repositioned in the park bench position with the operated side down. The patient is then tilted three-quarters prone and secured to the operating table with three inch tape. The patient's head is angled 45 degrees to the floor with the operated parietal occipital area on the inferior side. The patient's head is then tilted up 15 to 20 degrees and flexed. The head is secured in a Mayfield head holder with one set of points below the transverse sinus and the other in the left frontal region. An occipital parietal craniotomy is made with the medial limb over the sagittal sinus and the lateral limb descending behind the right ear to the transverse sinus. The bony margins are on the sagittal and transverse sinuses. With intraoperative ultrasound, if

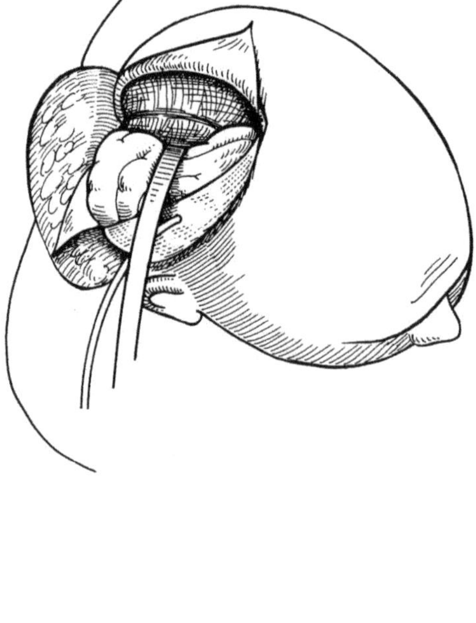

Fig. 1. New operative approach to pineal region

available, a cannula is placed through the dura into the right lateral ventricle. The dura is opened with a flap on each sinus. The occipital lobe should gradually fall away from the falx with gentle retraction as the spinal fluid escapes from the lateral ventricle. The tentorium cerebelli is identified and sectioned below and parallel to the straight sinus to the tentorial hiatus. The medial flap of the tentorium is lifted up and temporarily tacked to the falx with suture (Fig. 1). The microscope is then utilized to reach the pineal region. Should access to the third ventricle be required, a small, 2 to 3 mm, section of the splenium can be made to expose the internal cerebral veins and gain access between them to the third ventricle. Both the surgeon and the assistant are comfortably seated to perform surgery through the microscope for a prolonged period with limited fatigue. The drain is usually left in place upon closure and exits through a separate tunnelled drain site on the skin where it is left for several days after surgery to provide decompression and intracerebral pressure monitoring.

Results and Discussion

The position has been utilized without morbidity and mortality in six patients with lesions in the pineal tentorial region (Table 1).

In the supracerebellar approach to the pineal region popularized by Stein (1971), there are a number of disadvantages. The patient is in a sitting position which would increase the chance of air embolus. The position is uncomfortable for the surgeon as his arms must be extended above his shoulders to reach the pineal region. Prolonged work in this position is extremely tiring. Since the surgeon occupies the central portion of the operating field there is limited access for manual help. Access to the third ventricle is possible with this approach, however, this represents the most distal point in the operating field and at the limit of the operating instruments. No occipital lobe retraction is necessary with this approach.

To avoid the disadvantages of the sitting position Kobayashi et al. (1983) has introduced the Concorde position. The patient is prone with his neck flexed and the shoulders elevated but the head slightly tilted to the right to allow the surgeon to have access to this supracerebellar region. The position is still uncomfortable for the surgeon as he is operating from the patient's side. The chance of air embolus is diminished, although the head is still higher than the heart. By being in an opposite

Table 1. Lesions in pineal region

Lesions	*Location*
Germinoma	Pineal
Ganglioglioma Pineocytoma	Pineal
Glioma	Pineal
AVM	Splenium Medial parietal lobe
Meningioma	Tentorial notch
Lymphoma	Splenium and Hemispheral

position to the surgeon the assistant's access to the operating field is limited. The same criticisms about access to the third ventricle would apply in this as in the sitting position. There is no occipital lobe retraction in this approach either.

Reid and Clark (1978) have compared the supracerebellar and the occipital transtentorial approaches. In their proposal the patient is in the seated position, which includes the risk of air embolus. Retraction of the occipital pole, which is a disadvantage, could lead to a homonymous field defect. There is a wider operative field which allows more access for the surgeon and the assistant; however, the assistant is still to the side of the surgeon and the access to the operating field is still somewhat limited from this approach. To reach the third ventricle with the patient in this position, the operating table must be lowered or the surgeon must rise. This provides more convenient access to the third ventricle than in the supracerebellar approach but the direction movement required to reach this area is not optimal for the patient or surgeon.

To avoid these problems Sano (1983) suggested that the patient should be placed prone and the occipital transtentorial approach should be utilized. This position is comfortable for the surgeon, allows room for the assistant, and eliminates the risk of air embolus. Access to the third ventricle is improved over the supracerebellar approach but occipital lobe retraction is still required.

With the three-quarter prone position, the surgeon and assistant are seated comfortably and both have access to the entire operative field. The risk of air embolus is reduced although the head is still somewhat elevated. Access to the third ventricle is optimal as the splenium can be sectioned and the third ventricle adequately reached through this approach. Occipital lobe retraction is minimized. We feel that the three-quarter prone operated side down, occipital-parietal transtentorial approach provides the best alternative to reach the pineal region with elimination of the disadvantages of the other positions.

References

Kobayashi K, Sugita K, Tanaka Y, Kyoshima K (1983) Intratentorial approach to the pineal region in the prone position: Concorde position. J Neurosurg 58: 141–143

Reid WS, Clark WK (1978) Comparison of the infratentorial and transtentorial approaches to the pineal region. Neurosurg 3: 1–8

Sano K (1983) Pineal region tumors: Problems in pathology and treatment. Clin Neurosurg 30: 59–91

Stein B (1971) The infratentorial supracerebellar approach to pineal lesions. J Neurosurg 35: 197–202

Two Approaches to the Anterior Third Ventricle

I. Via the Velum Interpositum
II. Via the Lamina Terminalis and Sphenoid Sinus

R. H. PATTERSON, Jr. and M. H. LAVYNE, New York/USA

I. Via the Velum Interpositum

Attempts to remove a brain tumor in the anterior third ventricle are hampered by the surgeons inability to expose the cavity of the ventricle widely. An option is to enlarge the foramen of Monro posteriorly, but here the internal cerebral vein, which is formed by the joining of the thalamostriate and septal veins, is in the way. We believe that dividing either the septal vein or the thalamostriate vein carries no important risk because adequate collateral circulation exists between the superficial cortical and deep medullary venous systems that drain the posterior frontal and basal ganglion regions. Hirsch et al. as well as DeLandsheer et al. emphasize that one thalamostriate vein could be divided without risk (DeLandsheer et al. 1978; Hirsch et al. 1979). Our experience with fourteen third ventricle tumors operated on during the last five years supports the notion that this approach will give wide exposure to the third ventricle with safety (Lavyne and Patterson 1983).

Surgical Technique

Prior to surgery a bilateral carotid arteriogram with a venous phase is performed in order to identify the location of cerebral veins entering the sagittal sinus. We operate on the side of the head in which the venous drainage is most favorable for retraction of the cerebral hemisphere from the falx. We look for a spot in the region of the coronal suture that is free of veins so that no cortical vein will need to be divided in order to gain the required exposure.

The patient may be positioned on the operating table in one of two ways. The first possibility, which we have used for the most part, is to have the head straight with the nose pointed upwards. The approach then would be either on the right or left side along the falx to the region of the corpus callosum. The second possibility is to turn the head in a true lateral position with the side to be operated down and the unoperated side uppermost. The head is then tilted upwards and after a craniotomy is performed over the sagittal sinus and the dependent cerebral hemisphere, the brain falls by gravity away from the falx minimizing the amount of retraction that is necessary.

In either case, the bone flap measures about five cm square and exposes the appropriate cerebral hemisphere as well as the sagittal sinus. The dura is open, and if the bone flap has been well planned, it should be possible to retract the hemisphere from the falx without encountering any cerebral veins.

Spinal fluid is withdrawn from previously placed lumbar needles, and dissection is carried down to the corpus callosum and the pericallosal branches of the anterior cerebral arteries.

The corpus callosum is divided over a distance of two or three centimeters and the lateral ventricle is entered. The foramen of Monro is readily identified by following the choroid plexus. Retractors should not be placed deep in the body of the ventricle because the internal capsule passes in the wall of the ventricle and deep retraction may lead to a hemiparesis. A retractor can also be placed on the falx, but retraction must not be too heavy because a hemiparesis or speech defect can result from sagittal sinus occlusion.

The choroid plexus is coagulated and retracted superiorly and towards the opposite hemisphere. Dissection of the posterior margin of the foramen of Monro will reveal the thalamostriate and septal veins.

In case of a tumor of substantial size, the internal cerebral vein will be displaced laterally, and in this case it is usually appropriate to coagulate the septal vein and elevate the choroid plexus from the foramen of Monro posteriorly. This leaves the internal cerebral vein closely applied to the thalamus. In some cases it will be more appropriate to divide the thalamostriate vein, in which case the internal cerebral vein will be reflected superiorly with the choroid plexus. This affords a wide view of the inside of the third ventricle, including the posterior medial choroidal arteries, which are close to the internal cerebral vein. In some instances we have divided both the septal and thalamostriate veins without any harm to the patient. In these cases we observed a direct lateral vein that drains into the internal cerebral vein from the caudate nucleus in the mid-portion of the lateral ventricle. If this vein is present, it will cause enough flow in the internal cerebral vein that both the septal and thalamostriate veins may be divided without subsequent thrombosis of the internal cerebral vein (Fig. 1).

Despite removal of a tumor in the anterior third ventricle, some patients will still require a shunting procedure because of persistent hydrocephalus. If a shunt has not been performed prior to surgery, we generally leave a catheter in the lateral ven-

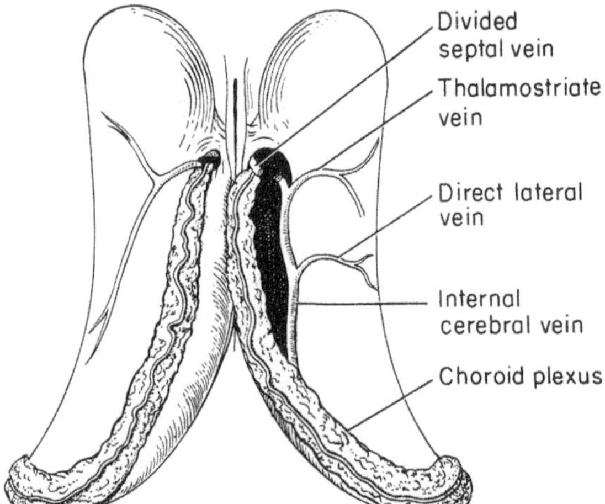

Fig. 1. The septal vein in the right lateral ventricle is divided and the choroid plexus has been elevated from the thalamus exposing the cavity of the third ventricle

tricle connected to an Ommaya's reservoir of a type that can be converted to a shunt. The reservoir attached to a catheter in the ventricle allows measurement of intracranial pressure in the postoperative period, allows aspiration of fluid if intracranial pressure is high, and may be readily converted to a shunt if necessary.

All our patients operated by this technique have done well postoperatively, though several required a shunting procedure.

One patient died two months following surgery as a consequence of a pulmonary embolus. Autopsy in this patient revealed no pathologic findings in the deep venous structures or in the basal ganglia that might be attributed to coagulation and division of the septal vein, which had been performed in this case.

II. Exposure of the Anterior Third Ventricle Through the Lamina Terminalis and Sphenoid Sinus

Exposure and removal of craniopharyngiomas located in the anterior third ventricle and suprasellar cistern is difficult because of the location of the tumor and also because in many cases the optic nerves are quite short with the optic chiasm nearly touching the tuberculum sellae. Many surgeons prefer to approach this tumor laterally along the sphenoidal ridge in order to gain access to the tumor behind the chiasm, but this is difficult because the internal carotid artery is in the way.

In these tumors we prefer a frontal approach along the line of the falx to expose the lamina terminalis. If the optic nerves are short, we advocate opening the sphenoid sinus and removing the tuberculum sellae to make room to remove the tumor without having to extract it between the optic tracts, which may be difficult if the tumor is large and calcified.

Surgical Technique

The operative approach can be through a small low unilateral bone flap on the right side that spans the distance between the falx and the temporal line just above the superior orbital ridge. The patient is positioned with the head in pin fixation and the nose pointed straight up. Lumbar spinal fluid drainage is also important to allow the brain to fall back from the roof of the orbit. If the orbital roof is tilted backwards approximately forty-five degrees, gravity will aid in the retraction. The region with the optic chiasm is then exposed, dividing the olfactory nerve. If retraction and exposure of the lamina terminalis is difficult, then the surgeon should extend the bone flap to the left side exposing the sagittal sinus. A bifrontal bone flap is probably appropriate in all cases in which the tumor is large, because one can anticipate that exposure of the lamina terminalis will be difficult. In this case the falx is divided just above the crista galli. In some cases it may be possible to preserve the olfactory tracts by dissecting them carefully from the underside of the frontal lobe. Dividing the falx then allows retractions of both frontal lobes not only posteriorly but also to either side, which will give excellent exposure of the lamina terminalis and the optic chiasm. Because the head is tilted backwards forty-five degrees, it is usually most convenient to use the operating microscope with straight eye pieces and to be seated using an armrest.

The first thing to do if the optic nerves are short is to remove the tuberculum sellae. This is done by creating a flap of dura over the tuberculum that is reflected anteriorly towards the crista galli. The sphenoid sinus is then opened using a mallet and chisel, or it can be opened by a high speed burr. In either case the sinus is opened from one optic nerve to the other and the bone of the tuberculum and the front of the sella turcica is removed either with the burr or with long, fine bone instruments. The dura, including the circular sinus, is then divided in front of the pituitary gland. This gives an excellent exposure between the optic nerves.

Attention is turned to the lamina terminalis, which can be distinguished from the optic nerves and chiasm by a red-colored blush of fine blood vessels. This is the appropriate place to push a blunt instrument through the lamina and expose the inside of the third ventricle.

Usually, craniopharyngiomas are firm, and the withdrawal of tumor from between the optic tracts means that the optic tracts are repeatedly brushed by each bit of tumor, which may lead to visual loss. All manipulation of the tumor should be done in a direction away from the optic nerves, chiasm, and tracts. Tumor fragments are pushed downwards into the sphenoid sinus and extracted from the sphenoid sinus without coming close to optic apparatus (Fig. 2).

After the tumor is removed, we take fat, which is usually obtained from another patient undergoing a general surgical operation, and put it in the sphenoid sinus after pushing the sphenoid mucosa downwards. When the fat fills the sphenoid sinus, we use a few sutures to reattach the dura over the fat so that it will not be extruded into the head if the patient sneezes or blows his nose. Spinal fluid is replaced, and the dura is closed.

Usually, the frontal sinuses will be widely open because of the saw cut flush with the roof of the orbit. We push the mucosa downwards and also fill these sinuses with fat. A small flap of pericranium is elevated from the underside of the scalp flap and sewn down to the dura to seal the opening to the frontal sinuses and to hold the fat in place. Then the bone plate is replaced and the scalp closed without drainage.

We have had experience with 125 operations for craniopharyngioma and used this in approximately 22 of these cases. We find the technique most helpful, and the

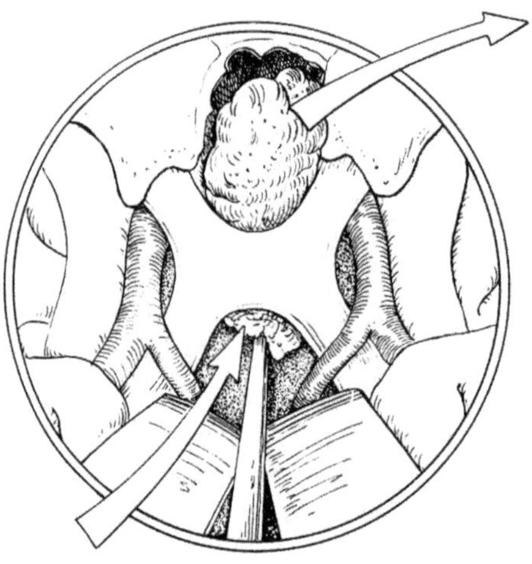

Fig. 2. Through a small bifrontal bone flap the lamina terminalis is exposed. The tuberculum sellae and front of the sella turcica has been removed. Tumor is pushed down and away from the optic chiasm (*A*) and extracted through the sphenoid sinus (*B*)

operative mortality in these 125 operations has been just 2. The first was in a patient who died in the postoperative period from upper gastrointestinal hemorrhage due to esophageal varices caused by an unrecognized malignant tumor of the liver. The second death occurred in a patient one week following surgery from a sudden cardiorespiratory arrest. The cause for this was not clear but since the patient was doing well and ambulatory, we believe that it may have had something to do with sudden change in intracranial spinal fluid dynamics (Patterson and Danylevich 1980).

Conclusion

In this paper we have presented two useful approaches to the two tumors in the anterior part of the third ventricle that we believe can be most helpful in dealing with tumors in this area.

References

1. DeLandsheer JM, Guyot JF, Jomin M, Sherpereel B, Laine E (1978) Acces au troisieme ventricle par voie inter-thalamo-trigonale. Neurochirurgie 24:419–421
2. Hirsch JF, Zouaoui A, Renien D, Pierre-Kahn A (1979) A new surgical approach to the third ventricle with interruption of the striothalamic vein. Acta Neurochir (Wien) 47:135–147
3. Lavyne MH, Patterson RH Jr (1983) Subchoroidal trans-velum interpositum approach to mid-third ventricular tumors. Neurosurgery Vol. 12, no. 1, 86–94
4. Patterson RH Jr, Danylevich A (1980) Surgical removal of cranio-pharyngiomas by a transcranial approach through the lamina terminalis and sphenoid sinus. Neurosurgery 7:111–117

Interhemispheric Trans-Lamina Terminalis Approach by Bifrontal Craniotomy to Tumor of the Anterior Part of Third Ventricle

J. SUZUKI, R. KATAKURA, T. KAYAMA, and T. YOSHIMOTO, Sendai/Japan

Introduction

Our surgical approach to tumors of the anterior portion of the third ventricle, namely the interhemispheric trans-lamina terminalis approach by bifrontal craniotomy, will be discussed [10].

This approach has several advantages. First, the main arteries can be exposed and the operative field is sufficiently wide to render the operative procedure safely. Second, cortical incision or excision is unnecessary. By cutting the lamina terminalis, which is usually thin and expanded as a result of hydrocephalus, even a large tumor can be removed. In addition, lethal complications are avoided, because this approach includes lesser risks of damage to the lateral wall of the third ventricle. In eighteen patients with a tumor in the third ventricle operation was performed via this approach. The operative technique and representative case will be reported.

Operative Method and Result

Various approaches to tumors of the third ventricle have been used (Fig. 1) since Dandy's right frontal excision. Whichever approach is taken, the substance of the brain, particularly the important tissue around the third ventricle, must not be damaged and cerebral vessels must not be sacrificed if the postoperative development of severe complications is to be avoided [2, 5]. To excise tumors from the third ventricle, it is inevitable that some damage will be done to the ventricular

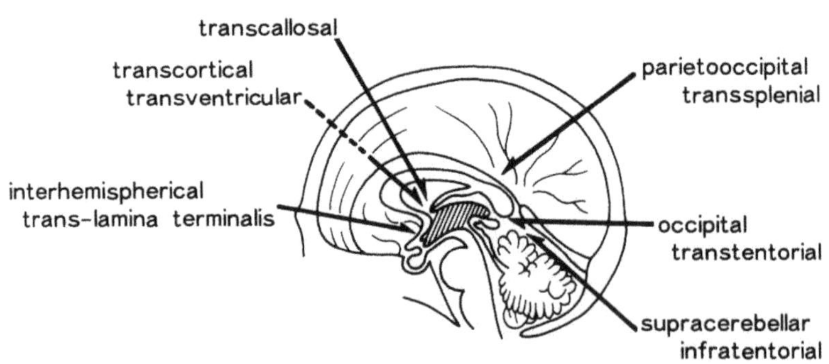

Fig. 1. Various operative approaches to a tumor of the third ventricle

wall; thus, it is relevant to note that its thinnest portion is at the lamina terminalis (Fig. 2) – that is, at the gap between the optic tracts posterior to the optic chiasm. In this region lie the hypothalamus and vital regulatory centers, such as the supraoptic nucleus and infundibular nucleus; in most cases, however, hydrocephalus is present due to the tumor and this region has become extremely thin and wide. In addition, hypothalamic functions are often found to be depressed. Before reaching a tumor that extends over the lamina terminalis, precautions must be taken regarding the anterior communicating artery. If this region is sufficiently dissected, however, the lamina terminalis can be passed through posteriorly, anterior to the anterior communicating artery, and the tumor removed. If a sufficient length of the anterior communicating artery is available for sectioning, it can be cut and the left and right A1 and A2 portions separated and displaced to the appropriate sides to produce a still wider operative field (Fig. 3). In cases in which irreversible changes have occurred in the optic chiasma because of the tumor, and recovery of visual defects is impossible, an anterior-posterior cut in the chiasm can render the field still wider.

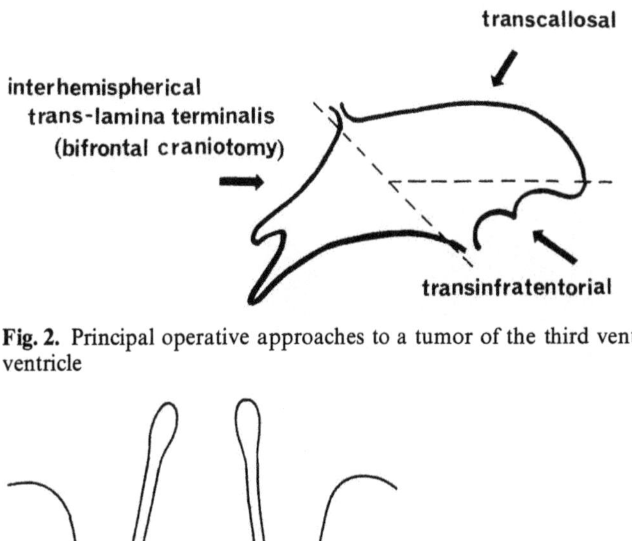

Fig. 2. Principal operative approaches to a tumor of the third ventricle in each portion of the ventricle

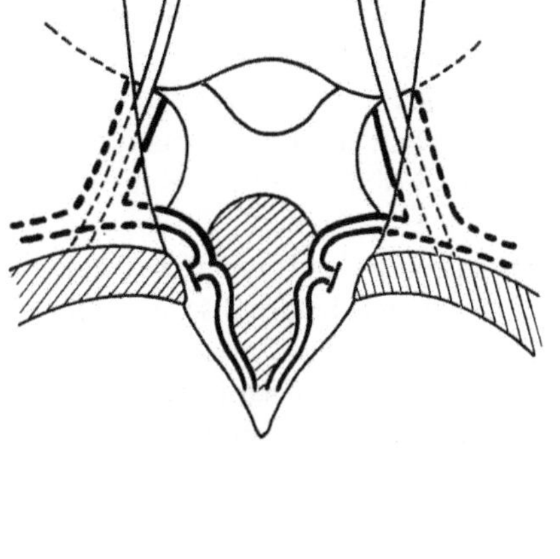

Fig. 3. If necessary, for a wider operative field, the anterior communicating artery can be cut

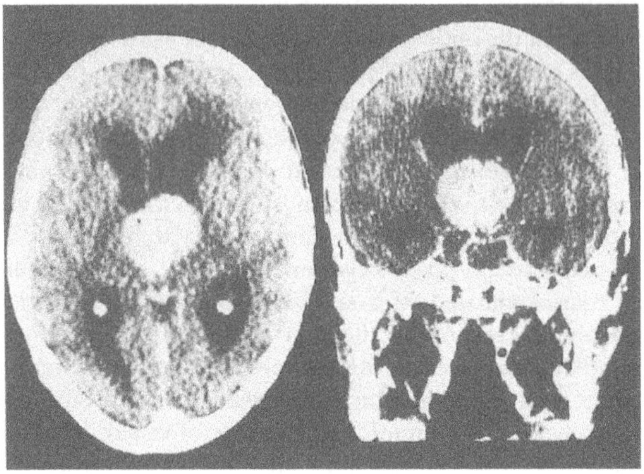

Fig. 4. Computed tomography scans with contrast medium enhancement. Preoperative CT scan with contrast medium enhancement, showing a giant tumor of the third ventricle

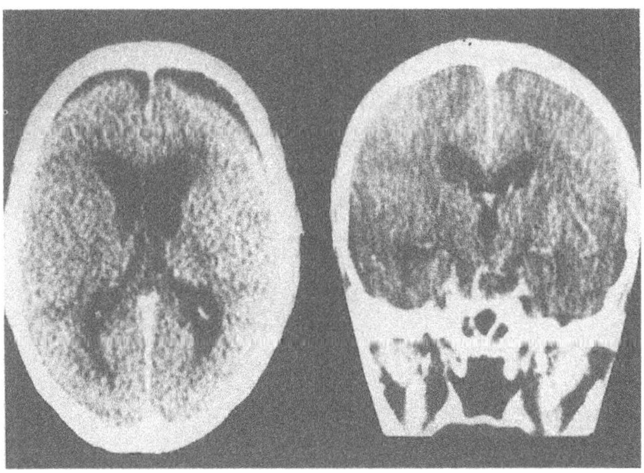

Fig. 5. Postoperative CT scan, showing that the tumor shadow has disappeared

Next a representative case is reported. The patient is a 37-year-old man who complained of headache and disturbance of visual field. Computed tomography scans with contrast medium enhancement showed a giant tumor of the third ventricle. So, we operated upon by our surgical method and the tumor was removed totally. Although he suffered from temporary diabetes insipidus, postoperatively, he was discharged in good condition (Figs. 4, 5).

Postoperative complications include diabetes insipidus and hypernatremia; in our experience, however, such symptoms have disappeared before discharge of the patient from the hospital. Compared with those of other surgical approaches, such complications are mild and infrequent. The complications and postoperative results in 18 cases that we have operated upon using this approach are shown in Table 1.

Table 1. Summary of cases undergoing operation by interhemispheric trans-lamina terminalis approach following bifrontal craniotomy

Pat. no.	Age (yr)	Sex	Diagnosis	Result of operation	Complication	Follow-up study
1	13	F	Craniopharyngioma	Total	Diabetes insipidus	7 yr 5 mo; died
2	43	F	Craniopharyngioma	Total		9 mo; died
3	40	M	Craniopharyngioma	Total		4 mo; died
4	7	M	Craniopharyngioma	Total	Diabetes insipidus	6 yr 60 mo; alive
5	29	M	Craniopharyngioma	Subtotal	Diabetes insipidus	10 yr; alive
6	39	M	Craniopharyngioma	Total	Diabetes insipidus	4 yr 5 mo; alive
7	56	F	Craniopharyngioma	Total	Diabetes insipidus	4 yr 3 mo; alive
8	13	M	Craniopharyngioma	Subtotal	Diabetes insipidus	4 yr 5 mo; alive
9	4	F	Craniopharyngioma	Total	Diabetes insipidus	4 yr 4 mo; alive
10	40	M	Craniopharyngioma	Partial	Diabetes insipidus	4 yr 5 mo; alive
11	10	M	Craniopharyngioma	Total	Diabetes insipidus	2 yr 8 mo; alive
12	31	M	Craniopharyngioma	Subtotal	Diabetes insipidus	1 yr 4 mo; died
13	8	F	Craniopharyngioma	Total	Diabetes insipidus; Hyperthermia	2 yr 1 mo; alive
14	24	M	Craniopharyngioma	Total	Diabetes insipidus	1 mo; alive
15	44	F	Oligodendroglioma	Total		4 yr 7 mo; alive
16	60	M	Pituitary adenoma	Total	Diabetes insipidus	1 yr 3 mo; alive
17	40	M	Cavernous angioma	Total	Diabetes insipidus	1 yr; alive
18	26	M	Arteriovenous malformation	Total		1 yr 5 mo; alive

This approach is suitable for tumors of the third ventricle, including those emerging from the anterior wall, the anterior portion of the foramen of Monro (even from the superior wall), the lateral wall connecting the foramen of Monro and the cerebral aqueduct, and the inferior wall.

Discussion

Various approaches for the surgical removal of tumors of the third ventricle have been attempted since Dandy's first report [1, 3, 4, 7, 8, 11]. Regardless of the approach used, it cannot be said that satisfactory results have been obtained, primarily because the third ventricle lies in a deep midline position and various autonomic nerve centers, the pineal gland, the pituitary gland, and other neuroendocrine nuclei lie close to its walls. Consequently, any damage to the tissue surrounding the third ventricle results in a poor postoperative recovery. We have surmised that an approach via the lamina terminalis would result in the least amount of damage to brain tissue, as direct cutting of the brain is avoided and the wall of the third ventricle is thinnest at this region. Furthermore, the thickness of the lamina terminalis is often reduced as a result of ventricular expansion caused by the brain tumor. By means of the bilateral frontal craniotomy reported herein, both olfactory nerves are preserved and the lamina terminalis is approached by bluntly separating the left and right frontal lobes [9]. Applications of this approach are therefore thought to be numerous. This surgical method is suitable for approaching not only tumors of the third ventricle but giant tumors at the anterior base of the brain and giant aneurysms of the anterior communicating artery as well. We believe our bilateral approach will prove more useful than the unilateral approach [6].

Conclusion

In the surgical removal of tumors of the third ventricle, we believe that the least amount of damage to brain tissue can be achieved by means of an approach through the lamina terminalis via a bifrontal craniotomy. We have so far operated upon 14 cases of craniopharyngioma and 1 case each of pituitary adenoma, cavernous angioma, oligodendroglioma, and arteriovenous malformation and have obtained favorable results.

References

1. Dandy WE (1921) An operation for the removal of pineal tumors. Surg Gynecol Obstet 33:113–119
2. Findler G, Cotev S (1980) Neurogenic pulmonary edema associated with a colloid cyst in the third ventricle. J Neurosurg 52:395–398
3. Hirsch JF, Zouaoui A, Renier D, Pierre-Kahn A (1979) A new surgical approach to the third ventricle with interruption of the striothalamic vein. Acta Neurochir (Wien) 47:135–147
4. King TT (1979) Removal of intraventricular craniopharyngiomas through the lamina terminalis. Acta Neurochir (Wien) 45:277–286
5. Lipton JM, Rosenstein J, Sklar FH (1981) Thermoregulatory disorders after removal of a craniopharyngioma from the third cerebral ventricle. Brain Res Bull 7:369–373
6. Patterson RH, Danylerich A (1980) Surgical removal of craniopharyngiomas by a transcranial approach through the lamina terminalis and sphenoid sinus. Neurosurgery 7:111–117
7. Poppen JL (1960) An atlas of neurosurgical techniques. Saunders, Philadelphia
8. Suzuki J, Iwabuchi T (1965) Surgical removal of pineal tumors (pinealomas and teratomas): Experience in a series of 19 cases. J Neurosurg 23:565–571
9. Suzuki J, Yoshimoto T, Mizoi K (1981) Preservation of the olfactory tract in bifrontal craniotomy for anterior communicating artery aneurysms, and the functional prognosis. J Neurosurg 54:342–345
10. Suzuki J, Katakura R, Mori T (1984) Interhemispheric approach through the lamina terminalis to tumors of the anterior part of the third ventricle. Surg Neurol 22:157–163
11. Van Wagenen WP (1931) A surgical approach for the removal of certain pineal tumors. Surg Gynecol Obstet 53:216–220

Microneurosurgical Anterior and Basal Interhemispheric Approaches for Lesions in and around the Anterior Third Ventricle

N. YASUI, A. SUZUKI, H. OHTA, H. KAMIYAMA, K. WATANABE, and K. SHINDO,
Akita/Japan

Summary

Anterior and basal interhemispheric approaches for the lesions in and around the third ventricle are reported. Interhemispheric dissection allows the least brain retraction and brain damage to approach in and around the anterior third ventricle. Surgical technique of our approaches are described in detail as well as clinical cases.

Author routinely uses the microsurgical anterior interhemispheric (AIH) approach [2, 14] for the cases with anterior communicating artery aneurysm. Through this approach, hematoma in the lamina terminalis cistern and the third ventricle could easily be removed with less brain retraction. Subarachnoid hematoma in the chiasmatic, interpeduncular and prepontine cisterns could be also removed with subchiasmatic route at the same approach. So microsurgical AIH approach has been applied to the lesions other than cerebral aneurysms situated in these areas. But, there are some differences in the surgical approach between cases with cerebral aneurysm and other lesions. In the latter cases, craniotomy should be situated more to the basal side because it is necessary to get the wider operative field at the area around the chiasma, lamina terminalis and subcallosal areas. Recently, craniotomy is extended from the mid-basal part of the frontal bone to the upper medial part of both orbits and some extent of the nasal bone. This approach is named basal interhemispheric (BIH) approach to be differentiated from usual AIH approach.

There are various operative approaches to lesions affecting the anterior third ventricle. Those are classified as transcortical [3, 9, 10], transcallosal [6, 10, 11], interhemispheric [13], subfrontal [4, 7, 10], transsylvian [10] and transsphenoidal [1, 5] approaches. In this paper, surgical technique of our approaches are described in detail as well as clinical cases.

Surgical Method

At first, surgical AIH approach for the area of anterior third ventricle is mentioned and then the different points of BIH approach are explained.

The patient is fixed in a supine straight head position. Bicoronal skin incision is made one or two centimeters behind the hairline. Lateral extent of incision is out-

---

Key words: Microneurosurgery, Anterior interhemispheric approach, Basal interhemispheric approach, Anterior third ventricle, Lamina terminalis

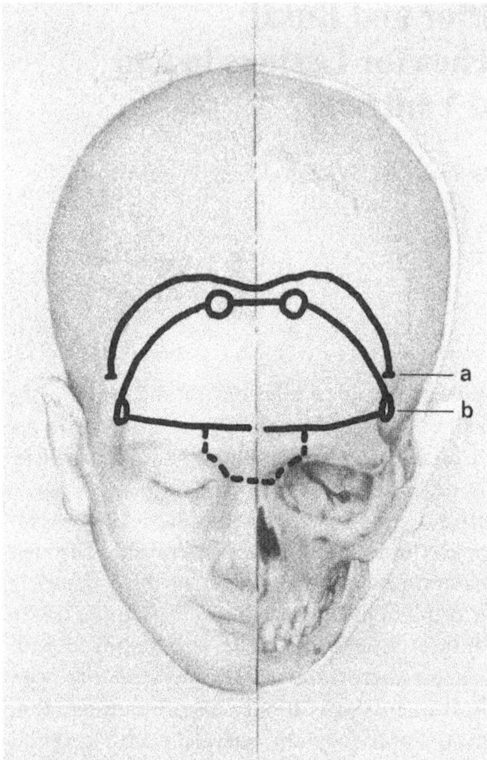

Fig. 1. Bicoronal skin incision and craniotomy. *Solid line (a):* line of skin incision. *Solid line (b):* burr holes and bone flap of the conventional bifrontal craniotomy. *Dotted line:* additional midfrontal craniotomy for basal interhemispheric approach

lined to preserve the branches of the facial nerve on each side. Subperiosteal dissection of the skin flap is performed to the upper ridge of the orbit. One or two burr holes are placed near the midline on one or both sides of the superior sagittal sinus (SSS) and the other two are placed at pterion. Bifrontal craniotomy is performed by neuroairtome. Bone cutting of the basal site is performed as close to the frontal base as possible from lateral burr hole to the midline on each side (Fig. 1). The frontal sinus is opened in most cases with third ventricular lesions, however, it is not necessary to extend the craniotomy so far in most of the aneurysm cases.

When the frontal sinus is exposed at the time of craniotomy, the mucous membrane is dissected, electro-coagulated and removed after being sterilized with 11% Povidone-iodine fluid. The internal lamina of the frontal sinus is removed to reduce the dead space. Operation is continued after covering the entire area with a cotton plaget soaked in antibiotics and Povidone-iodine fluid.

At the time of closure, the frontal sinus is packed with muscle and bone dust mixed with antibiotic powder to block the communication with the nasal cavity. After waterly tight closure of the dura, this area is covered by reflecting a flap of the periosteum or galea and stitching it to the dura mater according to the method of Pool [8].

In BIH approach, the head is dorsiflexed and craniotomy is extended by bone chisel into the anterior middle part of the frontal base. The dotted line in Fig. 1

shows the extent of the additional craniotomy in the frontal, and nasal bones. Lateral extent of craniotomy is just medial to the supraorbital foramen or notch and lower to the nasion. Crista gali is rongeured away as much as possible. Management of opened frontal sinus is similar to AIH approach.

Dura is incised in the shape of letter W and SSS and cut at the anterior end after ligation or bipolar coagulation in AIH approach. Dural incision parallel to SSS at the base side is added in BIH approach. The falx is usually cut at its anterior inferior end. When the bridging vein is under-developed in frontal pole, dural incision is performed in one side and it is not necessary to cut the SSS and falx.

Dissection of the interhemispheric fissure is performed under the operating microscope. There are three important anatomical key points, which should be defined during surgery, to get the good anatomical orientation in AIH approach. At first, pericallosal and/or callosomargical arteries are exposed at the level of the knee portion of corpus callosum. Next, dissection is continued toward the planum sphenoidal and then up to the tuberculum sellae. It is the most important procedure that interhemispheric fissure should be dissected sharply by a pair of microscissors as shown in Fig. 2. Maximum magnification of the operating microscope is necessary to confirm the vessels and arachnoid trabeculae and to make a sharp dissection. At the third step, dissection is performed posteriorly and superiorly to approach the area of lesions (Fig. 3). Head position is changed according to each operative step to get the natural operator's posture.

There are no necessities to approach the knee portion of corpus callosum in BIH. Dissection is performed directly toward the pre- and suprachiasmatic areas near the folded portion of arachnoid membrane.

When the chiasma is reached, lamina terminalis and/or subcallosal area, anatomical structures are confirmed and then operative procedures directed to the lesion are started through the appropriate route such as translamina terminalis, subchiasmatic and so on. Even if the tumor is large in size, it is not necessary to make extensive brain retraction. Repetitive dissection and extirpation are performed

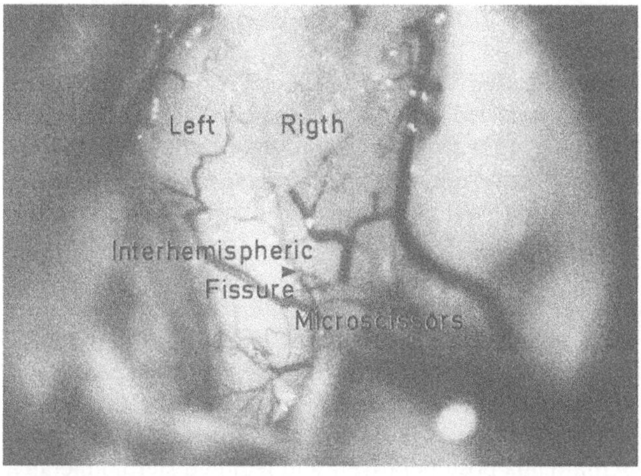

Fig. 2. Sharp dissection of the interhemispheric fissure

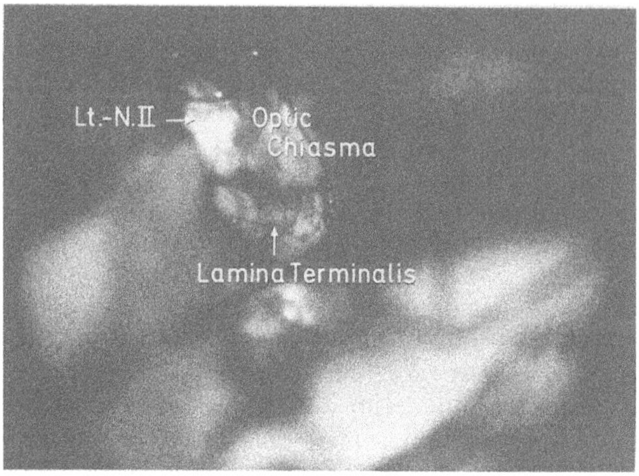

Fig. 3. Exposure of the optic chiasma and lamina terminalis

as follows: reduction of the mass is performed piecemeal and then the border of the tumor is dissected. In some cases, olfactory nerves are dissected from the frontal base according to the method of Suzuki et al. [12], to preserve the function of it.

After the intradural procedures, dura should be closed waterly tight, the opened frontal sinus is covered with periosteum as mentioned before, bone flap is secured at four points and then skin and galea are closed in the usual manner.

Case Reports

Case 1: Y.E., a 12-year-old boy, had undergone a subtotal removal of the craniopharyngioma by transsylvian approach 1½ years before. Residue of calcified tumor was left in the interpeduncular fossa because perforating arteries were involved in the tumor. Seventeen months after the first operation, he was readmitted to the hospital with an increasing visual field defect and disturbance of visual acuity in both eyes, especially at the right side. CT scan revealed a recurrence of the tumor extending to the anterior third ventricle (Fig. 4, left). Subtotal removal of the tumor and insertion of the cilicon tube connected with Ommaya's reservoir into the resected cavity was performed on June 7, 1983 by an interhemispheric approach. Postoperative CT scan revealed residual tumor in the interpeduncular fossa (Fig. 4, right). His visual acuity and field of both eyes improved and he now is doing fine as a school boy.

Case 2: A.S., a 10-year-old girl, complained of headache, nausea and vomiting without other neurologic signs including visual disturbance. Skull film showed calcified shadow in the suprasellar lesion. CT scan revealed marked hydrocephalus and large suprasellar mass with contrast enhancement. Total removal of the craniopharyngioma was performed two weeks after the ventriculo-peritoneal shunt operation. She had transient hypernatremia postoperatively and required steroid therapy. She was discharged without neurologic deficit.

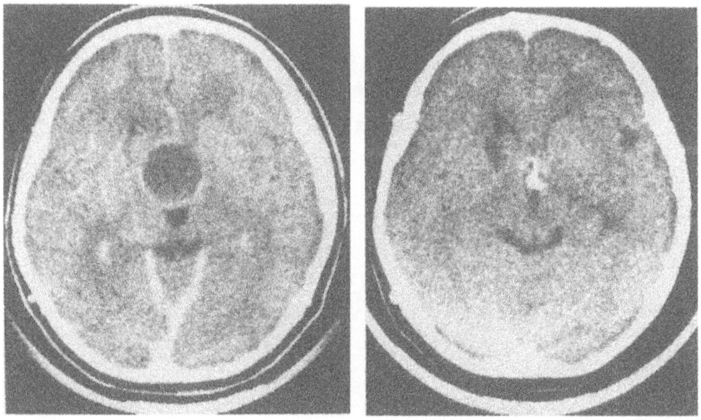

Fig. 4. Case-1: Craniopharyngioma. Preoperative enhanced CT scan shows cystic tumor extending to the anterior third ventricle (*left*). Postoperative plain CT scan reveals residual calcified tumor (*right*)

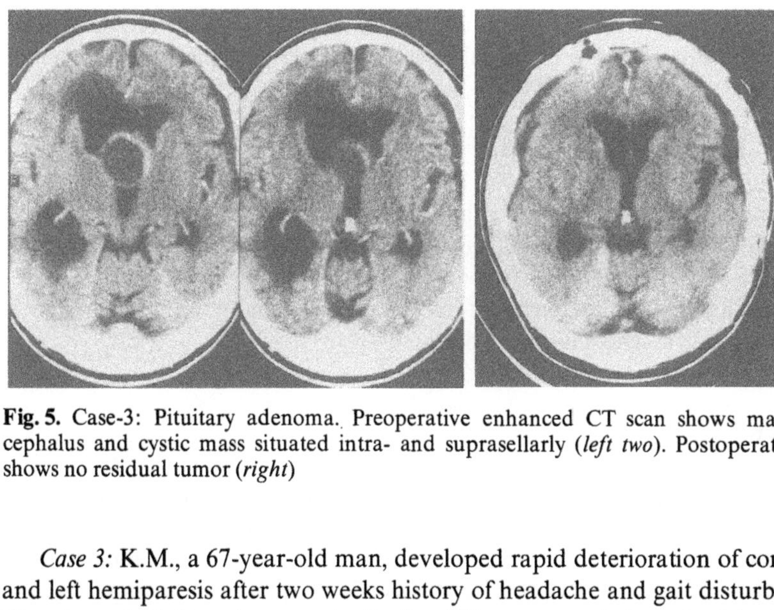

Fig. 5. Case-3: Pituitary adenoma. Preoperative enhanced CT scan shows marked hydrocephalus and cystic mass situated intra- and suprasellarly (*left two*). Postoperative CT scan shows no residual tumor (*right*)

Case 3: K.M., a 67-year-old man, developed rapid deterioration of consciousness and left hemiparesis after two weeks history of headache and gait disturbance. Skull film showed slight enlargement of sella. CT scan revealed marked hydrocephalus and partial intra- and suprasellar cystic mass mainly extending to the anterior third ventricle (Fig. 5, left). Total removal of the pituitary adenoma was performed by interhemispheric approach. Postoperative CT scan showed no residual tumor (Fig. 5, right). He complicated with pulmonary infection and then died with multiorgan failure following septic shock.

Case 4: M.S., a 56-year-old man, admitted to our hospital because of bilateral visual field defect with 3 week history of blurred vision. Skull film showed bone defect at the sellar lesion and suprasellar calcified shadow and CT scan revealed partial calcified sellar and suprasellar mass. A total removal of the chordoma was per-

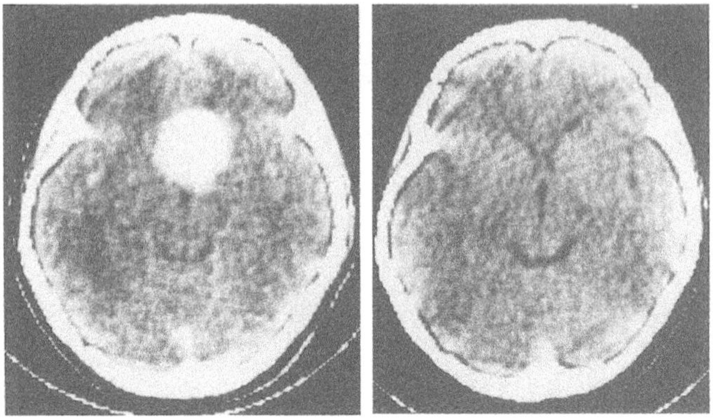

Fig. 6. Case-5: Tuberculum sellae meningioma. Preoperative enhanced CT scan reveals suprasellar enhanced mass (*left*). Tumor is totally removed in postoperative CT scan (*right*)

formed on November 20, 1984, by an interhemispheric approach. He required treatment of diabetus insipidus and his visual field defect showed slight improvement after the surgery.

Case 5: K.K., a 20-year-old female, developed bilateral visual field defect and headache. Blindness of the left eye with optic atrophy and temporal hemianopsia in the right eye were shown at admission and CT scan revealed suprasellar enhanced mass (Fig. 6, left). Tumor was totally removed by an interhemispheric approach (Fig. 6, right) and was diagnosed as tuberculum sellae meningioma. Her left blindness was unchanged postoperatively but right visual field acuity recovered normally and now, she is able to lead a normal working life.

Discussion

Several operative approaches have been reported for tumors situated in the area of anterior third ventricle. Translamina terminalis approach offers the least risk of brain damage for extirpating the anterior third ventricular tumor compared with other approaches such as transcortical or transcallosal approaches as described by Suzuki et al. [13]. When the tumor extends from the base to the anterior third ventricle, transsylvian, subtemporal and transsphenoidal approaches are also indicated. We perform the transsylvian approach especially in a case with marked lateral and posterior extension in this area but there are limitations of removal at the upward extended tumor. Tumors, which grow from the base and which are mainly located in the midline, are also good indications for interhemispheric approach. King (1979) [4] and Patterson and Danylevich (1980) [7] reported the approach through lamina terminalis with subfrontal route. Those approaches need more marked brain retraction compared with interhemispheric dissection.

Anterior interhemispheric approach reported here is about the same as Suzuki's approach to the third ventricle tumor [13], only with the difference that the author here recommends the sharp dissection of the interhemispheric fissure instead of blunt procedures. Pial membrane, arteries and veins are fixed tightly with arachnoid trabeculae at the interhemispheric fissure in which the arachnoid membrane is not covered, so that blunt procedures can easily result in the injury of pial membrane and small vessels. Precise and gentle procedures are essential when the arachnoid trabecula is cut to separate the fissure and vessels of each hemisphere under the maximum magnification of the operating microscope.

Recently, we develop the basal interhemispheric approach to the tumors in and around the anterior third ventricle and anterior communicating aneurysms situated high in position. Beneficial points of this approach are that the operative field is shorter from the cortex and lamina terminalis and the subcallosal area can be easier approached than by AIH approach. But there is a problem in this approach that additional craniotomy is more complicated compared with conventional craniotomy especially management of frontal sinus. It should be emphasized again that BIH approach needs less interhemispheric dissection and retraction of the brain compared with AIH and other approaches such as subfrontal or transsylvian approach.

References

1. Hardy J, Vezina JL (1976) Transsphenoidal neurosurgery of intracranial neoplasm. Adv Neurol 15:261–274
2. Ito Z (1982) The microsurgical anterior interhemispheric approach suitably applied to ruptured aneurysms of the anterior communicating artery in the acute stage. Acta Neurochir (Wien) 63:85–99
3. Kempe LG (1968) Operative Neurosurgery 1, Cranial, Cerebral, and Intracranial Vascular Disease. Springer, Berlin Heidelberg New York
4. King TT (1979) Removal of intraventricular craniopharyngiomas through the lamina terminalis. Acta Neurochir (Wien) 45:277–286
5. Laws ER Jr (1980) Transsphenoidal microsurgery in the management of craniopharyngioma. J Neurosurg 52:661–666
6. Long DM, Chou SN (1973) Transcallosal removal of craniopharyngiomas within the third ventricle. J Neurosurg 39:563–567
7. Patterson RH Jr, Danylevich A (1980) Surgical removal of craniopharyngiomas by a transcranial approach through the lamina terminalis and sphenoid sinus. Neurosurgery 7:111–117
8. Pool JL (1972) Bifrontal craniotomy for anterior communicating artery aneurysms. J Neurosurg 36:212–220
9. Poppen JL (1960) An atlas of neurosurgical techniques. WB Saunders, Philadelphia
10. Rhoton AL Jr, Yamamoto I, Peace DA (1981) Microsurgery of the third ventricle: Part 2, Operative approaches. Neurosurgery 8:357–373
11. Stein BM (1982) Transcallosal approach to third ventricular tumors. In: Schmiedek HH, Sweet WH (eds) Operative Neurosurgical Techniques, Indications, Methods, and Results, vol 1. Grune & Stratton, pp 575–584
12. Suzuki J, Yoshimoto T, Mizoi K (1981) Preservation of the olfactory tract in bifrontal craniotomy for anterior communicating artery aneurysms, and the functional prognosis. J Neurosurg 54:342–345
13. Suzuki J, Katakura R, Mori T (1984) Interhemispheric approach through the lamina terminalis to tumors of the anterior part of the third ventricle. Surg Neurol 22:157–163
14. Yasui N, Ito Z (1983) Microsurgical anterior interhemispheric approach for anterior communicating artery aneurysm. Neurosurgery 2:114–125

Interfornical Exposure of the Third Ventricular Chamber

M. L. J. Apuzzo, Los Angeles, CA/USA

Introduction

In 1944, Edward Busch (Busch 1944) described the development of the interfornical raphe following transcortical exposure of the lateral ventricular system. This maneuver offered him excellent exposure of six lesions of the third ventricular chamber. During the past 40 years a number of technical developments including introduction of the operating microscope, microinstrumentation, more effective retractor systems, and other innovations such as high potency glucocorticoids and better radiographic imaging have refined neurosurgical approaches to this region. These developments made it possible to establish narrow corridors of entry to this remote region with minimal physiologic impact. We have found the midline transcallosal interfornical approach to the third ventricular chamber to be a valuable corridor in management of third ventricular lesions affording rapid, safe access to the third ventricular chamber without the benefit of attendant hydrocephalus or large mass deformations to enhance the corridor or pathology's exposure (Apuzzo 1982; Apuzzo et al. 1982; Apuzzo and Giannotta 1987). This report will transmit our recent experience in 25 cases of third ventricular lesions managed by this technique.

Case Material

There were 25 cases approached by the midline interfornical technique. These include: 5 colloid cysts, 7 craniopharyngiomas, 3 intrinsic gliomas, 8 cysticercosis cysts, 1 artereovenous malformation, and 1 22-caliber-bullet. These lesions ranged in size from 1–4 cm and in texture from cystic with a filmy capsule to dense and fibrous type of masses. Five of the lesions involve not only the third ventricular region, but also the sellar and parasellar regions as well.

Radiologic definition was attained with high resolution CT scanning with attendant, metrizamide ventriculography when indicated. Magnetic Resonance Imaging has been employed in the later cases in the series. Care was taken to attain strict three dimensional contours of the lesions, especially in the sagittal plane (the plane of entry). Cerebral angiography was obtained in all cases.

Operative Techniques

All patients were operated on in the supine position with the head elevated 20° in pin fixation (Apuzzo 1982; Apuzzo and Giannotta 1987). A left frontal ventricular

Case material – I. Interfornical exposure

Location	Pathology
1. Ant. III	Colloid cyst (1.5 cm) V, *, T)
2. Ant. III	Colloid cyst (2 cm) (V, T)
3. Ant. III	Colloid cyst (1 cm) (T)
4. Ant. III	Colloid cyst (1.5 cm) (T)
5. III	Colloid cyst (2.5 cm) (V, *, T)
6. III	Craniopharyngioma (3 cm) (V)
7. III	Craniopharyngioma (2.5 cm) (V, T)
8. III	Craniopharyngioma (2.0 cm) (V, *, T)
9. III	Craniopharyngioma (2.5 cm) (V, T)
10. III	Craniopharyngioma (4 cm) (V, *)
11. III	Craniopharyngioma (3.0 cm) (V, *, T)
12. III	Craniopharyngioma (2.5 cm) (V, *)

V – Ventriculomegaly, * – Transient memory loss, T – Total excision (C.T.)

Case material – II. Interfornical exposure

Location	Pathology
13. FM ant. III	Cysticercosis (1.7 cm) (V, T)
14. FM ant. III	Cysticercosis (2 cm) (V, T)
15. FM ant. III	Cysticercosis (2 cm) (V, T)
16. FM ant. III	Cysticercosis (2 cm) (V, T)
17. Ant. III	Cysticercosis (2 cm) (V, *, T)
18. III	Cysticercosis (2.5 cm) (V, T)
19. III	Cysticercosis (2 cm) (V, T)
20. Post III	Cysticercosis (1.5 cm) (*, T)
21. III	Glioma (V)
22. III	Glioma (V)
23. III	Glioma (V)
24. FM III	AVM (*, T)
25. Post III	Bullet (22 cal)

FM – Foramen of Monro, V – Ventriculomegaly, * – Transient memory loss, T – Total excision (C.T.)

cannula was employed for pre- and postoperative monitoring and control of intracranial pressure. A 4×5 cm right-sided paramedian bone flap was employed in the pericoronal area with flap placement predicated on the cortical venous drainage as defined by angiography. A Budde retractor system was employed to maintain para falcine exposure with a 1 cm midline slot developed to the corpus callosum. With the operating microscope a 2–2.5 cm incision was made in the midline as defined by the falx. The fornix was identified and incision was completed in the midline raphe as defined by the attachment of the leaves of the septum pellucidum. Retraction of the columns of the fornix was occasionally maintained by a 5 mm retractor blade. Standard microsurgical techniques with occasional carbon dioxide laser adjuvents were employed to manage the pathologic lesion.

Ventriculostomies were maintained for 24–72 hours postoperatively.

Results

Excisability

Total excision was accomplished in 19 of the 22 potentially excisable lesions. This included 4 of 7 craniopharyngiomas where no evidence of tumor was apparent on postoperative imaging studies. Small to moderate tumor remnants were apparent in 3 cases where subfrontal parasellar extension of tumor existed and argues for consideration of a combined subfrontal and midline exposure in the event that parasellar extension of the mass is extensive.

Exposure was found to be adequate in all compartments of the chamber, especially in the anterior and middle third with posterior third lesions accessible with minor manipulations of head and microscope position. On a number of occasions the basilar artery and prepontine cisterns, or the sella contents were visualized upon completion of mass excision.

Complications

There were no deaths or incidence of gastrointestinal hemorrhage. There was no incidence of hemiparesis, alteration in endocrine status, preoperative visual status, or level of consciousness.

The major adverse observation was the development of a transient amnesic syndrome in 8 of 25 patients. This was characterized by an inability to retain recent events. The manifestation of the complaint was observed to be evident from 3 to 22 days postoperatively with 6 of the 8 patients being normal or returned to a preoperative baseline of mental status evaluation in seven days. At three months, postoperatively, no detectable amnesia or alteration in memory patterns was appreciated by patients, their families, or examining physicians.

Discussion

As one considers access to the third ventricular chamber, entry to the lateral ventricular system is the initial objective. Following lateral ventricular entry the surgeon is faced with the foramen of Monro which will vary in size dependent on the size and disposition of the lesion. At times this orifice is adequate for lesion excision, however, in general, it offers inadequate exposure for comfortable and successful lesion management and certainly inadequate visualization of the ventricular contents. It then becomes necessary to consider a number of alternatives, all of which require fornix manipulation. These include: (a) section of one or both fornical columns, (b) development of the choroidal fissure with lateral to medial retraction of the fornical complex, (c) development of the interfornical plane.

The interfornical approach is rapidly accomplished through the midline transcallosal corridor. It affords complete visualization of the third ventricle and its contents without sacrifice of normal anatomical structures. Our previously published data (Apuzzo et al. 1982) are coincident with those of others that a 2.5 cm callosal trunk section has insigificant physiological impacts; additionally, the controversial issues to the role of the fornix in memory function and amnesic syndrome deserve further study. Although this corridor does not alter fornical structures by section, but rather employs division of the natural raphe separation to enhance exposure, transient amnesic syndromes have been observed in approximately one third of the cases. It should be stressed that these are temporary phenomena and were not sustained for more than three weeks of time in any of our 25 cases. Moreover, no alteration of mentation was observed on clinical assessment, statements of patients or relatives at three months postoperatively. None of 6 patients who underwent formal neuropsychiatric assessment at three months manifested abnormal profiles (Apuzzo et al. 1982). The cause for this observation in the strictly physiologic sense is arguable, but probably relates to transmission of pressure to regions adjacent to the third ventricle during manipulation of the local pathology. Examination of these data would appear to imply that lesions of progressively firmer texture require greater manipulation and thus more local trauma. This would appear to be evident and our data with only 2 of 8 pliable cysticercosis cysts, but 4 of 7 dense craniopharyngiomas are manifesting postoperative memory dysfunction. No clear relation of the size of the lesion to observed incidence appears to exist.

In addition to the benefits of providing the surgeon with a corridor of minimum physiologic cost, this midline exposure offers the capability for simultaneous manipulation of the lesion not only through the 2 cm fornical exposure, but also simultaneously via both foramen of Monro, thus adding the technical opportunities for manipulation and lesion excision.

References

Apuzzo MLJ (1982) Transcallosal interfornical exposure of lesions of the third ventricle. In: Schmidek HH (ed) Operative neurological techniques: Indications and methods. Grune and Stratton, New York

Apuzzo MLJ, Chikovani OK, Gott PS, Teng EL, Zee CS, Giannotta SL, Weiss MH (1982) Transcallosal, interfornical approaches for lesions affecting the third ventricle: Surgical considerations and consequences. Neurosurgery 10:547–554

Apuzzo MLJ, Giannotta SL (1987) Interfornical approach. In: Apuzzo MLJ (ed) Surgery of the Third Ventricle. Williams and Wilkins (in Press)

Busch E (1944) A new approach for the removal of tumors of the third ventricle. Acta Psychiatr 19:57–60

Tumors in the Anterior Part of the Third Ventricle Removed by Right Transventricular Approach

H.-D. Herrmann and C. Kamm, Hamburg/FRG

During 5 years (1980–1984) 35 tumors of the third ventricle have been operated upon in the neurosurgical department of the University Hospital, Hamburg (UKE). These represented 5.3% of all supratentorial tumors operated upon during the same period of time. In this series no tumors were included which were only biopsied for histologic identification and radiotherapy.

Diagnostic Procedures

The localization and extension of the tumors were obtained in all cases by CT-scan without and with contrast enhancement. In only one case (Plexus papilloma) an additional Metrizamide ventriculography was found to be useful for the identification of the point of origin of the tumor. In all cases angiography was performed (transfemoral route). In those cases where the tumor was restricted to the anterior part of the ventricle bilateral carotid angiography was sufficient. In large tumors extending through the whole ventricle or in more posteriorly located tumors the basilary artery system was also visualized. The arterial phase of the angiograms revealed in few cases the site of vascularization of the tumor which was helpful during operation. In large tumors the operative approach (anterior or posterior approach) can be chosen according to the location of the vascular supply. In the venous phase attention should be paid to the bridging veins towards the superior sagittal sinus, if the transcallosal approach is considered, and to the displacement, the state of filling and possible collateral drainage of the veins surrounding the ventricle, the venous angle between septal and thalamostriate veins, the internal cerebral vein and vein of Galen.

Localization and Surgical Treatment

23 of the 35 tumors were either located or had their main extension, their point of origin or their main blood supply within the anterior portion of the third ventricle (Table 1). These tumors were approached by the right anterior transventricular route since all patients had dilated lateral ventricles suggesting a dilatation of the foramen of Monro also. A high transcortical approach was used at the typical site of frontal ventricular tap. If no ventricular drainage had to be performed preoperatively the ventricle was punctured after exposure of the cortex, and through a small cortical incision the ventricle was opened, guided by the puncture canal. After exposure of the foramen of Monro we used 3 alternative ways to enter the third ven-

Table 1. Tumors in the third ventricle operated 1980–1984. Neurosurg. Dept. UKE (University Hospital, Hamburg, FRG)

	Anterior part	Posterior part
Cysts	6	–
Astrocytomas	5	3
Oligodendrogliomas	2	–
Ependymomas	3	–
Plexus papillomas	2	–
Germinomas	1	9
Craniopharyngiomas	4	0
Total	23	12

Total = 35 tumors operated = 5.3% of all supratentorial tumors

tricle: Cystic or small tumors could be removed through the intact dilated foramen. If during tumor resection the exposure was found to be too restricted it was extended by the subchorioidal route (Delandsheer et al. 1978; Viale and Turtas 1980). In large tumors an interfornical approach has proved to be best (Rhoton et al. 1981). From the rather sagittal entrance to the lateral ventricle both fornix could be exposed after incision of the septum pellucidum. In most cases the septal vein had to be divided. By slight medial retraction of the incision the interfornical space could be incised, the fornix separated and the III. ventricle exposed.

In none of the cases neither the fornix nor the thalamostriate vein had to be divided for the benefit of the exposure. Resection of the tumors was performed with microsurgical technique. Throughout the past year the pulsed CO_2-Laser attached to the microscope (Cooper Variopulse, Donation of Deutsche Krebshilfe e.V.) has been a valuable additional tool. It eases the resection of tough fibrous tumors, but more important it was possible to "burn" tumors (pilocytic Astrocytomas) out of the superficial portion of the thalamus in such thin layers that no additional, clinically recognizable damage resulted.

At the end of the operation an external ventricular drainage was applied until CSF had completely cleared.

Results (Table 2)

Total removal of the tumor was assumed if at the end of operation and in the postoperative CT-scan with contrast enhancement no residual tumor could be detected. 3 of the 4 pilocytic astrocytomas arose from the subependymal layers (Casotto et al. 1985) and could be completely removed. From the recent experiences we anticipate that more of the pilocytic astrocytomas and ependymomas can be removed totally with the aid of the CO_2-Laser.

The 2 oligodendrogliomas originated from the septum pellucidum and could be totally removed without memory disturbances.

Table 2. Tumors in the third ventricle operated by anterior transventricular approach (1980–1984)

Type	N	Subtype	n	Removal					Permanent shunt	
				Male	Female	Total	Subtotal	Death	Preop.	Postop.
Cysts	6	Ependymal (colloid)	4	3	1	4			1 →	1 (8 mo) →
		Epidermoid	1	1		1				
		Arachnoid	1	1		1				
Astrocytomas	5	Pilocytic	4	2	2	3	1		1 →	
		Others, Grade I	1	1			1	1		
Oligodendrogliomas	2	Grade I, III		1	1	2				
Plexus papillomas	2			2		2				1 (2 mo) →
Ependymomas	3			1	2	1	2			2 →
Germinomas	1				1		1			
Craniopharyngiomas	4			3	1		(4)		3 →	1 →
Total	23			15	8	14	5 (9)	1	10	5 pre + postop. 5 postop.

Craniopharyngiomas could be removed totally out of the ventricle, however, a total removal of the tumor was not possible by this approach since they arose from the hypophyseal stalk – suprasellar region.

One patient died suddenly on the 4th postoperative day during ambulation. The cause of death could not be determined. 5 of the patients had an internal CSF-shunt before operation. These shunts were not removed. In addition 5 patients needed a shunt postoperatively inspite of free CSF passage through the III. ventricle. 2 of these patients had to be readmitted 2 and 8 months after a completely uneventful postoperative course with progressively enlarging ventricles. Neither by CT scan nor ventriculography a recurrence of the tumor could be found.

Postoperative radiotherapy was carried out in subtotally removed radiosensitive tumors (ependymoma, germinoma) and in one of the oligodendrogliomas grade III inspite of total removal. All patients are under regular neurologic and CT control. No recurrence could be detected up to now.

References

Casotto A, Buoncristiani P, Signorini E, Giordana MT (1985) Third ventricle gliomas. Report of 7 cases with benign clinical behaviour. Acta Neurochir (Wien) 74:43–48

Delandsheer JM, Guyot JF, Jomin M, Scherpereel B, Laine E (1978) Accés au troisieme ventricule par voie interthalamotrigonale. Neurochirurgie 24:419–422

Rhoton AL, Yamamoto J, Peace DA (1981) Microsurgery of the third ventricle: Part 2 Operative approaches. Neurosurgery 8:357–373

Viale GL, Turtas S (1980) The sub-chorioidal approach to the third ventricle. Surg Neurol 14:71–76

Intraventricular Tumors: With Special Reference of Those in and around the Brain Stem and Third Ventricle – Analysis of 125 Cases

L. BASAURI, Santiago/Chile

In order to have a panoramic view of intraventricular tumors that eventually can disturb the third ventricle and/or brain stem the patients with intraventricular tumors treated at the Neurosurgical Institute, Santiago – Chile, between 1970 and 1984 will be analysed.

Material and Methods

During the period 1970–1984 125 patients with ventricular tumors were treated at our Institute (see Tables 1, 2).

Age and Sex

Sixty percent of the patients were between the age of 0–15 years and 81% below 30 years. 85 patients were males, 32 patients females.

Location of Tumors

27% occupied the lateral ventricles, 24% the third and 49% the fourth ventricle.

Lateral Ventricles: 31 cases. Right side 22 cases and left side 9 cases. Ependymomas 18 (12 malignant). Choroid plexus tumors 5 patients (2 papillomas and 3 carcinomas). Astrocytomas 2 cases. Teratoma 1 case. Cisticercosis 5 cases.

Foramen of Monro: Two colloid cysts and 1 Cisticercosis.

Third Ventricle

Anterior Part: 17 cases. Astrocytomas 5, Teratomas 4, Cisticercosis 3, Ganglioneuroma 1 and Ependymoma 1 case. Glioma 1, Craniopharyngioma 2.

Table 1. Intraventricular tumors (N = 125)

Lateral ventricles	31 cases
Foramen of Monro	3
Anterior third ventricle	17
Posterior third ventricle	16
Fourth ventricle	58

Table 2. Intraventricular tumors. 125 cases

Histology	
Lateral ventricles:	31 cases
– Ependymoma	6
– Malignant	12
– Choroid plexus papilloma	2
– Choroid plexus carcinoma	3
– Astrocytoma	2
– Teratoma	1
– Cysticercosis	5
Foramen of Monro:	3 cases
– Colloid cyst	2
– Cysticercosis	1
Third ventricle:	33 cases
– Astrocytoma	7
– Teratoma	5
– Glioma	2
– Craniopharyngioma	2
– Ependymoma	1
– Pineocytoma	1
– Ganglioneuroma	1
– Cysticercosis	3
– No histology	11
Fourth ventricle:	58 cases
– Ependymoma	31
– Malignant	13
– Choroid plexus papilloma	7
– Choroid plexus carcinoma	1
– Medulloblastoma	3
– Dermoid cyst	1
– Cyst	1
– Cysticercosis	1

Posterior Part: 16 cases. We began operating tumors of the posterior part of the third ventricle 3 years ago. Before that we utilized the rationale of shunting hydrocephalus plus radiotherapy. Out of the 16 we have neuropathologic examination in 5 cases. 1 Teratoma, 1 Pineocytoma, 2 Astrocytoma (Grade II) and 1 Glioma.

Fourth Ventricle: 58 cases

Ependymoma was the common type with 31 benign and 13 malignant tumors, followed by choroid plexus tumors (8 cases). Despite the fact that 60% of the patients were below the age of 15 years in this particular group only 3 medulloblastomas were found.

Symptomatology

The most common symptoms and signs were intracranial hypertension, hydrocephalus and hemiparesis in tumors occupying the lateral ventricles, hypertension in those located at the foramen of Monro and hydrocephalus, hypertension, Parinaud syndrome and diabetes insipidus in patients harboring a third ventricle tumor and hydrocephalus associated to ataxia and cerebellar syndrome in the masses growing inside the fourth ventricle.

Diagnosis

It was based on the clinical picture plus angiography, brain scintigraphy and P.E.G. before 1977. In order to differentiate between an intraxial exophitic glioma vegetating inside the fourth and a true intraventricular tumor, we are still using in a small number of patients metrizamide ventriculography, alone or associated with a CAT Scan. M.R.I. looks promising to accomplish that goal.

Treatment

We will analyse the group as a whole and some special aspects mainly related to location.

The 58 patients with a posterior fossa tumor were operated upon. In all of them a radical excision was achieved. In 17 a shunt was inserted, either pre- or postoperatively. Sixteen cases received radiation therapy.

In 11 of the 17 cases located in the anterior part of the third ventricle a total resection was possible, in 5 a shunt was utilized and 4 were submitted to radiotherapy. In another 2 patients a stereotactically guided radioisotopic implantation was employed.

Five of the 16 posterior third ventricle tumors were approached directly using the supracerebellar/infratentorial approach (1 pineocytoma, 1 teratoma, 3 gliomas). The other 11 received radiotherapy combined with a shunt in 10 patients.

The rationale for tumors of the third ventricle can be summarized as follows:

a) Anterior Portion and/or Foramen of Monro: Transcallosal approach with preservation of the pillars of the Fornix in order to avoid amnestic sequelaes (Fig. 1) [6]. In those patients with a large hydrocephalus the transfrontal, transventricular route is used in some selected cases.

b) Posterior Portion:

B.1.– If the tumor is anterior to the central venous complex the interthalamic subtrigonal approach is used.

B.2.– If the tumor is posterior and/or inferior the supracerebellar/infratentorial route is preferable, with the patient in prone position, slightly seated and with his head flexed. The exact entrance of the microscopic light beam can be adjusted moving the table rather than the patient (Fig. 2).

The tumors occupying the lateral ventricles are usually approached through the posterior parietal lobe or transfrontally according to their location.

The general mortality was 28%, being nil for the lateral ventricle and anterior and posterior third ventricle, using the transcallosal and supracerebellar/infratentorial approach. There was no mortality and a low morbidity in the brain stem tumors submitted to open biopsy. The mortality was mainly due to posterior fossa surgery of very large tumors or terminal cases treated with a palliative VP shunt.

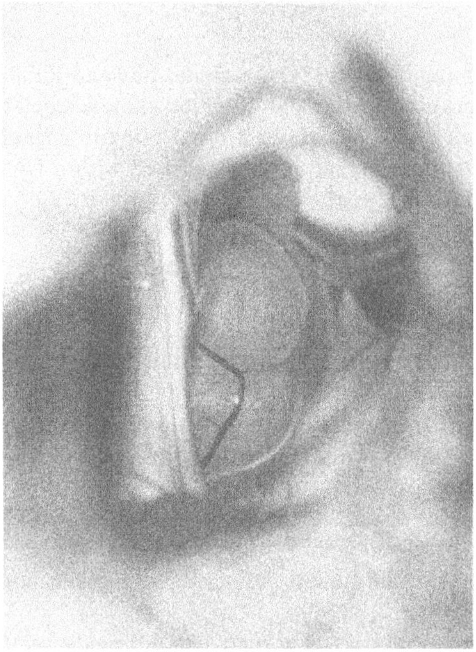

Fig. 1. Colloid cyst of the third ventricle emerging through the right foramen of Monro (Microphotography Zeiss × 18)

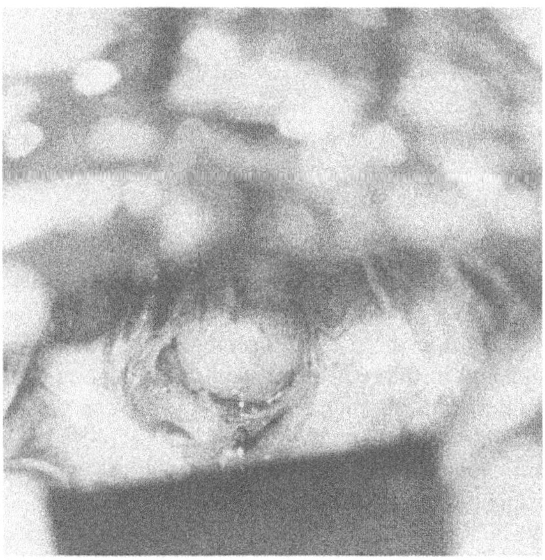

Fig. 2. Glioma of the posterior third ventricle supracerebellar/infratentorial approach

Comment

Intraventricular tumors very frequently disturb the CSF circulation giving origin to a secondary obstructive hydrocephalus. They also can invade the upper or lower brain stem or produce secondary compression due to cerebral herniations.

During the last 5 years the therapeutical management of the third ventricular tumors have become much more aggressive [1]. The direct surgical approach is recommended, using the transcallosal route [5, 6, 7, 8, 9, 10] for those of the anterior part, the supracerebellar/infratentorial for the tumors located posteriorly [11] and the interthalamic subtrigonal route for those situated anteriorly to the vein of Galen [2, 3, 4].

If the clinical profile is acute, the CAT Scan is suggestive of an immature tumor, the CSF biological markers are positive and the CSF cytology suggests a germinal tumor or a neuroblastoma, the trial of radiotherapy (2000 rads) followed by a control CAT Scan is judicious. If an important reduction in size is reached the full radiotherapeutic treatment is completed. In case the mass remains unchanged or gets bigger surgical exploration is mandatory.

The surgical exploration of intra-axial tumors, especially when a cystic or calcified portion exists, is used more often now [9]. M.R.I. [8] is more sensitive than CAT Scan [3] in demonstrating the response to treatment and disease relapse. M.R.I. gives a better information than CAT Scan in the relations to the floor of the fourth ventricle, and the exophytic portion but the presence of cystic or calcified regions is poorly demonstrated by M.R.I. and that is a drawback [8]. The modern neurooncological concepts for the adequate treatment of tumors combine the exact pathologic classification associated to the surgical diminution of the cellular population, before the use of radiation therapy or chemotherapy. In tumors deeply located in the cerebral hemisphere braquitherapy using stereotactic implantation is a good alternative.

The possibility of spinal seeding must be borne in mind in every tumor that has close relation with CSF pathways, as is the case in a intraventricular tumor floating in its compartment. Spinal axis radiation is mandatory as a complementary treatment [7].

References

1. Donat JF, Okazaki H, Gómez MR, Reagan TJ, Baker HL, Laws ER (1978) Pineal Tumors. A 53 year experience. Colloid cysts of the third ventricle. Arch Neurol 35:736–740
2. Jomin M, Lesoin F, Delandsheer JM, Laine E (1980) Intéret de la voie interthalamo-Trigonale dans le traitement des tumeurs du troisième ventricule et de la région épiphysaire. Neurochirurgie 26:171–177
3. Kendall B, Reider-Grosswasser I, Valentine A (1983) Diagnosis of masses presenting within the ventricles on computed tomography. Neuroradiology 25:11–22
4. Laine E, Blond S (1980) Les Tumeurs trigono-septales. Neurochirurgie 26:247–278
5. Long DM, Leibrock L (1960) The transcallosal approach to the anterior ventricular system and its application to the therapy of craniopharyngioma. Clinical Neurosurgery, vol 27. Chapter 10. Williams & Wilkins, Baltimore, pp 160–168
6. Michels LG, Rutz D (1982) Colloid cysts of the third ventricle. A radiologic-pathologic correlation. Arch Neurol 39:640–643

7. Neuwelt EA, Glasberg M, Freukel E, Kemp Clark W (1979) Malignant pineal regions tumors. A clinico-pathological study. J Neurosurg 51:597–607
8. Packer RJ, Zimmerman RA, Luerssen TG, Sutton LN, Bilaniuk LT, Bruce DA, Schut LA (1985) Brainstem gliomas of Childhood: Magnetic resonance imaging. Neurology 35:397–401
9. Reigel DH, Scarff TB, Woodford JE (1979) Biopsy of pediatric brain stem tumors. Childs Brain 5:329–340
10. Stein BM (1960) Third ventricular tumors. Clinical Neurosurgery, vol 27 – Chapter 17. Williams & Wilkins, Baltimore, pp 315–331
11. Stein BM (1979) Supracerebellar-Infratentorial approach to pineal tumors. Surg Neurol 11:331–337

Approach Problems in Anterior Third Ventricle Tumors: Review of 33 Cases

V. LUPRET and I. JELICIC, Zagreb/Yugoslavia

Introduction

In surgical treatment of anterior third ventricle tumors different approaches are used regarding the pathologic process and site (Stein 1977; Hirsch et al. 1979; Patterson and Danylevich 1980; Viale and Turtas 1980; Rhoton et al. 1981; Suzuki et al. 1984). Although anatomic tumor site determines surgical approach, we see from papers presented today and from publicated material that neurosurgeons use different approaches in treating tumors of same anatomic site with equal success (Long and Chou 1973; King 1979; Shucart and Stein 1978; Hirsch et al. 1979). That confirms the opinion that during tumor exposure and removal extremely precise microsurgical technique with preservation of vascular irrigation and drainage is of essential importance.

Clinical Material and Surgical Approaches

From October 1979 to December 1984 we operated at the Central Institute for Tumors and Allied Diseases of Zagreb 34 patients with primary or secondary tumors of anterior third ventricle, using three approaches: subfrontal and frontotemporal basal approach in 15 patients, transcortical-transventricular approach in 7 patients and anterior transcallosal approach in 12 patients (Figs. 1, 2, 3). The results of our analysis are summarized in Table 1.

Discussion

After carefully analysing the surgical possibilities and difficulties in these approaches, the microsurgical technique used and the postoperative results, we concluded that in some cases, where the tumor was very voluminous, no approach per se could lead us to a potentially radical tumor removal. In basal approaches sometimes we could not adequately visualize the upper tumor part which consequently made tumor removal despite careful dissection and preparation extremely difficult or impossible. Although intraoperatively we did not notice any vascular lesions, postoperative complications led us to the conclusion that some microvascular accidents must have actually happened. In transcortical-transventricular approach the neural tissue damage is inevitable and can lead to postoperative seizures. Generally,

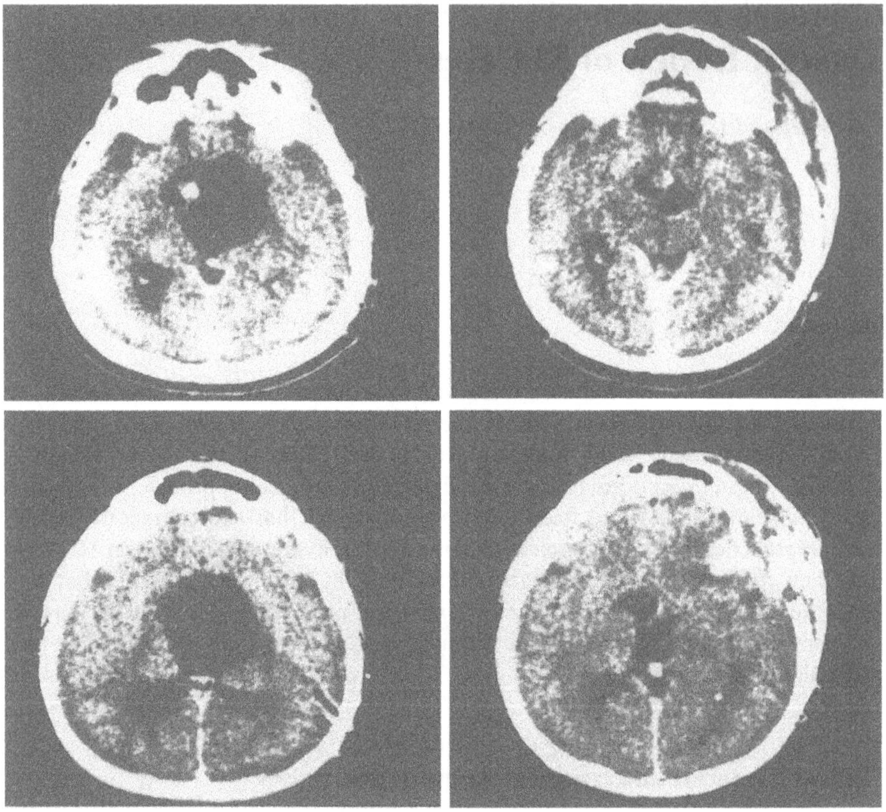

Fig. 1. Huge epidermoid of the third ventricle (*left*). Postoperative scan (*right*) shows rest of the tumor. Basal approach was used

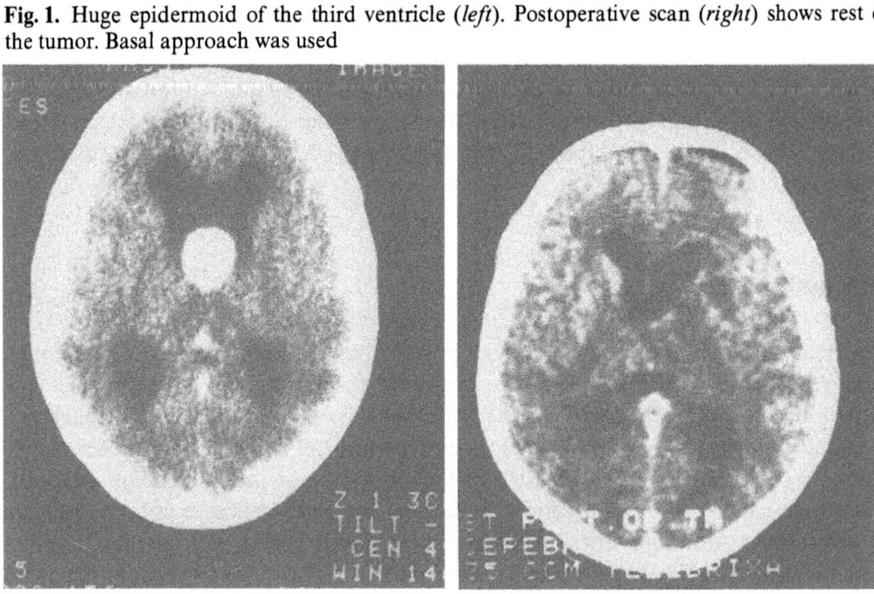

Fig. 2. Colloid cyst of the anterior part of the third ventricle. Transcortical-transventricular approach was used for removal of this mass

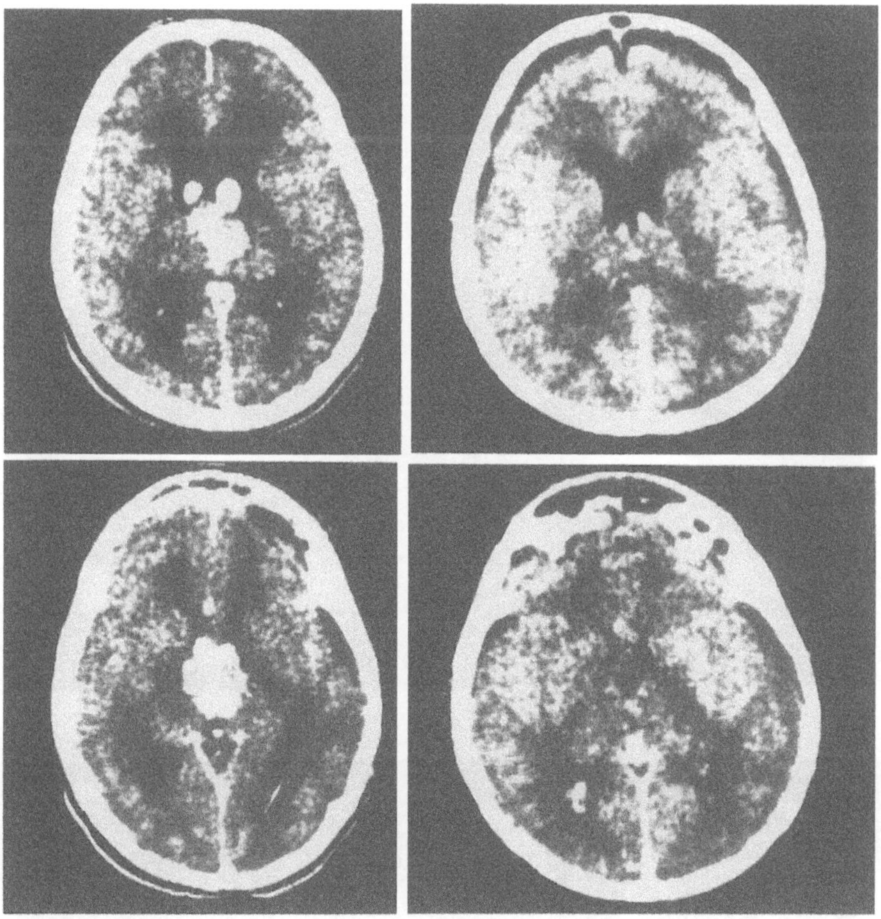

Fig. 3. Meningioma of the third ventricle removed using transcallosal approach

we found a widened foramen Monro which sometimes was not sufficient for radical tumor extirpation, and so it was necessary to widen the operative field incision of fornix (Rhoton et al. 1981). We find that the transcallosal approach is the procedure of choice in operative treatment of anterior third ventricle tumors. We used the median interfornical approach between internal cerebral veins. Consequently, the tumor visualization is very good and vascular hazard minimal. That is the reason why postoperative complications rarely occur. Still, in huge anterior inferior part of the third ventricle tumors dissection is difficult to perform because of tumor parts adhering to ventricle walls and total removal is therefore impossible. On account of difficulties we faced using particular approaches and due to postoperative complications in a specific case of a huge tumor we planned and performed a two stage surgery.

A 24-year-old female was diagnosed having a huge intra-ventricular craniopharyngioma compressing the chiasma and going to the right lateral ventricle (Fig. 4). We planned and performed a two stage surgery. Primarily we removed the

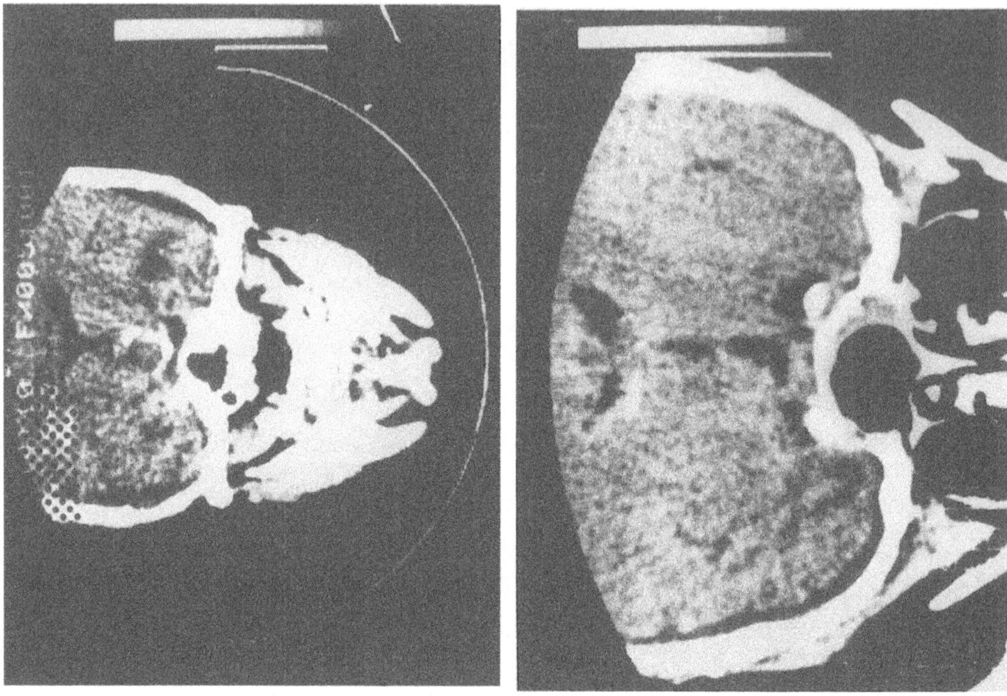

5

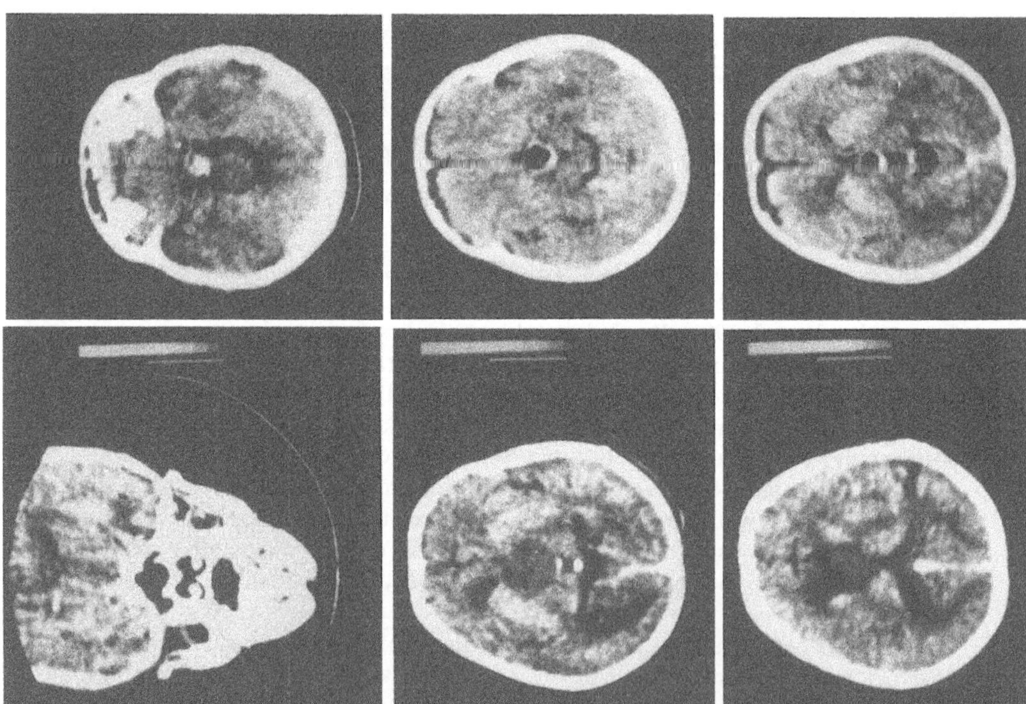

4

Table 1. Summary of cases operated by using three different operative approaches

Operative approach	Cases no	Diagnosis		Results of operation		Complications		Follow-up study	
Basal approaches (subfrontal, frontotemporal)	15	Craniopharyngiomas	8	Total excision	11	Death		Alive	11
		Epidermoids	3	Partial excision	4	Diabetes insipidus	9	Died (1–2,5 years later)	4
		Arachnoidal cysts	2						
		Hamartomas	2						
Transventricular approach	7	Colloid cysts	4	Total Excision	4	Hydrocephalus	1	Alive	6
		Glioma	1	Partial excision	3	Diabetes insipidus	1	Died (14 months later)	1
		Craniopharyngioma	1						
		Ectopic pinealoma	1						
Transcallosal approach	12	Craniopharyngiomas	3	Total excision	6	Hemiparesis	1	Alive	12
		Colloid cysts	3	Partial excision	6	Diabetes insipidus	1		
		Gliomas	3			Hydrocephalus	1		
		Meningioma	1						
		Ependymoma	1						
		Germinoma	1						

greater part of the tumor using transcallosal approach (Fig. 4). Fourteen days later we operated using the subfrontal approach through lamina terminalis and removed the rest of this tumor (Fig. 5). Eight days after the second operation the patient was discharged in excellent condition.

Fig. 4. Giant craniopharyngioma of the third ventricle (*left*) partially removed using transcallosal approach in first stage (*right*)

Fig. 5. The rest of the tumor removed in second stage using subfrontal approach through lamina terminalis

Conclusion

Although in most cases one stage surgery is sufficient in anterior third ventricle tumors, the proposed two stage surgery with no forced radical removing attempts and very low neural and vascular hazards could bring us to better operative results in some specific cases as discussed.

References

Hirsch JF, Zouaoui A, Renier D, Pierre-Kahn A (1979) A new surgical approach to the third ventricle with interruption of the striothalamic vein. Acta Neurochir (Wien) 47:135–147

King TT (1979) Removal of intraventricular craniopharyngiomas through the lamina terminalis. Acta Neurochir (Wien) 45:277–286

Long DM, Chou SN (1973) Transcallosal removal of craniopharyngiomas within the third ventricle. J Neurosurg 39:563–567

Patterson RH Jr, Danylevich A (1980) Surgical removal of craniopharyngiomas by a transcranial approach through the lamina terminalis and sphenoid sinus. Neurosurgery 7:111–117

Rhoton AL Jr, Yamamoto I, Peace DA (1981) Microsurgery of the third ventricle. Part 2. Operative approaches. Neurosurgery 8:357–373

Shucart WA, Stein BM (1978) Transcallosal approach to the anterior ventricular system. Neurosurgery 3:339–343

Stein BM (1977) Transcallosal approach to third ventricle tumors. In: Schmidek HH, Sweet WH (eds) Current techniques in operative neurosurgery. Grune and Stratton, New York, p 247–255

Suzuki J, Katakura R, Mori T (1984) Interhemispheric approach through the lamina terminalis to tumors of the anterior part of the third ventricle. Surg Neurol 22:157–163

Viale GL, Turtas S (1980) The subchoroid approach to the third ventricle. Surg Neurol 14:71–76

Suprasellar Lesions Affecting Third Ventricle

Endocrinological Disturbances Detected in Hypothalamic Lesions

R. Fahlbusch, M. Buchfelder, and U. Schrell, Erlangen/FRG

"Here in this well concealed spot almost all to be covered with a thumb-nail, lays the very mainspring of primitive existence – vegetative, emotional, reproductive, on which with more or less success man has come to superimpose a cortex of inhibitions."

Harvey Cushing, 1929 [1]

Introduction

Besides of vegetative, emotional and reproductive functions, the hypothalamus appears to be one of the central parts of neuroendocrine secretion connecting the central nervous system and the pituitary gland. But until recently the differentiation of primary hypothalamic and primary pituitary failure was hampered by the lack of neuroactive compounds acting at various stages of neuroendocrine regulation [2]. Since Guillemin et al. [3] have isolated growth-hormone releasing-hormone (hpGRH) from a human pancreatic islet tumor [10] and Vale et al. [11] have characterized the structure of corticotropin releasing hormone (CRH), new tools were made available for the differential diagnosis of primary hypothalamic and primary pituitary disease. By stimulating the pituitary directly by the means of exogenous hypothalamic releasing hormones or via the hypothalamus by the means of stress the defect can be localized at the pituitary or hypothalamic level [5].

Principles of Hypothalamo-Pituitary-Regulation

Hormone secretion of the anterior pituitary is under the control of neurohumoral stimulating and inhibiting factors released into the hypophyseal portal vessels. For each of the pituitary hormones there appears to be specifically reacting releasing and inhibiting hormones. But a pituitary hormone may also be regulated by different neurotransmitters.

It is known that a trophic peripheral hormone, e.g. cortisol, may be released in response to various stimuli. Physical or emotional stress or pain mediated via the central nervous system causes hypothalamic CRH release (Fig. 1). This exerts its effect on the pituitary's ACTH secretion. The cortisol secretion is elicited by the adrenal cortex by ACTH stimulation. When the glucocorticosteroid hormones reach the brain, the hypothalamus or the pituitary, their effect is inhibitory. This implies the existence of a negative feed-back mechanism that plays a part in regulating the output of releasing hormones and pituitary hormones. The circadian rhythm of

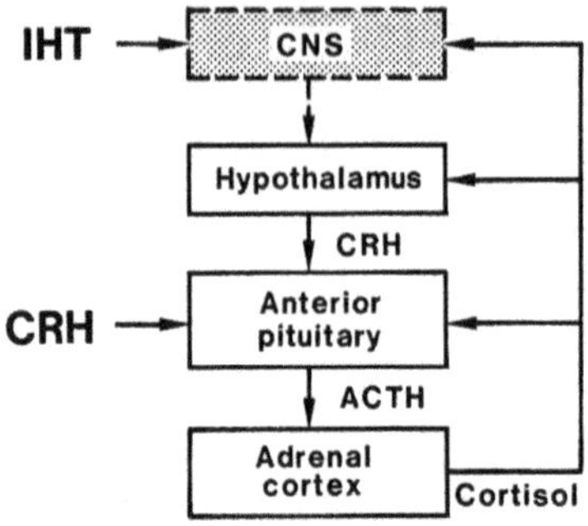

Fig. 1. Diagram showing the hypothalamic-pituitary-adrenal axis

ACTH and cortisol is mediated via the hypothalamus. The precise physiology of these mechanisms is still not fully understood.

This system can be challenged at various stages, enabling a differential diagnosis of lesions. In clinical endocrinological testing standardized stress situations can be generated by insulin-induced hypoglycemia (IHT). If the CRH secretion by the hypothalamus or its transport via the tuberoinfundibular system is damaged by a hypothalamic or pituitary stalk lesion, ACTH and cortisol secretion cannot be stimulated by insulin-induced hypoglycemia any more. However, in such cases exogenous CRH injection into a vein may replace the missing endogenous CRH in the hypothalamic-pituitary portal vessels and may lead to an ACTH-release by the pituitary, triggering cortisol release by the adrenal cortex. A missing ACTH and cortisol secretion following stress but a preserved ACTH and cortisol response to exogenous CRH application are indicative of hypothalamic or pituitary stalk damage and exclude primary pituitary failure.

A similar pathophysiologic mechanism is known about the growth-hormone axis. Stressing stimuli applied by insulin-induced hypoglycemia (IHT) cause the release of GH mediated by hypothalamic GRH secretion [13]. A missing response of GH to insulin-induced hypoglycemia associated with a GH-increase after exogenous GRH indicates hypothalamic failure.

This principle is not confined to the axis of the stress-hormones ACTH/cortisol and GH, but may in general also be applied to the hypothalamo-pituitary-thyroid axis or the hypothalamo-pituitary-gonadal axis. Thyreotropin (TRH) induced thyreoidea stimulating hormone (TSH) increase in patients with low basal thyroid hormones accounts for primary hypothalamic disorders while primary pituitary failure is more probable, when a TSH increase cannot be caused by exogenous TRH application [8].

On prolactin (PRL) secreted by the pituitary the hypothalamus exerts a predominantly inhibitory influence by a prolactin-inhibiting factor (PIF) which has to

Table 1. Endocrinological findings indicating hypothalamic or pituitary stalk lesions

1. Non-tumorous hyperprolactinemia (prolactin-levels are elevated slightly only)
2. TRH-induced TSH-increase in patients with central hypothyroidism (8)
3. CRH-induced ACTH/cortisol increase without ACTH/cortisol increase by IHT
4. GRH-induced GH increase without GH increase by IHT

date not been isolated but may be related to dopamine. Therefore the irritation of hypothalamic structures or the pituitary stalk may lead to hyperprolactinemia in contrast to the hyposecretion of all other pituitary hormones. Usually the hyperprolactinemia caused by the cessation of PIF-secretion results in prolactin-levels not more than 6-fold above the normal range. A summary of these principles is given in Table 1.

Endocrinological Methods

In our patients insulin-induced hypoglycemia testing (IHT) was performed by injection of 0.15 IU Insulin Actrapid per kg body weight. A blood glucose level below 40 mg/dl and clinical signs of stress were regarded to be adequate. A growth-hormone increase of at least 7 ng/ml and a cortisol increase of at least 12 μg/dl documented normal stimulation [2, 12]. The releasing hormone tests were performed by bolus injection of 100 μg ovine CRH and 50 μg hpGRH as described elsewhere [4, 6, 7, 9, 12, 13]. Blood was drawn over 120 minutes in 15 minute-intervals. ACTH, cortisol and GH were measured by radioimmunoassay. The normal range for basal ACTH-levels was between 20 and 50 pg/ml, for basal cortisol levels 10–21 μg/dl. Basal growth-hormone levels were normal up to 5 ng/ml. In addition basal prolactin and TSH levels were measured before and 30 minutes after injection of 200 μg TRH as were the peripheral thyroid hormones. Normal levels for serum prolactin ranged up to 500 μU/ml and basal serum TSH-levels ranged up to 5 μU/ml. Normal values for T3 were between 60 and 220 ng/dl and for T4 between 4.5 and 12 ng/dl.

Clinical Examples

Case 1: In a 15-year-old boy with a history of diabetes insipidus and a mild chiasma syndrome no clinical signs of puberty had developed. The CT scan showed an isodense tumor in the suprasellar cistern extending into the right hypothalamus (Fig. 2). The tumor was removed surgically via a craniotomy with exception of the tumor parts within the right lateral wall of the third ventricle. Histology revealed a germinoma. Endocrinologically the patient had non-tumorous hyperprolactinemia with prolactin-levels of 1089 μU/ml. This can be explained by a disturbed PIF secretion by the hypothalamus or transport via the pituitary stalk. Basal levels of the gonadotropins were low. Cortisol and growth-hormone could not be stimulated by IHT, but there was a considerable increase of cortisol and growth-hormone after injection of 100 μg CRH and 50 μg GRH intravenously (Fig. 3). Thus the endocrinological disturbances must be attributed to failure of the endocrine hypothalamus or pituitary stalk in this patient.

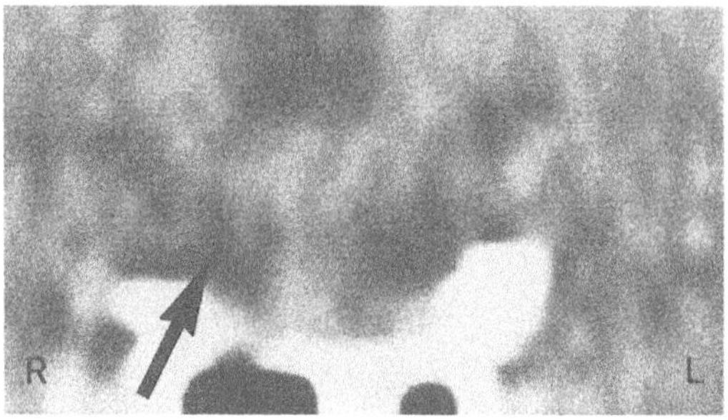

Fig. 2. Case 1: Suprasellar germinoma in the coronal reformation of thin-collimation CT sections. An isodense, not clearly confined tumor is visible in the right suprasellar cistern

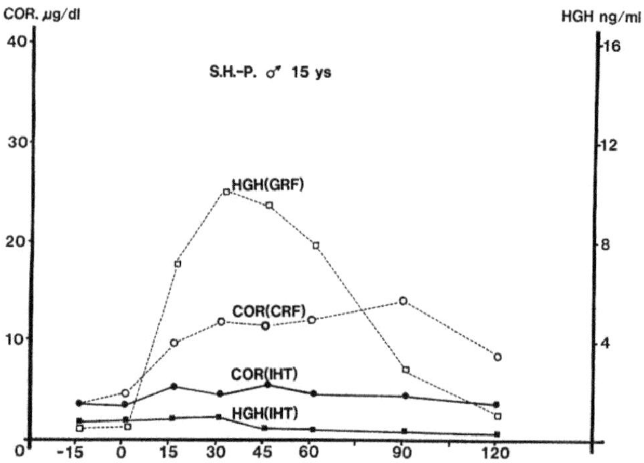

Fig. 3. Case 1: Secretion dynamics of cortisol and GH in the same case of suprasellar germinoma after IHT and CRH/GRH stimulation

Case 2: A 28-year-old man had a large, hypo to isodense suprasellar craniopharyngioma localized within the third ventricle (Fig. 4). After the transventricular surgical approach the cystic tumor had shrunk considerably. The preoperatively severe chiasma-syndrome had almost resolved. Three weeks later the solid tumor parts were removed by the transsphenoidal way. Clinically the patient had hypogonadism. In functional endocrinological testing serum cortisol could be stimulated normally by IHT and CRH (Fig. 5). In contrast GH could only be stimulated by GRH. Thus a partial hypothalamic or pituitary stalk defect, affecting the GRH-GH-axis only, must be suspected.

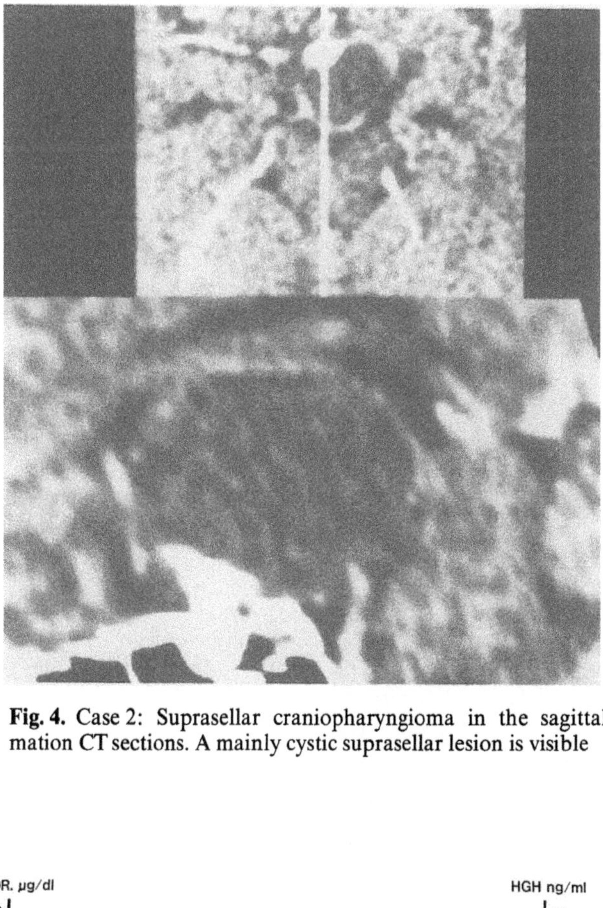

Fig. 4. Case 2: Suprasellar craniopharyngioma in the sagittal reconstruction of thin-collimation CT sections. A mainly cystic suprasellar lesion is visible

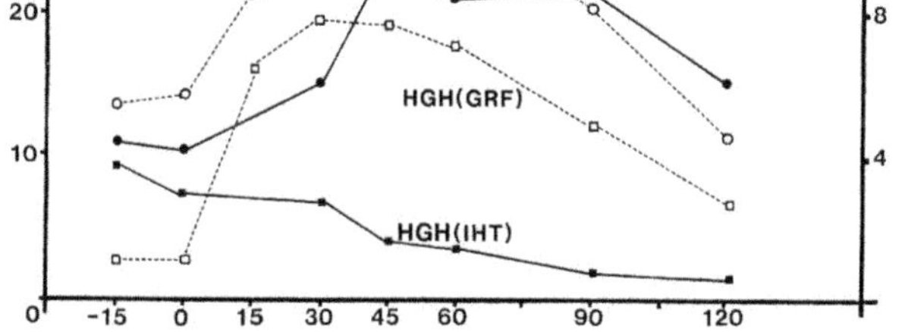

Fig. 5. Case 2: Secretion dynamics of cortisol and GH in the same case of suprasellar cystic craniopharyngioma after IHT and CRH/GRH stimulation

Case 3: In a 40-year-old man with a large calcified craniopharyngioma (Fig. 6) no endocrinological abnormalities could be detected clinically. Surgically only insertion of a ventriculo-atrial shunt system was performed because of obstructive hydrocephalus. He was in a poor vegetative condition and had a disturbed sleep-wake-rhythm. However endocrinological testing showed a normal secretion pattern of pituitary and peripheral gland hormones. Cortisol and GH could be stimulated normally by IHT as well as by CRH and GRH bolus injection (Fig. 7). Thus, even large lesions obviously located in the hypothalamic region need not necessarily be accompanied by hypothalamic or pituitary dysregulation.

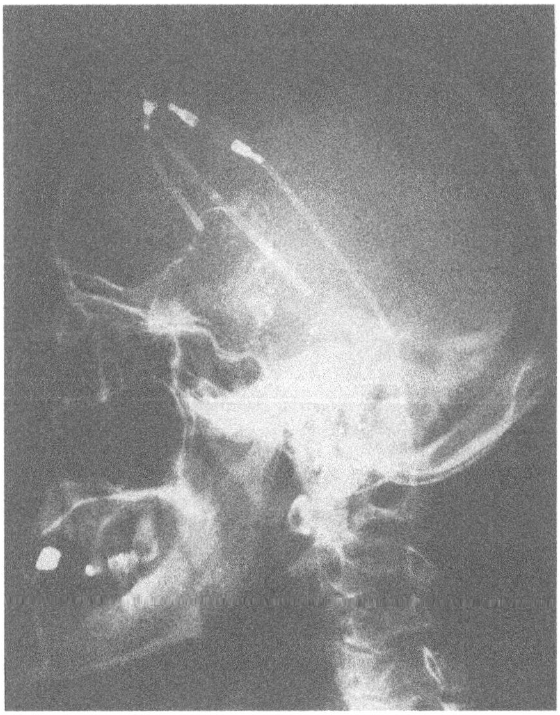

Fig. 6. Case 3: Suprasellar craniopharyngioma in the lateral skull X-ray. A huge calcified suprasellar mass extending into the 3rd ventricle is easily seen. A shunt-system was inserted for obstructive hydrocephalus caused by blockage of Monro's foramen

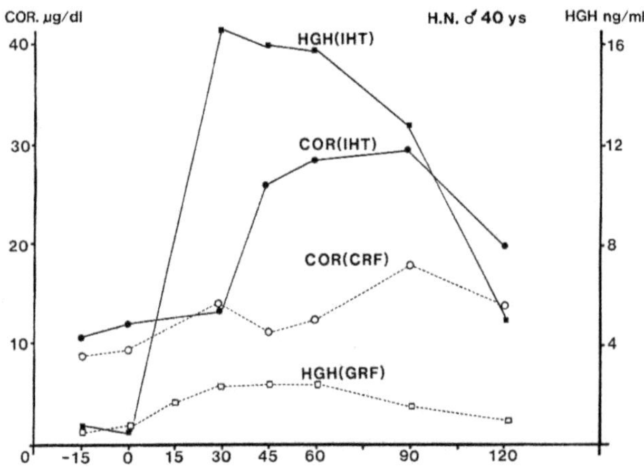

Fig. 7. Case 3: Secretion dynamics of cortisol and GH in the same case of calcified suprasellar craniopharyngioma after IHT and CRH/GRH stimulation. No abnormalities were detected despite the large lesion

Further Experience with Other Lesions

Altogether we have performed CRH and GRH stimulation tests in addition to conventional functional endocrinological assessment in 19 patients with lesions located in the suprasellar region or within the third ventricle (Table 2). Histologically 6 patients had craniopharyngiomas, 2 had germinomas, one had a glioma of the optic chiasma and another one had an infundibuloma. In 4 patients hydrocephalus caused by aquaeductal stenosis was diagnosed. No histological diagnosis could be obtained in these cases as well as in 3 patients in whom neoplastic or inflammatory lesions were suspected. In 11 out of the 19 patients the disease could be localized into the hypothalamic or pituitary stalk region by a lacking response of ACTH/cortisol and/or GH to IHT, but a positive response to exogeniously given CRH and GRH. It is remarkable that all 11 patients showed lacking stimulation of GH by IHT (1) but GRH induced GH increase, and in only 3 out of these 11 patients ACTH/cortisol could not be stimulated by IHT (2) but by CRH. In summary in most of the patients the endocrinological defect was diagnosed by a disturbance of the growth-hormone axis alone, which is known to be most sensitive for either mode of damage.

Table 2. Results of functional endocrinological testing in 19 patients with lesions located in the hypothalamic region or in the 3rd ventricle. (Aqu. stenosis = hydrocephalus caused by aquaeductal stenosis, Cort. = cortisol, CRH = corticotropin releasing hormone, Craniophar. = craniopharyngioma, F. = female, GH = growth hormone, GRH = growth hormone releasing hormone, M. = male, • clinical diagnosis not confirmed by histology) (1) (2) see text

Patient's initials	Sex	Age	Diagnosis	Insulin-Induced		GRH-Induced	CRH-Induced
				GH-increase	ACTH/cort. increase	GH-increase	ACTH/cort. increase
N. H.	M.	45	Craniophar.	sufficient	sufficient	sufficient	sufficient
L. P.	F.	62	Craniophar.	sufficient	sufficient	sufficient	sufficient
A. F.	F.	73	Craniophar.	subnormal	sufficient	subnormal	sufficient
G. F.	M.	27	Craniophar.	none (1)	sufficient	sufficient	sufficient
H. S.	M.	32	Craniophar.	none (1)	sufficient	sufficient	sufficient
S. A.	M.	36	Craniophar.	none	sufficient	none	sufficient
R. H.	M.	34	Inflammation •	subnormal (1)	sufficient	sufficient	sufficient
R. B.	F.	42	Infundibuloma	none (1)	sufficient	sufficient	sufficient
N. N.	F.	25	Lymphoma •	none (1)	sufficient	sufficient	sufficient
C. C.	M.	53	Epidermoid	none (1)	subnormal	sufficient	sufficient
W. R.	M.	23	Chiasma glioma	none (1)	none (2)	subnormal	subnormal
S. K.	M.	27	Germinoma	none (1)	none	sufficient	none
H. S.	M.	15	Germinoma	none (1)	none (2)	sufficient	sufficient
M. B.	F.	70	Metastasis •	none (1)	none (2)	sufficient	sufficient
G. F.	M.	41	Colloid cyst	sufficient	sufficient	sufficient	sufficient
S. V.	F.	31	Aqu. stenosis •	sufficient	sufficient	sufficient	sufficient
A. L.	M.	21	Aqu. stenosis •	sufficient	sufficient	sufficient	sufficient
I. M.	F.	28	Aqu. stenosis •	sufficient	sufficient	sufficient	sufficient
F. B.	F.	50	Aqu. stenosis •	subnormal (1)	sufficient	sufficient	sufficient

Conclusion

Low pituitary hormone levels of growth-hormone and ACTH, which increase after application of their releasing hormones GRH respectively CRH now can be used to document hypothalamic damage in contrast to primary pituitary failure. In these cases an adequate increase of the pituitary hormones by insulin-induced hypoglycemia is absent. This modern principle of differentiation, fills up the lacking diagnostic tools left by conventional endocrinological testing. The ability of localizing an endocrine disorder into the hypothalamus may be helpful in demonstrating tiny and isodense tumors hardly to be documented even by modern means of neuroradiologic evaluation as thin-collimation CT-scans. Possibly the findings of endocrinological tests will influence the indications for surgery in the hypothalamic and pituitary stalk lesions one day in a manner comparable to the value of present neuroendocrinology for pituitary surgery.

References

1. Cushing H (1929) The pituitary body and hypothalamus. Charles C. Thomas, Springfield
2. Fahlbusch R (1978) Endokrine Funktionsstörungen bei cerebralen Prozessen. Thieme, Stuttgart
3. Guillemin R, Brazeau P, Bählen P, Esch F, Ling N, Wehrenberg WB (1982) Growth-hormone releasing factor from a human pancreatic tumour that caused acromegaly. Science 218:585–587
4. Lytras N, Grossmann A, Perry L, Tomlin S, Wass JAH, Coy DH, Schally AV, Rees LH, Besser GM (1984) Corticotropin releasing factor: Responses in normal subjects and patients with disorders of the hypothalamus and pituitary. Clin Endocrinol (Oxf) 20:71–84
5. Müller EE (1985) Endocrinological differentiation of primary hypothalamic and primary pituitary disease. Acta Neurochir (Wien) 75:91–98
6. Müller OA, Losa M, Oeckler R, Werder v K (1984) CRF- and GRF-stimulation tests in patients with hypothalamic disorders. Acta Endocrinol [Suppl] (Copenh) 105:264, 33
7. Müller OA, Stalla GK, Hartwimmer J, Schopohl J, Werder v K (1985) Corticotropin releasing factor (CRF): Diagnostic implications. Acta Neurochir (Wien) 75:49–59
8. Pickardt CR, Geiger W, Fahlbusch R, Scriba PC (1972) Stimulation der TSH-Sekretion durch TRF-Belastung bei hypothalamischen und hypophysären Krankheitsbildern. Klin Wochenschr 50:42–52
9. Stalla GK, Hartwimmer J, Werder v K, Müller OA (1984) Ovine (o) and human (h) corticotropin releasing factor (CRF) in man: CRF-stimulation and CRF-immunoreactivity. Acta Endocrinol (Copenh) 106:289–297
10. Thorner MO, Perryman RL, Cronin MJ, Rogol AD, Draznin M, Johanson A, Vale W, Horvath E, Kovacs K (1982) Somatotrophic hyperplasia – successful treatment of acromegaly by removal of a pancreatic islet tumour secreting a growth-hormone releasing factor. J Clin Invest 70:965–977
11. Vale W, Spiess J, Rivier C, Rivier J (1981) Characterization of a 41-residue ovine hypothalamic peptide that stimulates secretion of corticotropine and β-endorphin. Science 213:1394–1396
12. Werder v K (1975) Wachstumshormone- und Prolaktinsekretion des Menschen. Urban & Schwarzenberg, München
13. Werder v K, Losa M, Stalla GK, Bock L, Müller OA (1985) Human pancreatic growth-hormone releasing factor (hpGRF): GRF- and GH-levels after bolus injection and infusion of hpGRF 1–44. Acta Neurochir (Wien) 75:81–87

Clinical and Surgical Management of Giant Pituitary Adenomas

A. Basso, M. Vitale, C. Yampolsky, A. Chervin, A. Kreutel, E. Caputi, and A. Guitelman, Buenos Aires/Argentina

Introduction

Giant pituitary adenomas are a difficult problem to deal with. They are herein considered as Grade IV of Vezina and Sutton, with a clear suprasellar expansion, producing visual defects, endocrinological disorders, increased intracranial pressure and in certain cases psychologic symptoms. So far surgical procedures regardless of their nature are associated with a great morbidity and mortality.

In 1972, Bromoergocryptine (BEC), a dopaminergic agonist, was introduced for the treatment of hyperprolactinomas of different etiologies (Besser et al. 1972; Del Pozo et al. 1974). Recently, several authors have described significant reduction in the size of prolactin secreting adenomas after administration of BEC, with improvement of the ophthalmologic and neurologic symptoms (Landolt et al. 1979; Thorner et al. 1980; Vaidya et al. 1978; Weiss et al. 1983). These effects would result from a selective inhibition of protein synthesis in prolactinic cells and a reduction of their cytoplasmatic volume and subsequently a lowering of serum prolactin levels. The use of BEC in Growth Hormone secreting adenomas as well as in non-secreting tumors, has not had a uniform response (Wass et al. 1979; Barrow et al. 1984).

Surgical procedures rarely produce complete removal of these adenomas, and the dopaminergic agonist lack tumoricidal effects. The isolated use of any of them has not produced satisfactory results.

The purpose of this paper is to report on our experience with a combined clinical and surgical approach to the management of these tumors.

Case Material and Methods

Twelve cases of giant pituitary adenomas were seen at Santa Lucia Hospital between November 1983 and January 1985. Three were male and nine were female. Their ages ranged from 17 to 38 years. Eleven patient had giant pituitary adenomas with high prolactin (PRL) levels, and one patient had acromegaly.

All the patients presented with headaches and visual defects (diminished visual acuity and/or visual field defects). Eight of them had secondary amenorrhea, one patient had primary amenorrhea, 10 had galactorrhea, three males had hypogonadism, and two patients had signs of severe intracranial hypertension (Table 1).

These cases were studied by skull x-rays, polytomography of the sellar region, computed tomography with axial and coronal sections, with and without contrast.

Table 1. Clinical and radiological findings in 12 pretreated patients

Case	Age	Sex	Headaches	Opthalmological findings	Radiological findings
1 RM	18	♀	Yes	Vision re: Amaurosis le: Fingers Left temporal hemianopsia	Macroadenoma grade IV with large lateral extension
2 EP	18	♂	Yes	Vision re: 20/20 le: 10/20 Left inferior temporal quadrantopsia	Macroadenoma grade IV with large lateral extension
2 EP	18	♂	Yes	Vision re: 20/20 le: 6/20 Left temporal hemianopsia	Macroadenoma grade IV
4 Mq de B	38	♀	Yes	Vision re: 20/20 le: 20/20 Bitemporal superior quadrantopsia	Macroadenoma grade IV
5 ME	37	♀	Yes	Vision re: 16/20 le: 16/20 Bitemporal hemianopsia	Macroadenoma grade IV
6 MC	19	♀	Yes	Vision re: 12/20 le: 20/20 Left temporal hemianopsia	Macroadenoma grade IV
7 FG	25	♀	Yes	Vision re: 20/20 le: 20/20 Left temporal inferior quadrantopsia	Macroadenoma grade IV
8 JM	17	♂	Yes	Vision re: Light perception le: Amaurosis	Macroadenoma grade IV with extension into the right cavernous sinus
9 M de O	21	♀	Yes	Vision re: 16/20 le. 20/20 Right temporal superior quadrantopsia	Macroadenoma grade IV
10 AY	38	♀	Yes	Vision re: 16/20 le: 14/20 Bitemporal inferior quadrantopsia	Macroadenoma grade IV
11 TR	31	♀	Yes	Vision re: 18/20 le: 20/20 Bitemporal inferior quadrantopsia	Macroadenoma grade IV
12 GOB	25	♀	Yes	Vision re: 20/20 le: 20/20 Right temporal inferior quadrantopsia	Macroadenoma grade IV

Bilateral carotid arteriography and in some cases Metrizamide cisternography, were also performed.

Endocrine function was assessed by measuring basal serum levels of PRL, GH, LH, FSH, TSH, T4 and cortisol by radioimmunoassay, and TRH test for PRL and TSH. Complete ophthalmologic evaluation was also carried out. To consider a suitable candidate for this approach an arbitrary minimum level of basal serum PRL of 100 ng/ml was established. Each patient was then started on progressive doses of BEC, based on their individual tolerance but without following a rigid schedule of dose or time of administration.

Bromocriptine was given for a period ranging from 2 to 43 weeks, with increasing doses between 5 and 35 mg a day. Prolactin levels were assessed during the drug treatment, 24 hours before surgery, one week after surgery and later on. Visual field measurement and tomography were performed before and after surgery. Surgery was indicated when a certain clinical stability was achieved, as judged by an improvement of endocrine and visual manifestation with a significant reduction of PRL levels and a diminution of both tumor volume and density, as established by CT densitometry.

In 10 cases surgery was performed by the transsphenoidal route and in the remaining two cases by the subfrontal approach. During the same time period another three patients (two females and one male) were not treated with Bromocriptine but operated through the subfrontal route by the same surgeon.

Pathologic examination using light microscopy, conventional staining and immunohistochemistry, using the immunoperoxidase method. P.A.P., as described by Sternberger, was performed in all cases. The postoperative management of these patients depended basically on their residual PRL levels. In all the cases where PRL levels remained over normal values, the treatment with BEC was restarted, although the doses were reduced to a level much lower than before surgery. In these series complementary radiotherapy was indicated only for the acromegaly case.

Results

After Bromocriptine treatment all patients reported the disappearance of their headaches and the recovery of vision with an improvement in both acuity and field measurements. Clinical improvement was observed prior to tomographic reduction of the size of the lesion. The BEC treatment produced a resumption of menses in three of the eight patients with secondary amenorrhea and a normalization in eight of the 10 patients with galactorrhea. Before treatment, the PRL range was between 105 and 5500 ng/ml, (mean 1232 ng/ml; ±464 SE). The patient with acromegaly had a basal PRL of 16 ng/ml, but it was decided nevertheless to include her in this study.

During BEC treatment the range was between 2 and 200 ng/ml, (mean 72.5 ng/ml; ± 16.9 SE). The reduction of tumoral mass after BEC administration, as evaluated by computer axial tomography, varied between 30 to 95%, with a mean of 72.5%; ± 5.9 SE (Fig. 1). Those tumors treated with BEC showed a clear diminution of their density, which was more remarkable in prolactinomas.

At surgery when the dura of the sellar floor was opened usually a spontaneous drainage of the sellar contents occurred. This consisted of an initial flow of a dense fluid carrying tissue debris, followed by a soft greyish tissue, which was easily removed by suction and ring curette. Bilateral jugular compression, performed by the anesthetist, facilitated the complete removal of the tumor by the transphenoidal ap-

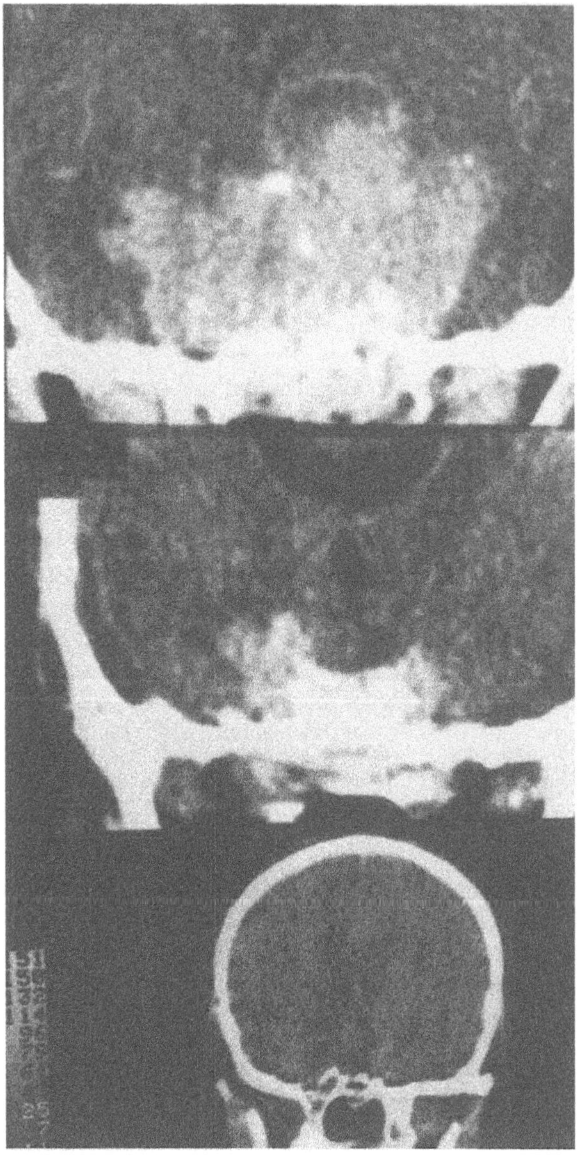

Fig. 1. Sequential high resolution CAT scan. *Upper:* Pretreated large macroadenoma. *Center:* After 19 weeks of BEC treatment. *Lower:* After Surgery

proach, and the exposure of the suprasellar arachnoid membrane as a result of the increased cisternal pressure.

These intraoperative findings did not depend on the duration of the previous BEC treatment, (minimum two weeks, maximum 43 weeks). They were directly related to the preoperative basal serum PRL levels; i.e., the lower the PRL level, the lower the tumoral density. In none of the cases in this series did we detect a fibrosis that made tumor removal difficult. The existence of an empty sella as well as a possible spontaneous rhinorrhea caused by the drastic drug-induced volume reduction

Table 2. Clinical and laboratory findings in 12 patients treated with bromocriptine and surgery

Case no.	Age	Sex	Pretreatment		Bromocriptine		One treatment with bromocriptine		Postsurgery	
			Clinical findings	PRL (ng/ml)	Dose (ng)	Period (weeks)	Clinical findings	PRL (ng/ml)	Clinical findings	PRL (ng/ml)
1 RM	18	♀	Acromegaly, 1° amenorrhea	16	25	5	Diffuse skin depigmentation	6	1° Amenorrhea	12
2 EP	18	♂	Hypogonadism, short height	820	5	2	No changes	114	No changes	37
3 CD	18	♂	Hypogonadism	5500	35	12	Without galactorrhea	68	No changes	49
4 MQ de B	38	♀	2° Amenorrhea, galactorrhea	788	5	2	2° Amenorrhea without galactorrhea	150	No changes	59
5 ME	37	♀	2° Amenorrhea, galactorrhea	105	5	8	Regular menses without galactorrhea	16	No changes	66
6 MC	19	♀	2° Amenorrhea, galactorrhea	280	7.5	20	No changes	16	Regular menses without galactorrhea	74
7 FG	25	♀	2° Amenorrhea, galactorrhea	150	5	4	Regular menses without galactorrhea	94	Regular menses without galactorrhea	81
8 JM	17	♂	Hypogonadism short height, galactorrhea	1100	35	19	Diffuse skin depigmentation without galactorrhea	53	No changes	76
9 M de O	21	♀	2° Amenorrhea, galactorrhea	247	5	5	No changes	66	Regular menses without galactorrhea	6.7
10 AY	38	♀	2° Amenorrhea, galactorrhea	2000	5	16	2° Amenorrhea without galactorrhea	200	Regular menses without galactorrhea	42
11 TR	31	♀	2° Amenorrhea, galactorrhea	3500	10	43	2° Amenorrea without galactorrhea	2	Regular menses without galactorrhea	44
12 GOB	25	♀	2° Amenorrhea, galactorrhea	280	5	5	Regular menses without galactorrhea	85	No changes	14

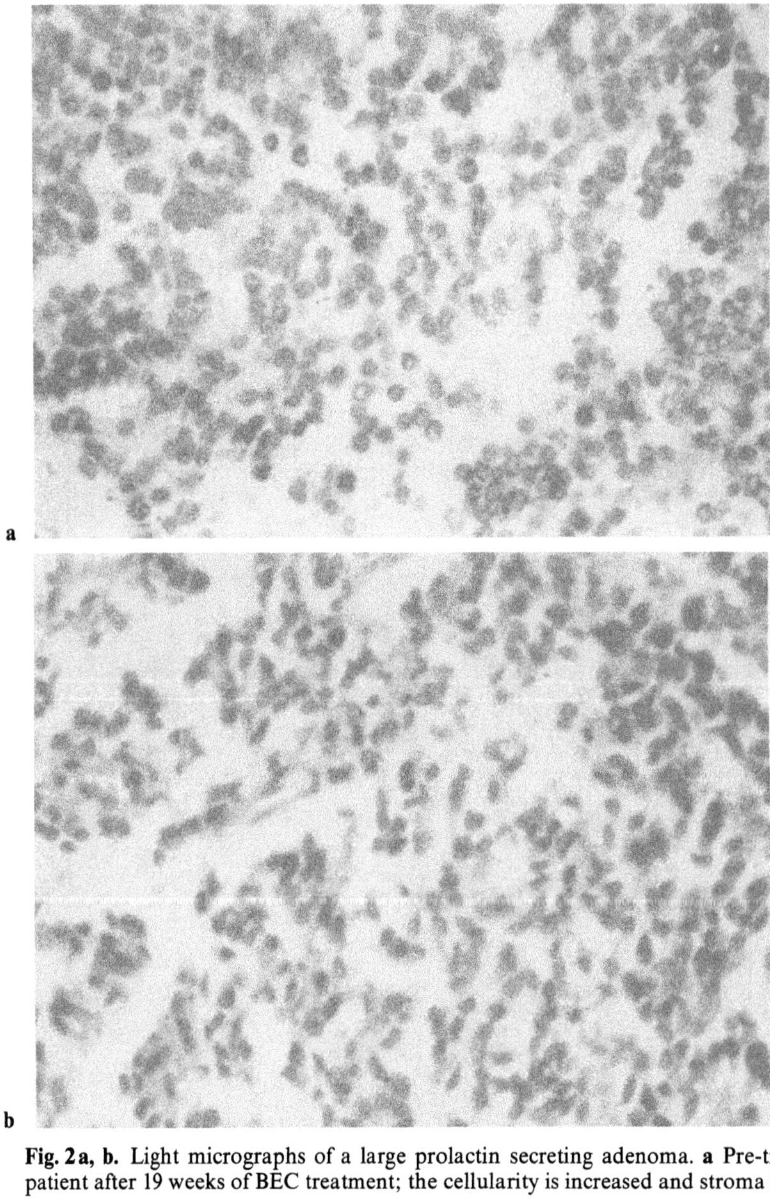

Fig. 2a, b. Light micrographs of a large prolactin secreting adenoma. **a** Pre-treated. **b** Same patient after 19 weeks of BEC treatment; the cellularity is increased and stroma is scarse

of the adenoma was solved in all cases by placing an intrasellar piece of muscle or fat tissue and then fitting a small piece of septum between the dura and the sellar floor, which is sealed with cyanoacrylate. In cases where the subfrontal approach was elected due to the lateral expansion of the adenoma, the removal of the tumor, greatly facilitated by its softness, was achieved by simple suction, with minimal brain retraction. Hemorrhage of the tumor cavity was therefore reduced to a minimum.

After surgery the patients remained free of headache and a progressive improvement in their ophthalmologic conditions was observed. Seven of the eight patients who had secondary amenorrhea resumed normal menstruation (Table 2). Basal PRL levels, one week after surgery, without treatment, showed a range between 6.7 ng/ml and 81 ng/ml (mean 46 ng/ml; ± 7.1 SE). Residual tumor was not detected by computed tomography after surgery, except in one case with a clear invasion of the right cavernous sinus. The three cases which had not had previous BEC treatment due to their absolute intolerance to the drug were operated on through the subfrontal route. The anatomic characteristics of these large invasive tumors make their separation from the surrounding neurovascular structures and their removal very difficult. Immediately after the operation, two of these cases showed signs of hypothalamic damage, marked hyperthermia and disturbance of consciousness, followed by coma and death.

Light microscopy studies of BEC treated tumors showed dense cell population with scarse and delicate stroma and with thin or sinusoid connective capillary septa (Fig. 2).

Discussion

Gerard Guiot, in his classic monograph of 1958 wrote: "When the pituitary adenoma has ceased to be intrasellar, when its proliferating nodules have penetrated the walls of the osteodural lodge in one or more places, trying to remove them can be difficult, impossible or dangerous." Presently there is no doubt that Bromocriptine, a specific agonist of dopaminergic receptors, has an action on PRL secretion, and therefore in the reduction of size and density of microprolactinomas (Bassetti et al. 1984). The same property has been used for the treatment of macrotumors, showing a dramatic improvement in both, the visual disturbances and neurologic disorders. The treatment of pituitary macrotumors only by pharmacologic means, especially in cases with suprasellar expansion or with chiasmatic or hypothalamic involvement, has been very limited, as these cases are usually considered a neurosurgical emergency. However, in 1980 Crossignani took the risk of medically treating a grade IV tumor of Vezina and Sutton even in the presence of a suprasellar expansion (Crossignani et al. 1980). This attitude could be extremely dangerous when reversible effect of Bromocriptine is considered (Thorner et al. 1981; Barrow et al. 1984).

Most reports point out that medical treatment is only a palliative resource, and clearly state that interruption of the drug treatment results in a fast recurrence of the tumor; on the other hand, the failure of surgical treatment of macrotumors due to the difficulty of their complete removal, further supported the medical approach. It is evident that these seemingly opposed therapeutic methods reach some concord as we search for better ways of removing tumors. The preoperative administration of BEC in cases of giant pituitary adenomas, with the dose and time required by each patient's particular tolerance, is in our experience an essential tool in the management of this pathology. A direct relationship between BEC dose, serum PRL level and tumor size was observed in every case of this series. The best results were clearly obtained in prolactinomas, but even in GH secreting adenomas an important diminution in tumor density was observed. A longer follow-up time of these patients will make it possible to demonstrate the real value of this approach.

References

Barrow DL, Tindall GT, Kovacs K, Thorner MO, Horvath E, Hoffman JC (1984) Clinical and pathological effects of bromocriptine on prolactin secreting and other pituitary tumors. J Neurosurg 60:1–7

Bassetti M, Spada A, Pezzo G, Gianasttasio (1984) Bromocriptine treatment reduces the cell size in human macroprolactinomas: A morphometric study. J Clin Endocrinol Metab 58:268–273

Besser GM, Parke L, Edwards CR, Forsyth IA, McNeilly AS (1972) Galactorrhea: Successful treatment with reduction of plasma prolactin levels by brom-ergocriptine. Br Med J (Clin Res) 3:669–672

Crossignani PG, Ferrari C, Malinverini A, Barbieri C, Matthei AM, Caldara R, Rochetti M (1980) Effect of central nervous system dopaminergic activation on prolactin secretion in man: Evidence for a common central defect in hyperprolactinemic patients with and without radiological signs of pituitary tumors. J Clin Endocrinol Metab 51:1068–1073

Del Pozo E, Varga L, Wyss H, Tolis G, Friesen H, Wenner R, Vetter L, Uehwiler A (1974) Clinical and hormonal response to bromocriptine (CB-154) in the galactorrhea syndromes. J Clin Endocrinol Metab 39:18–23

Guiot G (1958) Adenomes hypophysaires, Masson (ed), Paris, p 160–161

Landolt AM, Wuthrich R, Fellman H (1979) Regression of pituitary prolactinomas after treatment with bromocriptine. Lancet I:1082–1083

Thorner MO, Martin WH, Rogol AD, Morris JL, Perryman RL, Conway BP, Howard SS, Wolfman MG, McLeod RM (1980) Rapid regression of pituitary prolactinomas during bromocriptine treatment. J Clin Endocrinol Metab 51:438–445

Thorner MO, Perryman RL, Rogol AD, Conway BR, McLeod RM (1981) Rapid changes of prolactinoma volume after withdrawal and reinstitution of bromocriptine. J Clin Endocrinol Metab 53:480–483

Vaidya RA, Aloorkan SD, Rege NR, Maskati BT, Jahngir RP, Sheth AR, Pandya SK (1978) Normalization of visual fields following bromocriptine treatment in hyperprolactinemic patients with visual field constriction. Fertil Steril 29:632–636

Wass JAH, Thorner MO, Charlesworth MO, Moult PJA, Dacie JE, Jones AE, Besser GM (1979) Reduction of pituitary tumor size in patients with prolactinomas and acromegaly treated with bromocriptine. Lancet II:66–69

Weiss MH, Wycott RR, Yadley R, Gott P, Feldon S (1983) Bromocriptine treatment of prolactin secreting tumors. Surgical implications. Neurosurgery 12:640–642

The Effect of Suprasellar Lesions on Energy Balance

E. GROTE, Tübingen/FRG

The immediate and within seconds effective influence of the brain on peripheral glucose and energy supply is of neurogenic origin by way of the sympathetic and parasympathetic systems, whose most centrally located representation is in the hypothalamus. According to Ban 1966 (Fig. 1) the ventro-medial nucleus together with the lateral mamillary nucleus represent the sympathetic zone. The parasympathetic zone consists of a thin periventricular layer, the medial mamillary body and the ventro-lateral nucleus, which is in connection with the periventricular part in the septal region.

Neurogenic stimuli originating in the sympathetic zone immediately lead to glycogenolysis in the liver (Fig. 2), and at the same time to secretion of catecholamines,

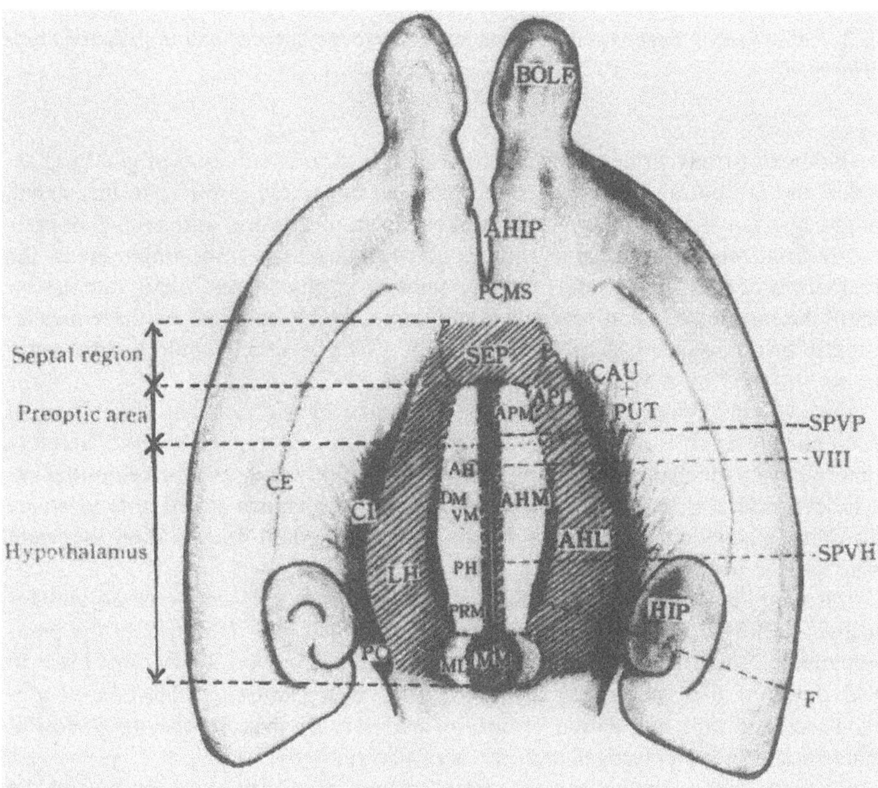

Fig. 1. Representation of autonomous nervous systems in the hypothalamus (Ban 1966)

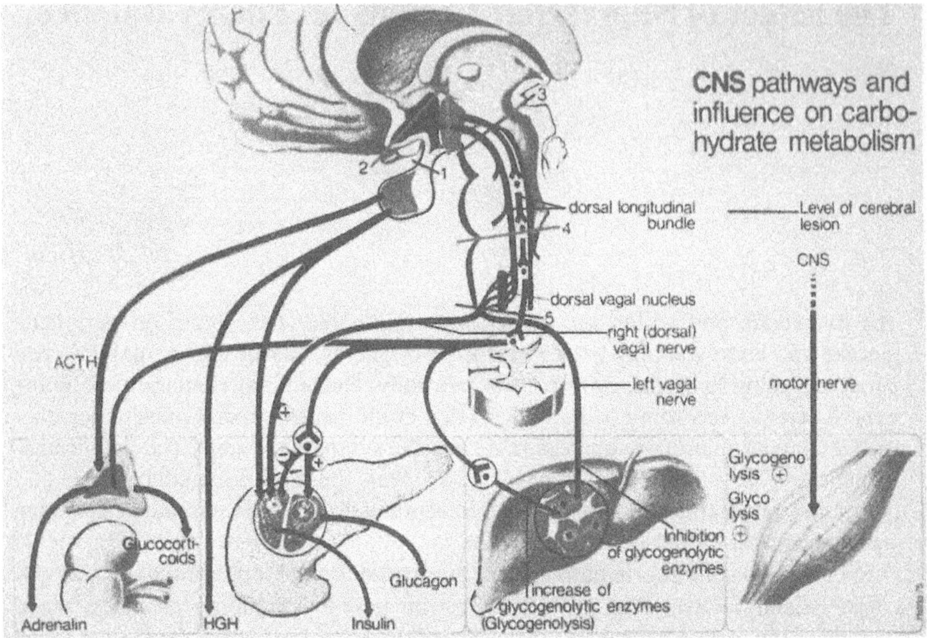

Fig. 2. Pathways and functions of the autonomous nervous systems to and in peripheral hormonal organs

break-down of triglycerides into free fatty acids and to stimulation of glucagon secretion and inhibition of insulin secretion. As an integrated response to this signal, blood sugar is elevated: glycogen is broken down to glucose, adrenalin mobilizes glucose from muscles, glucagon leads to glucogeneogenesis from amino acids, the break-down of triglyceride into free fatty acids saves glucose and finally the inhibition of the insulin secretion prevents that glucose, freshly supplied by these mechanisms, to be immediately stored in the form of glycogen, which would happen without nervous inhibition of insulin secretion (Grote 1981).

This system phylogenetically is to be explained by the fact that under normal conditions the brain is dependent upon glucose as its only energy source. Therefore it has to have a mechanism to supply this energy quickly and safely. Even under extreme cachexia and lack of fat and glycogen this mechanism is still able to create glucose by gluconeogenesis from proteins. After some days of starvation the brain tissue starts to utilize ketone-bodies.

This sympathetic mechanism, which at the same time leads to increased abilities for flight and fight may be almost completely inhibited by stimulation of the parasympathetic system (Shimazu 1967; Shimazu et al. 1965, 1966, 1968). This leads to break-down of the sympathetically modulated glycogenolysis, inhibition of glucagon secretion and stimulation of insulin secretion. By this mechanism glucose is stored back to fat and glycogen and free fatty acids to triglycerids.

This very fast sympathetically mediated system of energy break-down and the storage of these energy-forms under the effect of the parasympathetic system are substantiated and prolonged by hormonal effectors which are regulated from the hypothalamic area, too. GH and ACTH act with the same aim as the sympathetic system. Cortisol is necessary for the break-down of proteins and for gluconeogenesis, GH increases lipolysis and saves glucose. Therefore with the constantly increased supply of glucose in Cushing's disease and acromegaly the islet cells in the pancreas are no longer able to secrete high amounts of insulin and therefore a true diabetes mellitus occurs.

In anterior lobe insufficiency, however, these hormons are lacking. Therefore we find a very marked tendency to hypoglycemia; the lowest fasting blood sugar levels were found in these patients. Their extreme sensitivity to insulin induced hypoglycemia is known for decades.

There is no doubt that the neural as well as the hormonal effectors are monitored by glucosensible neurons of the hypothalamus (Fig. 3). According to Oomura et al. (1964, 1969), in the ventromedial hypothalamus neurons were stimulated by electro-osmotic application of glucose and depending on the dosage, their activity increased. On the other hand, in the lateral part of hypothalamus the activity of the neurons was elevated by lowering glucose. Only in the ventro-medial and lateral hypothalamus such neurons could be found, none were established in the cortex, thalamus or brain stem. Lowering of the blood glucose level in hypothalamus leads to immediate activity of sympathetic neural and hormonal systems, on the other hand hyperglycemia or local application of glucose into the 3rd ventricle lowers sympathetic activity and stops secretion of hormones.

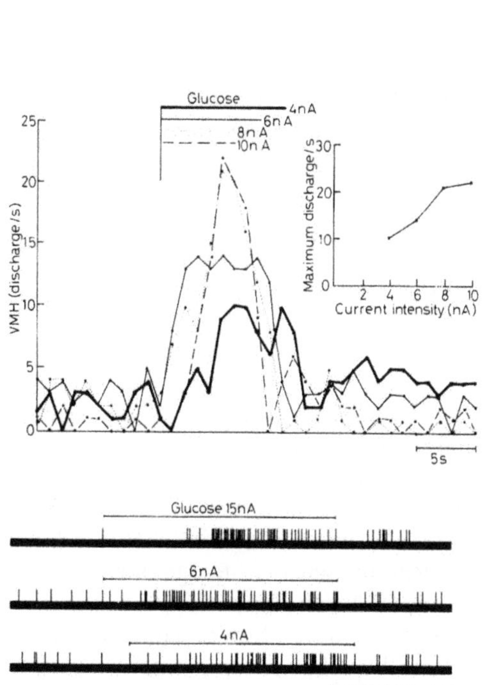

Fig. 3. Dose-dependent discharge of glucose-sensitive neurons in the hypothalamus after electroosmotic application (after Oomora)

On the contrary, slowly growing tumors compressing and displacing the hypothalamus never lead to hyperglycemia, but here often very low blood sugar levels are found, because only basic values of cortisol and GH are possible. Their stimulation and modulation are impaired because of the damaged axis.

Acute irritation of hypothalamus, however, leads to a marked hyperglycemia via the described mechanisms. The hypothalamus reacts as if intracellular glucopenia were present in its glucosensible neurons.

This behavior in spite of normo- or hyperglycemia can only be explained by derangement of the established point for glucose or by a true intracellular glucopenia in spite of hyperglycemia. Edema in hypothalamus after operation and irritation may lead to damaged transmembranous transport for glucose and to this reaction. The resulting hyperglycemia would be able to compensate for damaged membranous transport. In other words, the resulting hyperglycemia would be necessary for the survival of hypothalamic neurons.

Acute irritation after an operation of a large suprasellar pituitary adenoma, a meningioma or a craniopharyngioma not only leads to hyperglycemia, but all energy storage forms are broken down. Without actual need, fat and protein are broken down and supplied as fatty and amino acids. Even maximal external supply of nutrients does not stop the break-down of the stored forms of energy. Therefore, if hypothalamic irritation goes on for weeks or a dysregulated midbrain decerebrate rigidity exists, cachexia will result in spite of high external therapeutic supply. The so-called molar ratio of insulin and glucagon $\frac{\text{Insulin } \mu\text{U/ml}}{\text{Glucagon pg/ml}} \times 23.3$ (Unger 1972), decides whether the energy will be stored in the body or broken down. This molar ratio is highly influenced by irritation of the sympathetic nervous system. Normal values are between 5 and 10, meaning anabolic state, patients with hypothalamic irritation and in decerebrate rigidity show a very low value, between 0.2–2, being a pattern of catabolic state finally resulting in cachexia.

Glucose transfer measured by pharmacokinetic principles in gram/kg body weight/h (v. Hattingberg 1973) is more than doubled in hypothalamic irritation and midbrain herniation, in comparison to all other spontaneous and/or surgical conditions.

If the surgically induced hypothalamic irritation is of prolonged duration and the patient is constantly loosing weight, increasing the energy supply does not have a positive effect, but giving somatostatin is useful, because the result of high sympathetic activity on peripheral energy metabolism is then partially inhibited.

In summarizing, the hypothalamus decides about our energy balance. Bilateral destruction of the medial sympathetic zone in the ventromedial nucleus lowers general activity (Fig. 4), leading to decreased break-down of energy, and, because of the preserved ventrolateral parasympathetic system, to increased storage of energy. All these factors determine a hypothalamic obesity (Fröhlich 1901).

Only in those cases where both ventrolateral parts of hypothalamus are damaged and ventromedial parts are saved, true hypothalamic cachexia results, because these patients have preserved sympathetic activity, but have lost their capacity of storing energy. Because most neurosurgical suprasellar and hypothalamic diseases are in the midline, bilateral destruction of the ventromedial nuclei leading to

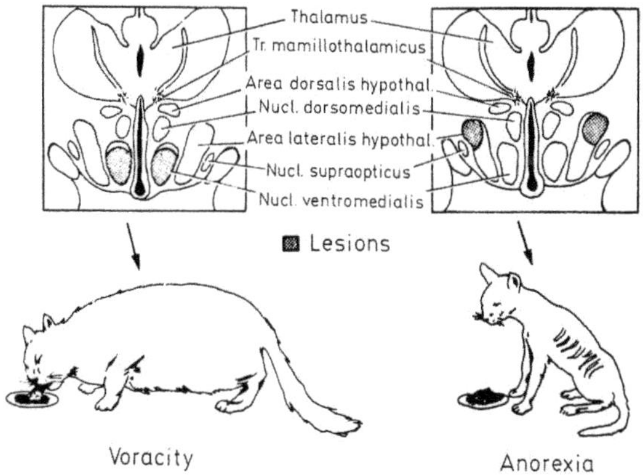

Fig. 4. Animal model of the sequelae of bilateral destroyal of ventromedial (*left*) and ventrolateral (*right*) hypothalamic nuclei (Courtesy of the Max-Planck-Institute of Psychiatry, Munich, Prof. Ploog)

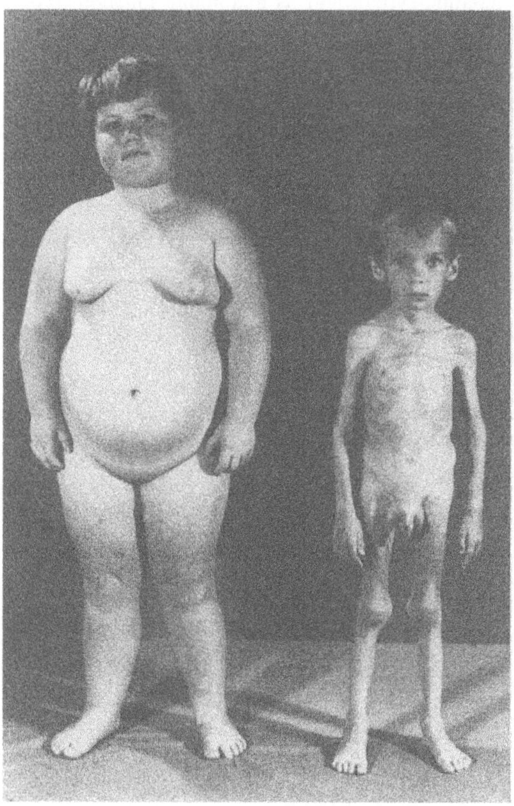

Fig. 5. See text

true hypothalamic obesity is much more often than cachexia. This latter only occurs with destroyed ventrolateral and partially preserved ventromedial nuclei which is obviously a much rarer condition.

Two clinical examples:

An 8-year-old girl suffered from a hamartoma of the medial infundibulum resulting in hypothalamic obesity and precocious puberty (Fig. 5).

A 6-year-old boy suffered from a craniopharyngioma destructing almost all the hypothalamic neurons but with some ventromedial parts preserved, as proven by sympathetic activity and hormone control.

The concentration of Adrenalin and Noradrenalin in the draining vein of the adrenal medulla is markedly reduced after an increase in the systemic glucose level or local application of glucose in the 3rd ventricle. After denervation of the medulla, concentration of catecholamines drops even more. The fatigue after a big meal is due to this mechanism. The satiated (person) has been deprived of his sympathetic effectors and abilities.

References

Ban T (1966) The septo-preoptico-hypothalamic system and its autonomic function. Progr. Brain Res, vol 21 A, Elsevier: Amsterdam, p 1–43

Fröhlich A (1901) Ein Fall von Tumor der Hypophysis cerebri ohne Akromegalie. Wiener Klin Rundschau 15:383

Grote E (1981) The CNS Control of Glucose Metabolism. Acta Neurochir [Suppl] (Wien) 31

v Hattingberg HM (1973) Mathematische Verfahren zur Auswertung von pharmakokinetischen Untersuchungen. Arzneimittelforsch 23:1646

Oomura Y, Kimura K, Ooyama H, Maeno T, Iki M, Kuniyoshi M (1964) Reciprocal activities of the ventro-medial and lateral hypothalamic areas of cats. Science 143:484

Oomura Y, Ono T, Ooyama H, Wayner MJ (1969) Glucose and osmosensitive neurones of the rat hypothalamus. Nature 222:282

Shimazu T (1967) Glycogen synthetase activity in liver: regulation by the autonomic system. Science 156:1256

Shimazu T, Fukuda A (1965) Increased activities of glycogenolytic enzymes in liver after splanchnic nerve stimulation. Science 150:1607

Shimazu T, Fukuda A, Ban T (1966) Reciprocal influence of the ventromedial and lateral hypothalamic nuclei on blood glucose level and liver glycogen content. Nature 210:1178

Shimazu T, Amakawa A (1968) Regulation of glycogen metabolism in liver by the autonomic nervous system. II. Neural control of glycogenolytic enzymes. Biochim Biophys Acta 165:349

Unger RH (1972) Insulin/glucagon ratio. Isr J Med Sci 8:252

Removal of Craniopharyngioma by a Unilateral Interhemispheric Trans-Lamina Terminalis Approach: Operative Procedures and Postoperative Management

N. Arita, S. Mori, T. Ikeda, T. Hayakawa, Y. Ushio, and H. Mogami, Osaka/Japan

Introduction

The majority of craniopharyngiomas is located in the suprasellar region and extends toward the third ventricle behind the chiasm. The retrochiasmal portion of the tumor cannot be removed under direct observations by an ordinary pterional or subfrontal approach alone. We have experienced 42 craniopharyngiomas in adults during the 15 years from 1970 to 1984. Biopsy or partial removal of the tumor followed by irradiation has been our standard treatment. Among 37 cases treated by this regimen, 14 deaths (38%) have occurred during the follow-up period of one year to 15 years. Recently, we have used a unilateral interhemispheric trans-lamina terminalis approach to attempt radical excision of craniopharyngiomas. The operative procedures and postoperative management of the patients are described.

Surgical Procedures

The scalp is incised in a semicoronal fashion with the patient in the supine position. A low right frontal craniotomy based on the supraorbital ridge is made. The bone flap is 6 cm in anteroposterior width, and one cm to the left of the midline. The frontal sinus is often opened. We pack a piece of the temporal muscle soaked in saline containing an antibiotic after the mucosa is coagulated and removed, and then a flap of the periostium is created and sutured to the dura to close the sinus. The dura is incised parallel to the supraorbital rim. Contusion to the frontal lobe when retracting the brain is carefully avoided in this approach. We open the right Sylvian fissure to drain the cerebrospinal fluid until the brain becomes well retracted. By this maneuver, we consider that a right unilateral approach is sufficient for the following procedures, instead of the bifrontal craniotomy and incision of the falx. A dural incision is added parallel to and 2 cm away from the superior sagittal sinus. Then an interhemispheric dissection of both frontal lobes is started; first, the genu of the corpus callosum is exposed, and then the anterior cerebral arteries are followed proximally to the chiasmal region. The tuberculum sellae, prechiasmatic cistern, chiasm and anterior communicating artery are visualized. The tumor cannot be seen in the prechiasmatic cistern when the chiasm is prefixed (Fig. 1). The lamina terminalis is a thin anterior wall of the third ventricle between the upper margin of the chiasm and the anterior commissure. It consists of gray matter and pia mater, and 10 mm in average length in normal subjects (Yamamoto et al. 1981). The organum vasculosum of the lamina terminalis, one of the circumventricular organs, is located just above the chiasm. The physiologic function of this in human is not well under-

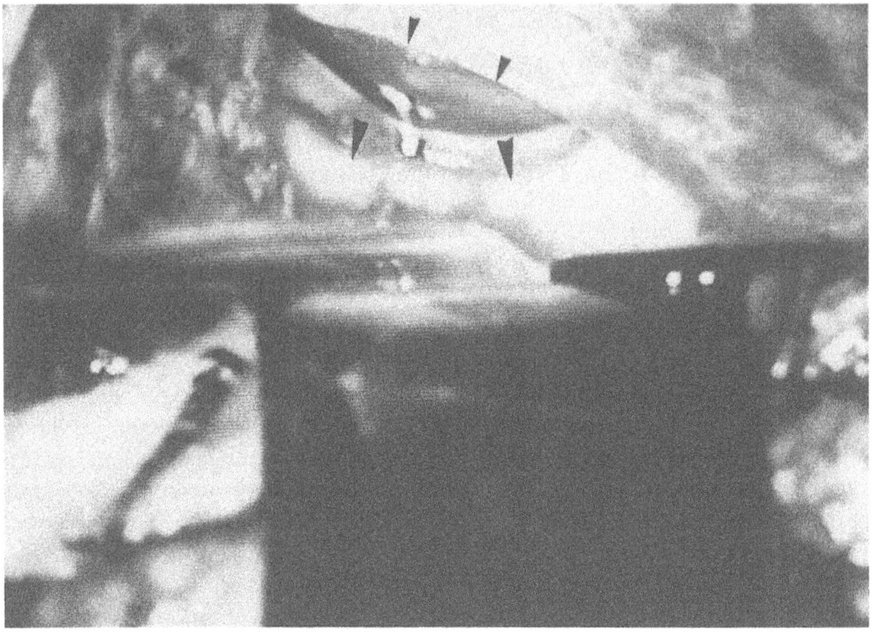

Fig. 1. Operative microphotograph of subfrontal exposure of the chiasm (*large arrow-heads*), prechiasmatic cistern and tuberculum sellae (*small arrow-heads*) in a 35-year-old male with a craniopharyngioma. The chiasm was prefixed, and the tumor was not visualized at all

stood (Weindl and Sofroniew 1978). It is stretched and even protruded in the presence of a retrochiasmal extension of a craniopharyngioma (Fig. 2). Several small vessels run over it. We puncture the lamina terminalis on its avascular part with a 23 G needle (Fig. 3), and a small amount of the fluid is aspirated if the tumor is cystic. Even removal of 1 or 2 ml fluid produces space for dissection to render later procedures more easily. Incising the lamina terminalis allows dissection while directly observing the retrochiasmal portion of the tumor from the hypothalamus. Except for the intraventricular craniopharyngioma reported in the literatures, the tumor grows upwards by pushing up the floor of the third ventricle. Accordingly, when the lamina terminalis is incised, the tumor is still covered by the stretched floor of the third ventricle which is inevitably incised to enter the inside of the tumor. If the tumor contains solid portions, intracapsular decompression is performed first. Sharp dissection is considered to be mandatory to separate the capsule of the tumor from the surrounding structures (Fig. 4). For this procedure, metrizamide CT cisternography offers useful and precise information about the extent of the tumor and its relationship with the hypothalamus and midbrain (Fig. 5). Coagulation by bipolar forceps is avoided as much as possible to prevent damage to the hypothalamus. Any small amount of bleeding is controlled simply by pressing with a cottonoid. We consider that the continuity between the median eminence and pituitary stalk should be preserved on either side to maintain the pituitary functions. And we try to find the stalk when dissecting the wall of the tumor from the floor of the third

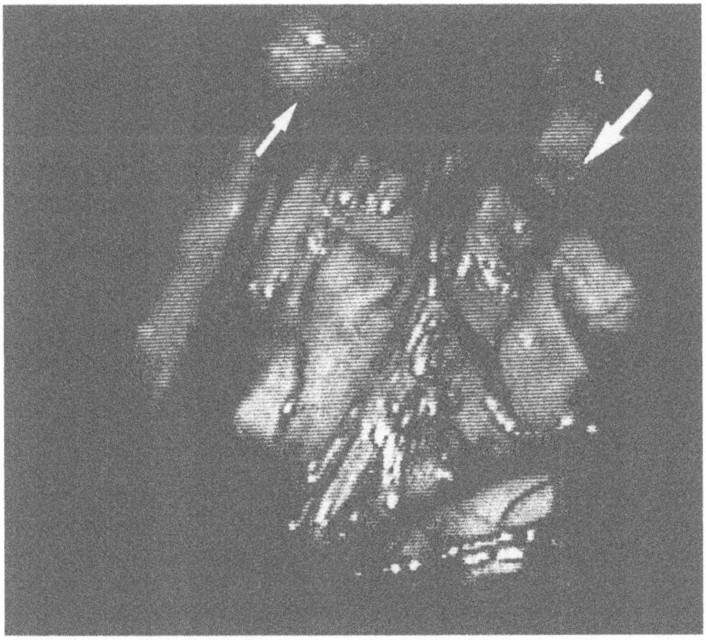

Fig. 2. Operative microphotograph of interhemispheric exposure of the lamina terminalis in the same case as in Fig. 1. *Large arrow,* anterior communicating artery; *small arrow,* left anterior cerebral artery

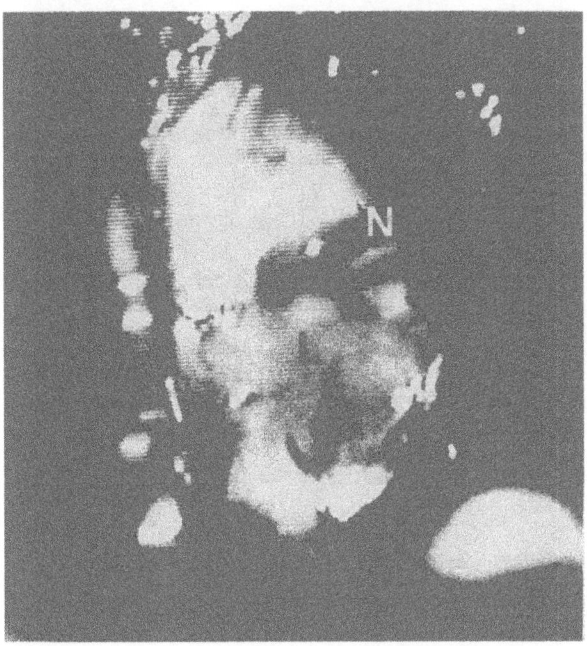

Fig. 3. Operative microphotograph demonstrating puncture (N = needle) of the lamina terminalis (L) in a 33-year-old female with a craniopharyngioma

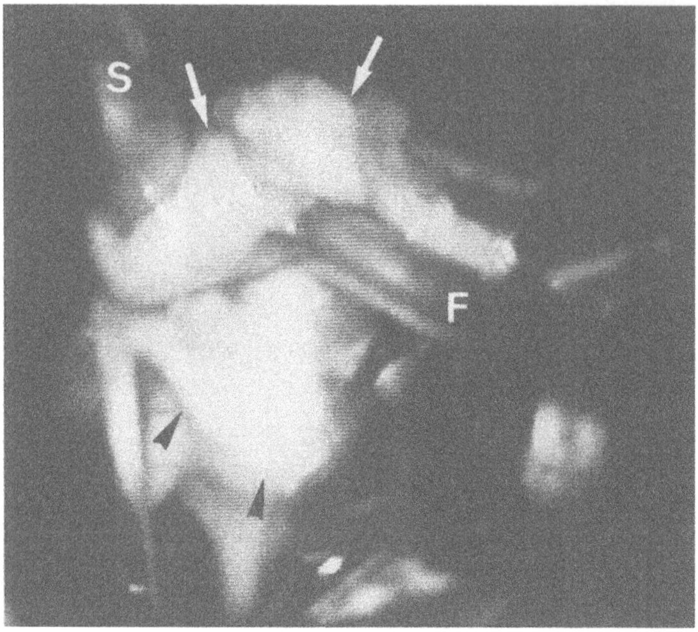

Fig. 4. Operative microphotograph showing sharp dissection of the tumor (*arrows*) from the floor of the third ventricle (*arrow-heads*) in the same case as in Fig. 3. F = tumor forceps; S = suction tube

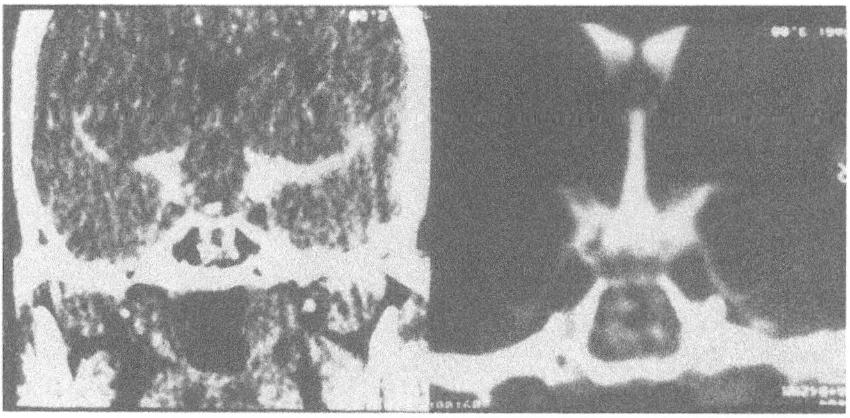

Fig. 5. Metrizamide CT cisternographs obtained before (*left*) and after (*right*) the operation in the same case as in Fig. 3. Metrizamide did not fill in between the hypothalamus and upper portion of the tumor. After removal of the tumor, the floor of the third ventricle descended and the suprasellar cistern was filled with metrizamide

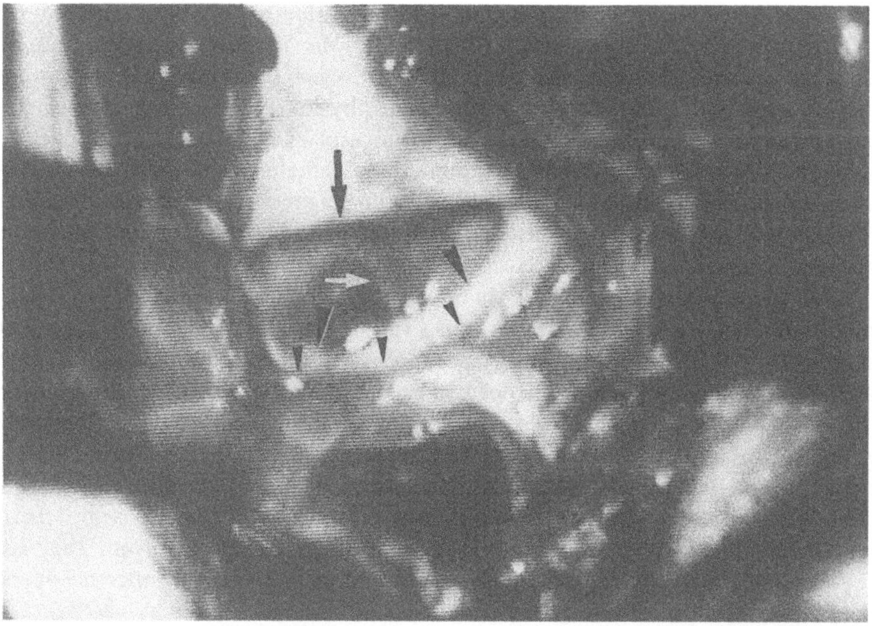

Fig. 6. Operative microphotograph obtained after total removal of a craniopharyngioma in the same case as in Fig. 3. The pituitary stalk (*white small arrow*) was preserved. *Large arrow:* tuberculum sellae; *large arrow-heads:* chiasm; *small arrow-heads:* anterior communicating artery

ventricle. The remaining part of the tumor is usually not as firmly adherent to the surrounding structure as to the floor, and it can be removed either through the lamina terminalis or the prechiasmatic space (Fig. 6).

Results and Postoperative Management

Five adult patients underwent removal of a craniopharyngioma by this approach. Microscopic total resection of the tumor was achieved in 4 patients, while the remaining patient had pulmonary tuberculosis, and a subtotal resection was made. We have experienced no operative deaths. Postoperative radiotherapy was not given in these patients. All 5 patients are still alive and have returned to their preoperative daily activities 6 months to 3 years and 6 months after the operation. Visual disturbance experienced by 4 patients before the operation disappeared or was much improved by the surgery. Diabetes insipidus developed in all cases within 2 to 13 hours after surgery. We have not administered vasopressin preparations in the immediate postoperative period. In general, the urinary output exceeds 300 ml/hour for 2 consecutive hours or 500 ml/hour, and the hourly fluid intake and output are recorded. If the patient is alert and thirsty, he is allowed to drink tap water as he wishes. Intravenous fluid is given to balance the output. Initially, only 5% dextrose water solution is used. In the absence of endogenous vasopressin, the urinary output reaches over 950 ml/hour when the glomerular filtration rate is 125 ml/minute. Accordingly, when the urinary output reaches this volume, osmotic diuresis by hyperglycemia due to a large amount of infusion of the 5% dextrose solution usually accompanies simple diabetes insipidus. Therefore, when the urinary output becomes large, a hypotonic solution with one half of the physiologic osmolality, consisting of sodium, chloride, and dextrose, is given for fluid replacement instead of 5% dextrose solution. To avoid hemolysis by hypotonicity, a catheter inserted to the superior vena cava is used for an intravenous route. By this regimen, the serum levels of electrolytes are maintained quite constant during the period of polyuria, and no serious systemic complications have occurred. The water balance should be maintained hourly. Hyponatremia may occur in the early postoperative period due to administration of vasopressin preparations. This is more difficult to manage than simple polyuria. Non-vasopressin preparations which are considered to cause release of endogenous vasopressin, for example carbamazepin and clofibrate, were not very effective in reducing the urinary output in the immediate postoperative period of this radical excision of the tumor. In 3 patients, diabetes insipidus was transient, and the urinary output decreased to less than 3000 ml/day about one week after operation. The remaining 2 patients continued to have a large urinary output, and DDAVP (1-desamino-8-D-arginine vasopressin) was given. They still required this for 8 months, and 2 years and 6 months, respectively, after the operation.

Endocrinological assessment was carried out in all the patients before and after the operation. As replacement therapy for the anterior pituitary function, hydrocortisone and/or thyroxine were required in 4 of the 5 patients.

Conclusion

No definite evaluation of this surgical approach can be made since the follow-up period is still short in our cases, and recurrence of tumors were reported years after radical excision (Katz 1975).

Radical excision of craniopharyngiomas has been achieved with excellent results by other surgical approaches (Matson and Crigler 1969; Aiba and Yamada 1980), including the transtemporal approach with anterior temporal lobectomy (Symon and Sprich 1985) and the transsphenoidal approach (Laws 1980). Removal of a craniopharyngioma through the lamina terminalis is by no means a new approach. When the chiasm was prefixed, the lamina terminalis was incised in the case of craniopharyngioma in children (Hoffman et al. 1977). In the series including both children and adults, the tumor was removed through the lamina terminalis in 23 of the 37 patients (Sweet 1976). Radical excision by a transcranial approach via the lamina terminalis and sphenoid sinus was also reported (Patterson and Danylevich 1980). Dissection of the tumor from the hypothalamus is the crucial point of the surgical excision of craniopharyngiomas, since firm adhesion of the tumor to the floor of the third ventricle exists in most cases. Incising the lamina terminalis allows direct observation to fascilitate dissection of this part of the tumor. We believe that this approach is a good method for the radical excision of craniopharyngiomas, even in adults in whom total resection of the tumor was not used to be attempted.

Acknowledgment: The authors are grateful to all the staff in the Department of Neurosurgery, Osaka University Medical School.

This investigation was supported by a Grant-in-Aid from the Ministry of Welfare.

References

Aiba T, Yamada S (1980) Surgery of craniopharyngiomas in adults – with special reference to their operative indications from the viewpoint of follow-up results and microsurgical radical resection of the tumors preserving the pituitary stalk. Neurol Med Chir (Tokyo) 20:439–451 (in Japanese)

Hoffman HJ, Hendrick EB, Humphreys RP, Buncic JR, Armstrong DL, Jenkin DT (1977) Management of craniopharyngioma in children. J Neurosurg 47:218–227

Katz EL (1975) Late results of radical excision of craniopharyngiomas in children. J Neurosurg 42:86–90

Laws ER Jr (1980) Transsphenoidal microsurgery in the management of craniopharyngioma. J Neurosurg 52:661–666

Matson DD, Crigler JF Jr (1969) Management of craniopharyngioma in children. J Neurosurg 30:377–390

Patterson RH, Danylevich A (1980) Surgical removal of craniopharyngiomas by a transcranial approach through the lamina terminalis and sphenoid sinus. Neurosurgery 7:111–117

Sweet WH (1976) Radical surgical treatment of craniopharyngioma. Clin Neurosurg 23:52–79

Symon L, Sprich W (1985) Radical excision of craniopharyngioma. Results in 20 patients. J Neurosurg 62:174–181

Weindl A, Sofroniew MV (1978) Neuro-hormones and circumventricular organs. In: Scott DE, Kozlowski GP, Collins F, Weindl (eds) Brain-endocrine interaction. Neural hormones and reproduction. Karger, Basel, p 117–137

Yamamoto I, Rhoton AL Jr, Peace DA (1981) Microsurgery of the third ventricle: part 1. Microsurgical anatomy. Neurosurgery 8:334–356

The Transpetrosal-Transtentorial Approach and Its Application in the Therapy of Retrochiasmatic Craniopharyngiomas

A. HAKUBA, Osaka/Japan

Our experience with the transpetrosal-transtentorial approach [1, 2, 3] for retrochiasmatic craniopharyngiomas is herein reviewed and the operative technique is described. Excellent exposure of the retrochiasmatic and suprasellar regions is gained with minimum retraction of the temporal lobe and cerebellum. Our transpetrosal approach is a simplified modification of the translabyrinthine approach [4]. However, it is completely different from the latter in that respect that hereby hearing on the operated side can be preserved [3]. The author has experienced 9 patients with retrochiasmatic craniopharyngiomas extending into the posterior hypothalamus, radically operated on by the transpetrosal-transtentorial approach with relatively good results.

Clinical Materials

Seven of the nine patients were male (Table 1). The patients' ages ranged from 6 to 62 years with an average age of 29. The symptoms and signs present before the operation were pan-hypopituitarism in six cases, intracranial hypertension in five, failing vision in three and bitemporal hemianopsia in two. Duration of the symptoms ranged from 3 months to 7 years with an average of 2.5 years. One patient (Case 8) had two previous operations and another one (Case 9) had one previous operation. Radiologic examination of these patients showed that eight (Cases 1, 2, 3, 4, 5, 6, 7, 9) had suprasellar tumors, growing both intraventricularly into the third ventricle and extraventricularly into the interpeduncular fossa, and the remaining one had a large tumor extending suprasellarly, laterally into the middle fossa and also posteriorly into the posterior fossa. Either total or extensive radical excision was successfully accomplished in six patients (Cases 1, 2, 3, 4, 8, 9).

Operative Technique

The operation is performed usually on the right side. The patient is placed on his left side in the "park bench" position. The skin incision starts at the upper margin of the zygomatic arch about 1 cm anteriorly to the external auditory meatus, and runs upward and then backward around the ear lobe, and then downward one finger breadth behind the posterior margin of the mastoid process to the mastoid tip (Fig. 1). The skin flap is turned laterally. The posterior temporal fascia and muscle are divided in the line of the crista supramastoidea and the lateral suboccipital muscles are divided in the line of the skin incision, and are elevated subperiosteally and turned with the skin flap below the crista supramastoidea, and the mastoid process and the retromastoideal suboccipital bone are exposed. Multiple burr holes are made in the suboccipital and temporal regions. Then a mastoidectomy is accomplished and the sigmoid sinus is exposed in full length as low as the jugular bulb (Fig. 2). The suboccipital-temporal bone flap is elevated, and hinged on the temporal muscle. Trautman's triangle is now well exposed. While the subtemporal dura mater is retracted forward and the posterior petrosal dura mater and the sigmoid sinus are retracted medialward by self-retaining retractors with Sugita's tapering

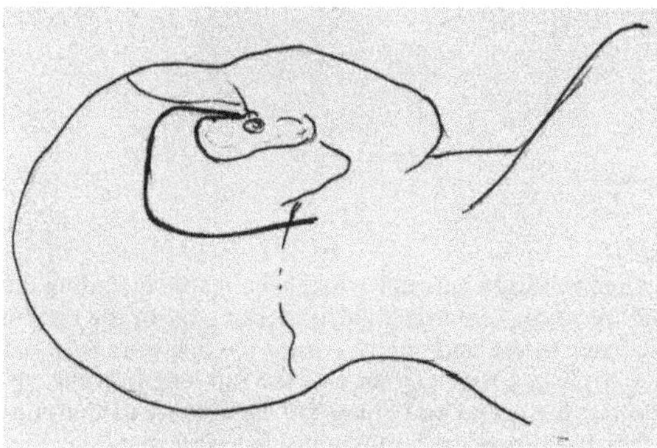

Fig. 1. Positioning and skin incision

Table 1. Summary of the 9 cases

Case no.	Age	Sex	Symptoms and signs	Treatment	Type of tumor	Result
1	7	M	Raised ICP	1) Total removal 2) VP shunt	Infundibulum Infundibulum	Excellent Excellent
2	6	M	Bitemp. hemianop. panhypopituitarism	1) Subtotal removal 2) Radiotherapy	Infundibulum Infundibulum	Excellent Excellent
3	10	M	Raised ICP panhypopituitarism	Total removal	Infundibulum	Excellent
4	22	M	Raised ICP	Extensive radical removal	Infundibulum	Excellent
5	62	F	Failing vision panhypopituitarism	Total removal	Infundibulum	Good
6	40	M	Bitemp. hemianop.	Total removal	Infundibulum	Vegetative
7	62	M	Raised ICP panhypopituitarism somnolence	1) VP shunt 2) Radiotherapy 3) Total removal	Infundibulum	Died
8	19	F	Failing vision panhypopituitarism	Total removal	Stalk	Excellent
9	34	F	Raised ICP failing vision panhypopituitarism	1) Transsphenoidal approach and drainage of cyst fluid 2) Total removal	Stalk	Excellent

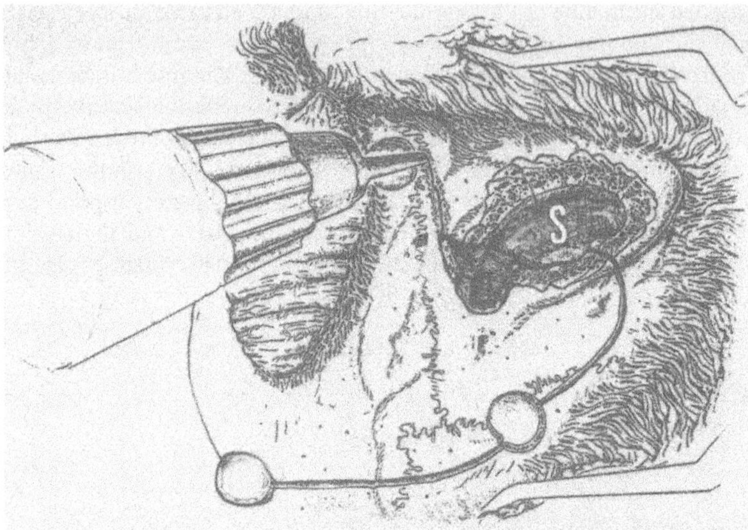

Fig. 2. The skin flap had been elevated and multiple burr holes had been made, including the first burr hole at the asterion, the second burr hole centered at the posterior edge of the base of the mastoid process and third burr hole made at the mid point between the first burr hole and inion. A radical mastoidectomy was accomplished with exposure of the full length of the sigmoid sinus (*S*) and the dura mater located for a few mm along the sigmoid sinus both anteriorly and posteriorly and then the suboccipital temporal craniotomy was performed

brain spatulas, the posterior part of the petrosal bone restricted to 1 cm depth from the petrosal ridge is removed up to the level of the internal auditory meatus the roof of which is partially removed, and 5 mm in depth anteriorly to it up to the tip of the petrosal bone (Fig. 3). The subtemporal dura is opened as far anteriorly as possible toward the superior petrosal sinus and the posterior petrosal dura is opened along the superior petrosal sinus and sigmoid sinus. After clipping and dividing the superior petrosal sinus anteriorly to the entrance of the petrosal vein (Fig. 4), the tentorium is divided to the hiatus, right behind the dural entrance of the right trochlear nerve. The trochlear nerve is retracted downward and the arachnoid membrane of the ambient cistern is opened. The lower margin of the hypothalamus is separated from the capsule of the tumor while the right third cranial nerve, and the posterior communicating artery (P-com) and its anterior perforators are carefully preserved. Then, further dissection is made in order to separate the ventral part of the tumor from the ventral margin and inferior medial wall of the hypothalamus. Internal decompression of the isolated part of the tumor is made. Then the posterior inferior part of the tumor which is usually extraventricular, is separated from the basilar tip and also the proximal portions of the ipsilateral posterior cerebral artery and superior cerebellar artery, and further internal decompression of this isolated portion of the extraventricular tumor is performed. Thereafter, the tumor capsule is removed piece-meal. The A-1 portion of the right anterior cerebral artery, and the medial and posterior walls of both internal carotid arteries can be visualized directly through this approach and separated from the tumor capsule. Through this ap-

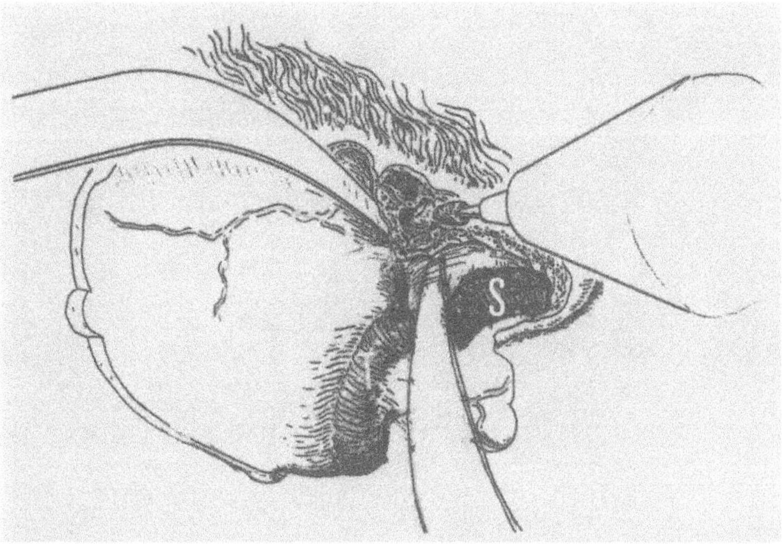

Fig. 3. The suboccipital temporal bone flap which had been elevated and hinged on the temporal muscle was omitted in this picture. While the subtemporal dura mater was retracted forward and the posterior petrosal dura mater as well as the sigmoid sinus (*S*) were retracted medially by self-retaining retractors, the postero-medial part of the petrosal bone was removed with an air drill. T: transverse sinus

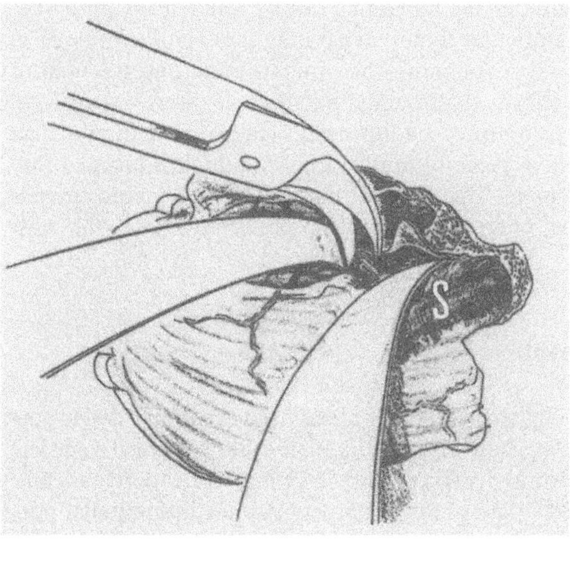

Fig. 4. The subtemporal dura mater was opened as far anteriorly as possible, and the posterior petrosal dura mater was divided along the sigmoid sinus and then along the superior petrosal sinus. Two Weck clips were applied to the superior petrosal sinus between the petrosal vein and root of the trigeminal nerve. A tentoriotomy started at this point

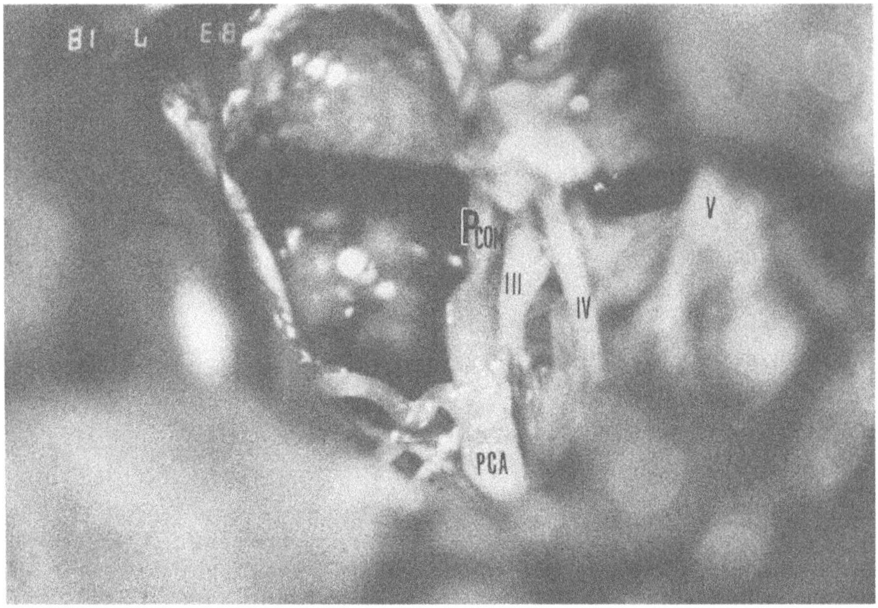

Fig. 5. Case 5. Through the transpetrosal-transtentorial approach the tumor had been removed totally. *Pcom* = posterior communicating artery, *III* = oculomotor nerve, *IV* = trochlear nerve, *V* = trigeminal nerve, *PCA* = posterior cerebral artery

proach, one is also able to see directly the remaining deeper walls of the third ventricle while dissecting the intraventricular tumor. Separating the tumor capsule from the anterior inferior part of the hypothalamus, the pituitary stalk and the inferior surface of the optic chiasma is performed also under microscopic direct vision. Total removal of the tumor can be accomplished by this means (Fig. 5). The dural defect is closed using a fascia lata graft. A piece of muscle from the thigh is inserted into the bony defect of the petrosal bone. The exposed portion of the sigmoid sinus is covered by pieces of thin cortical bone which has been preserved during the mastoidectomy.

Operative Findings and Result

In five patients (Cases 1, 2, 3, 5, 7) the tumors originated from the infundibular portion of the hypothalamus, growing both intraventricularly into the third ventricle through a large defect in its floor and extraventricularly into the interpeduncular fossa. In two cases (Cases 4, 6) the origin of the tumor was also the infundibular portion and the mass grew upward into the third ventricle through a hole in the elevated and invaginated floor of the ventricle and extraventricularly into the interpeduncular fossa. One case (Case 8) originated from the pituitary stalk, extended suprasellarly with marked elevation of the third ventricle, laterally into the middle fossa and posteriorly into the posterior fossa. The remaining one (Case 9) was also originated from the pituitary stalk and extending suprasellarly with marked elevation of the third ventricle and right posterolateral displacement of the pituitary stalk.

Follow-up examinations at 6 months after surgery showed five patients (Cases 1, 2, 3, 4, 9) had normal function of the central nervous system (CNS), normal intelligence and visual acuity, and one patient (Case 8) had normal CNS function, intelligence and visual acuity but she continued to have defects in the visual fields, and one patient (Case 5) who was almost blind preoperatively had normal intelligence with mild weakness of the legs, but she became blind postoperatively. One patient (Case 6) in this series was in poor neurologic condition due to hemorrhage from a traumatic aneurysm which appeared at the repaired site of the P-1 segment of the right posterior cerebral artery. The remaining patient who had a giantic solid craniopharyngioma with marked posterior hypothalamic dysfunction remained in the same neurologic condition and died of pneumonia 7 months after the operation. Postoperative CT scans showed no residual tumor in any of the patients except for one (Case 2) (Fig. 6, a, b). The postoperative endocrinological study in these patients showed panhypopituitarism in 8 cases. The remaining one patient (Case 1) showed normal pituitary function. Three children were showing normal growth without hormonal treatment.

a

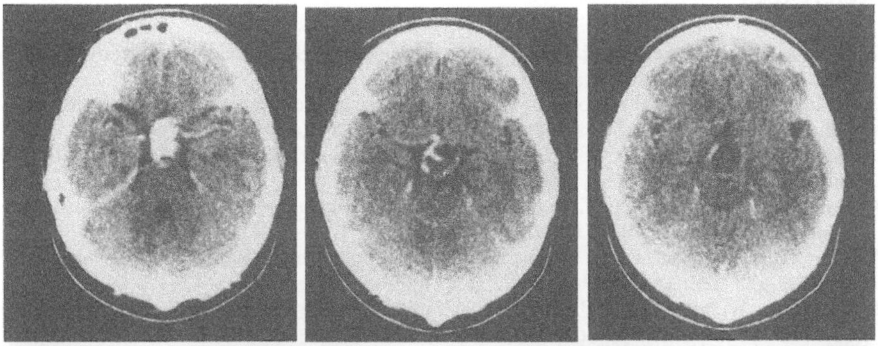

b

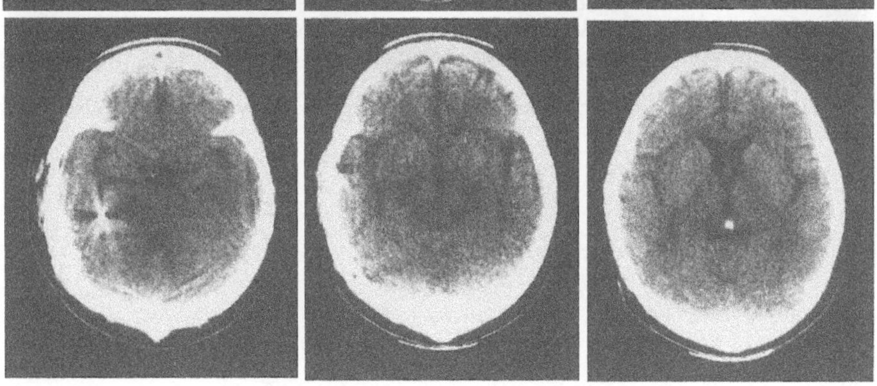

Fig. 6 a, b. Case 9. **a** Preoperative CT scan. **b** Postoperative CT scan

Discussion

Morrison and King [6] have reported a translabyrinthine transtentorial approach for cerebello-pontine angle tumors. In their approach, the labyrinthus including the middle ear, has to be destroyed. In our transpetrosal approach, the opening of the antrum is limited and the ear ossicles are not even touched, and it is not necessary to remove the labyrinth except for the posterior semicircular canal and the medial part of the horizontal semicircular canal. Adequate hearing was preserved in seven out of nine cases in this series. Postoperative oculomotor palsy was recognized in all of the patients as an operative complication. However, all of them improved within 3 to 6 months after the surgical intervention. Recognizing the excellent results of Sweet and others through a transfrontal route [5, 7, 8] we nevertheless feel that a transpetrosal-transtentorial approach may provide a better anatomic appreciation of the retrochiasmatic craniopharyngioma and its surrounding structures. However, we realize that this operation is technically more demanding and we do not have experience with this operative approach in sufficient numbers of craniopharyngioma cases to determine whether this surgical method offers a definite advantage in terms of mortality and morbidity over previous operative approaches, and also the postoperative follow-up periods of these patients are not long enough yet to determine the radicality through this approach, but we are encouraged by our results to date.

References

1. Hakuba A, Nishimura S et al. (1977) Clivus meningioma: Six cases of total removal. Neurol Med Chir (Tokyo) 17:63–77
2. Hakuba A (1978) Total removal of cerebello-pontine angle tumors with a combined transpetrosal-transtentorial approach. Neurol Surg 6:347–354 (in Japanese)
3. Hakuba A, Nishimura S (1981) Total removal of clivus meningiomas and the operation results. Neurol Med Chir (Tokyo) 21:59–73
4. House WF (1964) Monograf. Transtemporal bone microsurgical removal of acoustic neuromas. Arch Otolaryngol 80:599–756
5. King TT (1979) Removal of intraventricular craniopharyngiomas through the lamina terminalis. Acta Neurochir (Wien) 45:277–286
6. Morrison AW, King TT (1973) Experiences with a translabyrinthine-transtentorial approach to the cerebello-pontine angle. J Neurosurg 38:382–390
7. Patterson RN, Danylevich A (1980) Surgical removal of craniopharyngiomas by a transcranial approach through the lamina terminalis and sphenoid sinus. Neurosurgery 7:111–117
8. Sweet WH (1976) Radical surgical treatment of craniopharyngioma. Clin Neurosurg 23:52–79

Surgery of Processes Affecting Midbrain and Basal Ganglia

Surgery of Processes Along the Pyramidal Tract and the Internal Capsule

U. EBELING, H. J. REULEN, and P. HUBER, Bern/Switzerland

The subject of this workshop is centered on brain stem and basal ganglia. One of the important anatomic structures is the fiber tract of the motor system, usually called the pyramidal tract. The localization and functional representation of the motor cortex is well known. Very little, however, is known about the exact course of this fiber tract from the cortex down to the internal capsule. In addition no study exists on the extent of displacement of the fibers of the pyramidal tract by pathologic processes such as tumors located anteriorly or posteriorly in the neighborhood of this fiber tract.

The subject of the investigation was to gain some data as to the localization of the pyramidal tract in patients with brain tumors or brain abscesses near or in the course of the pyramidal tract. The preliminary results, the methods and the surgical conclusions will be presented.

Anatomic Remarks to the Pyramidal Tract

The pyramidal tract predominantly originates in the area 4 and 6. The fibers pass through the white matter of the centrum semiovale to the internal capsule [2, 4, 7, 8, 11–14, 16, 19, 21]. The fibers of the face, arm and leg show an arrangement like a fan, which opens against the cortex and shuts when approaching the posterior limb of the internal capsule [3, 20, 22]. When comparing the motor cortex and the posterior limb of the internal capsule both structures show a nearly 90 degree angle (Fig. 1). The fan of the fiber system has to rotate from its former oblique anterior–posterior position to one completely turned by 90 degree. The face now is located anteriorly, followed by the fibers of the hand and arm, while the leg is located most posteriorly. This typical arrangement has been demonstrated both in anatomic (retrograde degeneration) as well as electrophysiological studies (stimulation) [5, 6]. A good short review about the controversial results and opinions about the arrangement of the fibers of the pyramidal tract in the posterior limb of the internal capsule was given by Englander in 1975 [10].

Methods and Results

1. As a first step we have tried to gain some measures on the depth and thickness of the fan, generated by the pyramidal tract using the fiber preparation method of Klingler in formalin fixed human brains [17]. If only the fibers of the precentral motor area (area 4 and 6) are considered, where about 60% of pyramidal tract fibers

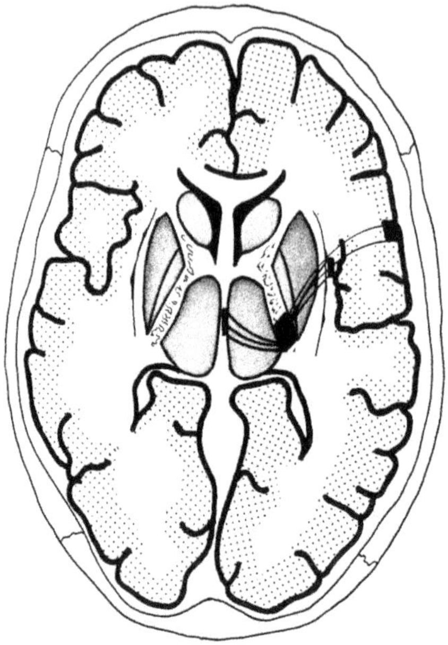

Fig. 1. Schematic representation of the course of the pyramidal tract from the motor area to the posterior limb of the internal capsule

originate in the human, the approximate thickness amounts only to 3–6 mm. The radius of the fan was estimated about 40–50 mm.

2. The precentral gyrus and the pyramidal tract were localized in the CT-Scan, in order to have some geometric relations to a tumor laying in the neighborhood of this tract or in the tract itself. In the CT the precentral sulcus and gyrus show a typical configuration [18]. According to Kido the junction between the superior frontal and precentral sulcus marks the anterior border of the gyrus precentralis and is very constantly to be identified in CT-scans closest to the vertex [9, 15]. The posterior border of the gyrus precentralis is marked by the central sulcus. The angle between the precentral sulcus and the midline averages 63–68 degrees [9, 15].

3. As a basis for any measurement some landmarks are needed. We have used the coronal suture as a bony landmark, which can be seen in the CT-Scan as well as in the conventional lateral X-ray film of the skull, respectively [1]. If the coronal sutures are connected with a straight line, the distance to the central sulcus can be measured at any point and amounts to about 60 mm near the midline in the CT. This distance becomes smaller towards the lateral end of the central sulcus.

4. In contrast to the precentral sulcus the fiber system of the pyramidal tract cannot be directly visualized in the CT. Additionally it can be displaced by a mass lesion. It may be determined indirectly by using the grid-system developed by Tailarach and Szikla [22] (Fig. 2). The location and the course of the various parts of the pyramidal tract – face, arm and leg – through the white matter were determined by Tailarach by electric stimulation during stereotactic operations [22]. By using this grid-system the location of the pyramidal tract can be determined on a normal lateral X-ray film of the skull in patients with a mass lesion. In the grid-system we transformed the measures of the coronal sutures.

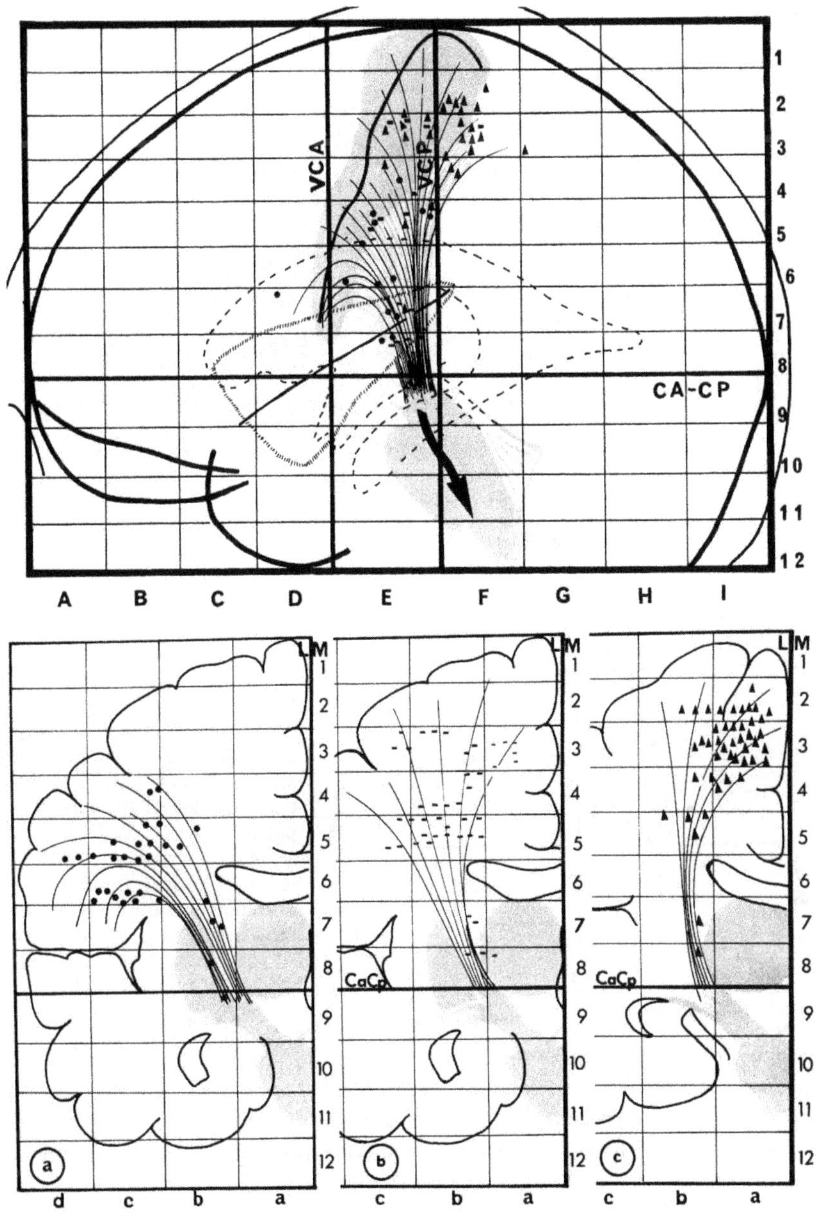

Fig. 2. The origin and course of the fibers of the pyramidal tract from the Atlas of Tailarach [22]. *VCA* = Linea verticalis anterior (tangential to the posterior edge of the anterior commissure); *VCP* = Linea verticalis posterior (tangential to the anterior edge of the posterior commissure); *Ca Cp* = Interconnecting line through the superior edge of the anterior commissure and inferior edge of the posterior commissure

- • face and tongue responses
- – upper limb responses
- ▲ lower limb responses

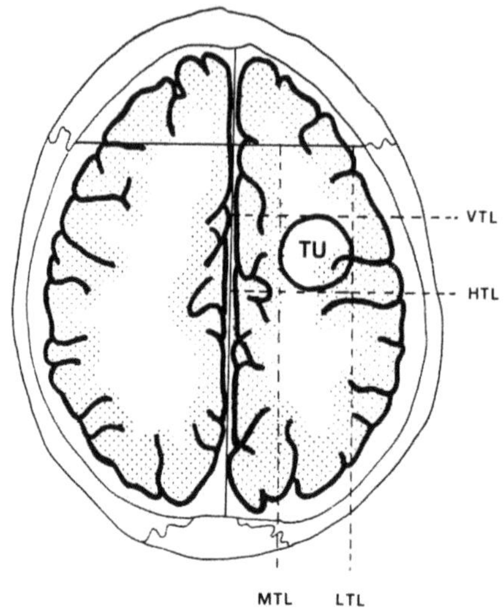

Fig. 3. The Fig. shows the necessary measurements. The margins of the tumor and the coronal suture are drawn in. The distance between the posterior and anterior margin of the tumor and the coronal suture are measured. *VTL* = anterior tumor limit, *HTL* = posterior tumor limit, *MTL* = medial tumor limit, *LTL* = lateral tumor limit

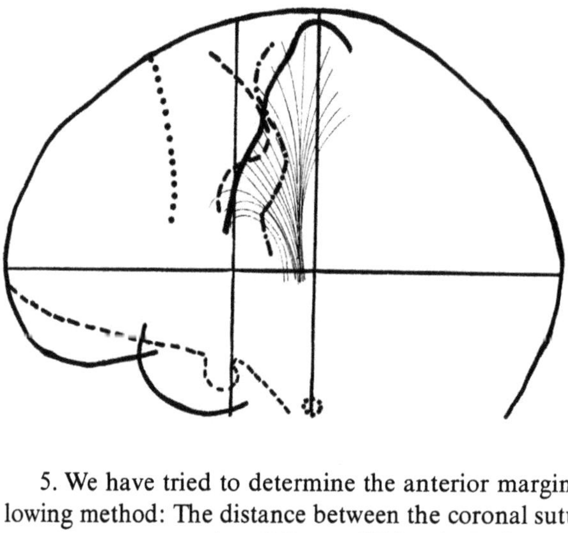

Fig. 4. This Fig. shows the coronal suture and the normal course of the pyramidal tract after Tailarach [22]. The posterior border of the tumors of patients with and without a motor deficit are drawn in. ··· = Coronal suture. - - - = Posterior margin of the tumors without a motor deficit. -·-·-· = Posterior margin of the tumors with a motor deficit

5. We have tried to determine the anterior margin of the pyramidal tract by following method: The distance between the coronal sutures and the dorsal border of a tumor was measured at different CT-levels. Patients with such a tumor, but without a motor deficit were compared with patients with a motor deficit, such as mono- or hemiparesis. Only well defined lesions (12 small glioblastomas, 9 metastasis, 2 brain abscesses) were used for this evaluation (Fig. 3).

The points obtained at various CT-levels in the deep white matter were compared with normal localization of the pyramidal tract [22] (Fig. 4). It becomes evident that the pyramidal tract can be displaced posteriorly by a tumor by some 10 mm. The line corresponding to the posterior tumor margin in patients without a motor deficit is 5–10 mm behind the normal localization of the pyramidal tract. In the patients with a motor deficit this line lies a few mm posteriorly. Thus the motor system may be shifted posteriorly about 5–10 mm by tumors located anteriorly to this system.

Conclusions

This line may be considered as a safety zone, which should not be crossed when resecting such lesions. However, at the moment we are not yet able to give the exact averages and the variations of this line since our results are based only on 23 patients. We need more data. It is our hope that by collecting more data, we will be able to remove lesions with more safety.

References

1. Ahmadi J et al. (1982) Localisation of intracranial lesions utilizing the coronal suture as a landmark on axial computed tomography. Surg Neurol 17:209–212
2. Barr LM (1972) The human nervous system. An anatomical viewpoint. Harper, Intern Ed, p 316–330
3. Beevor CE (1890) An experimental investigation into the arrangement of the excitable fibres in the internal capsule of the bonnet monkey. Phil Trans Roy Soc (London) 181 (B):49–88
4. Bennett AH (1885) Case of brachial Monoplegia due to lesions of the internal capsule. Brain 8:78–84
5. Bertrand B et al. (1966) Stimulation during stereotactic operations for dyskinesias. J Neurosurg 24:419–423
6. Bertrand G et al. (1965) Electrical exploration of the internal capsule and neighbouring structures during stereotactic procedure. J Neurosurg 22:333–343
7. Brodal A (1969) Neurological anatomy – In relation to clinical medicine. Sec ed. University Press New York Oxford London Toronto
8. Carpenter MB (1976) Human Neuroanatomy. 7. ed. Williams & Wilkins Comp, Baltimore
9. Ebeling U et al. (1986) Localization of the precentral gyrus in the computed tomogram and its clinical application. J Neurol 233:73–76
10. Englander RN et al. (1975) Location of the pyramidal tract in the internal capsule. Anatomic evidence. Neurology (NY) 25:823–826
11. Everett NB (1971) Functional anatomy. 6. ed. Lea & Febinger, Philadelphia
12. Flechsig P (1881) Zur Anatomie und Entwicklungsgeschichte der Leitungsbahnen im Großhirn. Arch Anat Physiol: 12–75
13. Flechsig P (1887) Über Systemerkrankungen im Rückenmark. Arch Heilk 18:101, 289 ff.
14. Foerster O, Bumke O (1936) Handbuch der Neurologie. 6. Band. Springer, Berlin, S 1–357
15. Kido DK et al. (1980) Computed tomographic localization of the precentral gyrus. Radiology 135:375–377
16. Lassek AM (1954) The pyramidal tract. Its status in medicine. C.C. Thomas, Springfield, Ill
17. Ludwig E, Klingler J (1956) Atlas Cerebri Humani. Karger, Basel New York
18. Matsui T et al. (1978) An Atlas of the human brain for computerized Tomography. Fischer, Stuttgart, Igaku-Shoin, Tokyo
19. Nathan PW et al. (1955) Long descending tract in man. 1. review of present knowledge. Brain 78:248–303
20. Pfeiffer RA (1934) Myelogenetisch-anatomische Untersuchungen über den zentralen Abschnitt der Taststrahlung, Pyramidenbahn, der Hirnnerven und zusätzlicher motorischer Bahnen. Nova Acta Leop. Carol. 1, 341–473
21. Quensel F (1910) Über den Stabkranz des menschlichen Stirnhirnes. Folia Neuro-Biol 4:319–334
22. Tailarach J, Szikla G (1967) (eds) Atlas of stereotaxic anatomy of the Telencephalon. Masson & Cie, Paris

Management of Tuberculoma in the Brain Stem and the Thalamus

S. N. Bhagwati, Bombay/India

Surgical management of intrinsic space-occupying lesions of the thalamus and brain stem pose several inherent problems of approach because of the likely damage that may occur to the vital structures around the lesion if total excision were attempted. A good anatomic delineation and morphologic evaluation of the lesion as shown by a CT Scan, therefore, becomes necessary, both to correctly diagnose the cases and to plan the modality of treatment.

The incidence of tuberculoma in the thalamus and the brain stem has been reported to be around 5%–6% of all intracranial tuberculomas in the pre-scan era [4]. This is the incidence of histopathologically verified tuberculomas either after surgery or autopsy. The incidence would be higher if one would include unverified thalamic and brain stem lesions that were diagnosed on air-study and responded to antitubercular line of treatment. With the advent of CT Scan, we are more definite about the diagnosis of tuberculomas and their response to treatment.

A large number of tuberculomas appear as iso- or mildly hyperdense lesions with a fair amount of edema around it. On contrast administration, the tuberculoma may appear as a ring enhancing lesion with a central area of necrosis or as a conglomeration of multiple ring enhancing lesions or as a disc lesion with uniform enhancement [3, 6]. When the lesion is less than a centimeter in size, it is designated as a microtuberculoma. At times, the lesion may be patchy, more so when there is an encephalitic process, and may be mistaken for a glioma. In case of a tubercular abscess, the ring enhancing lesion would have a hypodense center. Nearly three-fourths of the patients with tuberculoma have either a ring enhancing lesion or a disc lesion with a fair amount of edema around it.

A history of pyrexia, tuberculous contact or tuberculosis in the past, presence of an elevated Erythrocyte Sedimentation Rate, positive tuberculin test and existence of concomitant tuberculous lesion would be additional evidence in favor of the diagnosis of tuberculoma [1, 2, 5].

As soon as the diagnosis of a tuberculoma is made, a 3 drug regime of bactericidal antitubercular drugs like Streptomycin, Isoniazide and Rifampicin is started along with steroids. In over three-fourths of the cases, there is a good response to the medical regime and the tuberculoma resolves without any surgery [1, 2, 9, 11]. In those cases, with an associated hydrocephalus, ventriculo-peritoneal shunt is inserted. A frequent clinical and CT Scan monitoring is carried out to see the response of the lesion to the drugs [1, 2, 7, 11]. Surgery is carried out if the lesion fails to respond to medication or if the mass lesion poses a threat to life or vision.

In the last two and a half years we have treated three thalamic and three brain stem tuberculomas; two of these were intrinsic brain stem tubercular abscesses. Two of the thalamic and one of the brain stem tuberculomas were in the first decade, one thalamic was in the second decade, one brain stem was in the third decade whereas one brain stem tuberculoma was in the fourth decade. Except for one, a six year old female child with a thalamic lesion, all were males. Mantoux test was positive in three cases. Erythrocyte Sedimentation Rate was 32 mm in one case, 62 mm in another and 100 mm in the third. It was normal in the rest of the cases. One had concomitant miliary tuberculosis as well as tubercular meningitis.

Of the thalamic tuberculomas, one was in a boy of 18 years who had headache and progressive right-sided hemiparesis for 3 months with bilateral papilledema. CT Scan showed an irregular enhancing lesion in the left thalamus with some edema around it. Though his Erythrocyte Sedimentation Rate was only 20 mm and Mantoux test was negative, he was put on antitubercular line of treatment. Gradually, his condition started improving and neurologic deficit disappeared over the next three months. Repeat CT Scans over the next six months showed a complete disappearance of the lesion. The second was in a girl of 6 years who had a rather rapid development of left-sided weakness with spastic athetoid spasms and pyrexia of 25 days duration. The Erythrocyte Sedimentation Rate was 62 mm. Possibility of tubercular meningitis with vasculitis was thought of but lumbar CSF did not show any abnormality except for elevation of proteins to 70 mgm%. CT Scan showed a conglomeration of ring enhancing lesions in the right thalamic region (Fig. 1). She started improving with antitubercular drugs and when seen 10 weeks later, her left sided weakness and spastic athetoid spasms had significantly reduced. CT Scan showed a marked reduction in the size of the ring enhancing lesion (Fig. 2). The third was in a boy of 6 years with headache, vomiting, drowsiness, bilateral papilledema, upward conjugate gaze impairment and mild left-sided weakness of 8–10 days duration. CT Scan showed a ring enhancing lesion in the right thalamic region with a moderate degree of hydrocephalus. Ventriculoperitoneal shunt was inserted and antitubercular drugs were started. He showed a steady improvement, his papilledema cleared up and left sided weakness regressed. Unfortunately, we have not

1
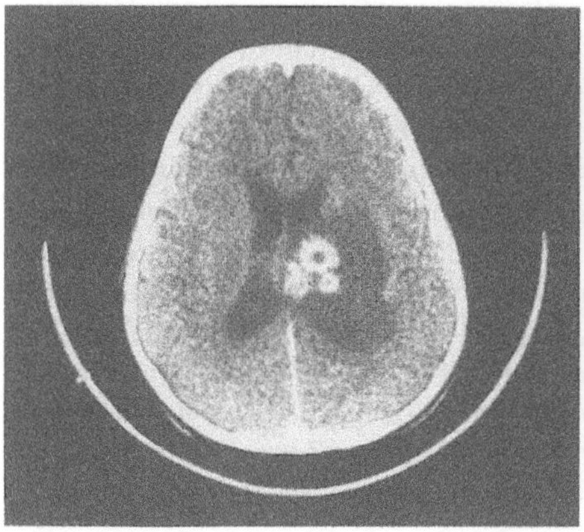

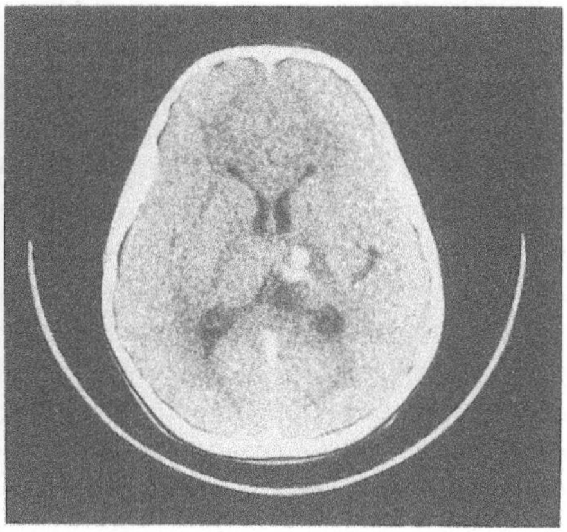
2

Fig. 1. CT Scan with contrast shows a conglomeration of ring enhancing lesions

Fig. 2. CT Scan with contrast shows marked reduction in the size of the lesion been able to repeat his CT Scan. Thus, in these three patients who had thalamic tuberculoma, the response to medication was excellent. The tuberculomas disappeared and neurologic deficit regressed significantly.

There were three cases of brain stem tuberculoma during this period. One of them had an uniformly enhancing solid lesion that protruded out into the cerebellopontine angle. It was about 3.5 cm × 3.0 cm × 3.0 cm in size. Though the Erythrocyte Sedimentation Rate was 40 mm and Mantoux test was positive, it was considered to be an ependymoma and a craniotomy was performed. The lesion was approached postero-laterally. The cerebellum had to be incised before it was visualized. A total excision was carried out with relative ease. The patient had a good postoperative course but his facial weakness and minimal pyramidal deficit have persisted. The second patient had been treated for tubercular meningitis and miliary tuberculosis for 2 months before his clinical condition became worse. He was admitted in a semi-comatose condition with a right facial weakness and a right spastic hemiparesis. Erythrocyte Sedimentation Rate was 100 mm and Mantoux test was positive. X-ray of the chest showed persistence of miliary infection. CT Scan showed a large, mildly hypodense lesion with ring enhancement in the brain stem, the lesion continuing through the crus into the thalamus on the left side as a small solid enhancing lesion (Fig. 3). He had an associated hydrocephalus. Ventriculoperitoneal shunt was inserted and antitubercular drugs were continued. He showed an improvement in his level of consciousness but the rest of the neurologic deficit persisted. CT Scan was repeated 3 months later, when the lesion in the brain stem was found to have increased in size. The central area of necrosis was more hypodense (Fig. 4). It was, therefore, felt that surgical excision or evacuation should be carried out. A midline posterior fossa craniectomy was performed. The cerebellar tonsils were separated, when a bulge in the floor of the 4th ventricle could be seen on the left side. Aspiration with size 18 BD needle resulted in evacuation of about 20 ml of pus. An attempt to open up the abscess with bipolar diathermy had to be given up because of brain stem disturbances. Tubercle bacilli were seen on smear examination of the pus. The patient started showing a gradual improvement but died 7 days later of severe pulmonary infection. The third patient was a male child of 8 years who presented with progressive giddiness, ataxia, slurred speech, impaired conjugate deviation of the eyes, bilateral facial weakness, impairment of swallowing and bilateral pyramidal signs. CT Scan showed a large, well delineated area of low attenuation with enhancement only at one spot peripherally within the brain stem (Fig. 5). The possibility of drainage of a cystic lesion coming up to the surface of the roof of the fourth ventricle was considered and midline posterior fossa craniotomy was carried out. Separation of cerebellar tonsils again showed a bulge in the floor of the fourth ventricle in the midline. Aspiration yielded about 12 ml of pus which showed the presence of tubercule bacilli on smear examination. The child was put on antitubercular drugs. There was a rapid improvement in his condition. External ocular movements became fuller, swallowing improved, spasticity was relieved, coordination improved and he could start walking without support. CT Scan, repeated 3 weeks later, showed an almost total disappearance of the lesion.

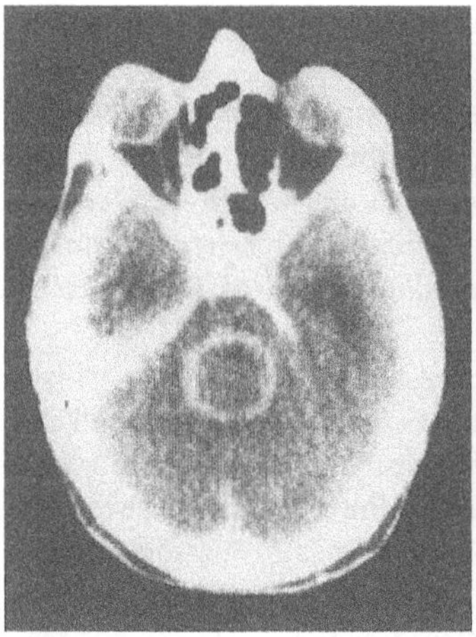

3

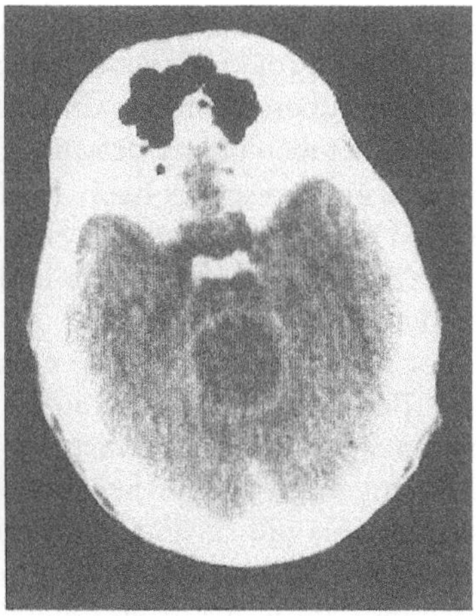

4

Fig. 3. CT Scan with contrast shows a minimally hypodense ring enhancing lesion in the brain stem

Fig. 4. CT Scan with contrast shows a more hypodense lesion in the brain stem which has also enlarged in size

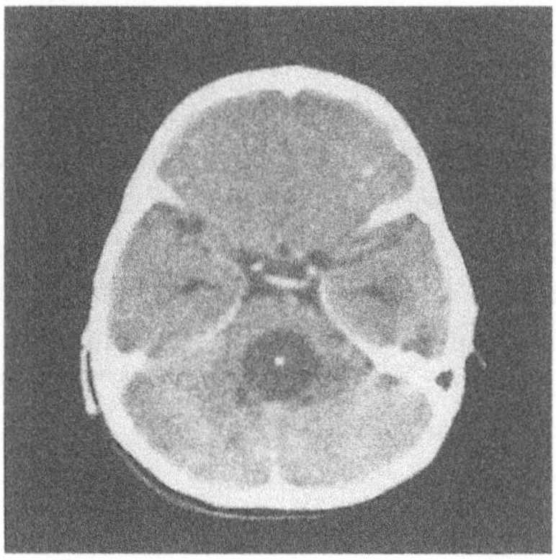

Fig. 5. CT Scan with contrast shows a large cystic lesion in the brain stem that has split and pushed the fourth ventricle backwards

Discussion

This experience with the management of thalamic and brain stem tuberculomas shows that many of them do respond well to medication and that drug therapy should be the primary mode of treatment. A successful medical management obviates the need for surgical excision in an area like the thalamus or the brain stem with its attendant risks of neurologic deficit. Insertion of a ventriculoperitoneal shunt may be necessary if there is an associated hydrocephalus. Monitoring of the patient by repeated clinical examination and CT scanning at intervals of 6–8 weeks is essential to determine the response of the lesion to medication. If the lesion fails to reduce in size or tends to enlarge, the possibility of a mistaken diagnosis or resistant tuberculoma has to be taken into account. Stereotaxic biopsy of the thalamic lesion would be the safest way of knowing its pathologic nature.

In case of brain stem tuberculomas again a similar approach is desirable. Had the patient with the solid tuberculoma protruding into the cerebellopontine angle been treated with drugs alone, very probably the tuberculoma would have resolved completely with a good regression of the neurologic deficit. Its presence was not suspected and a direct recourse to surgery was undertaken; some of the neurologic deficits did persist after surgery.

Drug therapy alone does not seem to be effective enough in patients with tuberculous abscesses. The patient with concomitant tubercular meningitis and miliary tuberculosis continued to deteriorate inspite of antitubercular drugs and a supportive regime. CT Scan showed a further increase in the size of the lesion. Hypodensity of the central area did suggest the possibility of pus formation [8, 10]. It was obvious that the lesion was not responding to the drugs, either because the organisms had become resistant to the drugs administered or the drugs did not reach the core of the lesion in sufficient concentration [12]. Probably a distended abscess caused compression of the vessels at the periphery with resultant ischemia and poor drug delivery. The response to aspiration seemed to be excellent, especially in the child, the subsequent CT Scan showing an almost total clearance of the lesion.

The tuberculous abscess can be tapped either by splitting the vermis and approaching it from the region of the floor of the fourth ventricle when situated posteriorly or through the region of the cerebellopontine angle when located posterolaterally or through subtemporal approach when it occurs antero-laterally. Tapping of the abscess can be safe and beneficial provided it is fairly large and has reached the surface. Aspiration can also be performed by stereotaxic procedure. Similarly, solid tuberculomas in such situations can be partially excised so long as they have reached the surface. Often, a total excision is not necessary as the drugs seem to act well after a biopsy. Total disappearance of the lesion is known to occur thereafter with drugs alone.

Summary

To conclude, thalamic and brain stem tuberculomas are best treated initially with the drug regime. Most of them do respond to drug therapy alone. Ventriculoperitoneal shunt insertion may be necessary when tuberculoma is associated with hydrocephalus. Tuberculous abscess may not respond to medication alone and would need to be aspirated either by a craniotomy or by stereotaxic procedure. Solid tuberculomas that fail to respond to medication alone can be partly excised when they have reached the surface; they seem to respond to medication better thereafter.

References

1. Bhagwati SN (1982) Management of Intracranial Tuberculoma – Paper presented at the Annual Conference of the Neurological Society of India
2. Bhagwati SN (1985) Management of Intracranial Tuberculoma in Children. Under publication in Child's Nervous System

3. Bhargava S, Tandon PN (1980) Intracranial Tuberculomas – A CT Study. Br J Radiol 53:935
4. Dastur DK et al. (1968) Pathological Analysis of Intracranial Space-Occupying Lesions in 1000 cases including Children. J Neurol Sci 6:575–592
5. Dastur HM (1972) A Tuberculoma Review with some Personal Experiences (Part I – Brain) Neurology India 20:111
6. Du Boulay G (1979) Computerized Tomography of the Brain. In: Lodge Sir T, Science RE (eds) Recent Advances in Radiology and Medical Imaging No. 6. Churchill Livingstone, New York, p 17–35
7. Haskitt JR Jr, Branch CE Jr (1979) Brainstem Tuberculoma – Value of Sequential Computed Tomography. Ann Neurol 6:275
8. Leblanc R (1981) Tuberculous abscess – Report of a case with CT correlation. Neurosurgery Vol 8 (1):88–91
9. Pandya SK et al. (1982) Caseative Liquefaction within Brainstem Tuberculoma under Drug Therapy with simultaneous regression of Cerebral Tuberculosis. Vol. 30, 2 Neurology India, p 121–128
10. Reichenthal E et al. (1982) Tuberculous abscess and its appearance on computed tomography. J Neurosurg 56:597–619
11. Tandon PN et al. (1981) Medical treatment of intracranial tuberculomas. Abstracts in Vol. on 'The National Seminar of CNS Infections' held at AIIMS, New Delhi
12. Whitner DR (1978) Tuberculous Brain Abscess – Report of a case and review of the literature. Arch Neurol 35:148–155

Neurosurgical Aspects of Processes at the Tentorial Margin

M. SAMII, Hannover/FRG

The surgical processes encountered at the Tentorial Margin would be principally those arising from the various anatomic structures present in this complex region.

a) From the tentorium itself we would have
   1. Meningiomas:
      i) tuberculum sella
      ii) medial wing of the sphenoid
      iii) petroclival
   2. Arteriovenous malformations have also been reported to arise from the tentorium.

b) From the circle of Willis and its outflow:
   1. Aneurysms
   2. Angiomatous malformations

c) From the cranial nerves:
   Schwannomas can arise from any of the cranial nerves having the Schwann's sheath, but most commonly in this region we would have the acoustic and less commonly the trigeminal neurinomas. Rarely neurinomas have also arisen from III, IV and VI cranial nerves.

Significantly all of these tumors appear in the vicinity of the tentorial margin. Occasionally there may be patients with Von Recklinghausen's disease who may have multiple neurinomas. Such patients are also known to have accompanying meningiomas or gliomas.

d) Primary tumors from existent brain tissue:
   1. Optic chiasma gliomas
   2. Hypothalamic tumors
   3. Massive extrasellar extensions of pituitary adenomas
   4. Posterior third ventricular tumors

e) Tumors of 'congenital' etiology:
   1. Craniopharyngiomas (Rathke's pouch tumors)
   2. Epidermoid tumors
   3. Teratomas

f) Secondary deposits

Except for the vascular processes which generally present acutely in the form of subarachnoid hemorrhage (SAH) and its consequences, tentorial margin space-occupying lesions are notorious for their delayed detection. This may seem surprising when one considers the complicated anatomy of numerous cranial nerves, blood channels and the presence of some of the most sensitive areas of the brain. Obviously their possible involvement is both tardy and to an extent compensatory, considering the slow growth of these lesions which are more often benign, and the presence of several small and large neighboring cisterns which on being compressed could provide the extra space without significant disturbance of the patient's health. As a result these growths are allowed to assume often frightful proportions yet with relatively few deficits. In recent times CT scan and MRI have contributed in providing not only a relatively earlier diagnosis but also details with respect to their exact extent and location, and perhaps the probable pathology.

Despite the facility offered by CT scans and MRI, appropriate cerebral angiography is an essential adjunct. It is in fact the only diagnostic test for vascular disorders. But it would be an underestimation if its utility was merely restricted to the study of such conditions. It is an invaluable tool for the study of tumors: Arterial, capillary and venous phases, all should be done. Unless clearly irrelevant, it is often advantageous to complete the whole 4 vessels' study instead of restricting it to only the carotid or the vertebrobasilar systems. Besides providing the clue of the feeding and draining vessels of tumors, it gives information on the condition of surrounding vessels, whether only stretched and displaced, narrowed or even engulfed. Hypertrophy of the tentorial artery of Bernasconi and Cassinari in AP and lateral views is pathognomonic for a tentorial meningioma.

Principles

A three dimensional image of the process and its juxtaposition with other vital structures should be formed by the surgeon in planning the various possibilities of approaching a tentorial lesion. The tentorial margin may be reached from above or below the tentorium. Sometimes a combined supra- and infratentorial approach is necessary.

The rigid tentorial margin surrounding the brain stem, cranial nerves and blood vessels may appear to limit the surgical activity to the compartment from which the operation commences. This is a discouraging concept. This tough ring can be transected to offer greater view and orientation of the surrounding structures. Moreover, with progressive enlargement of the tumor, these vital structures are compressed, displaced and distorted. The nerves and blood vessels undergo a further linear stretch. By piecemeal intracapsular tumor removal more room is created which also permits the surgeon the liberty to move from one compartment to another through the same craniotomy, a situation which would be inconceivable in a normal anatomic state. Yet another way to increase the working space would be by drilling the apex of the petrous bone to which the tentorium is attached.

Finally, there has been indisputable proof that microtechniques have reduced the morbidity and mortality following surgery in this region. Processes at the tentorial margin are often entangled with critical neural and vascular structures. The microscope provides brillant illumination of these deep areas and stereoscopic vision and magnification of every millimetre of the delicate tissues the surgeon handles, dissects, retracts or cuts. Combined with sound microtechnique it permits him a good opportunity to meticulously dissect the offending lesion whilst safeguarding several fine vessels to the diencephalon, the mesencephalon and the basal ganglia. Above all, it allows the neurosurgeon to operate through a small opening with minimal brain retraction, thus minimizing brain damages.

Surgical Approaches to the Tentorial Margin

A. Supratentorial approaches
   1. Subfrontal subchiasmatic
   2. Pterional and subtemporal
   3. Medial occipital
B. Infratentorial approach
   1. Lateral suboccipital
   2. Supracerebellar (supravermial)
C. Combined supra- and infratentorial approach
   Combined subtemporal lateral suboccipital approach

A. Supratentorial Approaches

1. The Subfrontal Subchiasmatic Approach

This approach is chosen in cases of suprasellar lesions with parasellar and particularly retrosellar extension. The common tumors that can be excised using this route are suprasellar adenomas, craniopharyngiomas and tuberculum sella meningiomas. These tumors when they reach large sizes elevate the suprasellar structures and widen the parasellar space. This may lead to a retrofixed chiasma with opening of the angle between the optic nerves and the chiasma. In particular cases the tumor can separate the supracavernous part of I.C.A. from the optic nerve giving sufficient distance for lateral approach of the tumor. In these situations a subchiasmatic or a laterochiasmatic appraoch can be performed. If the distance between the tuberculum sella and optic chiasma is not large enough for total removal, a retrochiasmatic approach through the lamina terminalis should be accomplished.

The choice of the frontal craniotomy, whether right or left or bifrontal, depends on the extension of the tumor to the parasellar and retrosellar region.

In case of midline tumors with no extreme lateral extension, a right frontal craniotomy is performed. With parasellar extension we prefer to make the approach on the opposite side to the maximum parasellar extension of the lesion into the tentorial margin. This is important as it gives a better subchiasmatic visual access to the structures at the tentorial margin (Figs. 1a–b). Tumors that extend bilaterally are usually better approached by using a bifrontal craniotomy. The craniotomy should be quite basal extending to the roof of the orbit without respect to the frontal sinus. The sinus mucosa is removed and the sinus is temporarily packed with a gauze impregnated in antibiotic. The superior sagittal sinus will be ligated and the attachment of the falx to the crista galea is transected in the bifrontal approach.

After the dura is opened, the frontal lobe is gradually retracted to expose the sellar region. With microsurgical dissection the olfactory nerve can be preserved (Suzuki 1981; Samii 1981) (Figs. 2a–b). Our strategy for excising the tumor will depend

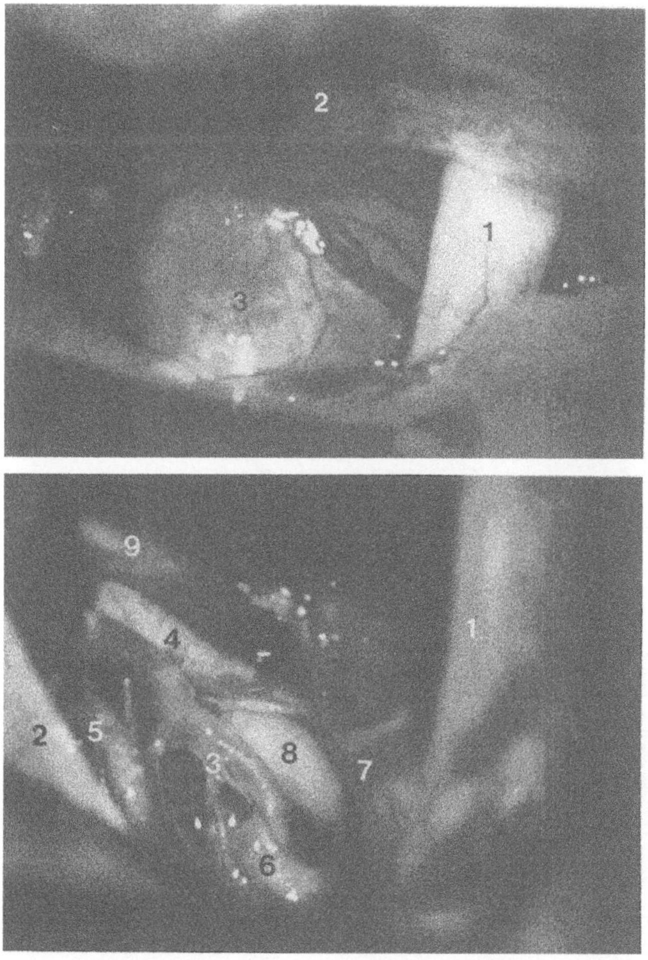

a

b

Fig. 1. a Subchiasmatic view of a large pituitary adenoma exposed by a right subfrontal craniotomy. *1* Right optiv nerve, *2* Tuberculum sella, *3* Tumor. **b** Subchiasmatic view of structures at the left tentorial margin after excision of a large pituitary adenoma using a right subfrontal approach. *1* Right optic nerve, *2* Left optic nerve, *3* Left posterior communicating artery, *4* Left oculomotor nerve, *5* Left anterior choroidal artery, *6* Left posterior cerebral artery, *7* Infundibulum, *8* Left abducens nerve, *9* Dorsum sella

on the manner of its growth. Usually the tumor grows gradually, compressing and displacing the surrounding structures in all possible directions. In such a case all important structures are localized around the capsula. Gradual resection and debulking of the tumor will make the capsula collapse giving more space. The capsula is then easily detached from the optic nerves and chiasma. The vessels related to the capsula are carefully dissected; these include the carotid arteries, the posterior communicating arteries and small perforating branches to the diencephalon. Under the microscope it is possible to distinguish between vessels that merely pass across the capsula and those that contribute to its blood supply. The latter are coagulated and

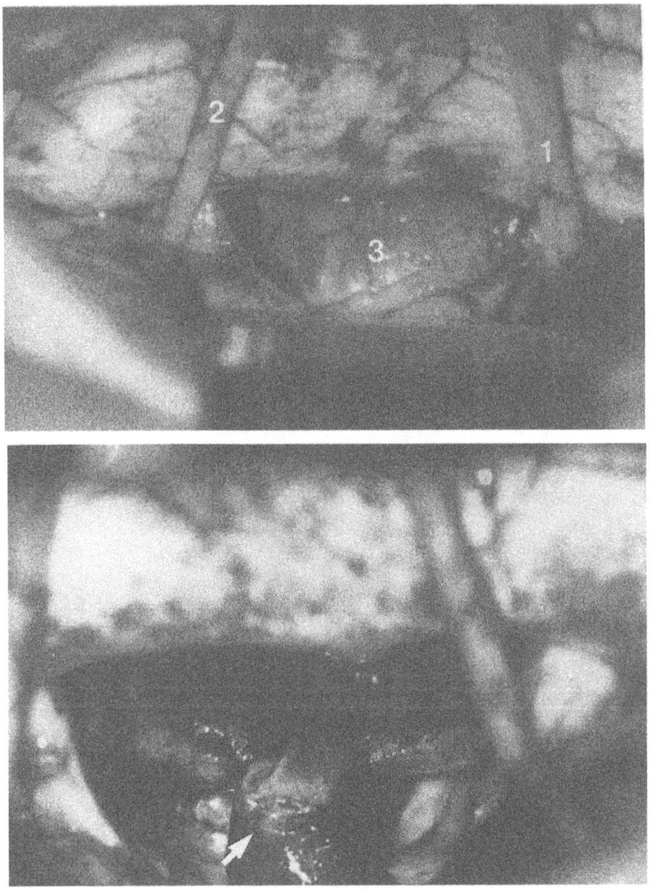

a

b

Fig. 2. **a** Bifrontal approach of a pituitary adenoma with preservation of both olfactory nerves. *1* Right olfactory nerve, *2* Left olfactory nerve, *3* Tumor. **b** The two olfactory nerves are still preserved after tumor excision. The *arrow head* shows the infundibulum

divided. In contrast to this group we are sometimes confronted by a second group of tumors which grow and then engulf the surrounding structures, as in case of some meningiomas growing in this area. In handling these tumors one must start at definite clear anatomic landmarks, beginning where the surrounding vital structures are not involved. The first few millimetres of the I.C.A. are used as a landmark and the tumor is followed around the vessels, sparing the perforating arteries. The optic and oculomotor nerve are freed in a similar fashion. If the tumor involves the floor of the third ventricle or cannot be removed completely subchiasmatically, a retrochiasmatic approach through the lamina terminalis is done. After total excision one can have a very good view of the interpeduncular and prepontine cistern (Figs. 3 a–b).

Finally, one should mention that care should be taken to preserve the infundibulum as this reduces the postoperative occurrence of diabetes insipidus.

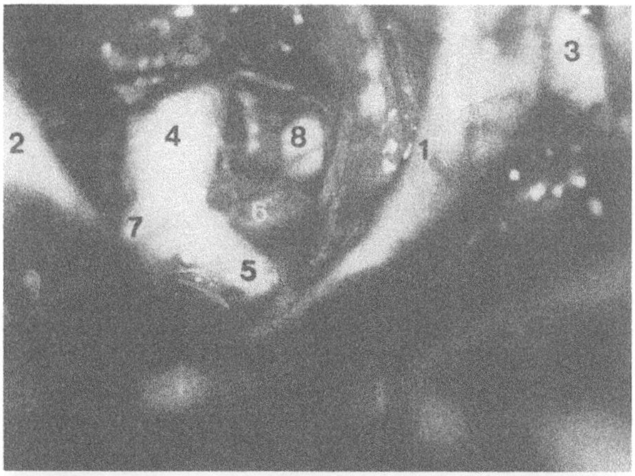

a

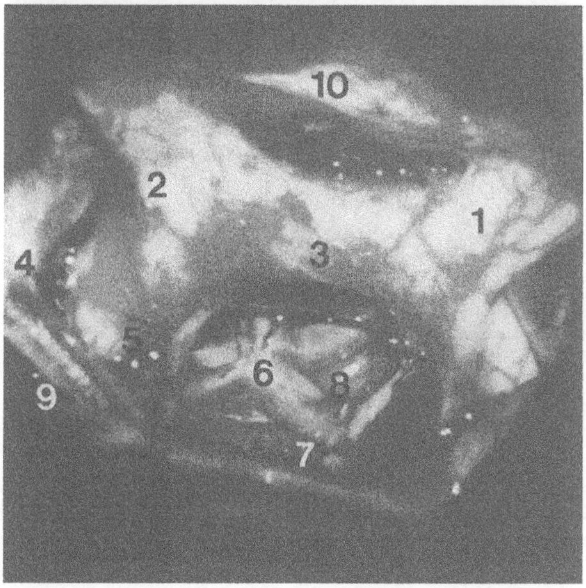

b

Fig. 3. **a** Subchiasmatic view of the interpeduncular and prepontine cistern after excision of a large pituitary adenoma. *1* Right optic nerve, *2* Left optic nerve, *3* Right carotid artery, *4* Basilar artery, *5* Right posterior cerebral artery, *6* Right superior cerebellar artery, *7* Left posterior cerebral artery, *8* Pons. **b** Retrochiasmatic view through the prepontine space after excision of a large craniopharyngioma. *1* Right optic nerve, *2* Left optic nerve, *3* Optic chiasma, *4* Left internal carotid artery, *5* Optic tract, *6* Basilar artery, *7* Right posterior cerebral, *8* Right superior cerebellar, *9* Left anterior cerebral artery, *10* Tuberculum sella

During closure the frontal sinus is sealed out by reflecting a flap of periosteum down from the under-side of the scalp and suturing it to the closed dura.

Case: (Figs. 4a–c)

A nine-year-old female child presented in a somnolent state with a past history of headache and gradual deterioration of visual acuity. Ophthalmologic examination

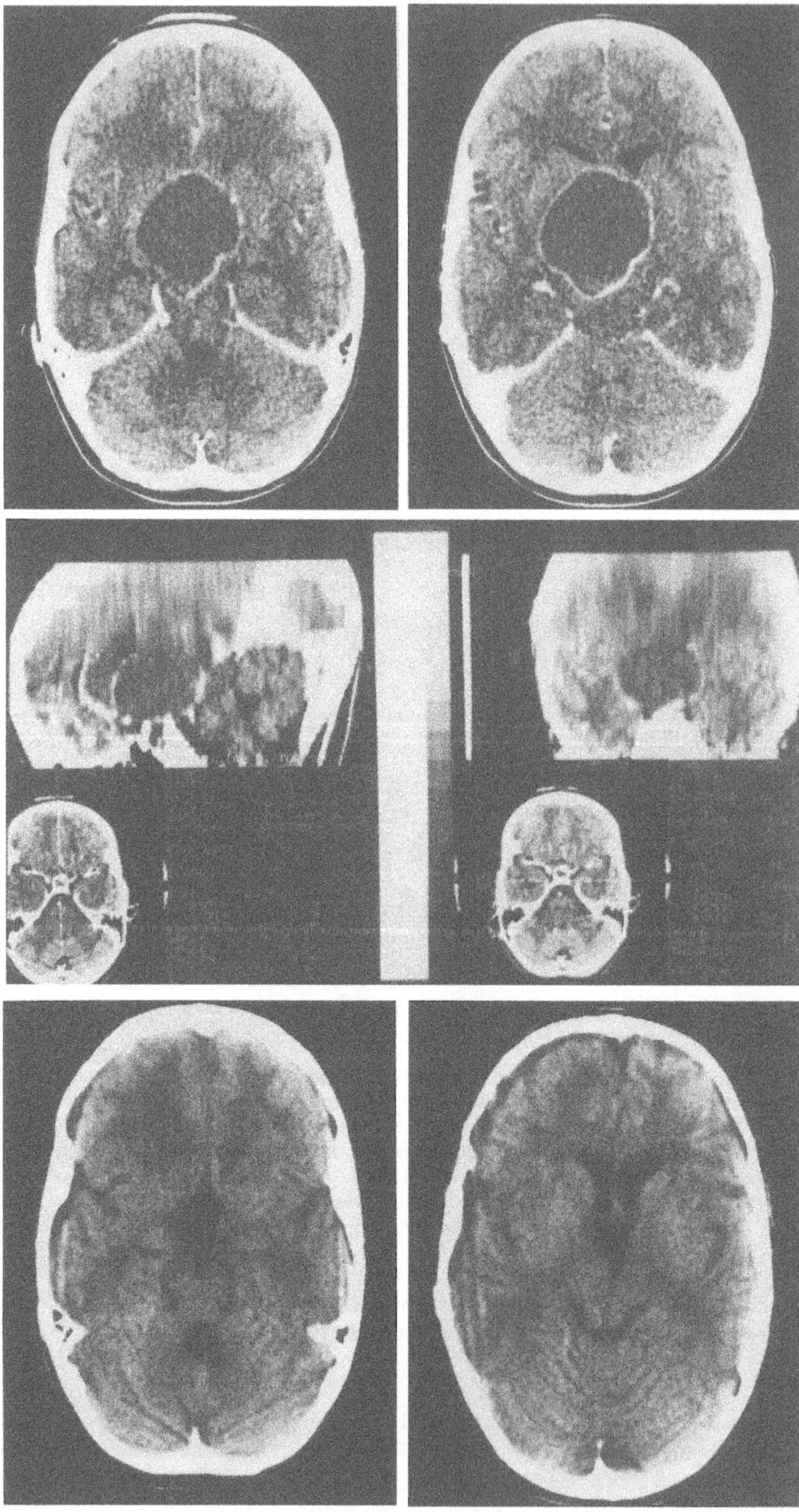

a

b

c

revealed central tubular vision in the left eye and perception of light in the right eye, as well as bilateral primary optic atrophy. Computerized axial tomography (Figs. 4a, b) showed a large suprasellar cystic craniopharyngioma with a small solid sellar part. The tumor filled the third ventricle, occluding the foramen of Monro and producing obstructive hydrocephalus. A ventriculoperitoneal shunt was done to improve the level of consciousness by relieving the obstructive hydrocephalus. Two weeks later a bifrontal osteoclastic craniotomy was carried out and the anterior part of the tumor exposed. The tumor was punctured and the cyst aspirated.

Gradual resection of the tumor capsule from the left and right optic nerves and carotid arteries was done. The majority of the capsule and the tumor could be removed subchiasmatically, but there was still a tumor remnant left behind the chiasma and in the third ventricle. The third ventricle was opened through the lamina terminalis and the tumor was totally excised. After total removal we had a good view of the pons, interpeduncular fossa as well as the basilar artery and its tributaries.

In the early postoperative period the child suffered from a transient D.M. and was for three days somnolent.

The patient was discharged five weeks after surgery in a very good general condition. Her visual deficit was the same. Postoperative control C.T. scan showed complete excision of the tumor (Fig. 4c).

2. Pterional and Subtemporal Approach

This approach is recommended for lesions in the region of the anterior and middle third of the tentorial notch. So, it is useful for aneurysms of the anterior circulation and upper basilar artery as well as tumors in the lesser wing of sphenoid, retro-orbital, parasellar, dorsum sella and prepontine areas.

A curved frontotemporal incision is made inside the hairline and running 1 cm anterior to the tragus. In this way one secures an adequate approach to the lesser wing of the sphenoid and the floors of the anterior and middle fossae.

After raising a small frontotemporal flap and removing the lateral part of the lesser wing, the approach is continued intradurally along the sphenoid wing, in the direction of the anterior clinoid process by gradually opening the cisterns and removing CSF. This procedure must not be rushed, so that by constant aspiration of CSF and gentle retraction the frontal and temporal lips of the Sylvian fissure can be gradually opened without any undue pressure on the brain.

After exposure of the optic nerve and the further opening of the cisterns along the edge of the tentorium the internal carotid, the posterior communicating, the anterior choroidal arteries and also the oculomotor nerve are exposed in the anterior third of the tentorial notch. By further dissection along the free margin of the middle third of the tentorium in a posterior direction, the trochlear nerve and the

Fig. 4. a CT-scan showing a large cystic craniopharyngioma with suprasellar extension. **b** CT-scan with sagittal and coronal reconstruction showing extension of the tumor posteriorly to the interpeduncular and prepontine spaces. Superiorly the tumor extends to the foramen of Monro. **c** Postoperative CT-scan after total removal of the tumor (case I)

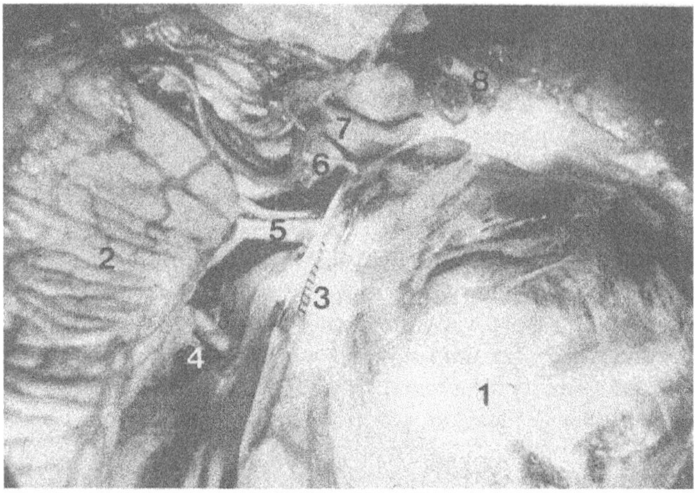

a

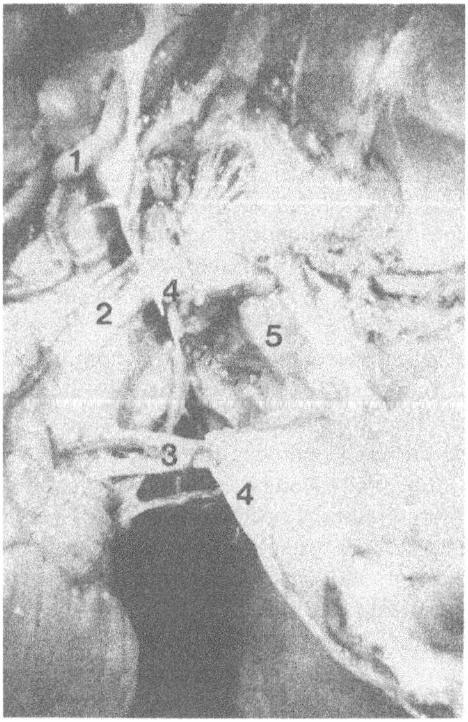

b

Fig. 5. **a** Anatomic specimen showing the region of the petrous apex and cerebellopontine angle from above. The temporal lobe and tentorium are removed (Courtesy of Prof. J. Lang, Würzburg/FRG). *1* Middle cranial fossa, *2* Cerebellum, *3* Superior petrosal sinus, *4* Vestibulocochlear and facial nerves, *5* Trigeminal nerve, *6* Trochlear nerve, *7* Oculomotor nerve, *8* Optic nerve. **b** Anatomic specimen showing the view from the middle fossa into the cerebellopontine angle after the petrous apex is removed. *1* Oculomotor nerve, *2* Trigeminal nerve, *3* Vestibulocochlear and facial nerves, *4* Transected superior petrosal sinus, *5* Carotid artery in petrous bones

junction of the posterior communicating artery with the posterior cerebral artery become visible, as well as its origin from the basilar artery. After incising the margin of the tentorium and stitching it back in its middle third one has a very good view into the depth of the infratentorial space. Further, our surgical strategy will depend on the anatomic variations of the tentorial notch (Lang 1985). In some individuals the tentorial notch is narrow. In such a situation the exposure of the tentorial margin does not permit any view to the infratentorial region. The above mentioned incision of the tentorium can be a good help in certain circumstances, but would still not be sufficient for those giant tumors which extend infratentorially in the cerebellopontine angle and prepontine space. In order to avoid a second stage surgery through a lateral suboccipital approach, we coagulate and transect the superior petrosal sinus and expose the petrous apex. This can carefully be removed by a high speed diamond drill up to the internal auditory meatus (Figs. 5a, b).

The seventh and eighth cranial nerves are now visible and can be dissected free from the lesion. The manner in which we deal with the fifth nerve will depend on the clinical findings and morphologic behavior of the tumor. If there is no functional deficit and it is only compressed by the tumor all efforts are undertaken to preserve the nerve (Figs. 6a–h). In cases of functional deficit and infiltration of the nerve fascicles, e.g. invasive meningioma, it is recommendable to sacrifice the nerve for a more radical removal of the tumor. The most important facts in such giant tumors at the tentorial margin are their relation to vessels supplying the brain stem and the severe adhesion of the tumor to this very delicate area. According to my personal experience one can decompress the brain stem by gradual resection of the tumor from lateral to medial in a piecemeal manner until the tumor is completely removed. During dissection some small arteries can be sacrificed without compromising the blood supply to the mesencephalon.

As the circle of Willis demonstrates a tremendous degree of variation we are not able to determine in each individual case the exact blood supply and collateral circulation of the brain stem (Mitterwallner 1955). There are no fixed criteria to be taken into consideration for this special problem. The outcome of all the operated cases has shown that many of those vessels which are supplying the tumor and additionally the brain stem, can be sacrificed without any postoperative consequences. It seems that it is more dangerous to apply traction to brain stem vessels by pulling

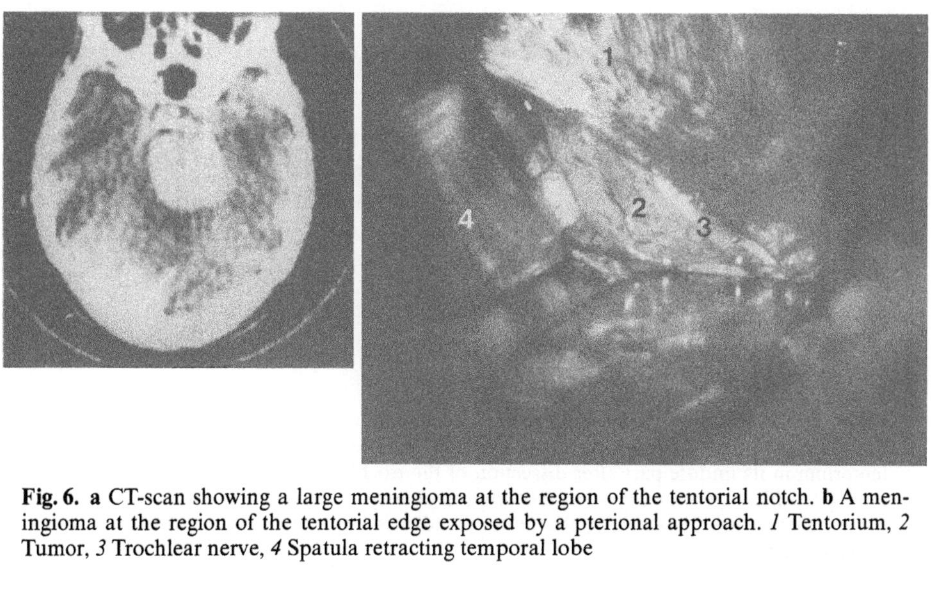

a b

Fig. 6. **a** CT-scan showing a large meningioma at the region of the tentorial notch. **b** A meningioma at the region of the tentorial edge exposed by a pterional approach. *1* Tentorium, *2* Tumor, *3* Trochlear nerve, *4* Spatula retracting temporal lobe

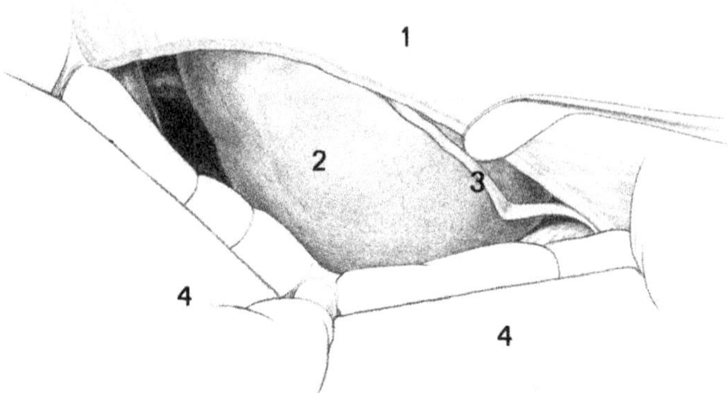

c

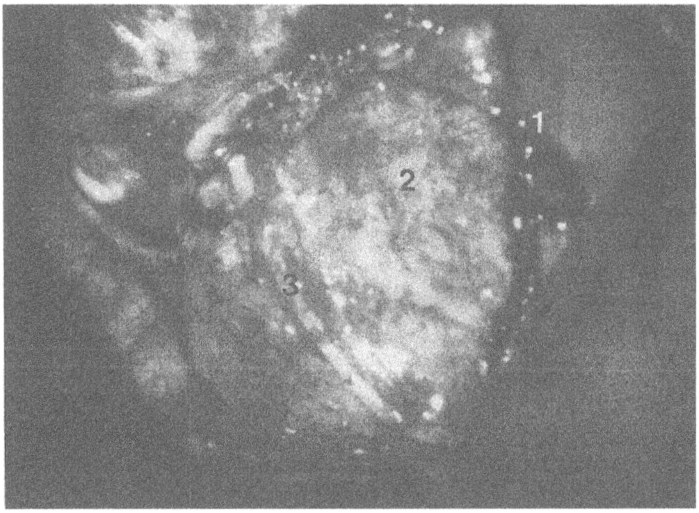

d

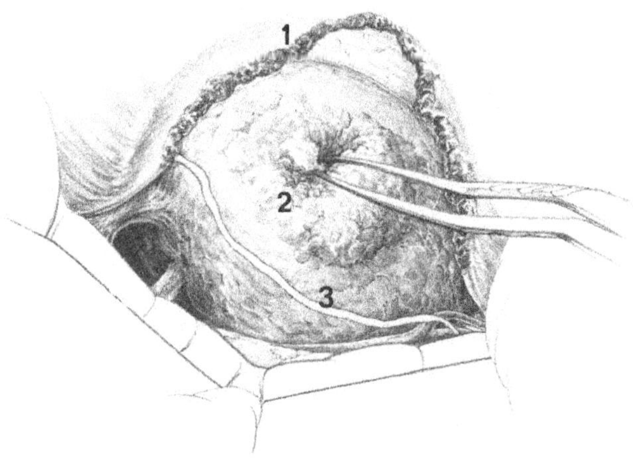

e

Fig. 6. c Diagram showing the surgical view after brain retraction in the pterional approach. *1* Tentorium, *2* Tumor, *3* Trochlear nerve dissected from tentorial edge, *4* Spatula. **d** Incising the tentorium in its middle part after dissection of the trochlear nerve. *1* Incised tentorium, *2* Tumor, *3* Trochlear nerve. **e** Diagram showing tumor removal after the tentorium is incised. Note the wide exposure given when the tentorial edge is cut. *1* Incised tentorium, *2* Tumor, *3* Trochlear nerve.

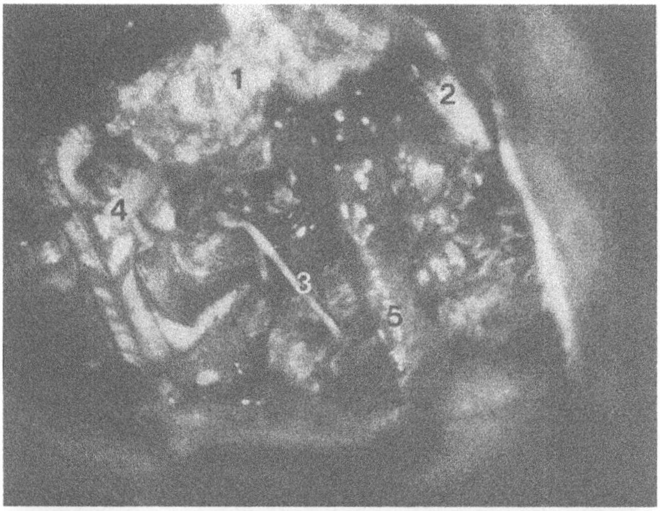

f

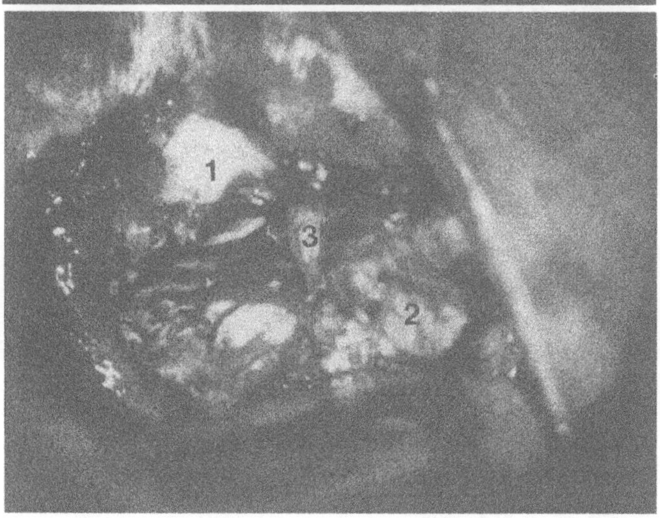

g

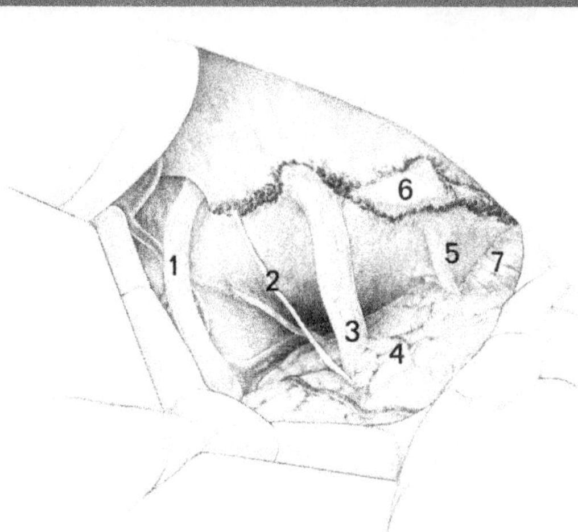

h

Fig. 6. f Surgical view after the tumor is excised. *1* Tentorium, *2* Site of removed petrous apex, *3* Trochlear nerve, *4* Oculomotor nerve, *5* Trigeminal nerve. **g** Surgical view of the cerebellopontine angle after removal of the petrous apex and excising the infratentorial part of the tumor. *1* Petrous bone, *2* Pons, *3* Vestibulocochlear and facial nerves. **h** A drawing demonstrating the operative field after total removal of the tumor. *1* Oculomotor nerve, *2* Trochlear nerve, *3* Trigeminal nerve, *4* Pons, *5* 7th and 8th cranial nerves, *6* Site of removed petrous apex, *7* Cerebellum

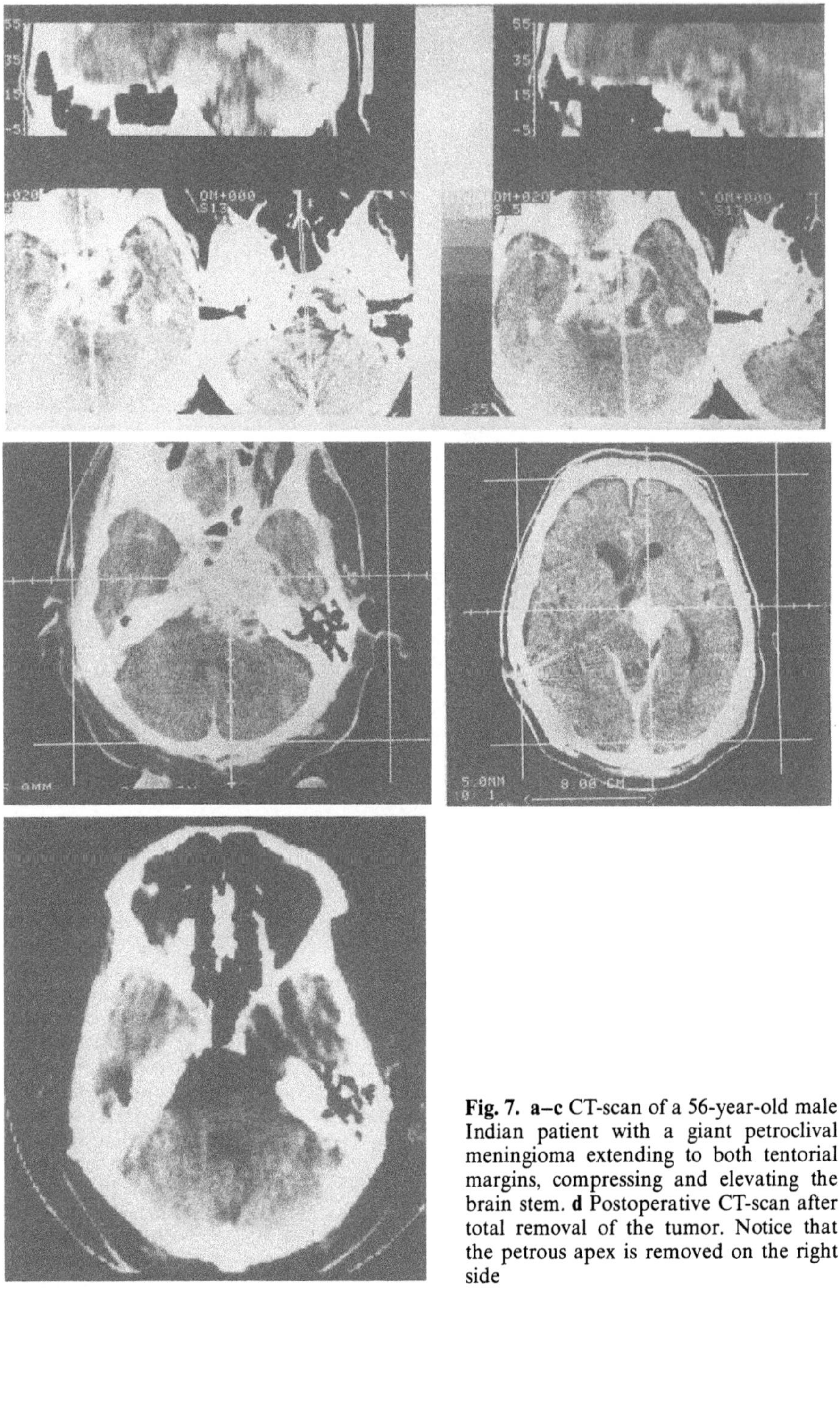

a b c d

Fig. 7. a–c CT-scan of a 56-year-old male Indian patient with a giant petroclival meningioma extending to both tentorial margins, compressing and elevating the brain stem. **d** Postoperative CT-scan after total removal of the tumor. Notice that the petrous apex is removed on the right side on the tumor. Traction of any vessel at the brain stem can lead to interstitial rupture and bleeding which causes severe brain stem lesions and marked neurologic deficits. It seems wiser to coagulate and cut such vessels when needed on the tumoral side.

Case (Figs. 7a–d)

A male Indian patient, 56 years old, complained of gradually progressing left hemiparesis of six months' duration. This was accompanied by emotional instability and a complete fifth cranial nerve lesion. His CT scan showed a petroclival mass destroying the clivus and the petrous apex and compressing the third ventricle producing secondary obstructive hydrocephalus (Figs. 7a–c). A ventricular shunt was performed in India. After verification of the benign nature of the tumor (meningioma) through a stereotaxic biopsy, the patient was referred to our clinic. The modified pterional approach was carried out for total removal of the tumor. After removal of the supratentorial part, the tentorium was incised, superior petrosal sinus was coagulated and transected and the petrous apex was drilled out to the internal auditory meatus. Due to the previous clinical loss of the trigeminal nerve function and its infiltration by the tumor the trigeminal as well as the trochlear nerves were sacrificed to enable complete removal of the tumor. The patient had an uneventful postoperative course. He left the hospital four weeks later with complete recovery of his hemiparesis (Fig. 7d).

3. Medial Occipital Approach

This approach may be recommended for medially situated space-occupying lesions in the posterior part of the tentorium and at its junction with the cerebral falx. The commonest lesion in this part is meningioma. It is also used for tumors in the pineal region when they are mainly located above the tentorial edge if there is no major extension to the posterior fossa or opposite side. Angiomas at the region of vein of Galen can also be managed using this approach.

The patient is placed in a semisitting position modified from Jannetta (Jannetta 1977). The osteoplastic flap is fashioned so that the medial limit of exposure is formed by the superior sagittal sinus and the inferior limit by the transverse sinus. The dura is opened in a triradiate fashion, the edges held by stay suture. The merit of this approach is the nearly complete absence of important veins between the occipital lobe and either the tentorium or the posterior part of the sagittal sinus. The approach is made along the falx cerebri (Dandy 1936; Krause 1926) and on the tentorium (Poppen 1966) by lifting up the occipital pole and holding aside the occipital lobe avoiding pressure (Figs. 8a–d). A wide approach to the infratentorial lesions in the posterior part of the third ventricle can be achieved by incising the tentorium parallel to the straight sinus (Lapras et al. 1973). The superior cerebellar veins entering the straight sinus commonly do so within 3–4 mm of the midline and most may be preserved by leaving the cut between 5 mm–1 cm from the midline (Symon 1982). The free edges of the incised tentorium are retracted with sutures. The arachnoid is incised allowing inferior displacement of the vermis. The exposure provides a view to the superior vermis, the precentral vein, the internal cerebral and basal veins at the junction with the vein of Galen, the collicular plate, the splenium, the

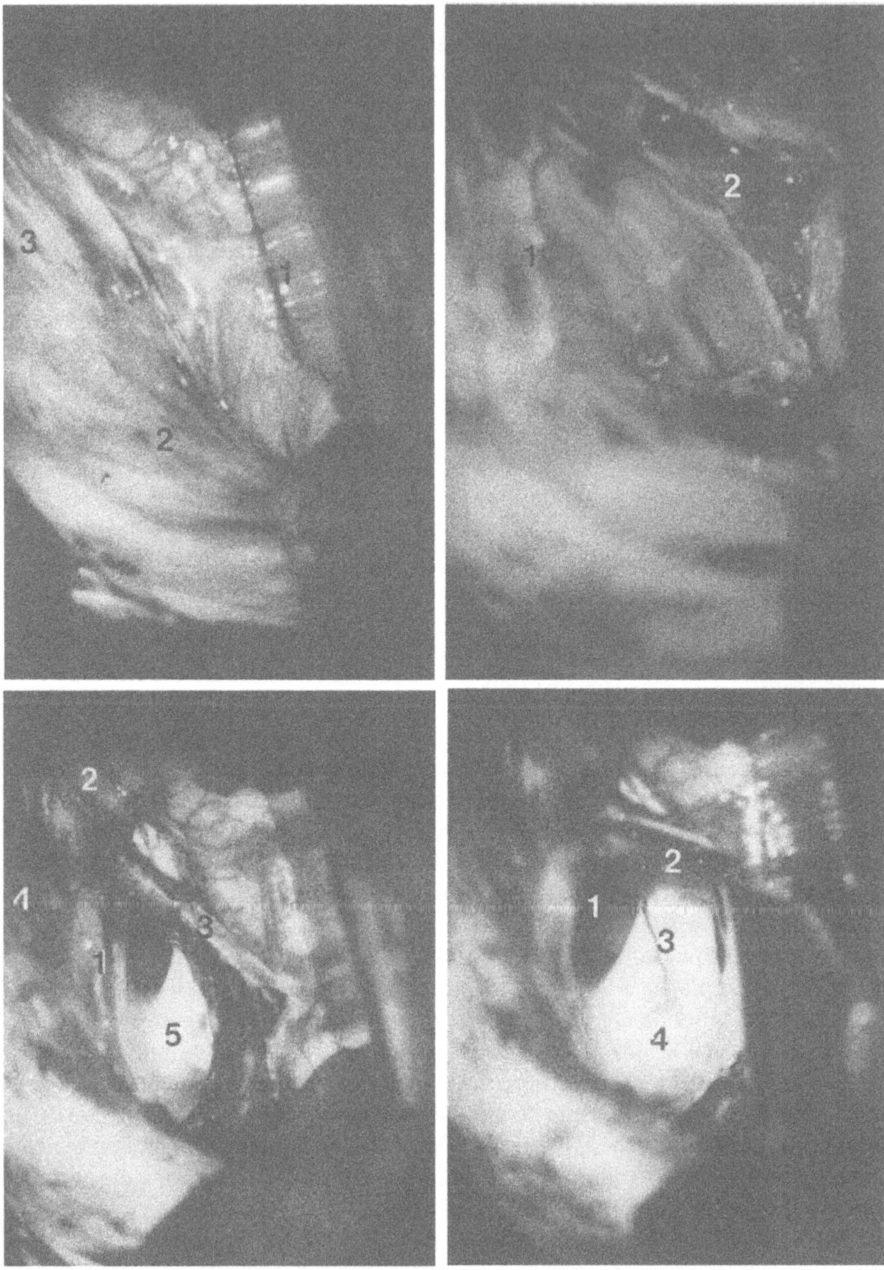

a b c d

Fig. 8. **a** Figure showing medial occipital supratentorial approach in a case of pineal germinoma. *1* Spatula retracting right occipital lobe, *2* Tentorium, *3* Straight sinus. **b** The tentorium is incised a few millimetres parallel to the straight sinus. *1* Incised tentorium, *2* Tumor. **c** Condition after tumor removal, view through the posterior wall of third ventricle. *1* Incised tentorium, *2* Great vein of Galen, *3* Basal vein of Rosenthal, *4* Straight sinus, *5* Third ventricle. **d** View in the third ventricle after removal of the pineal tumor. *1* Left foramen of Monro, *2* Choroid plexus, *3* Fornix, *4* Anterior commissure posterior third ventricle, the opposite tentorial edge and branches of the superior cerebellar artery. Care should be taken to avoid injury of the medial occipital vein draining into the basal vein shortly before its confluence with the great vein of Galen. Injury of this vein may be responsible for development of homonymous hemianopia which may complicate such an exposure.

B. Infratentorial Approaches

1. The Lateral Suboccipital Approach

We use this approach in case of lesions extending from the cerebellopontine angle into the tentorial notch (acoustic neurinomas, meningiomas, epidermoids and other rare tumors).

The semisitting position is used. The head is fixed in a three point Mayfield apparatus with slight extension, forward flexion and lateral rotation of about 30° to the side of the lesion. This permits a direct approach along the pyramid to the cerebellopontine angle and the edge of the tentorium. A linear skin incision is made 2 cm posterior to the mastoid and extending from just above the superior nuchal line to the upper part of the neck. The craniotomy is about 3 cm across made in such a way to expose the transverse sinus above and the sigmoid sinus laterally. The previously used enlargement of the craniotomy in medial direction up to the midline and caudally by opening the foramen magnum and resecting the arch of the atlas is no longer necessary when using microsurgical techniques (Rand and Kurze 1965; Yaşargil 1978; Samii 1979). In this approach the exposure up to the sigmoid sinus, by gradual removal of the mastoid is of special importance. With the aid of a high speed diamond drill it is possible to remove bone easily to the medial margin of the sigmoid sinus and in addition, to avoid the danger of opening the venous pathways. The danger of air embolism is considerably reduced by using the semisitting position, combined with elevation of the lower extremities. A doppler probe is used to detect even small quantities of air entering the vascular system and also makes it possible if necessary to stop immediately and completely any air inflow by means of an indwelling catheter in the right atrium.

The dura is opened about 2–3 mm from the sinus with a curved incision medially, right up to the transverse and sigmoid sinus. The cerebellum is gradually retracted medially and slightly upwards. The cisterna magna is opened and C.S.F. is allowed to drain giving more space. In cases of acoustic tumors the dura around the internal auditory canal is coagulated and excised off the petrous bone. A burr is used to drill away the posterior and superior aspects of the auditory canal. Solution is continuously used to prevent excessive heating which may injure the structures in the canal. At the first indication of soft tissue the rest of the bone is removed by a dissector. During drilling care should be taken in the inferior part of the canal, as in some cases the jugular bulb is high and may be injured if one is not careful enough. Rhoton (1974) has cautioned against drilling beyond the extent of the crista falciformis to avoid injury of structures of the inner ear if hearing is preserved. The position of the jugular bulb and the posterior semicircular canal should be preoperatively carefully recognized using a high resolution CT-scan. Starting from a

5–10 mm opening of the capsula, debulking of the tumor is performed. The tumor capsula loses its primary tension and can be dissected from the overlying arachnoid. The caudal cranial nerves and anterior inferior cerebellar artery are identified at the inferior pole of the tumor and freed from the capsula. An immediate identification of the facial nerve in the cerebellopontine angle, when the tumor is large, is impossible. The nerve is almost always pushed by the tumor anteriorly. With more debulking of the tumor the capsula gradually collapses and the superior pole can be dissected from the petrosal vein and the trigeminal nerve. The medial portion of the capsula is then gradually dissected from the brain stem. Here the facial nerve can be identified. Any direct manipulation of the nerve will almost lead to postoperative loss of function. The nerve must not be detached from the capsula, but the tumor must be carefully dissected from the nerve. The most adherent part is usually a few millimetres from the internal auditory canal. A successful excision is done when this is the last part to be dissected from the capsula. Thus, first the intrameatal part of the tumor is removed and the nerve is identified and followed medially to this point. In case of dissection of the nerve only from one direction preservation of function and continuity is very difficult. When the nerve has lost its continuity, we are faced with different possibilities. When the proximal and distal ends are identified, they can be sutured either directly or, if not possible, using a sural graft (Samii 1980). If only the proximal stump is identified, then it is sutured to the nerve distal to the geniculate ganglion using a sural graft (Samii 1980). If the proximal stump is not available, we prefer to do a facial hypoglossal anastomosis at a second stage.

After total excision of the tumor the petrosal vein, superior cerebellar artery and the trigeminal nerves and cochlear nerves are to be seen in the superior anterior pole of the field, the caudal cranial nerves and anterior inferior cerebellar artery in the inferior pole.

The air cells in the petrous bone are closed by bone wax and the canal is sealed by a piece of muscle using a few drops of fibrin glue. This is very important to prevent postoperative C.S.F. fistula. The dura is closed in a water-tight manner.

In case of trigeminal neurinomas with extension into the C.P.A., the 7th and 8th C.N. are compressed downwards, the 3rd and 4th are usually elevated. The brain stem is compressed and displaced to the contralateral and posterior direction.

The operative exposure is the same as described above without opening of the I.C.A. (Figs. 9a–h).

2. Supracerebellar Approach

The posterior third of the tentorial margin around the territory of the pineal region can be reached by the supracerebellar approach. The pineal region may show a wide variety of pathologic processes, ranging from the most malignant to the most benign (Sano 1983). These tumors indent the posterior aspect of the third ventricle or infiltrate its wall, finally the ventricular cavity.

The commonest tumors in this region are the so-called germinomas or pinealomas of the two-cell-pattern type PTC (Sano et al. 1981). Other pathologies that may sometimes reach huge sizes are falco-tentorial meningiomas, teratomas and pineoblastomas. The strategy for management of these pathologic processes is still a matter of controversy. Germinomas or two-cell-pattern type of pinealomas are radio-

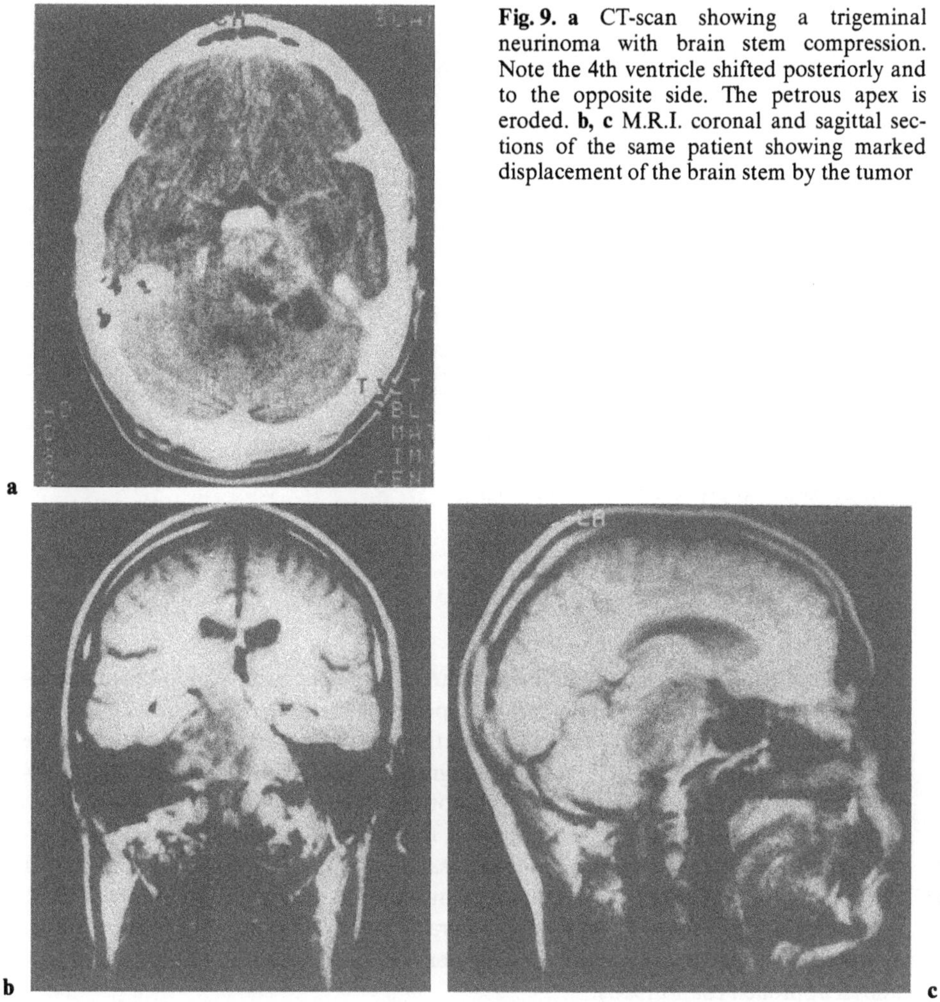

Fig. 9. a CT-scan showing a trigeminal neurinoma with brain stem compression. Note the 4th ventricle shifted posteriorly and to the opposite side. The petrous apex is eroded. **b, c** M.R.I. coronal and sagittal sections of the same patient showing marked displacement of the brain stem by the tumor

sensitive. Therefore some advocate radiation alone or radiation plus ventricular shunting are the established treatments. The greatest criticism against direct surgery is the anticipated significant operative mortality and the increased probability of dissemination metastases in the CSF. However, we believe that with the recent advances in the technology of diagnosis, pre- and postoperative managements and perfection of operative techniques no significant operative risk is encountered when dealing with these tumors.

It seems also that reduction of the bulk of neoplasm by direct surgery, even if that neoplasm is radiosensitive, is important for the effectiveness of radiotherapy. Sano (1981, 1985) also reported no increased incidence of dissemination metastases in his series of patients operated on such tumors. One should also not forget that by using that conservative line of management we can miss those patients harboring benign pathologies which could be completely cured by a direct attack.

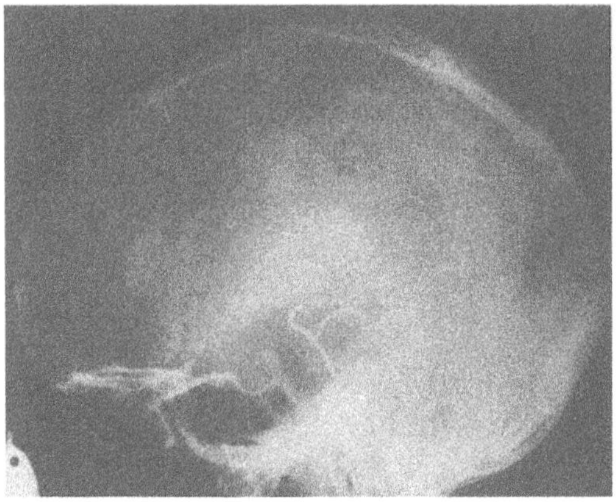
d

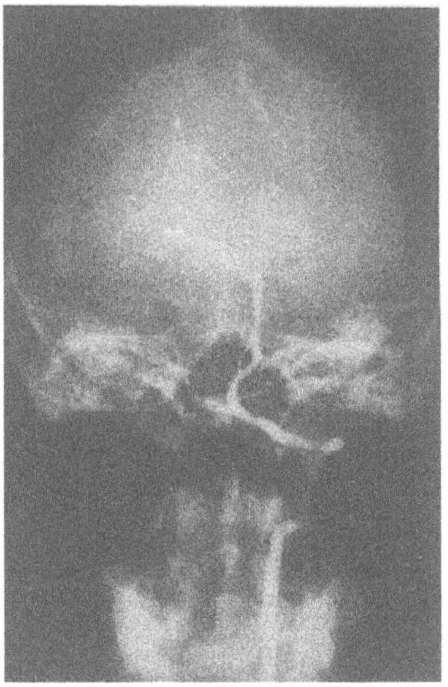
e

Fig. 9. d Left vertebral angiography. Lateral view showing bowing and posterior displacement of basilar artery. **e** Left vertebral angiography A.P. view showing lateral displacement of the basilar artery with elevation of both superior cerebellar and posterior cerebral arteries

In our clinic we manage these cases by direct surgical attack. The following treatment (radiotherapy, chemotherapy) will depend on the pathologic character of the tumor. Usually a preliminary idea of the pathology of the tumor is obtained before surgery from radiography (CT scan, angiography, MRI) and hormonal assay (Alphafetoprotein, AFP, human chronic gonadotrophin HCG) in the serum and CSF.

Several approaches have been proposed for excision of tumors in the pineal region. These include: the parietal transcallosal (Dandy 1921; Suzuki and Iwabuchi 1965), the occipital or parieto-occipital transtentorial (Poppen and Marino 1968; Ausman et al. 1985), the infratentorial supracerebellar (Krause 1926; Stein 1977), the posterior transventricular (Van Wagener 1931), the frontal or anterior transcallosal approach (Sano 1985).

The infratentorial supracerebellar approach is preferred for most tumors invading the pineal region because, hereby, the access is not obstructed by the deep venous system that caps the dorsal and lateral aspects of the pineal tumors. (The occipital transtentorial approach is only used for tumors above the tentorial edge if there is no major extension to the posterior fossa or opposite side and for those located above the vein of Galen.) In the infratentorial supracerebellar approach the surgery is done in the semisitting position. Some surgeons prefer the concorde position (Kobayashi et al. 1983). The head and neck is flexed to bring the tentorium near the horizontal plane. A vertical midline incision is used. The suboccipital craniotomy extends above the lower edge of the torcular and both transverse sinuses. The dural incision extends up to the inferior margin of the transverse sinus. Gravity assists the cerebellum in falling down away from the tentorium cerebelli. The straight sinus and tentorium may be elevated with a retractor and the vermis is retracted gently inferiorly. Bridging veins over the superior surface of the cerebellum may be coagulated and transected without risk. Incision of the arachnoid over

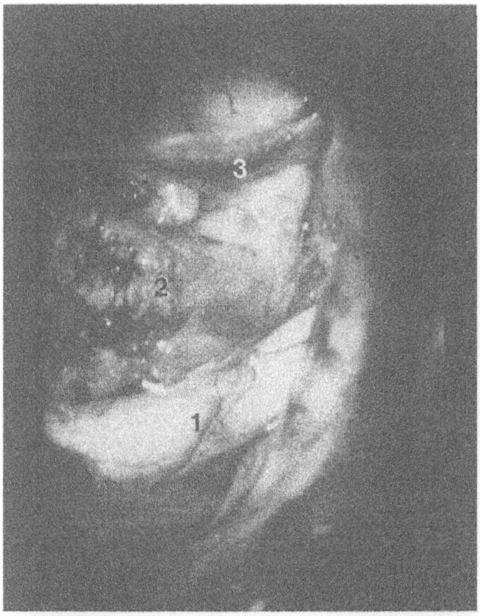

f

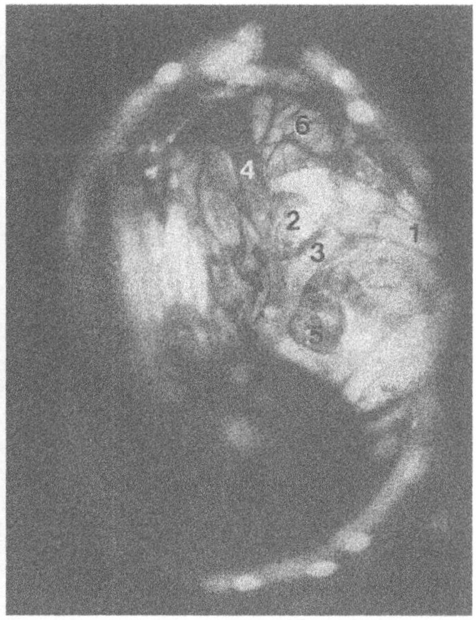

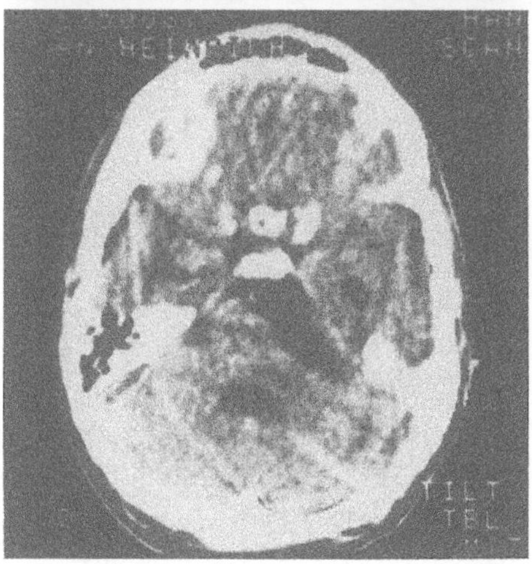

h

Fig. 9. f Removal of a trigeminal neurinoma using a lateral suboccipital approach. *1* 7th and 8th nerve. Note that they are displaced caudally by the tumor. *2* Tumor, *3* Petrosal vein. **g** Surgical field after total excision of the tumor. *1* Right oculomotor nerve, *2* Left oculomotor nerve, *3* Right posterior cerebral artery, *4* Right superior cerebellar artery, *5* Left superior cerebellar artery, *6* Brain stem. **h** Postoperative CT-scan after excision of the tumor

the quadrigeminal cistern brings the tumor and deep venous system in view (Figs. 10a–c). The vein of Galen and the internal cerebral veins are above the tumor. The precentral vein is posterior, – the thalamus, the medial posterior choroidal and posterior cerebral arteries and basal veins lateral. The superior cerebellar arteries and veins are below.

Case:

A male patient, 15 years old, presented with a stuporous state. His condition started two years previously with headache, diabetes insipidus followed by bilateral hearing disturbance. On examination the patient had bilateral papilledema, positive Parinaud's sign. CT-scan showed a hyperdense space-occupying lesion in the pineal re-

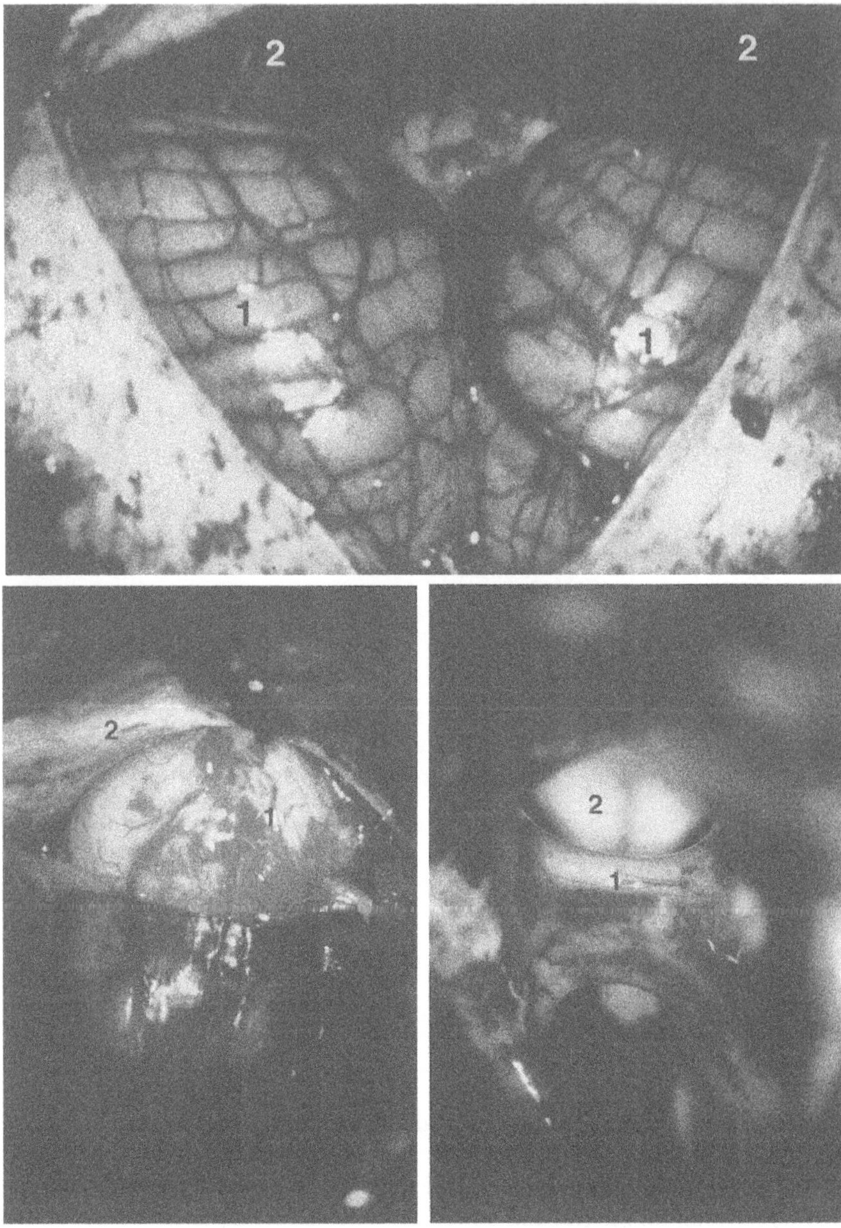

a

b

Fig. 10. a Infratentorial supracerebellar approach. *1* Cerebellar hemisphere, *2* Transverse sinus. Note that without retraction there is a sufficient space between the tentorium and cerebellum. **b** Exposure of the tumor in the pineal region. *1* Tumor, *2* Tentorium. **c** View in the third ventricle after removal of the tumor. *1* Interthalamic connection, *2* Fornix

a

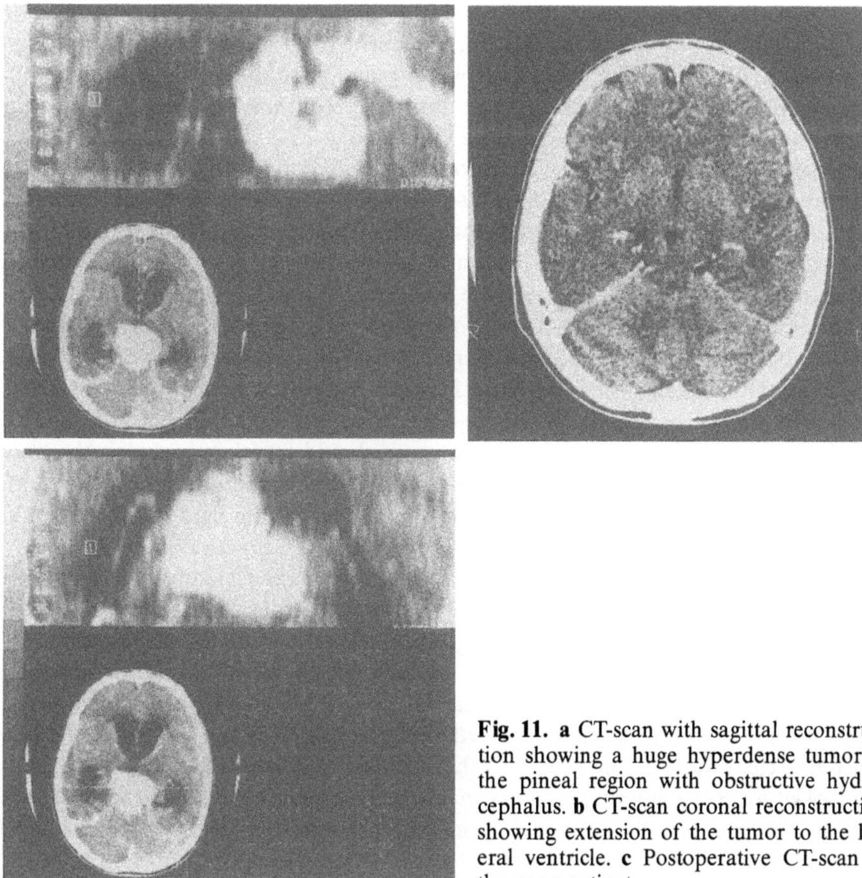

c

b

Fig. 11. **a** CT-scan with sagittal reconstruction showing a huge hyperdense tumor in the pineal region with obstructive hydrocephalus. **b** CT-scan coronal reconstruction showing extension of the tumor to the lateral ventricle. **c** Postoperative CT-scan of the same patient

gion with hydrocephalus (Figs. 11a, b). A ventricular shunt was done. Following the improvement of his general condition, excision of the tumor was accomplished through a supracerebellar subtentorial approach. Postoperatively the patient showed an excellent recovery, his follow-up CT-scan demonstrated complete excision of the tumor (Fig. 11c). The tumor excised was histopathologically verified as a teratoma with malignant changes. The patient received postoperatively deep X-ray therapy as a supplementary treatment.

C. Technique of Combined Subtemporal Suboccipital Approach

The patient lies in the park bench position, the head is rotated about 30° away from the side of the tumor with the neck flexed and the face directed towards the floor.

A retromastoidal skin incision is extended in a curved fashion towards the temporal region. A temporal craniotomy is performed extending downwards as low as possible to the floor of the middle fossa and posteriorly to the transverse sinus. If the tumor extends to the parasellar region, the trepenation should extend anteriorly to the pterion. The bone flap is kept attached to the temporal muscle and both are retracted frontally. A suboccipital craniectomy is performed exposing the transverse sinus and extending laterally to expose the sigmoid sinus. The bone over the proximal part of the sigmoid sinus is removed by a diamond drill. The bone drilling should extend to remove the lateral 10–15 mm of the petrous bone with avoidance of destruction to the inner ear structures. This is quite important especially when aiming to approach the dorsum sella and clivus. The upper surface of the petrous bone can also be drilled away to reduce retraction applied to the temporal lobe.

The dura is opened about 2 mm posterior to the sigmoid sinus. The transverse sinus is ligated and transected at its junction with the sigmoid sinus preserving the drainage for Labbé's vein. The dural incision is directed medially just below the transverse sinus. The tentorium is incised near its attachment to the petrous bone till the incisura. During opening the incisura care should be taken to define the trochlear nerve. Usually when the tumor is large enough to extend through the tentorial hiatus the nerve is pushed laterally, thus hanging across the field during tumor excision. The preservation of the trochlear nerve in such cases is usually impossible.

Now the temporal lobe together with the tentorium and the transverse sinus can be retracted upwards. Care should be taken not to obstruct the drainage of the Labbé's vein with the brain spatula. The sigmoid sinus is laterally retracted using a dural stay suture. The cerebellum is retracted medially to expose the cerebellopontine angle. In most cases the laterally displaced 7th and 8th cranial nerves can now be seen. These nerves are usually dissected from the tumor in ease, owing to the presence of a clear arachnoidal sheath. If these nerves cannot be identified, they should be looked for in the internal auditory meatus. The trigeminal nerve may be engulfed by the tumor especially in cases of meningioma and its functional preservation is sometimes impossible. During removal of the upper lateral part of the tumor care should be taken to avoid injury of the oculomotor nerve. This is usually displaced laterally. The nerve is prepared from the tumor with ease due to its arachnoidal covering.

The tumor excision is continued in a piecemeal manner gradually exposing the brain stem. Care should be taken to avoid injury of the basilar artery and its branches. The relation of the artery to the tumor should be carefully speculated from the preoperative angiography with a clear idea of whether the artery is only displaced or also engulfed by the tumor.

After tumor excision the incised tentorium is repaired; if this is not possible, it can be left open. The supratentorial and infratentorial dura is closed and the defect over the lateral sinus is patched by a piece of temporal fascia. Any opened air cells are sealed by bone wax and a piece of muscle fixed either with fibrin glue or a couple of stitches. This will avoid the occurrence of any CSF fistula.

Using this approach, one can have a good exposure to the dorsum sellae, clivus, to structures lying posterior to the petrous apex and those in the midline.

When the craniotomy is extended to the pterional region, the surgeon has a good view of the structures extending from the optic chiasma to the dorsum sella and downwards till the foramen magnum. The ocular cranial nerves can be followed from their origin till their entrance in the cavernous sinus. The retraction both to the

a b c

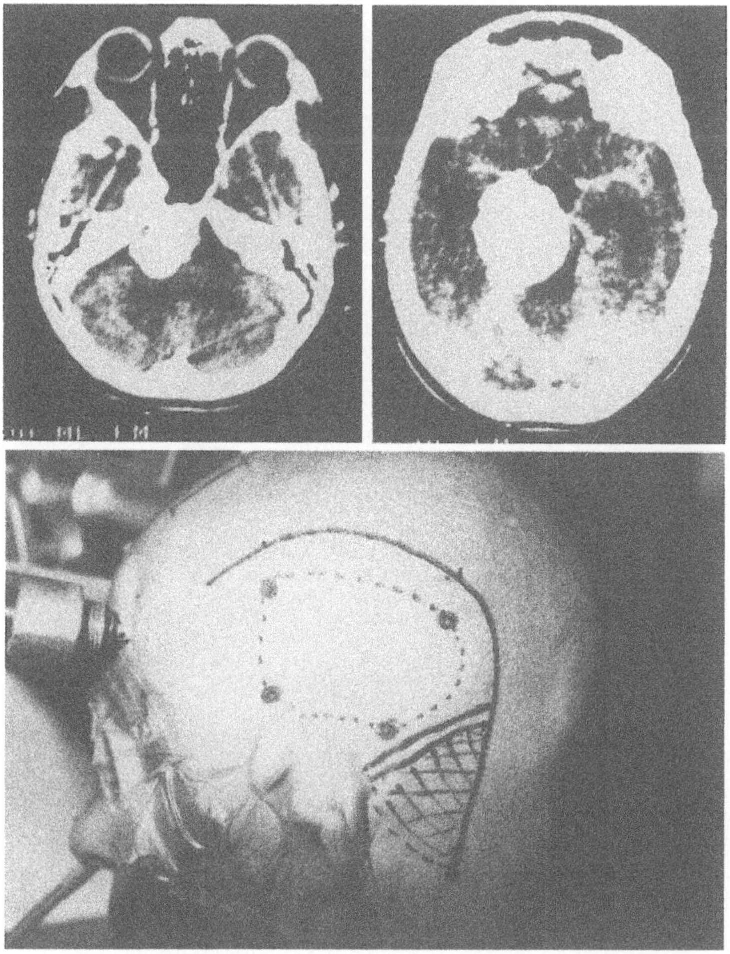

Fig. 12. a, b CT-scan of a left petroclival meningioma extending both supra- and infratentorially. **c** The skin incision, the temporal craniotomy and suboccipital craniectomy in the combined supra- and infratentorial approach. The site of the transverse sinus in between is marked

cerebellum and temporal lobe is minimized by drilling the outer surface of the petrous bone.

Hakuba (1978) extended the translabyrinthine transtentorial approach of Morrison and King (1973) to include a suboccipital subtemporal craniotomy. He reported that using this approach he was able to excise meningiomas at the clivus region (Hakuba et al. 1977).

Symon (1982) recommended using this approach especially in three conditions; clivus and petrous apical tumors (chordomas or meningiomas), difficult or complex upper basilar aneurysms and cholesteatomas extending through the tentorial hiatus.

When the hearing function is intact, we reject a petrosectomy or labyrinthectomy to improve the exposure.

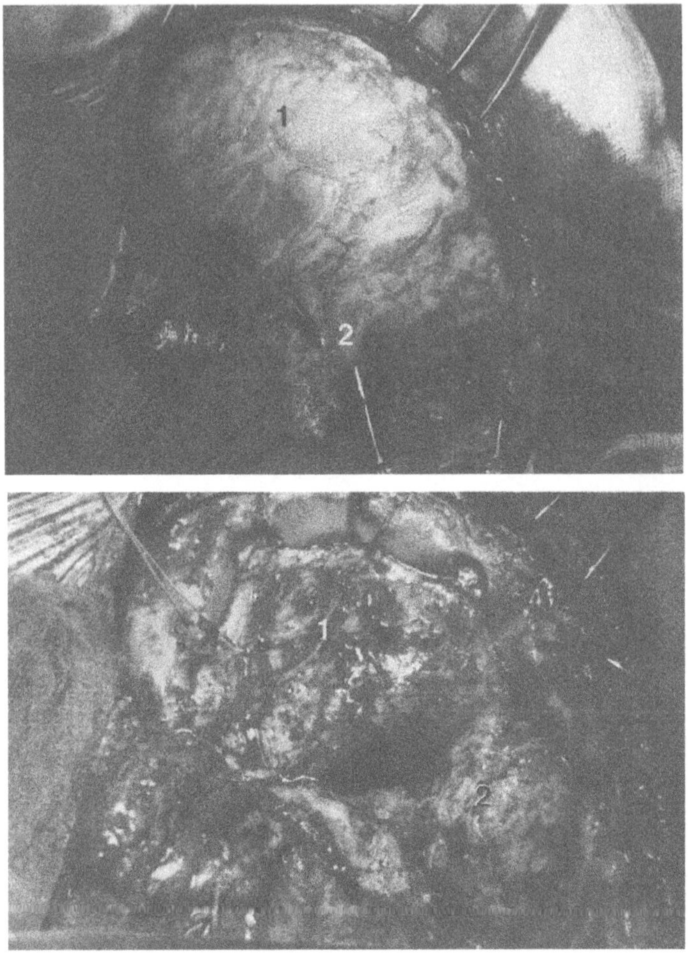

d

e

Fig. 12. **d** View after reflection of the skin and muscle flap. *1* Squamous part of temporal bone, *2* Mastoid process. **e** Condition after left temporal craniotomy and lateral suboccipital craniectomy. *1* Temporal dura, *2* Cerebellar dura

We believe that the combined operative technique is the best when total excision of a tumor cannot be performed using only supra- or infratentorial approaches. The surgeon should be flexible and ready to extend his suboccipital or subtemporal approach to a combined one when total removal of a tumor cannot be achieved by only one approach.

Case:

A 39-year-old male patient presented with a right hemiparesis and left trigeminal hypesthesia of a gradual onset and progressive course. His condition deteriorated after he developed an obstructive hydrocephalus, and a ventriculoperitoneal shunt

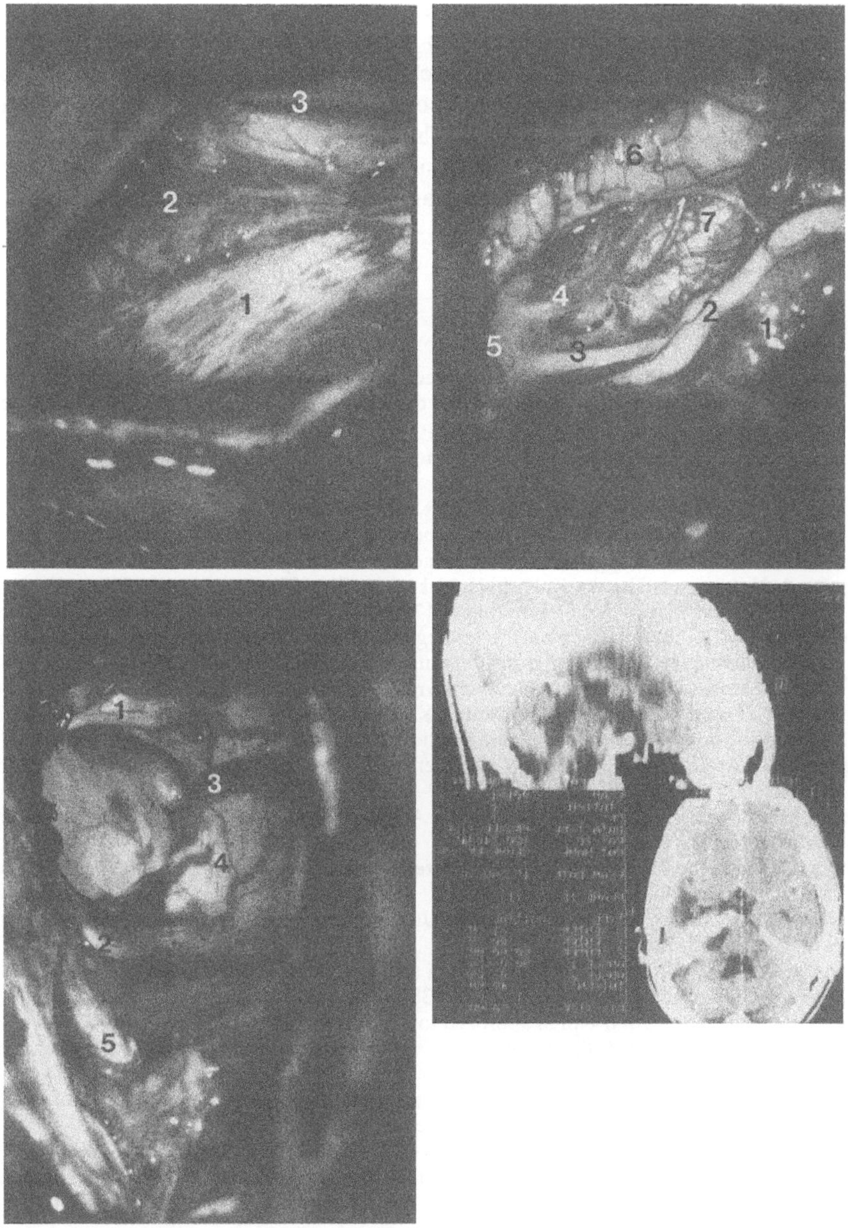

Fig. 12. **f** Retraction of the temporal lobe and exposure of the supratentorial part of the tumor. *1* Tentorium, *2* Tumor, *3* Retracted temporal lobe. **g** Surgical view after excision of the supratentorial part of the tumor. *1* Tumor (infratentorial part), *2* Oculomotor nerve, *3* Posterior communicating artery, *4* Anterior choroidal artery, *5* Internal carotid artery, *6* Temporal lobe, *7* Brain stem. **h** Surgical view of the cerebellopontine angle after excision of the infratentorial part of the tumor. *1* Oculomotor nerve, *2* Trigeminal nerve, *3* Superior cerebellar artery, *4* Brain stem, *5* 7th and 8th cranial nerves. **i** Postoperative CT-scan with sagittal reconstruction

was needed. Regarding the position and extension of the tumor (Figs. 12a–b), the combined approach was chosen aiming to radical excision of the tumor. The above mentioned technique was used in approaching this tumor without ligation and excision of the left transverse sinus (Figs. 12c–h). Postoperatively the right hemiparesis increased and the patient developed a facial weakness. After one month his facial weakness disappeared and his hemiparesis showed marked improvement. Figure 12i shows a follow-up CT-scan after 1½ years following the tumor excision.

References

Ausman J et al. (1985) A new operative approach to the pineal region. In: Samii M (ed) Surgery in and around the brain stem and the third ventricle. (1986) Springer, Berlin Heidelberg New York, pp 326–328

Dandy WE (1921) An operation for the removal of pineal tumors. Surg Gynecol Obstet 33:113–119

Dandy WE (1936) Operative experience in cases of pineal tumor. Arch Surg 33:19–46

Hakuba A (1978) Total removal of cerebellopontine angle tumors with a combined transpetrosal-transtentorial approach. Nashmkeigeka 6:347–354

Hakuba A, Nishmura S, Tanaka K, Kishi H, Nakamura T (1977) Clivus meningioma: Six cases of total removal. Neurol Med Chir (Tokyo) 17:63–77

Jannetta PJ (1977) Observations on the etiology of trigeminal neuralgia, hemifacial spasm, acoustic nerve dysfunction and glossopharyngeal neuralgia. Definitive microsurgical treatment and results in 117 patients. Neurochirurgia (Stuttg) 20:145–154

Kobayashi S, Sugita K, Tanaka Y, Kyoshima K (1983) Infratentorial approach to the pineal region in the prone position: Concorde position. J Neurosurg 58:141–143

Krause F (1926) Operative Freilegung der Vierhügel nebst Beobachtungen über Hirndruck und Dekompression. Zentralbl Chir 35:2812–2819

Lang J (1985) Anatomy of the tentorial margin. Advances in Neurosurgery 13. Springer, Berlin Heidelberg New York, p 173–182

Lapras C, Dechaume JP, Deruty R (1973) Traitement des tumeurs de la region pineale. Lyon Chir 69:196–198

Mitterwallner FV (1955) Variationsstatistische Untersuchungen an den basalen Hintergefäßen. Acta Anat (Basel) 24:51

Morrison AW, King TT (1973) Experiences with a translabyrinthine-transtentorial approach to the cerebellopontine angle. J Neurosurg 38:382–390

Poppen JL (1966) The right occipital approach to a pinealoma 25, p 706–710

Poppen JL, Marino RJ (1968) Pinealomas and tumors of the posterior portion of the third ventricle. J Neurosurg 28:357–364

Rand RW, Kurze T (1965) Microneurosurgical resection of acoustic tumors by a transmeatal posterior fossa approach. Bull Los Angeles Neurol Soc 30:17–20

Rhoton A (1974) Microsurgery of the internal acoustic meatus. Surg Neurol 2:311–318

Samii M (1979) Neurochirurgische Gesichtspunkte bei der Behandlung der Akustikusneurinome mit besonderer Berücksichtigung des N. Facialis. Laryngol Rhinol Otol (Stuttg) 58:97–106

Samii M (1980) Nerves of the head and neck. In: Omer GE, Spinner M (eds) Management of peripheral nerve problems. WB Saunders, Philadelphia, pp 507–547

Samii M (1981) Olfactory nerve. In: Samii M, Jannetta PJ (eds) The Cranial Nerves. Springer, Berlin Heidelberg New York, pp 66–73

Sano K (1983) Pineal region tumors: Problems in pathology and treatment. Clin Neurosurg 30:39–91

Sano K (1985) Microsurgery of tumors in the pineal region. Microneurosurgery 3rd ed. In: Rand RW (ed) C.V. Mosby Company, Saint Louis, p 391–397

Sano K et al. (1981) Brain tumor registry in Japan, vol 3

Sano K, Matsutani M (1981) Pinealoma (germinoma) treated by direct surgery and postoperative irradiation: a long term follow up. Child's Brain 8:81–87

Stein BM (1977) The intratentorial supracerebellar approach to pineal lesions. J Neurosurg 35:197–202

Suzuki J (1981) Preservation of the olfactory tract in bifrontal craniotomy for anterior communicating artery aneurysms and functional prognosis. J Neurosurg 54:342–345

Suzuki J, Iwabuchi T (1965) Surgical removal of pineal tumors: experience in a series of 19 cases. J Neurosurg 23:565–571

Symon L (1982) Surgical Approaches to the Tentorial Hiatus. Adv Techn Standards Neurosurg 9:69–112

Van Wagener WP (1931) A surgical approach for the removal of certain pineal tumors: report on a case. Surg Gynecol Obstet 53:216–220

Yaşargil MG (1978) Mikrochirurgie der Kleinhirnbrückenwinkel-Tumoren. In: Kleinhirnbrückenwinkeltumoren. Springer, Berlin Heidelberg New York, pp 215–257

Laser Surgery on and Within the Neuraxis

F. Heppner, R. W. Oberbauer, and P. W. Ascher, Graz/Austria

Neurosurgical operative technique with the CO_2-Laser was for the first time introduced by the Universitätsklinik für Neurochirurgie Graz in 1976, taking into account the specific biophysical properties of this type of laser (Heppner and Ascher 1976). The tissue is divided by heat without causing penetrating field lines as in diathermy. Coagulation is also effected by heat, but contrary to bipolar coagulation forceps no electric circuit is closed. These advantages are especially noticeable in operations within or close to the brainstem, because the risk of interference with neurovegetative regulating centers is markedly diminished.

Another advantage operating with the CO_2-Laser is the possibility to adjust the penetration depth of the laser beam exactly to fractions of millimeter, being relative to the output energy, the focussing of the beam and the exposition time. Investigations of one of us (Ascher 1977) have shown that conventional instruments used for the cutting of nerval tissue (spatula, suction or diathermy) will finally always result in tearing of tissue, while the cutting effect of the CO_2-Laser consists in denaturising the cell proteins causing a smooth walled cut, with diminished tendency to the formation of scar tissue (Fig. 1). These properties make the CO_2-Laser, rather than conventional techniques eminently suitable for operative explorations into the inner of the pons or the medulla oblongata, especially for removing a circumscribed neoplasma, a microangioma or the evacuation of a hemorrhagic cyst (Heppner

Table 1. Cerebral tumors of midline and adjacent structures in the own material. Expanding lesions of extracerebral origin (such as craniopharyngiomas, meningiomas, metastases) are not included (Autochthonous midline lesions of the brain 1950–1984)

	Medulla obl.	Vermis	Pons	IIIrd. ventricle	Pineal region	Corpus call.	Total
Glioblastoma			0-0-1	14-2-2		3-0-1	23
Astrocytoma	2-1-1	0-1-0	4-0-1	8-0-2		5-0-0	25
Oligodendroglioma		1-0-0		4-0-0			5
Spongioblastoma	1-0-0	7-0-0	3-0-0	1-0-0			12
Ependymoma	16-0-1	1-0-0	1-0-0	6-1-0			26
Medulloblastoma	12-3-4	14-2-1	2-0-0			0-0-1	39
Pinealomas, teratomas et al.					27-1-0		28
Not classified variants (angiomatous neoplasms)	8-3-4	1-3-0	8-25-19	19-22-47	3-0-6		168
Op. – pall. – cons.	39-7-10	24-6-1	18-25-21	52-25-51	30-1-6	8-0-2	326

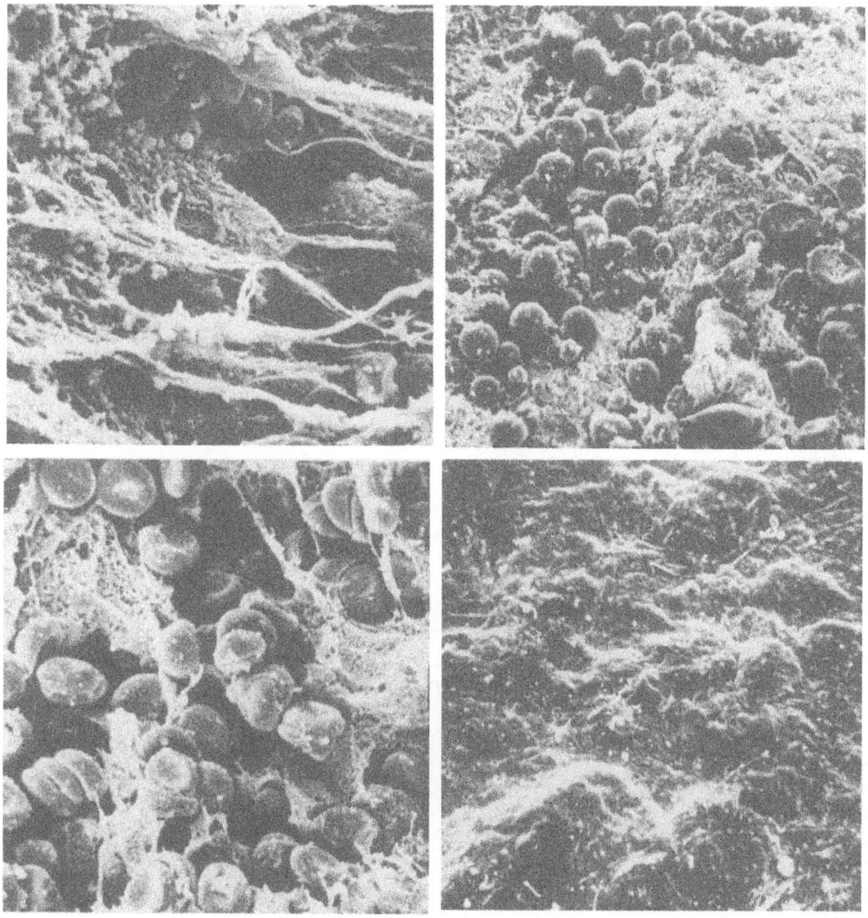

Fig. 1. Scanning electron microphotography of cutting planes in the brain performed by 4 different means: spatula (*left above*); sucker (*right above*); diathermy (*left below*); CO_2-laser beam (*right below*). Note the smooth surface of the laser cut

1981; Ascher and Heppner 1981; Heppner and Ascher 1982; Heppner et al. 1982; Heppner 1984; Heppner et al. 1984).

From October 1950 until October 1984, 1337 gliomas of the cerebrum were operated, 326 were located close to or within the midline structures (Table 1). (During the same period 53 intramedullary tumors of the spinal cord were operated.)

Operations of midline lesions with the CO_2-Laser were first started in 1976. Those cases are listed in Table 2 (Craniopharyngiomas have been excluded). Exactly in one half of the cases, i.e. in 39 patients, the lesion was situated in or close to pons and medulla oblongata (Table 3).

Table 2. Tumors of the brainstem that had been dealt with by means of lasers (July 1976–December 1984)

Histology	
Astrocytoma	20
Ependymoma	11
Medulloblastoma	11
Meningioma	9
Pineal tumor	6
Angiomatous lesion	6
Spongioblastoma	3
Cholesteatoma	1
Papilloma	2
Lipoma	1
Sarcoma	1
Glioblastoma	1
Not classified	2
Metastasis	4
Total	78

Table 3. Tumors of pons and medulla oblongata that underwent laser surgery

Site	Pons	Rhomb-encephalon	Cerebellum pons	Cerebellum rhomb.	
Medulloblastoma	1	5	–	7	13
Astrocytoma	1	3	1	1	6
Spongioblastoma	1	–	–	1	2
Ependymoma	1	6	1	1	9
Papilloma	–	1	–	–	1
Sarcoma	1	–	–	–	1
Angioma	1	1	1	–	3
Metastasis	–	–	2	1	3
Not classified	–	–	–	1	1
Total	6	16	5	12	39

Results

When an intervention in regions formerly thought to be inaccessible is dared the operative mortality is of primary interest. At operation no death occurred. In the postoperative period, i.e. within 3 weeks, we lost 6 patients: 3 due to brain edema, 2 due to pulmonary embolism, 1 due to pneumonia. This postoperative mortality rate of 15% in those desperate cases is fairly low proving the capability of the CO_2-Laser in such areas.

Dependent on the specific histology which includes also medulloblastomas a survival time of less than 6 months was attained in 7 cases; in another 10 cases clinical cure was achieved, whilst the remaining group of 22 cannot be judged with certainty, as in some cases the time of postoperative observation has been too short, while from other patients who came from abroad further information was sometimes difficult to obtain.

One case is important to mention. It was an 8-year-old boy suffering from a medulloblastoma invading pons and rhombencephalon. The tumor was resected by means of the Neodymium-YAG-Laser in contrast to all other cases where the CO_2-Laser was used. After operation the patient was and remained apallic until death occurred 8 months later during which time he received megavolt- and Chemotherapy. No autopsy was performed.

Especially notable was the success after operative removal of intramedullary tumors of the spinal cord with the CO_2-Laser beam.

Discussion

We believe that in operations within the basal parts of the *third* ventricle the CO_2-Laser will only offer an advantage over the more conventional techniques when a microsurgical approach to these difficult regions becomes possible. Technical improvements like fiber glass optics in combination with an endoscope would also be of considerable help in handling the laser beam in diencephalic regions.

Diffuse growing gliomas of the pons will still remain inoperable. An exact preoperative differential diagnosis using Computerized Tomography and PEG is therefore of utmost importance. An additional investigation with NMR (Nuclear Magnetic Resonance) would be a further safety factor.

Although the advantages of the Neodymium-YAG-Laser in operation of highly vascular lesions within the cerebrum have been proved (Beck 1981), its use in operations on the neuraxis demands careful consideration as, differing from the CO_2-Laser, the beam of the Neodymium-YAG-Laser penetrates deeper into the tissue, where it exerts a scattering effect. In the vicinity of the third ventricle its careful use can sometimes be beneficial as the successful operation of an AV-malformation within the thalamus of one of our patients, a 9-year-old girl, demonstrates.

Operation with the Neodymium-YAG-Laser on the brainstem as has been done in one case of our series should be avoided for the above mentioned reasons.

Our expectations that the CO_2-Laser could safely be used within the pons and the medulla oblongata were fully confirmed, always provided that vegetative and circulatory trends observed early by an experienced anesthetist were passed on to the operating surgeon.

References

1. Ascher PW (1977) Der CO_2-Laser in der Neurochirurgie. Molden, Wien München Innsbruck Zürich
2. Ascher PW, Heppner F (1981) Neurosurgical laser techniques. In: Biomedical laser-technology and clinical applications. Springer, Berlin Heidelberg New York, 17:219–227
3. Beck OJ (1981) Vergleichende Untersuchungen hinsichtlich des Lasereinsatzes in der Neurochirurgie. 221. Colloquium der Med. Fakultät der Univ. München. MBB-AT, Information 2

4. Heppner F, Ascher PW (1976) Über den Einsatz des Laserstrahls in der Neurochirurgie. Acta Medicotechn 24:424–426
5. Heppner F (1981) Der Laser in der Neurochirurgie. In: Dinstl K, Fischer PL (Hrsg) Der Laser. Springer, Berlin Heidelberg New York, S 143
6. Heppner F, Ascher PW (1982) The CO_2-laser in neurosurgery. In: Liss AR (ed) Int. advantages in surgical oncology, vol 5, New York
7. Heppner F, Ascher PW, Oberbauer RW (1982) Surgery of brain-stem tumours in children. Proc. 33rd Annual meeting of the "Deutsche Gesellschaft für Neurochirurgie" in Kiel 1982. Acta Neurochir (Wien) 62:132
8. Heppner F (1984) Die medizinischen Laser – heute. Öst Ärzteztg 39, 11:811
9. Heppner F, Oberbauer RW, Ascher PW (1985) Direct surgical attack to pontine and rhombencephalic lesions. In: Koos W (ed) Proc European Society for Paediatric Neurosurgery. Vienna, Oct 10–13. Acta Neurochir Suppl 35:123–125

Advanced Technologies for the Treatment of Brain Stem Tumors

V. A. FASANO, R. URCIUOLI, and R. M. PONZIO, Turin/Italy

Summary

Very few cases of surgical treatment of brain stem neoplasms have been registered in the literature. The intrinsic tumors are often treated by radiation therapy only without biopsy which is considered too hazardous, treatment being limited to few cases (evacuation of an intrinsic cyst). In the tumors originating from the brain stem and bulging out from the axis only the extrinsic part is generally removed. More recently the introduction of new technologies (NMR, intraoperative ultrasonography, Laser, CUSA) has modified the surgery of these kinds of tumors. The main advantages offered are: a) a safe aggression of the brain stem; b) the possibility to perform a correct histologic diagnosis; c) a reduction of the fields and doses of postoperative radiation therapy.

Our series consisted of 9 operated tumors: 5 intrinsic (4 solid and 1 cystic) and 4 protruding out from the axis. Histology revealed a pilocytic astrocytoma in 4 cases, an anaplastic astrocytoma in 4 cases and a metastasis in one case. All patients were submitted to X-ray therapy after surgery.

Patients with anaplastic astrocytoma died between 5 to 12 months after treatment. Patients with pilocytic astrocytoma are still alive after 5 and 3 years and 1 year and able to return to school.

The results of a comparative group treated only with radiation therapy shows a survival time similar to that of operated patients, ranging from 15 to 47 months, however, a remarkable period of time for clinical improvement is required (Bray et al. 1958).

Introduction

The vast majority of brain stem gliomas arise in the pons extending cephalad and caudally for a variable distance. In exceptional cases they may arise in the mesencephalon, medulla or upper cervical spinal cord. Two distinct groups exist:

1. tumors producing an enlargement of the brain stem and a shift of the floor of the 4th ventricle;
2. tumors arising from the brain stem and protruding with exophytic nodules into the cerebellopontine angle and 4th ventricle.

Key words: Brain stem tumors, Laser, NMR, Intraoperative ultrasonography, CUSA Radiotherapy.

The prognosis of these tumors has been generally considered almost invariably bad.

Matson [5] stated 1968: "Should any patient still be alive 18 months after diagnosis, re-investigation and surgical exploration is indicated as some other lesion is probably present. Regardless of specific histology brain stem gliomas must be all classified as malignant tumors since their location in itself renders them inoperable." He therefore concluded that exploration for confirmation should be avoided if possible, since such surgery is useless.

However, already in 1968, Pool [7] described three cases of confirmed astrocytoma of the brain stem, in which the lesions were intrinsic in one case and bulging out into liquoral spaces in two cases. The patients survived for long periods after decompressive surgery and radiotherapy.

In 1971, Lassiter et al. [4] carried out a surgical exploration in 34 patients with brain stem gliomas suspected by air study. In 6 patients it was possible to take a biopsy safely or to remove subtotally the tumor which protruded into the 4th ventricle or fungated anterolaterally from the pons. In 5 patients a large neoplastic cyst in the brain stem was evacuated by needle aspiration and this contributed to long term survival in 4 cases. For this reason the author suggested an exploration of all brain stem gliomas before giving radiotherapy in the hope of identifying a cystic tumor. This is in accordance with Milhorat [6] who observed in a case of a cystic pontine glioma an immediate clinical improvement following evacuation of the cyst and a survival time of 15 years.

Four years later, Reigel et al. [8] stressed the importance of obtaining biopsy verification to permit more accurate correlation of treatment results with pathology.

In 1980, Hoffman et al. [3] reported the results of the surgery in 10 patients with brain stem tumors protruding into the floor of the 4th ventricle. The experience of this author confirms the value of an aggressive approach, surgical resection leading to excellent long term results. It is noticeable that 5 of these patients did not receive any X-ray therapy after surgery, none showing clinical or CT evidence of tumor growth during a follow-up of 1 year to 5 years.

The introduction in the very recent years of new diagnostic (NMR imaging, intraoperative sonography) and surgical devices (Laser, CUSA) contributes to change the attitudes towards the management of these kinds of tumors [2]. The advantages offered by these technologies are discussed in this paper.

Series of Cases and Results

Our series included 9 brain stem tumors divided in the 2 groups described above according to CT or NMR findings. Five cases belonged to the 1st group and 4 to the 2nd (Figs. 1, 2).

Five were children (average age: 6,2 years) and 4 adults (average age: 34 years). Eight cases were solid tumors, 1 (1st group) showed an intratumoral hemorrhage.

The neurologic examination at admission showed in all cases deficit of long pathways with involvement of cranial nerves in 8 cases. Surgery was performed through the floor of the 4th ventricle (median approach) in 5 cases (3 of the 1st

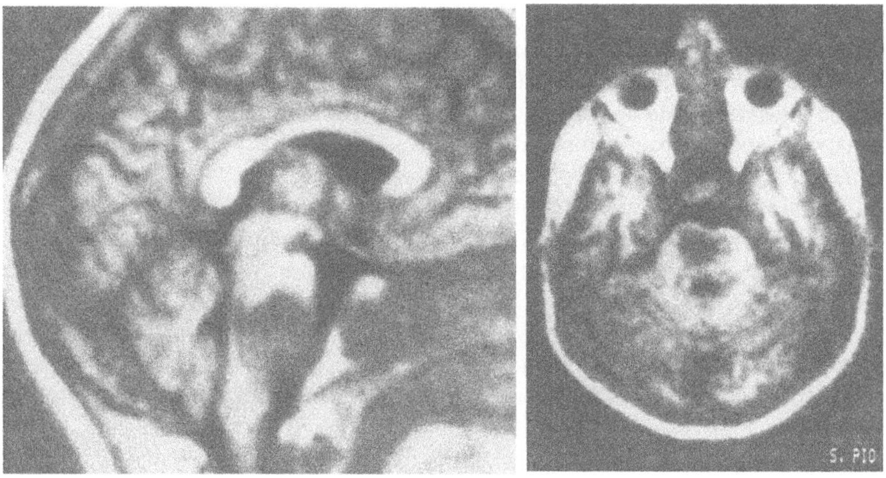

a b

Fig. 1 a, b. Intrinsic tumor of the brain stem (pons) reaching the floor of the 4th ventricle. **a** Lateral NMR scan. **b** Axial NMR scan

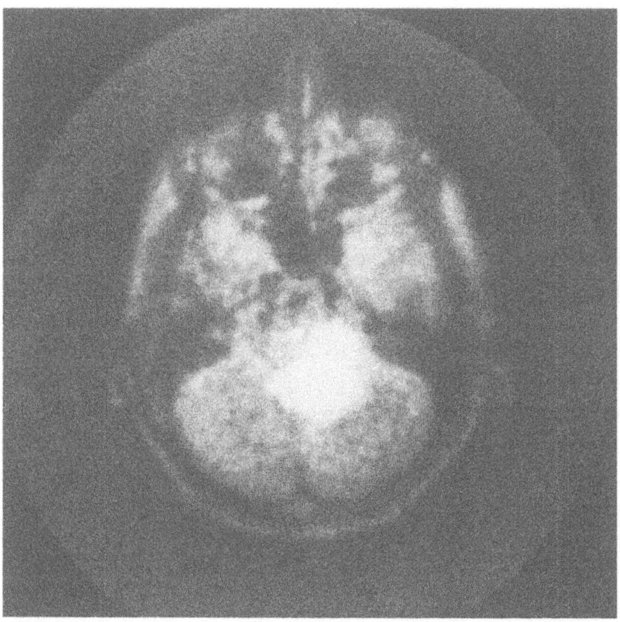

Fig. 2. Brain stem tumor protruding from the axis and blocking the CSF spaces. Axial NMR SE scan

group and 2 of the 2nd) or through the cerebellopontine angle (lateral approach) in 4 cases (2 of the 1st group and 2 of the 2nd).

Histologic examination revealed a pilocytic astrocytoma in 4 cases, all children (2 of the 1st group and 2 of the 2nd), an anaplastic astrocytoma in 4 cases, 3 adults and 1 child (2 of the 1st group and 2 of the 2nd), a metastasis in an adult (1st group).

A postoperative worsening of the neurologic status never appeared. In 4 an immediate clinical improvement was noticed.

All cases were submitted to radiotherapy after surgery. The patients with anaplastic astrocytoma died during a period of 5 to 12 months after operation. All patients with pilocytic astrocytoma are still alive after 5 and 3 years, and 1 year; these patients are able to attend school leading a useful life.

A comparative study was performed in 5 children with brain stem tumor demonstrated on CT scan, submitted to X-ray therapy without biopsy.

Four cases belonged to the 1st group and one to the 2nd. The average age was 6.4 years.

At admission all patients showed involvement of long pathways and four presented mono- or bilateral cranial nerve palsy.

A worsening was noticed in one case. Two patients improved their neurologic status.

Concerning the survival time one patient treated in 1980 is still alive and leads a useful life. In the remaining 4 cases, at 12 months' follow-up, all patients are alive and one of them is able to attend school.

Discussion

In the past, surgery has been limited to the excision of the portion of the tumor protruding out from the axis or to the evacuation of an intrinsic tumoral cyst.

Our experience demonstrates that a direct approach has become possible also in intrinsic solid tumors.

NMR and intraoperative real time ultrasonography give more precise informations about the volume, the localization and the extension of the lesion (ventral or dorsal with lateral or bilateral involvement of the brain stem).

The A-scan ultrasonograph operating at 8 MHz is able to detect the depth of the tumor, and operating frequencies of 15 MHz make it possible to distinguish the pathologic tissue from the normal, thus enabling to increase the selectivity of the tumoral excision (Fig. 3).

The computerized superpulsed CO_2 laser affords a safe incision of the brain stem and a layer by layer exfoliation of the mass. CUSA is used to remove the extraaxial portion if present. Tumors localized dorsally are easier to be removed through the roof of the 4th ventricle, these intrinsic tumors are the most common and show clinical and surgical problems similar to upper cervical cord tumors. The lateral approach is limited to intrinsic tumors with marked lateralization or to tumors spreading into the cerebellopontine angle.

The main advantages of the surgical treatment of the brain stem tumors are:

a) Possibility to obtain an exact histologic diagnosis. Stereotactic biopsy does not often reach the same results because of the small fragments of tissue. Moreover the tumor can vary from region to region showing clear polar spongioblastic features in some areas and marked malignancy in others. Sometimes biopsy may fail because it is performed in perilesional tissues.
b) Reduction of the fields and doses of postoperative radiotherapy. This is especially important since many patients are children, who, after excessive ir-

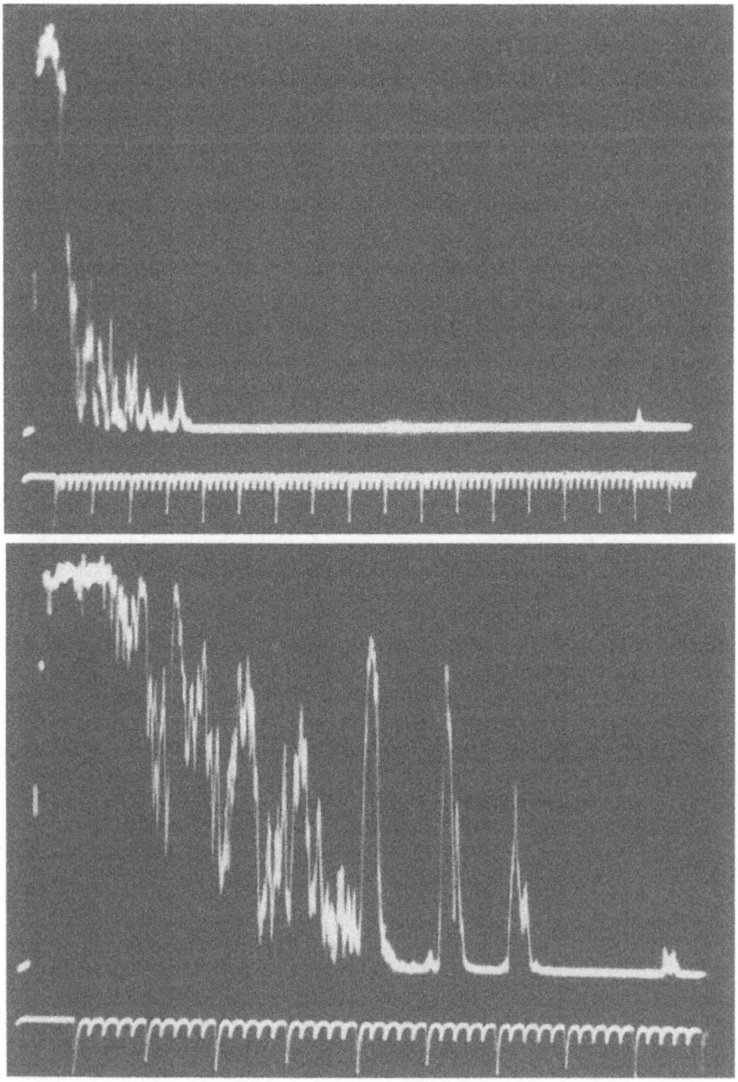

a

b

Fig. 3a, b. A-scan ultrasonography in cerebral tumors. **a** The sharp saw-toothed waves (on the left) indicate a dishomogenous structure with prevalent glial component (astrocytoma); the regular line (on the right) indicates a homogeneous hypercellular tissue (normal cerebral parenchyma). **b** The markedly irregular diagram indicates a dishomogenous tissue followed by single spikes (fibrous structure): meningioma and capsula

radiation, may be affected by complications. Moreover the removal enhances the effectiveness of radiotherapy stimulating the transition of the tumoral cells from G_0 to metabolic active phase.

c) Possibility to obtain a clinical improvement either in cystic or solid tumors. This must be confirmed on a large series of cases.

Regarding the relations between surgery and radiotherapy the clinical experience shows that the association of both gives similar survival rate (ranging from 15 to 47 months) and useful life (in 40% of the treated patients) compared to X-ray therapy only, without worsening of the morbidity. After radiotherapy, however, prognosis is determined only by the responsiveness to treatment and moreover a remarkable period of time is always required to improve the clinical status. Bray et al. [1] reported that most of his patients showed an improvement in between 3 to 6 weeks after therapy had begun.

Prognosis does not change in intrinsic tumors and in tumors bulging out from the axis. Results confirm the strict link existing between the histologic pattern and the clinical prognosis, survival time becoming in the classic pilocytic astrocytoma longer than in high-grade astrocytomas characterized by necrosis, hemorrhage and mitosis.

References

1. Bray PF, Carter S, Taveras JM (1958) Brain stem tumors in children. Neurology (NY) 8:1–7
2. Fasano VA, Lombard GF, Ponzio RM (1983) Preliminary experiences with the use of three lasers (CO_2, Nd:YAG, Argon) in some posterior fossa tumors in childhood. Child's Brain 10:26–38
3. Hoffman HJ, Becker L, Craven MA (1980) A clinically and pathologically distinct group of benign brain stem gliomas. Neurosurgery 7:243–248
4. Lassiter KRL, Alexander E jr, Davis CH jr, Kelly DL jr (1971) Surgical treatment of brain stem gliomas. J Neurosurg 34:719–725
5. Matson DD (1968) Neurosurgery of infancy and childhood, 2nd ed. Charles C. Thomas, Springfield, Ill, pp 469–477
6. Milhorat TH (1975) Pontine glioma. JAMA 232:595–596
7. Pool JL (1968) Gliomas in the region of the brain stem. J Neurosurg 29:164–167
8. Reigel DH, Scarff TB, Woodford JE (1979) Biopsy of pediatric brain stem tumors. Child's Brain 5:329–340

Posterior Fossa: IV Ventricle, Clivus, Foramen Magnum

The Removal of the Petrous Pyramid to Improve Neurosurgical Access to the Brain Stem

J. HELMS and K. SCHÜRMANN, Mainz/FRG

The removal of tumors at the brain stem below the level of the tentorium is mainly achieved by the suboccipital approach. This procedure involves at least some pressure against the cerebellum and the brain stem.

Extensive tumors in this region frequently cause damage of the labyrinthine nerves, with loss of hearing and sometimes vestibular function. The facial nerve and the vagus nerve group remain functionally intact over a longer period of time.

The appropriate surgery aims at avoiding additional damage and preserving the remaining nervous function where possible.

During the last 8 years of continuous collaboration with the neurosurgical department of our university this aim was achieved. The removal of greater parts of the temporal bone and pyramid including the labyrinth made this possible.

The surgical team work with extended temporal bone resection included 7 meningiomas, 3 chondromas, 3 glomus tumors, 1 cholesterol granuloma and 1 aneurysmatic bone cyst of the pyramid protruding into the cerebellum.

Independent oto-neurosurgical collaboration [2] has led simultaneously to similar ideas in the Pittsburgh Group as Dr. Sekhar [3] illustrated during the last international conference on Skull Base Surgery in Mainz, 1984.

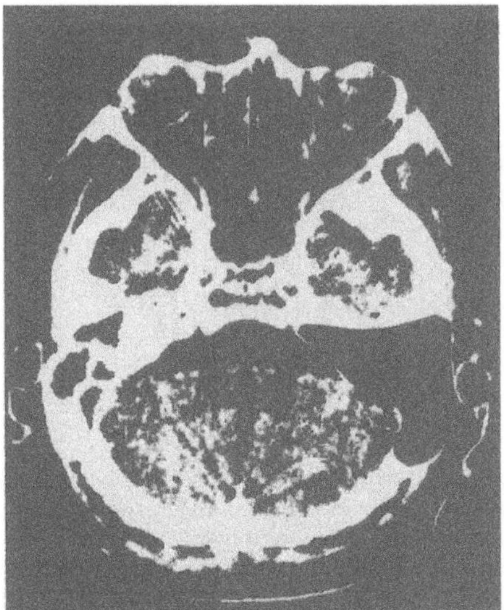

Fig. 1. Principles of pyramid removal to improve neurosurgical access to the brain stem. The pyramid area of a normal CT of the skull was darkened to demonstrate the effect of the surgery

The principles of the intervention are described in Fig. 1 and technical details in Figs. 2 a–d.

If possible a one stage combined neck-neuro- and otosurgical intervention is performed for removal of tumors at the area of the tip of the pyramid. If facial function is still present the nerve is transposed anteriorly to enlarge access to the deep parts of the temporal bone (Fisch and Pillsbury [1]). In the new position it runs from the geniculate ganglion over the Eustachian tube, medial and posterior aspect of the mandibular joint to the parotid gland. The outer ear canal, middle ear and labyrinth are removed until the internal auditory meatus is reached.

The superior petrosal nerve is dissected at the geniculate ganglion and the facial nerve may be placed downwards to the jugular bulb and the floor of the pyramid. After slowly drilling the bone at the anterior area of the pyramid the internal carotid artery is identified in its vertical and horizontal part and the tip of the pyramid is

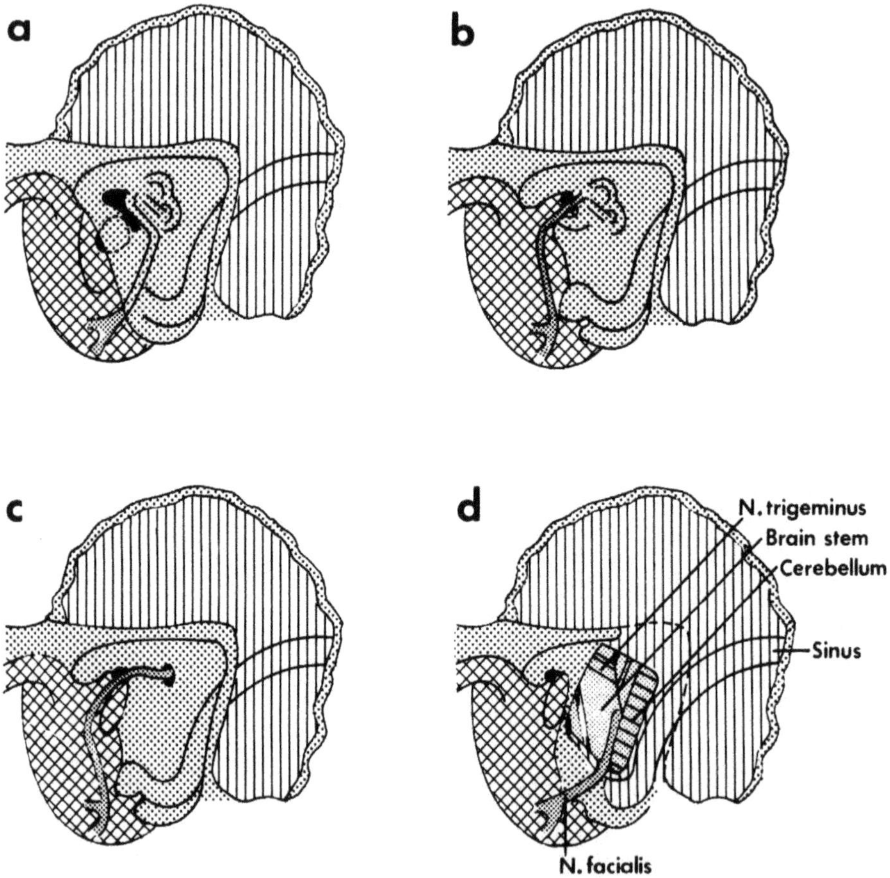

Fig. 2a–d. Lateral aspect of pyramid removal operation. **a** Initial situation. **b** The facial nerve is dislocated anteriorly. **c** The labyrinth is removed and only thin bone is covering the roof and the posterior wall of the pyramid. **d** The bone at the roof and the posterior wall of pyramid has been removed and the dura is opened. The facial nerve is positioned downwards to give access to the tip of the pyramid

removed posterior to the foramen lacerum. The roof and the posterior wall of the pyramid are thinned out by diamond burr drilling so that only paper like bone remains on the dura, at least at the area of the sinuses.

The neurosurgeon, who takes over when this stage of the intervention is achieved, is thus able to identify the necessary anatomic landmarks without distortion of the soft tissues. As required in each specific case he will ligate the sinuses, open the dura thus obtaining an improved access from an anteriorly rotated angle to the brain stem.

The basic principles of these interventions for the removal of extended diseases in the pyramid were worked out by Denecke [4].

References

1. Fisch U, Pillsbury HC (1979) Infratemporal fossa approach to lesions in the temporal bone and base of the skull. Arch Otolaryngol 105:99–107
2. Helms J, Schürmann K (1984) Interdisciplinary approach to benign tumors of the lateral skull base. Int. Congr. Skull Base, Mainz, 1984
3. Sekhar N, Samii M (1984) Petroclival meningiomas. Int. Congr. Skull Base, Mainz, 1984
4. Denecke HJ (1966) Chirurgie der Erkrankungen in der Felsenbeinpyramide unter Berücksichtigung der horizontalen Anteile der A. carotis int. Arch Ohr-Nas-Heilk 187:656

The Posterolateral Approach to the Foramen Magnum

A. PERNECZKY, Vienna/Austria

Introduction

The region of the foramen magnum creates a number of diagnostic problems since processes located in this region are easily misjudged for a considerable variety of atypical symptoms (Symonds and Meadows 1937; Rubenstein 1938). Mostly, the morphologic diagnosis provides the expected clarification only when a process of the foramen magnum has been localized by the clinical examination (Margolis 1976). Surgery performed at the occipitocervical junction is a challenging task both from an anatomic and a functional point of view (Drake 1973). The present paper discusses the posterolateral approach to the foramen magnum.

Surgical and Anatomic Remarks

Processes dorsal or lateral to the medulla oblongata are approached via the suboccipital route with an additional laminectomy from C1. The surgical options are different if the target of surgical exposure is ventral to the medulla. In this case, three approaches may be selected:

1. transoral approach (Mullan et al. 1966; Sano et al. 1966; Sano 1973)
2. transcervical approach (Fox 1967, 1983; Stevenson et al. 1966)
3. dorsolateral approach (Koos et al. 1985)

The first two approaches are the most direct and at the same time shortest approaches to ventral extradural tumors. However, in the intradural dissection this does not afford the same overview of the anatomic structures as provided by the dorsolateral approach (Drake 1969; Fox 1983; Koos et al. 1985).

The dorsolateral approach must be performed as far lateral as possible, being the only way to avoid intraoperative retraction and compression of the brain stem. Accordingly, three key points have to be considered in the dissection:

1. Retromastoid craniotomy with opening of the foramen magnum in its dorsolateral quadrant
2. Drilling of the jugular tubercle
3. Exposure of the vertebral artery between C0 and C1.

In the following, the individual operative steps for the exposure of ventrally situated processes of the foramen magnum are described.

1. *Patient's position:* sitting or semi-sitting or modified parkbench position.
2. *The skin incision* is an extension of that skin incision we use in the exposure of the cerebellopontine angle. The extension line courses along the border of the trapezius up to the level of C2 (Fig. 1).
3. The muscle layers are mainly severed in the directions of the fibers (Lang and Wachsmuth 1979) (trapezius muscle, splenius muscle of head and neck). This causes no functional impairment of the muscles after closure of the wound.
4. The exposure of the bony structures, aside from the exposure of the retromastoid region, also includes dissection of the ipsilateral portion of the posterior arch of the atlas, of the atlanto-occipital joint as well as the ipsilateral lamina of C2. This allows visualization of the posterior atlanto-occipital membranes and of the extradural portion of the vertebral artery between C0 and C1. Removal of the exposed portion of the arch of the atlas is rarely required.
5. The craniotomy is performed retromastoidly so as to remove the posterior lateral circumference of the foramen magnum as well. In doing so the border of the sigmoid sinus has to be followed in the direction of the jugular tubercle with a diamond drill before opening the dura (Fig. 2), since the bony prominence would obstruct the view of the ventral region of the foramen magnum. The opening of the foramen magnum is extended laterally only so far as not to hurt the atlanto-occipital joint.
6. The dural opening courses about 5 mm beside the border of the sigmoid sinus. Inferiorly, it courses dorsally past the point of passage of the vertebral artery. Here, dural arteries originating from the vertebral artery may be encountered. Suturing the lateral border of the dura to the periosteum may visualize the anterior foramen magnum region. The medial portion of the dura remains above the cerebellar hemisphere as a protective layer during surgery.
7. The ipsilateral tonsil of the cerebellum and the cerebellar hemisphere must be a little retracted, which affords a ventral view past the medulla oblongata.

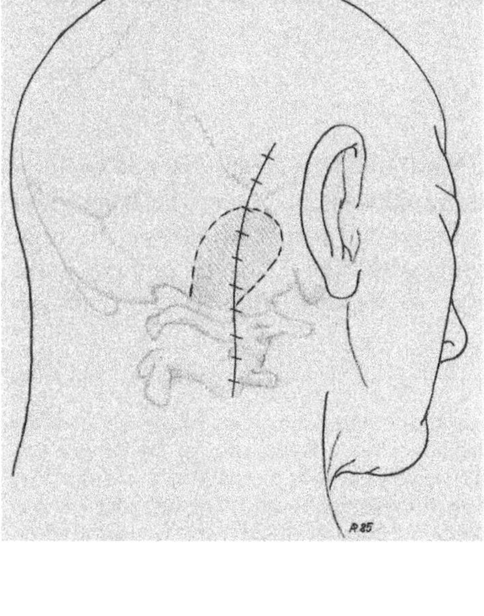

Fig. 1. Skin incision and area of craniotomy. Note the removal of the dorsolateral margin of the foramen magnum

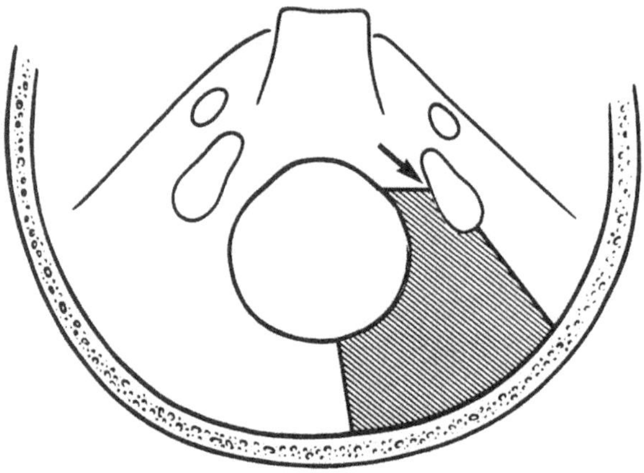

Fig. 2. Scheme demonstrating the extension of the craniotomy. Note the removal of the jugular tubercle (*arrow*)

According to the pathologic process, the choice of approach is different:

1. Ventral intradural space-occupying processes (mostly meningiomas, more rarely neurinomas, cholesteatomas etc.) (Yasuoka et al. 1978; Dodge et al. 1956) are approached from the side where the tumor mass is more pronounced. The described dorsolateral approach provides an excellent view from C1 to the dorsum sellae. During removal of the tumor ventral structures of the contralateral side become visible and may be dissected (Fig. 3). The displacement of the brain stem caused by the tumor eases the dissection, since additional retraction of the medulla is not necessary.
2. In ventral non space-occupying processes (mainly aneurysms of the vertebral artery or the vertebrobasilar junction), the process is exposed through the dorsolateral approach with an excellent overview of the surrounding anatomic structures. In aneurysms of the midline we choose the approach from the side where the vertebral artery is weaker (Fig. 4). The dissection is made intradurally along the vertebral artery up to the basilar artery. If the approach were from the side of the stronger-caliber vertebral artery, it would hide the aneurysm together with the basilar artery.

Conclusion and Summary

Processes of the foramen magnum located ventrally may be approached on three routes: the transoral, the transcervical and the dorsolateral route. The latter offers the best overview of the structures ventral to the brain stem. Due to the wide-angle view to caudal and rostral the region is overlooked from C1 to the pituitary stalk. Consequently, the following structures may be exposed through this approach (Table 1, Fig. 5).

Fig. 3 A–D. Meningioma of the ventral portion of the foramen magnum. Approach from the left side. **A** CT-scan demonstrates the large ventral tumor mass. **B** Elevation of the left cerebellar tonsil. The spinal portion of the accessory nerve is dislocated and expanded upward by the tumor. **C** After removal of the main tumor mass the left vertebral artery and the left hypoglossal nerve are prepared. **D** After total tumor removal one can see the opposite vertebral

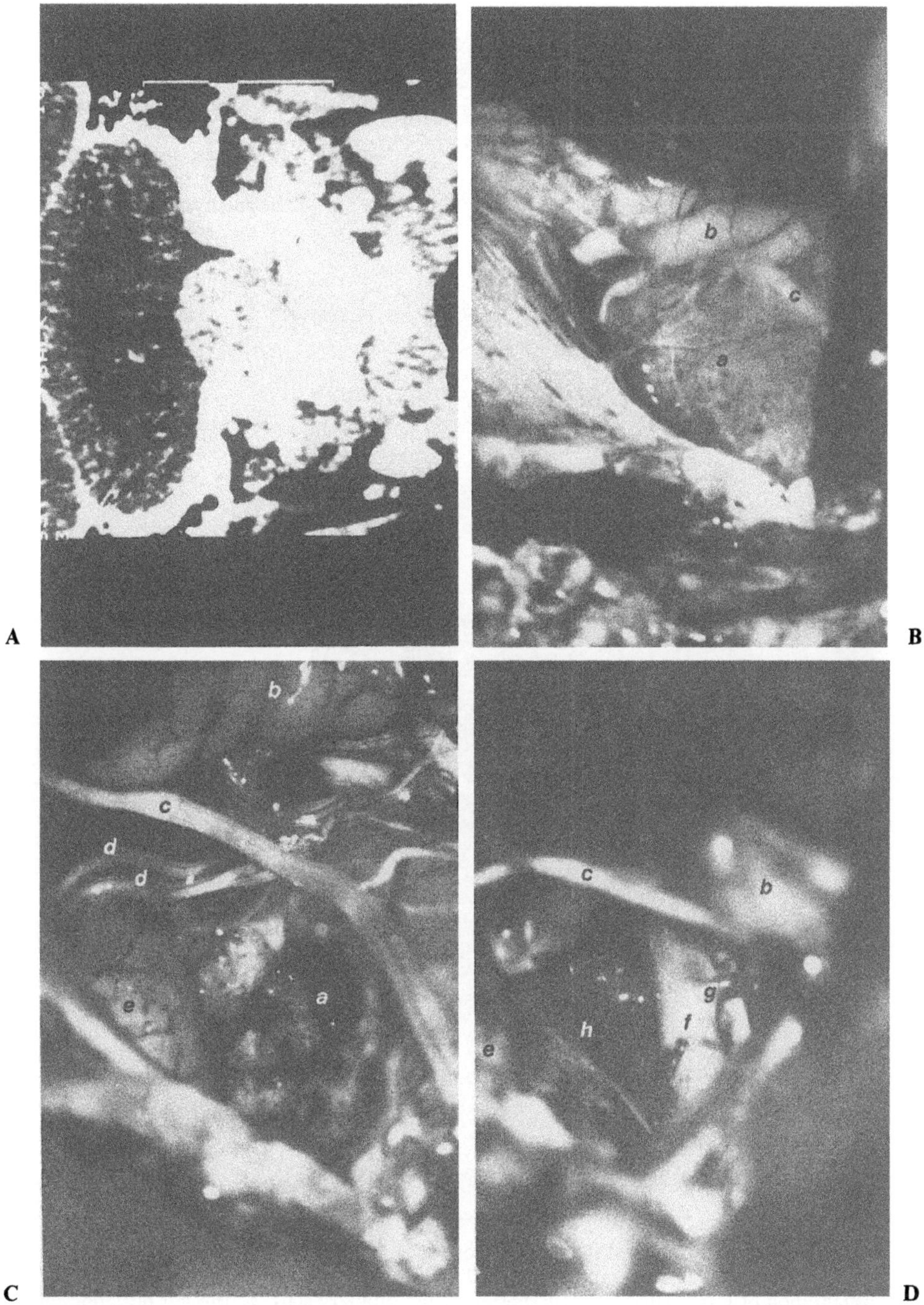

artery and the origin of the right PICA. *a* = Tumor, *b* = left cerebellar tonsil, *c* = spinal radix of the left accessory nerve, *d* = fibers of the left hypoglossal nerve, *e* = left vertebral artery, *f* = right vertebral artery, *g* = origin of the right PICA, *h* = anterior margin of the foramen magnum (tumor attachment)

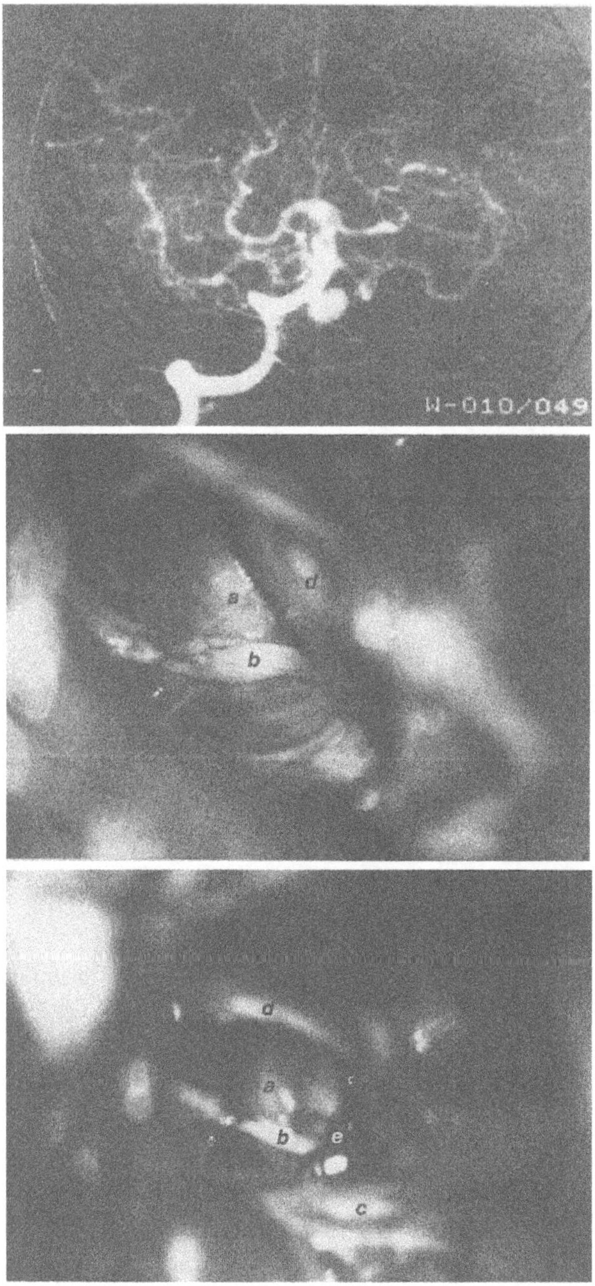

A

B

C

Fig. 4A–C. Aneurysm of the vertebrobasilar junction with dominant right vertebral artery. Approach from the left side. **A** Digital subtraction angiography, A-P view. **B** The left abducent nerve is adherent to the surface of the aneurysm. **C** After clipping of the aneurysm the abducent nerve is decompressed. *a* = aneurysm, *b* = left, abducent nerve, *c* = left glossopharyngeal and vagus nerves, *d* = brain stem, *e* = clip

Fig. 5A–D. Demonstration of the extensive overview by the dorsolateral approach to the foramen magnum. Approach from the right. Diagnosis: Cholesteatoma of the clivus region. **A** Visualization of tuber cinereum. **B** Exposure of the pituitary stalk. **C** The left posterior communicating artery and the left oculomotor nerve. **D** Overview of the vertebrobasilar junction. *a* = right vestibulocochlear and facial nerves, *b* = right trigeminal nerve, *c* = tuber cinereum, *d* = pituitary stalk, *e* = left optic tract, *f* = left posterior communicating artery, *g* = left oculomotor nerve, *h* = right abducent nerve, *j* = pons, *k* = medulla oblongata, *m* = basilar artery, *n* = right vertebral artery, *o* = left vertebral artery

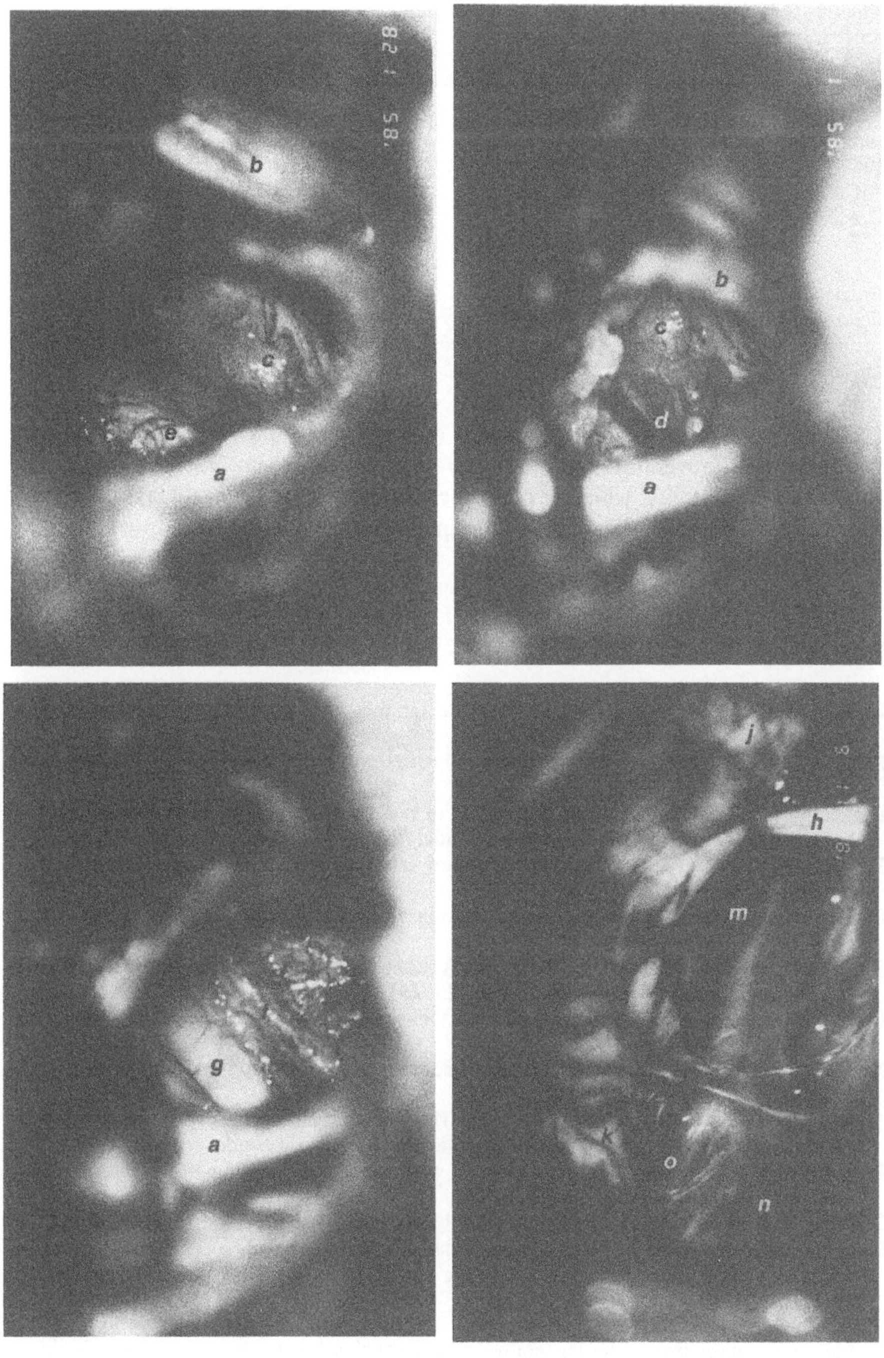

A B C D

Table 1. Structures exposed through the dorsolateral approach to the foramen magnum

Ipsilateral	Median	Contralateral
Vertebral a. (intra-extradural) PICA AICA Cranial nerves IV–XII	Basilar a. Clivus Tuber cinereum Pituitary stalk	Vertebral a. (intradural) PICA (origin) Cranial nerves III, VI (optic tract) Posterior communicating a.
Brain stem Ventrolateral		(posterior cerebral a.)

The drilling of the jugular tubercle is of particular importance for exposing the structures in the ventral region of the foramen magnum, aside from the retromastoid craniotomy, which is performed far lateral. Through the approach ventral intradural tumors as well as vascular malformations of the vertebrobasilar junction may be exposed.

References

Dodge HW Jr, Love JG, Gottlieb CM (1956) Benign tumors of the foramen magnum. Surgical considerations. J Neurosurg 13:603–617

Drake CG (1969) The surgical treatment of vertebral-basilar aneurysms. Clin Neurosurg 16:114–169

Drake CG (1973) Management of aneurysms of posterior circulation. In: Youmans JR (ed) Neurological Surgery, vol 2. Saunders, Philadelphia, pp 787–806

Fox JL (1967) Obliteration of midline vertebral artery aneurysm via basilar craniectomy. J Neurosurg 26:406–412

Fox JL (1983) Intracranial Aneurysms. Springer, Berlin Heidelberg New York Tokyo, pp 786–791

Koos WTH, Spetzler RF, Pendl G, Perneczky A, Lang J (1985) Color atlas of microneurosurgery. Thieme, Stuttgart New York, pp 118, 125–134

Lang J, Wachsmuth W (1979) Praktische Anatomie. Springer, Berlin Heidelberg New York, vol 1/B, S 309–430

Margolis MI (1976) A simple myelographic maneuver for the detection of mass lesions at the foramen magnum. Radiology 119:482–485

Mullan S, Naunton R, Hekmatpanah J (1966) The use of an anterior approach to ventrally located tumors in the foramen magnum and vertebral column. J Neurosurg 24:536–543

Rubenstein JE (1938) Astereognosis associated with tumors in the region of the foramen magnum. Arch Neurol Psychiatr 39:1016–1032

Sano K (1973) Aneurysms of the vertebral and basilar arteries. Neurol Surg (Tokyo) 1:193–199

Sano K, Jimbo M, Saito I (1966) Vertebro-basilar aneurysms with special reference to the transpharyngeal transclival approach to the basilar artery aneurysm. Brain Nerve (Tokyo) 18:1197–1203

Stevenson GC, Stoney RJ, Perkins R-K (1966) A transcervical transclival approach to the ventral surface of the brain stem for removal of a clivus chordoma. J Neurosurg 24:544–551

Symonds CP, Meadows SP (1937) Compression of the spinal cord in the neighborhood of the foramen magnum. Brain 60:52–84

Yasuoka S, Okazaki H, Daube J (1978) Foramen magnum tumors: analysis of 57 cases of benign extramedullary tumors. J Neurosurg 49:828–838

The Transoral Surgical Approach to the Craniocervical Junction

M. N. Hadley and R. F. Spetzler, Phoenix, AZ/USA

Introduction

The transoral approach is the most direct surgical approach to anterior pathology of the lower clivus and the superior cervical spine. The approach is not new, yet its use has been limited by technical difficulty and concerns over inadequate exposure and postoperative complications. In recent years a number of surgeons have developed considerable experience with the approach and have reported their refined surgical techniques [3–5, 10, 11]. We find that with the use of [1] the McGraver retractor, [2] the operating microscope, [3] intraoperative radiography and, [4] intraoperative spinal cord and brain stem monitoring, a safe, reliable surgical procedure with minimal morbidity and mortality can be accomplished [4, 9, 10]. Our series of 20 patients with atlantoaxial or clival pathology treated surgically via the transoral route is summarized.

Clinical Material and Methods

Twenty patients aged 9 to 70 years (median 42 years) were treated surgically by the senior author (RFS) utilizing the transoral approach through the posterior pharyngeal wall. There were 7 males and 13 females.

Fifteen patients had pathology involving the axis-odontoid complex. Six of these had a severe degenerative disease due to rheumatoid arthritis, five had congenital craniovertebral junction anomalies and three patients had traumatic C-1–C-2 subluxation with an associated Type II odontoid fracture. The final patient had epidural compression from neoplastic replacement of the bodies of C-2 and C-3 from metastatic tumor (Table 1).

Five patients had other pathology at the level of the inferior clivus and/or anterior superior cervical spine. Three patients had extradural tumors (chordomas), one had an intradural epidermoid of the inferior clivus and one young male had a high anterior intradural cervical AVM with an associated pseudoaneurysm.

All patients were examined in detail and underwent extensive radiologic evaluation. All twenty patients were studied with plain radiographs, myelography and either AP and lateral tomography or computerized tomography of the posterior fossa and/or cervical spine. Seven patients had angiograms and three underwent three dimensional computerized tomography in an attempt to clearly define the extent of craniovertebral junction pathology. Two patients had Magnetic Resonance Imaging (MRI) studies which confirmed the clinical diagnosis of basilar invagination.

Table 1. Outline of pathology at the craniovertebral junction treated via transoral approach

Craniocervical junction pathology		
Odontoid pathology:	15	
Congenital		5
Rheumatoid arthritis		6
Traumatic C_{1-2} sublux.		3
Neoplasm C_2, C_3		1
Other Pathology:	5	
Extradural tumor		3
Intradural tumor		1
AVM with pseudoaneurysm		1
Total	20	

Surgical Approach

Following induction of general anesthesia, a flexible oral endotracheal tube is inserted. In the supine position, the patient's head is secured in a Mayfield fixation device, unless a preexisting Halo vest immobilizer is in use. A self-retaining McGraver three-ring retractor is inserted. This allows the tongue and endotracheal tube to be depressed caudally. Two red rubber catheters are inserted through the nostrils into the nasopharynx and sutured to the uvula. The uvula and soft palate are retracted into the nasopharynx by placing traction on the two rubber catheters and tying them to the McGraver apparatus. This combination of retraction affords a wide operative exposure of the posterior pharyngeal wall [4, 9, 10].

The patient's mouth and pharynx are prepared with iodine solution and the operating microscope with a 300 mm lens is brought into position. By using the tubercle of the axis as a landmark, a longitudinal midline incision is made through the posterior pharyngeal tissues (Fig. 1). For odontoid pathology the incision is made directly over the tubercle and extended approximately 2.5 cm superiorly and inferiorly. For pathology at the lower clivus, a more cephalad incision is made extending upward through the posterior wall of the nasopharynx. The soft tissues of the posterior pharynx are retracted laterally with traction sutures or a large lid retractor. The C-1-2 and C-2-3 interspaces may be defined utilizing intraoperative radiography.

A high speed drill is used to perform the bone work, either superiorly through the clivus or inferiorly at the bodies of C-1, C-2 or C-3. The depth of bone dissection can be clearly delineated by placing contrast material into the resected cavity and obtaining lateral, and if necessary, AP cervical radiographs. This technique allows an accurate estimate of the depth and width of bone removal. A fine diamond tip burr is used to resect the remaining cortical bone layer to expose the posterior longitudinal ligament, (dura at the clivus resection).

When performing this procedure for odontoid resection, we open the posterior longitudinal ligament if it is thick and calcified or if it does not bulge into the drill cavity following odontoid excision. The dura mater then assumes a more normal po-

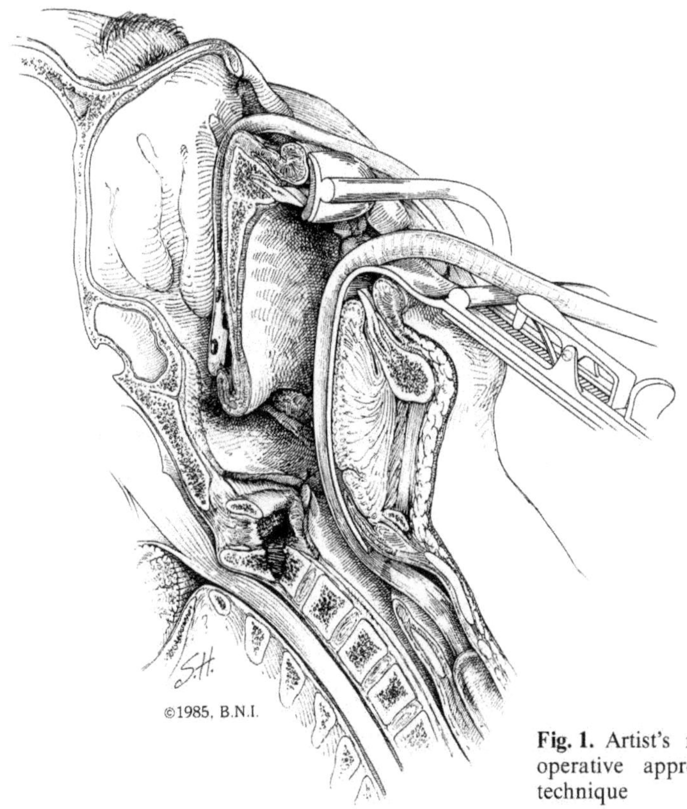

Fig. 1. Artist's representation of the operative approach and retraction technique

sition, a change which can be documented radiographically. The wound is irrigated with antibiotic solution and the posterior pharyngeal wall is closed in a single or double layer.

For tumor removal at the inferior clivus, this approach allows an extensive anterior exposure for excision or biopsy. With the utilization of microneurosurgical techniques, we have removed three clival chordomas without operative morbidity or mortality. For anterior intradural lesions, this exposure again is excellent. The transoral approach afforded a generous exposure to both an anterior epidermoid at the pontomedullary junction and an arteriovenous malformation with venous aneurysm at the C-2–C-3 level. The dura mater is incised in the midline, and following tumor removal or pseudoaneurysm clipping the dura mater is approximated with 6.0 nylon sutures when possible. Fascia lata is then placed over the dural closure and secured in place. The posterior pharyngeal wall tissues are closed. The difficulty in obtaining a water tight closure must be emphasized. The posterior pharyngeal wall adjacent to the sphenoid sinus is very thin and fragile, making a good closure difficult [6]. We are presently experimenting with a laser fused dural closure that appears promising in providing a water tight dural seal. A lumbar drain is inserted following any transoral-transdural procedure and spinal fluid is drained continuously to a level that keeps ICP at zero at the craniovertebral junction.

Somatosensory cortical evoked responses and brain stem auditory evoked potentials are recorded throughout these procedures. Computerized display screens are utilized intraoperatively to observe the minute-to-minute somatosensory cortical and brain stem auditory responses. A hard copy can be generated for comparison to previous recordings. All data are stored on digital cassettes for further analysis postoperatively.

Results

We performed 20 transoral-transclival surgical procedures on patients over an 8-year period (1977–1985).

Fourteen procedures were performed for odontoid resection (Figs. 2–4). Three transclival operations were for extradural tumor (chordoma), one was for an intradural tumor (epidermoid). One patient had debulking of extensive epidural metastatic tumor from C-2 and C-3 (Figs. 5–8) and the final patient had an intradural repair of a pseudoaneurysm associated with an AVM.

None of the eighteen patients with extradural pathology had a significant postoperative complication or death from their transoral procedure. [One patient died from a massive pulmonary embolus following a second surgical procedure to fully correct her craniocervical junction pathology performed six weeks after the initial transoral procedure] (Table 2).

Both patients who had intradural pathology died, one eight weeks and the other 6 months postoperatively. The first patient was a young male who bled from a C-2

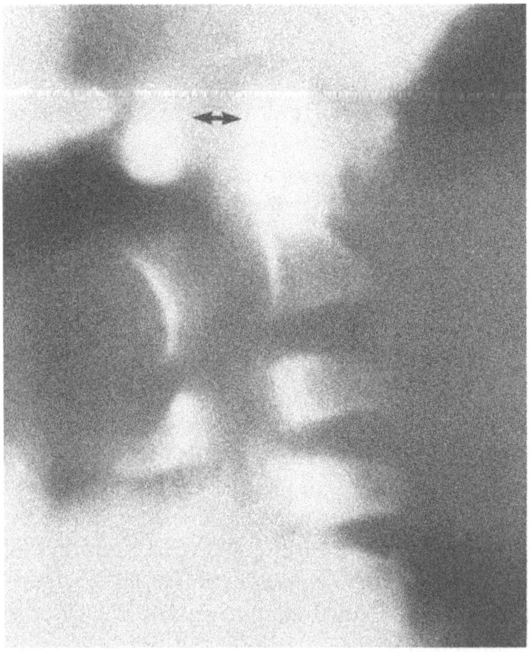

Fig. 2. Lateral tomogram of a young female patient with congenital abnormalities of the CVJ. Note marked narrowing of high cervical canal by the posteriorly displaced odontoid process (*black arrows*)

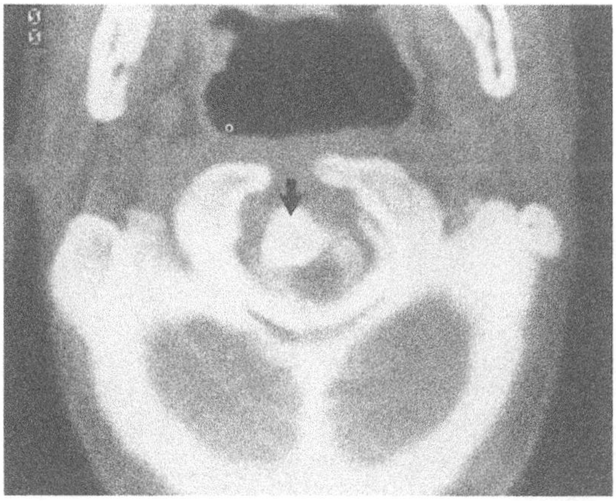

Fig. 3. Metrizamide CT scan demonstrating marked cervicomedullary compression by the posteriorly located odontoid (*black arrow*)

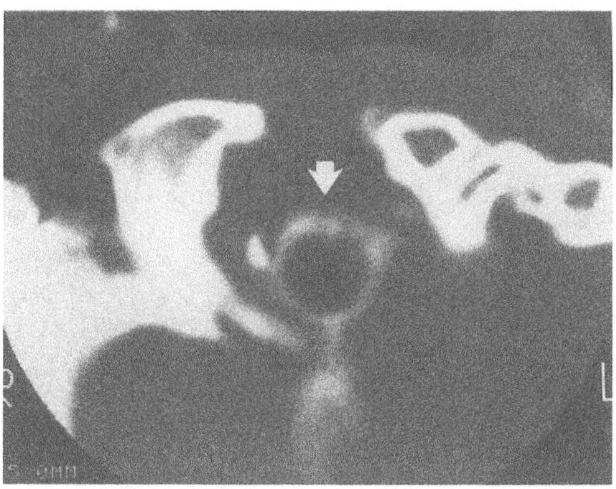

Fig. 4. Postoperative metrizamide CT scan demonstrating resection of the dens (*white arrow*) and elimination of cervicomedullary compression

Table 2. Outcome of twenty patients treated surgically via the transoral approach

Follow-up transoral approach	Morbidity	Mortality
Odontoid pathology:		
Congenital	0	0
Rheumatoid	0	0
Traumatic C_{1-2} sublux.	0	0
Neoplasm C_2, C_3	0	Pulmonary embolus 7 weeks
Other pathology:		
Extradural tumor	0	0
Intradural tumor	0	Brain infarction 6 months
AVM with pseudoaneurysm	Meningitis	Rupture of basilar mycotic aneurysm 8 weeks

(Median follow-up 3.0 years)

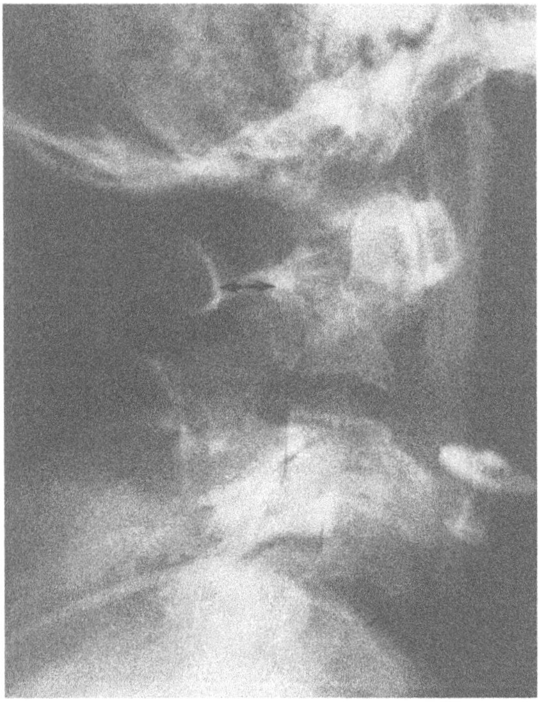

Fig. 5. Preoperative lateral radiograph in an elderly female demonstrating severe degeneration with multiple subluxations caused by neoplasm involving C-2 and C-3. Note narrow cervical canal at C-1-2 (*black arrows*)

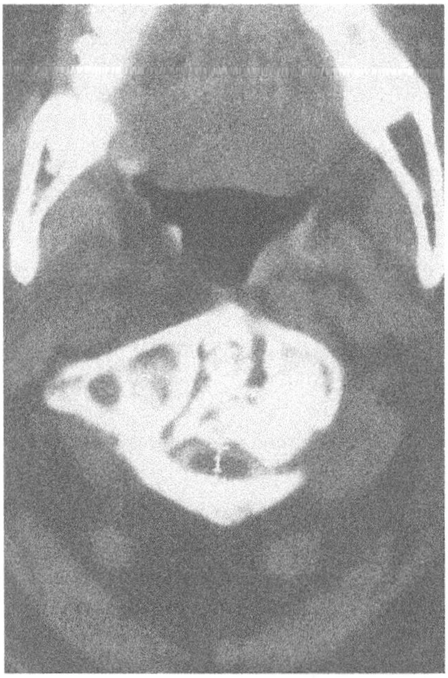

Fig. 6. Preoperative metrizamide CT study demonstrating compression of the cervical cord.

7 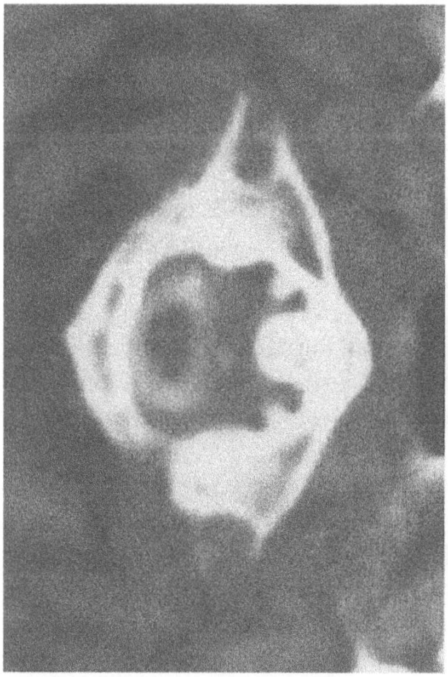 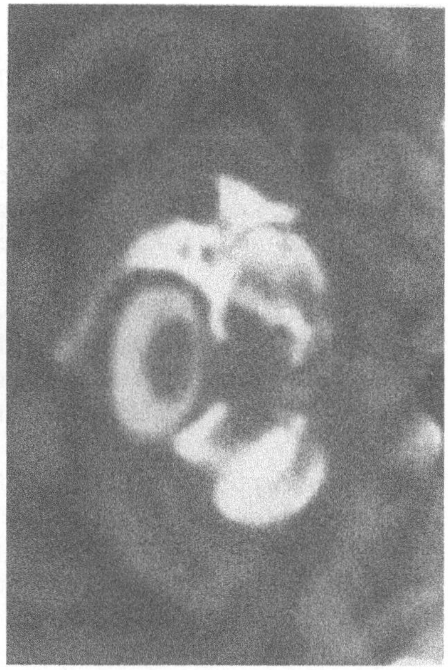 8

Figs. 7, 8. Postoperative metrizamide CT studies demonstrating decompression of the cervical cord after transoral debulking of the epidural metastatic tumor from the C-2 and C-3 levels. (This patient died from a massive pulmonary embolus 6 weeks later after a posterior fusion procedure)

level AVM. We repaired a large associated pseudoaneurysm via the transoral-transdural approach. He developed purulent meningitis without evidence of wound dehiscence and died 8 weeks postoperatively of a new mycotic basilar artery aneurysm which ruptured. The second patient (pontomedullary junction epidermoid) improved dramatically after tumor excision and brain stem decompression. Four months postoperatively she developed meningitis of unknown etiology. She did not develop a CSF leak or evidence of wound dehiscence and recovered with antibiotic therapy. Two months later (6 months following the initial surgery), she presented with significant brain stem dysfunction. CT scan revealed tumor recurrence with brain stem and cerebellar compression. A posterior fossa craniotomy was performed to debulk the tumor and relieve compression. She died one week later of massive brain stem infarction. At autopsy the dural closure was intact. There was no postmortem evidence of infection.

The surviving 17 patients have all shown improvement or stabilization of their preoperative neurologic deficits. The three patients with clival chordomas have received postoperative radiotherapy and are being followed regularly for signs of tumor recurrence.

Discussion

Several key points regarding the transoral surgical procedure need to be emphasized:

1. The choice of a surgical approach to the craniovertebral junction must be made carefully. Selection of the procedure or combination of procedures must be individualized to achieve the most beneficial result. In most cases the location of the pathology and the mechanism of brain stem or spinal cord compression is the influencing factor [1, 3, 5, 11]. Ventral craniovertebral junction (CVJ) pathology should be approached anteriorly; dorsal pathology is best treated from a posterior approach. If instability exists following decompression then a stabilization procedure with fusion should follow. A number of patients, particularly those with craniovertebral junction anomalies will require a combination of surgical approaches [5, 11].

2. In the past, significant morbidity and mortality have been reported following the transoral-transclival surgical procedure – factors which have limited its general acceptance and application. We believe that refinements in microneurosurgical techniques combined with proper retraction, intraoperative neurophysiologic monitoring and intraoperative radiography result in a safe and efficacious surgical procedure [4, 9, 10].

We routinely use a flexible oral endotracheal tube secured caudally by the McGraver 3-ring retractor. This combination, with the use of the red rubber catheters to retract the uvula and soft palate superiorly, provides a wide exposure of the posterior pharyngeal wall and obviates the need to perform a tracheostomy or split the mandible, tongue and palate. The endotracheal tube is left in place for at least 24 hours postoperatively to avoid potential respiratory compromise from glottic swelling. A tracheostomy tray is placed at the bedside following removal of the endotracheal tube as a precautionary measure, should respiratory compromise occur. We have had no airway complications in our series.

Somatosensory cortical and brain stem auditory potential recordings are sensitive intraoperative neurophysiological monitoring techniques when performing neurosurgical procedures of high risk [2, 4, 7–9, 10]. Our experience has demonstrated their predictive value in instances of potential spinal cord or brain stem injury and their correlation between observed intraoperative responses and clinical outcome.

The use of intraoperative radiography (both AP and lateral planes) is an important surgical adjunct [4, 9, 10]. The depth and width of bone dissection and decompression can be accurately assessed, particularly in combination with contrast material which is placed into the resection cavity. Intraoperative fluoroscopy can document the adequacy of spinal cord decompression by the degree of dural elevation following odontoid resection.

3. The integrity of the dura mater remains an obstacle and a challenge for the successful outcome of a transoral surgical procedure. In the eighteen procedures we performed for extradural pathology we had no significant morbidity and zero mortality. In each case the dura mater remained intact. Both patients on whom we performed transoral procedures for intradural pathology died: one eight weeks, the other six months following surgery. Both patients developed meningitis, one of

which occurred four months after surgery and was treated uneventfully. Neither patient had evidence of wound dehiscence. The dura mater was approximated with a primary closure in the young male patient, while a fascia lata patch was secured with both suture and glue in the woman with the brain stem epidermoid. She was treated for seven days following surgery with head elevation and CSF lumbar drainage.

While our experience is limited, we feel the transoral approach is a viable alternative in the treatment of intradural pathology at the lower clivus or anterior superior cervical spine. Best results can be obtained by using the surgical adjuncts and monitoring techniques outlined above with close attention to sterile microneurosurgical techniques. Meticulous closure of the dura mater and posterior pharyngeal wall with postoperative CSF decompression will result in proper wound healing. We believe further experience with intradural lesions and dural closure techniques will result in the refinement of the transoral approach for intradural pathology, reducing the operative morbidity and mortality to that experienced with extradural lesions.

References

1. Apuzzo MLJ, Weiss MH, Heiden JS (1978) Transoral exposure of the atlantoaxial region. Neurosurgery 3(2):201–207
2. Croft TJ, Brodkey JS, Nulsen FE (1972) Reversible spinal cord trauma: a model for electrical monitoring of spinal cord function. J Neurosurg 36:402–406
3. Di Lorenzo N, Fortuna A, Guidetti B (1982) Craniovertebral junction malformations. J Neurosurg 57:603–608
4. Masferrer R, Hadley MN, Bloomfield S, Spetzler RF (1985) Transoral microsurgical resection of the odontoid process. BNI Quart 1(3):34–40
5. Menezes AH, VanGilder JC, Graf CJ, McDonnell DE (1980) Craniocervical abnormalities: A comprehensive surgical approach. J Neurosurg 53:444–455
6. Mullan JF (1981) Comment: Combined transoral and median labiomandibular glossotomy approach to the upper cervical spine. Neurosurgery 8(6):674
7. Nash CL Jr, Brodky JS, Croft TJ (1972) (Abstract) A model for electrical monitoring of spinal cord function in scoliosis patients undergoing correction. J Bone Joint Surg [Am] 54:197
8. Owen MP, Brown RH, Spetzler RF, Nash CL Jr, Brodkey JS, Nulsen FE (1979) Excision of intramedullary arteriovenous malformation using intraoperative spinal cord monitoring. Surg Neurol 12:271–276
9. Selman WR, Spetzler RF, Brown R (1981) The use of intraoperative fluoroscopy and spinal cord monitoring for transoral microsurgical odontoid resection. Clin Orthop 154:51–56
10. Spetzler RF, Selman WR, Nash CL, Brown RH (1979) Transoral microsurgical odontoid resection and spinal cord monitoring. Spine 4(6):506–510
11. VanGilder JC, Menezes AH (1982) Craniovertebral abnormalities and their treatment. In: Schmiedek HH, Sweet WH (eds) Operative Neurosurgical Techniques. Grune and Stratton, New York

Transoral Surgery in Craniocervical Ventral Extradural Processes

E. Pásztor, J. Vajda, P. Piffkó, and I. Gádor, Budapest/Hungary

The number of publications advocating transoral approach in ventrally placed space-occupying processes of the craniocervical region has increased lately. Advantages of anterior transoral decompression of the clival and upper cervical region has been emphasized mostly in cases of extradurally localized lesions such as: i) in cases of craniocervical malformation with upwardly invaginated odontoid into the medulla at the level of foramen magnum and atlanto-axial dislocation (Pásztor et al. 1980; Menezes et al. 1980a, b; Di Lorenzo et al. 1982; Miller and Parent 1984). ii) in cases of odontoid fracture and antero-posterior dislocation with anterior compression of the cord (Spetzler et al. 1979; O'Laoire and Thomas 1982). iii) in some cases of inflammatory processes, mostly in rheumatoid arthritis and tuberculosis with bulbar and spinal cord lesion (Wang 1981; Fang et al. 1983; Menezes 1984; Crockard et al. 1985a, b). iv) in cases of extramedullary tumors of the clivus and upper cervical vertebrae (Wood et al. 1980; Delgado et al. 1981; O'Laoire and Thomas 1982; Pásztor et al. 1984).

The success of transoral surgery in extradural processes encouraged some authors to reconsider its possible role in cases of intradural lesions at the foramen magnum and clival region. Formerly it had been performed sporadically and then abandoned because of high incidence of postoperative infectious complications (CSF fistulas). Efforts have been made recently to make closure of the dura and other layers after clipping a basilar aneurysm or resection of an intradural tumor capable to prevent CSF leakage (Hayakawa et al. 1981; Litvak et al. 1981; Hitchcock and Cowie 1983; Crockard and Bradford 1985).

Surgery

Our microsurgical technique of transoral anterior decompression is described in detail elsewhere (Pásztor 1985).

Results

13 patients have been operated on by transoral route. Six were female, 7 male, the youngest 22 and the oldest 57 years of age.

Clinical data are summarized in Table 1.

Table 1. 13 cases

Sex	Age	Site of lesion	Duration of symptoms	Follow-up, length	
Basilar impression (4 cases)					
M	46	Odontoid	15 years	Excellent	7 yrs
F	41	Odontoid	8 years	Improved	2 yrs
F	44	Odontoid	4 years	Improved	1.5 yrs
F	34	Odontoid	4 years	Excellent	0.5 yr
Tumors (8 cases, 10 operations)					
M	29	Osteoblast C_{2-3}	5 years	Excellent died of other cause	5 yrs
M	27	Osteoblast odont. C_2	3 months	Excellent	5 yrs
M	41	Osteoblast odont. C_2	3 months	Excellent	3 yrs
F	27	Chordoma clivus	5 years	Improved died of tumor	2 yrs
F	57	Chordoma C_{2-4}	5 years	Excellent	3 yrs
	60	Chordoma recid		Died of pneumonia and meningitis	
M	46	Chordoma odont. clivus	2 years	Excellent	2 yrs
	48	Chordoma recid		Improved	1 yr
M	44	Chordoma clivus	5 months	Excellent	2 yrs
F	22	Ectopic nasopharynx thyroid adenoma	1 year	Excellent	3 yrs
Trauma (1 case)					
M	30	Odontoid fracture	1 month	Excellent	1 yr

Case Report

The history of the patient up to the recurrency of the chordoma is reported elsewhere (Pásztor et al. 1984). A 48-year-old man was operated on 2 years before recent admission because of difficulties in moving his tongue and pains in the nape of the neck. A mass of chordoma was removed apparently completely via transoral approach from the clivus and C_1–C_2 bodies. Postoperative epipharyngeal irradiation of 6000 cGy was instituted. The patient was symptom-free and back at work. He was readmitted in August 1983 because of nasal speech and reappearance of difficulty in swallowing. Examination revealed a mass intumescence into the nasopharynx mainly on the left, paresis of the left XIIth cranial nerve, mild nystagmus at horizontal gaze to the right and typical nasal speech.

CT showed tumorous hyperdensity in the left oral area of the posterior fossa and marked further destruction of the clivus which was also notable on cranial tomograms (Figs. 1, 2). Right retrograde brachial angiograms demonstrated invasion of an epipharyngeal space-occupying lesion into the posterior fossa (Fig. 3). A transoral reoperation was performed with retracheostomy. A double shifted retropharyngeal incision was used to explore the necrotic mass that was subsequently removed by suction. X-ray intraoperative control helped to estimate the depth of the surgical cavity close to the bulbar surface (Fig. 4). The postoperative period was uneventful.

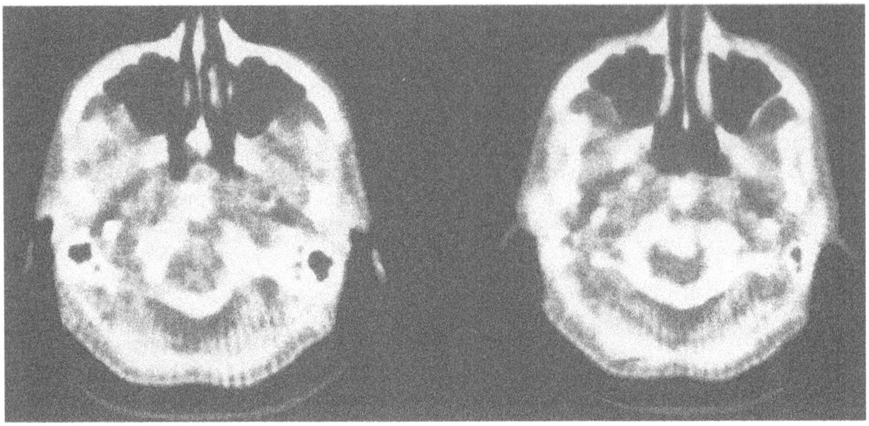

Fig. 1. CT scans at the level of the foramen magnum (*left*) and atlas (*right*) show penetrating destruction of the ventral part of the occipital bone and clivus on the right side and also massive destruction of the anterior arch of the atlas around the odontoid

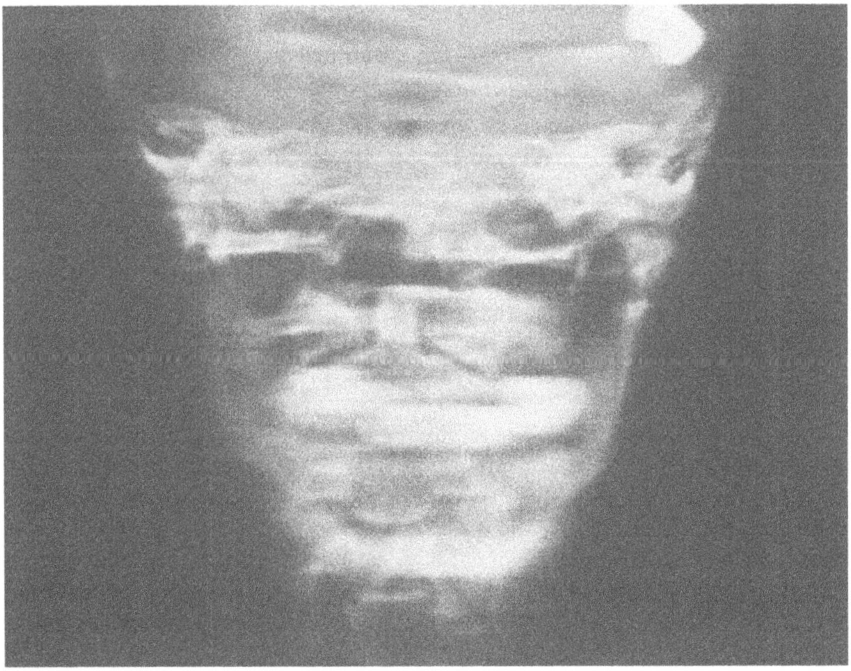

Fig. 2. AP tomogram of the craniocervical region demonstrates the disappearance of bony structure around the right side of the clivus

Fig. 3. Preoperative right retrograde brachial angiogram in lateral view shows an extreme dislocation of the proximal basilar artery and the vertebral junction. The chorioideal point of the fourth ventricle and vertebral artery are pushed backwards

Fig. 4. Intraoperative lateral X-ray film shows the surgical instrument touching the ventral dura at the foramen magnum once the tumor in front of it has been removed transorally

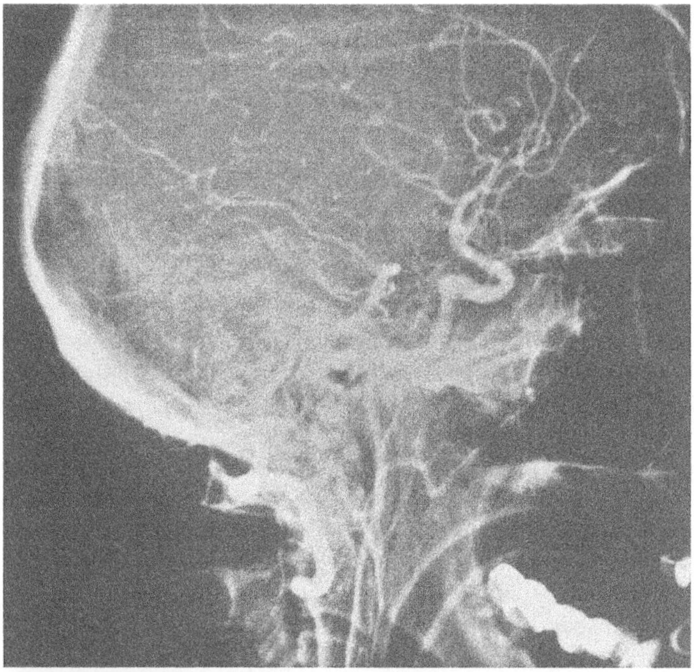

3

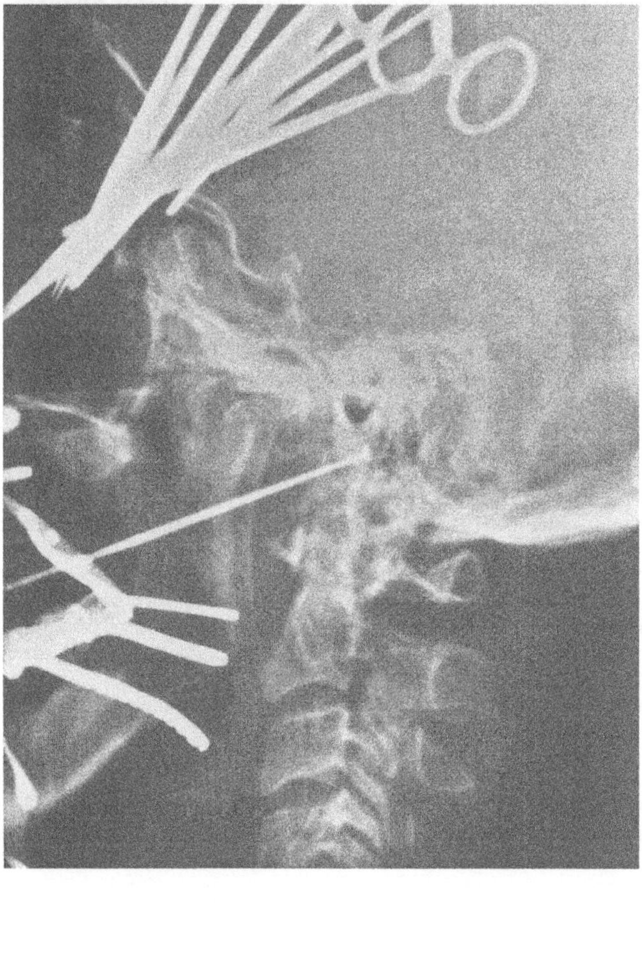

4

Perfect healing of wounds was observed. His symptoms were eased considerably. Second term of irradiation was commenced. He is doing well again and is back at work.

Discussion

We feel that our increasing experiences in transoral surgery for extradural craniocervical abnormalities, trauma, tumor are convincing in favor of this special kind of neurosurgical approach. Recent developments in the surgical technique has satisfactorily made it safe by achieving better wound-healing. Even in our two cases of transoral reoperation no difficulties in finding anatomic guides and layers were encountered and perfect wound-healing could be gained for the second time. Except for one clinically substantially deteriorated cachexic case of recurrent chordoma with postoperative meningitis without any sign of CSF accumulation or leakage, no complication of infection occurred. Method of incision and suturing retropharyngeal layers in parallel lines seems here of paramount importance. Surgery for intracranial chordomas is discouraging though, but with the aid of safe transoral approach recurrencies can be handled better for a longer period of time.

We also found internal bony autograft using even bits and pieces to fill tumorous cavity up for fixation rather valuable in our tumor cases where destruction of statically important spots might be put at risk. In this way shorter spells of inevitable immobilization can be achieved and better functional recovery can be expected.

With promising results of transoral surgery in different extradural craniocervical lesions we believe neurosurgeons are at a stage to make steps to apply its advantages again in intradural or even subarachnoid lesions.

References

1a. Crockard HA, Pozo P, Ransford A, Essigman W (1985) Transoral surgery for anterior cranio-cervical compression in rheumatoid arthritis. J Neurol Neurosurg Psychiatry (in press)
1b. Crockard A, Bradford R (1985) Transoral transclival removal of a schwannoma anterior to the craniocervical junction. J Neurosurg 62:293–295
2. Delgado TE, Garrido E, Harwick RD (1981) Labiomandibular, transoral approach to chordomas in the clivus and upper cervical spine. Neurosurgery 8:675–679
3. Di Lorenzo N, Fortuna A, Guidetti B (1982) Craniovertebral junction malformation. J Neurosurg 57:603–608
4. Fang D, Leon JCY, Fang HSY (1983) Tuberculosis of the upper cervical spine. J Bone Joint Surg [Br] 65:47–50
5. Hayakawa T, Kamikawa K, Ohmishi T, Yoshimine T (1981) Prevention of postoperative complications after a transoral transclival approach to basilar aneurysms. J Neurosurg 54:699–703
6. Hitchcock E, Cowie R (1983) Transoral-transclival clipping of a midline vertebral artery aneurysm. J Neurol Neurosurg Psychiatry 46:446–448
7. Litvak J, Summers TC, Barron JL, Fisher LS (1981) A successful approach to vertebrobasilar aneurysm. Technical note. J Neurosurg 55:491–494
8a. Menezes AH, Graf CJ, Hibri N (1980) Abnormalities of the cranio-vertebral junction with craniomedullary compression. Child's Brain 7:15–30

8b. Menezes AH, Van Gilder JC, Graf CJ, McDonell DE (1980) Craniocervical abnormalities. A comprehensive surgical approach. J Neurosurg 53:444–455
9. Menezes AH (1984) "Cranial settling" in rheumatoid arthrosis. Contemp Neurosurg 6, 16:1–8
10. Miller J, Parent AD (1984) Microscopic decompression of the anterior upper cervical spine: a case of odontoid malunion to the atlas. Neurosurgery 14:583–587
11. O'Laoire SA, Thomas DGT (1982) Transoral approach to the cervical spine: Report of four cases. J Neurol Neurosurg Psychiatry 45:60–63
12. Pásztor E, Vajda J, Piffkó P, Horváth M (1980) Transoral surgery in basilar impression. Surg Neurol 14:473–476
13. Pásztor E, Vajda J, Piffkó P, Horváth M, Gádor I (1984) Transoral surgery for craniocervical space-occupying processes. J Neurosurg 60:276–281
14. Pásztor E (1985) Transoral approach for ventral craniocervical pathological processes. In: Symon L (ed) Advances and technical standards in neurosurgery, vol 12, pp 125–170
15. Spetzler RF, Selman WR, Nash CL, Brown RH (1979) Transoral microsurgical odontoid resection and spinal cord monitoring. Spine 4:506–510
16. Wang LX (1981) Peroral focal debridement for treatment of tuberculosis of the atlas and axis. Chin J Orthop 1:207–209
17. Wood BG, Sader ES, Levine HL, Dohn DF, Tucker HM (1980) Surgical problems of the base of the skull: An interdisciplinary approach. Arch Otolaryngol 106:1–5

Posterior Fossa Transtentorial Route to Basal Perisellar Space-Occupying Lesions

P. C. Potthoff, Gelsenkirchen-Buer/FRG

Introduction

Access to perisellar basal space-occupying lesions via a lateral suboccipital and occipital approach through the posterior fossa has only recently been reevaluated by Symon (1982): "There is no approach which gives as extensive an exposure of the clivus from the posterior clinoids to the foramen magnum as this combined supra- and infratentorial exposure, ...".

This access is facilitated even more in such tumors that occupy the middle as well as the posterior fossa with unilateral extension through the tentorial hiatus to one cerebellopontine angle. With such an anatomic tumor extension, the tumor itself forms a trail for its systematic dissection and removal from behind in anterograde fashion.

Our own experience in five of such cases is presented.

Operative Technique

The patient is in a sitting or semi-sitting position. The head is fixed in a sharp head holder in straight forward direction. This orthograde head position is preferred for optimal three-plane spacial orientation along and above the skull base.

Skin incision is vertical, parietal to nuchal in generous extension, paramedian to the tumor side. Trephination is performed in the suboccipital region on the side of predominant tumor extension within the posterior fossa. Bone resection is enlarged across the transverse sinus to the occipital region. The dura is opened infratentorially, the transverse sinus is left intact. The transverse sinus may be divided and/or the occipital dura may be additionally opened later if necessary.

The microscope is applied. With self-retaining retractors, access is gained to the lateral posterior fossa and cerebellopontine angle. Tumor dissection is begun here and is facilitated especially with cystic space-occupying lesions. After the tentorium has been reached, it is divided generously. It has then to be decided if additional opening of the occipital dura or even additional division of the transverse sinus is necessary to gain sufficient exposure.

The tumor is followed through the tentorial incisura and resected in its lateral, basal and medial extension. Cranial nerves may be heavily distorted by the tumor and must be spared. The basilar artery and its ramifications may have close relations to the tumor and must be taken care of. Ascending tumor resection is now carried forward to the retroclival, retrosellar, perisellar, suprasellar, and diencephalic region with exposure of the circle of Willis up to the carotid syphon, of the pituitary stalk and the optic chiasm. The dissection of the contralateral carotid artery may be hindered to a certain extent by the hypophyseal stalk. Irregular tumor extension or its infiltration in the perisellar region may impede complete dissection and resection.

Case Reports

Five operated cases with different space-occupying lesions are tabulated with results in Table 1.

Table 1. Suboccipito-occipital combined transtentorial operations in five cases

Patient	Diagnosis	Operation	Result 1985
1. F. A. M 7 yrs	Arachnoidal cyst	Left side May 24, 1978	Visits special school, minor headache, dystaxia left side
2. T. A. F 55 yrs	Epidermoid	Left side Aug. 11, 1980	Died from postoperative hemorrhage Aug. 13, 1980
3. B. F. M 46 yrs	Meningioma	Right side Feb. 10, 1982	No deficit, working full time
4. St. E. F 15 yrs	Craniopharyngioma	Right side Aug. 26, 1982	No neurologic deficit, died 1 year postoperatively, infection + hypopituitarism
5. T. B. F 8 yrs	Craniopharyngioma	Right side Nov. 22, 1984	Well, with oculomotor and trochlear palsy right

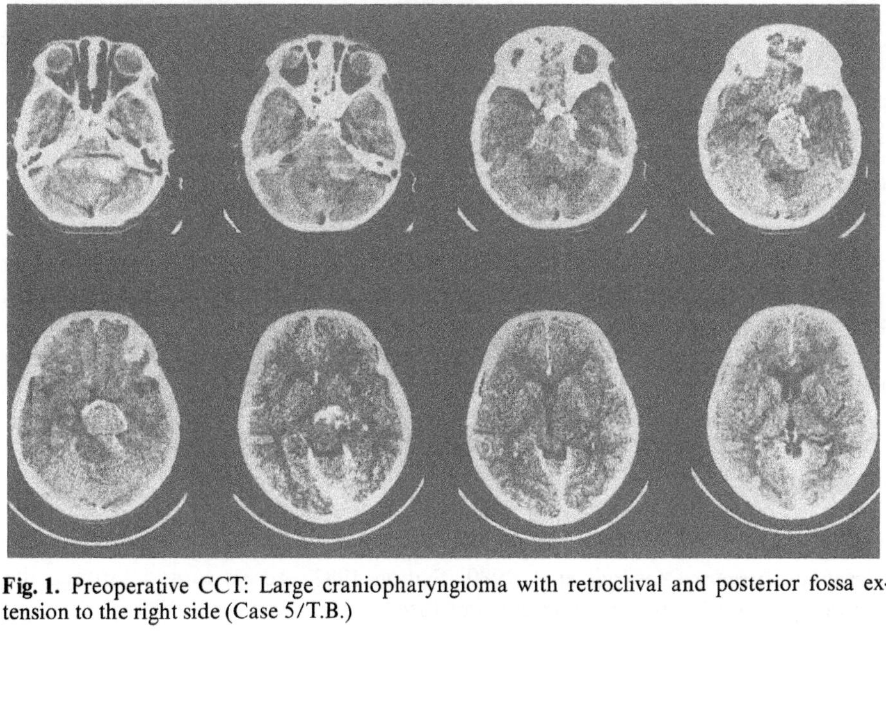

Fig. 1. Preoperative CCT: Large craniopharyngioma with retroclival and posterior fossa extension to the right side (Case 5/T.B.)

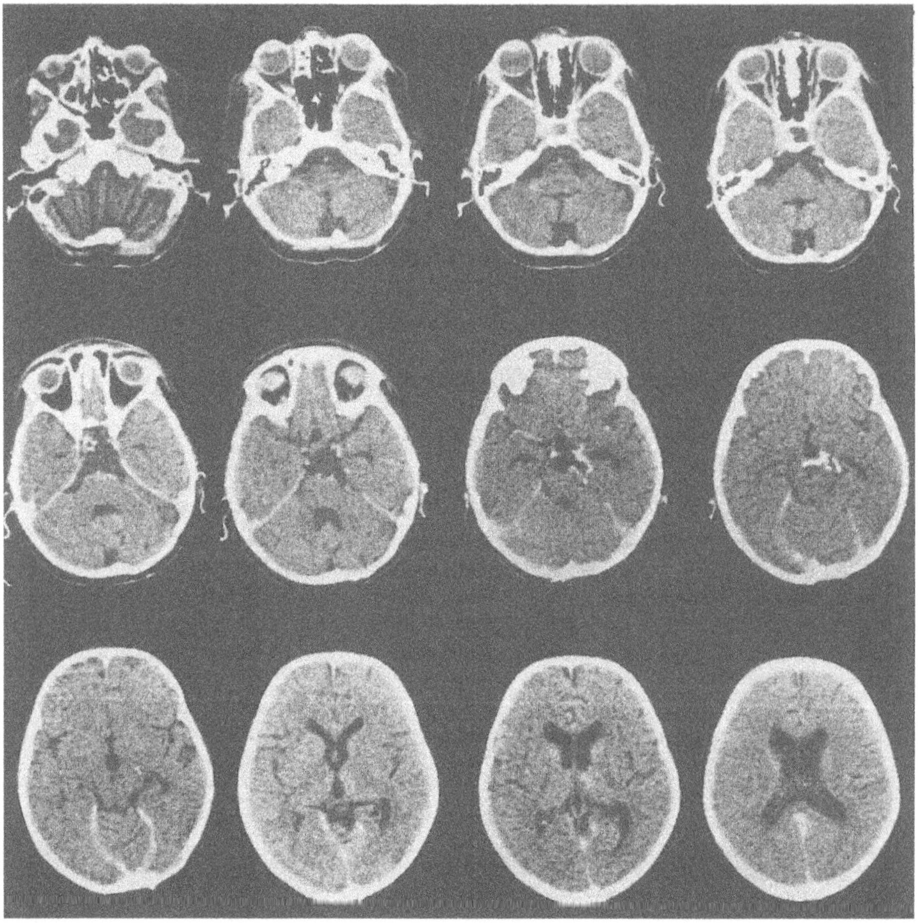

Fig. 2. Postoperative CCT after microneurosurgical subtotal removal via combined suboccipito-occipital transtentorial approach to same craniopharyngioma as Fig. 1: Basal, retroclival and perisellar parts completely resected, invasive calcified capsular remnants on the right side above tentorium (Case 5/T.B.)

In cases 1 and 5 subtotal, and in cases 2, 3 and 4 total resection was accomplished.

Figures 1 and 2 represent case 5 pre- and postoperatively, a case of giant craniopharyngioma.

Discussion

With increased anatomic knowledge (Ono et al. 1984) and improved techniques of microneurosurgery (Yasargil et al. 1980; Symon 1982), access to and through the tentorial incisura has become a safer procedure.

Table 2. Suggested advantages of posterior fossa transtentorial route to basal perisellar space-occupying lesions

Advantages
Posterior fossa transtentorial route to basal perisellar tumors extending to posterior fossa
1. With asymmetrical extension, ipsilateral cerebellopontine angle approach is facilitated.
2. Transtentorial tumor growth through the hiatus performs axis of anterograde resection –
3. – with exposition of brain stem and cranial nerves *in longitudinal direction.*
4. In cystic lesions, optimal *caudal* drainage decompression is achieved.
5. In multiloculated craniopharyngiomas optimal exposure and *resection of basal matrix* is possible.

Tumors that occupy the middle *and* the posterior fossa can be resected with optimal exposure from a combined suboccipital-occipital trephination by a transtentorial route.

Advantages of this technique are:

1. In tumors with club-like asymmetrical extension into the posterior fossa, exposure is facilitated from the ipsilateral cerebellopontine angle into which the tumor protrudes.
2. By its transtentorial extension, the tumor itself has performed a natural axis of anterograde resection that can be followed in straight posterior-anterior direction (Compare "petro-clival line", Yasargil et al. 1980). In this direction, tumor exposition is maximalized by tentorial splitting (and resection) on the side of predominant tumor extension. (Thus angulated tumor resection as from a subfrontal, pterional or subtemporal approach is avoided.)
3. On the same way, exposition of the brain stem and of cranial nerves on the predominant side of the asymmetrical tumor growth becomes possible *in longitudinal direction,* i.e. along their natural anatomic course. This facilitates their preparation considerably from brain stem origin to skull base foramina.
4. For cystic lesions an optimal caudal exposure and resection may be essential for optimal continuous caudal drainage decompression.
5. In multiloculated craniopharyngiomas the combined suboccipital-occipital transtentorial approach (not taken into consideration in the recent compilation of Konovalov 1981) appears the best way for exposure and resection of the basal matrix of such craniopharyngiomas in order to avoid early recurrent tumor growth and/or recurrent cyst formation.

Summary

In microneurosurgery, certain supra-perisellar/diencephalic space-occupying lesions at the skull base are probably best attacked via a combined suboccipital-occipital approach through the posterior fossa. This recommendation applies preferably to tumors occupying the middle as well as the posterior fossa with unilateral extension through the tentorial incisura to one cerebellopontine angle. Five operated cases (arachnoid cyst, epidermoid, meningioma, two craniopharyngiomas) are reported. The technique of the combined microneurosurgical operation via cerebellopontine angle, with tentorial splitting and with ascending basal tumor resection is described. The operation is performed in the sitting position. The main advantage is complete exposure of the brain stem and of cranial nerves on the side of the predominant asymmetrical tumor growth *in longitudinal direction,* i.e. along the natural anatomic course of these neurofunctionally important structures.

References

Konovalov AN (1981) Operative management of craniopharyngiomas. In: Krayenbühl H et al. (eds) Advances and technical standards in neurosurgery, vol 8. Springer, Wien New York, p 281–318

Ono M, Rhoton AL Jr, Barry M (1984) Microsurgical anatomy of the region of the tentorial incisura. J Neurosurg 60:365–399

Symon L (1982) Surgical approaches to the tentorial hiatus. In: Krayenbühl H et al. (eds) Advances and technical standards in neurosurgery, vol 9. Springer, Wien New York, p 69–112

Yaşargil MG, Mortara RW, Curcic M (1980) Meningiomas of basal posterior cranial fossa. In: Krayenbühl H et al. (eds) Advances and technical standards in neurosurgery, vol 7. Springer, Wien New York, p 3–115

Tumors of the Fourth Ventricle and the Aquaeductus

R. LORENZ, Frankfurt/FRG

A wide variety of special tumors can be observed in the fourth ventricle and the aquaeductus, arising from the floor, the peduncles or velum, the roof of the fourth ventricle or subependymally (Tsuboi et al. 1983; Wilcke 1984; Gökalp et al. 1981; Pascual-Castroviejo et al. 1982; Rosario et al. 1981). Others are not to be considered as tumors in a strict sense, as arachnoid cysts (Korosue et al. 1983) or hemangiomas (Kobayashi et al. 1984; Occhiogrosso et al. 1983).

The corresponding points of all these affections are the role of a certain space-occupying lesion and their tight connection to the aquaeductus and the fourth ventricle, allowing to speak about them as a group. Morphologically, these space-occupying lesions can either easily be isolated for instance as an angioblastoma or have to be carefully separated from the adjacent tissues as a spongioblastoma, arising from the posterior velum.

Material

In a 5-year period among 282 operations on the posterior fossa we have observed 20 space-occupying lesions of the fourth ventricle and the aquaeductus (Table 1), two thirds of the patients being under 25 years of age. These tumors could be differentiated in eight special histologic groups (most frequently spongioblastomas and medulloblastomas, followed by plexuspapillomas, ependymomas and microan-

Table 1. Age distribution and histologic classification of tumors of the fourth ventricle and the aquaeductus

Age (years)	No	–5	–10	–15	–20	–25	–30	–35	–40	–45	–50	–55	–60	–65
Medulloblastoma	4	2			1					1				
Spongioblastoma	4	2		1		1								
Plexuspapilloma	3								1		1			1
Ependymoma	3				1	2								
Microangioma with hematoma	3		1					1	1					
Angioblastoma	1							1						
Oligodendroglioma	1				1									
Epidermoid	1					1								
Total	20	4	1	1	3	4	–	2	2	1	1	–	–	1

Table 2. Origin of space-occupying lesions in the 4th ventricle and the aquaeduct

Ventral	2
Ventrolateral	5
Lateral	4
Dorsal	9
Total	20

giomas with capsuled hematoma). Their origin was mainly in the dorsal parts (anterior or posterior velum), 7 being located in the ventral region (Table 2).

Results

In all but two of them tumor resections were done (Table 3). In 8 cases a complete removal was possible, in 9 (mainly in medulloblastomas and spongioblastomas) only subtotal resection could be established. In 2 probe excisions were done, tumors being localized in the medulla and pons respectively.

We used a symmetric midline approach with a midline skin incision (18×) or a flap (2×). Positioning of the patient was: lying on the side, prone position or sitting, depending on the enlargement of ventricles, raised intracranial pressure, age and general condition (Luyendijk 1976). The point of preparation of the fourth ventricle differed corresponding to the size and the localization of the process. For the lower parts an approach through the Foramen Magendi with dissection of the posterior velum uni- or bilateral was used, for the upper parts and the aquaeductus an incision at the Pyramis-Uvula-point was done (Seeger 1980).

The final outcome (Table 4) as listed shows improvement in 12, no change in 5, impairment in 2 and death in 1 case. 14 patients (Table 5) had no or only slight neurologic deficit, in no sense being handicapped. 3 suffered from moderate symptoms, two needed help because of severe ataxia and discoordinations.

Table 3. Operative management

Operative procedures	No.	Tumor resection			Symptomatic (shunt procedure)
		Complete removal	Subtotal removal	Probe excision	
Medulloblastoma	4	–	4	–	–
Spongioblastoma	4	–	2	1	1
Plexuspapilloma	3	1	1	–	1
Ependymoma	3	2	1	–	–
Microangioma with hematoma	3	3	–	–	–
Angioblastoma	1	1	–	–	–
Oligodendroglioma	1	–	1	–	–
Epidermoid	1	1	–	–	–
Total	20	8	9	1	2

Table 4. Final outcome respecting the general result

Final outcome	No.	Improved	Unchanged	Impaired	Dead
Medulloblastoma	4	3	1	–	–
Spongioblastoma	4	2	2	–	–
Plexuspapilloma	3	2	–	1	–
Ependymoma	3	1	–	1	1
Microangioma with hematoma	3	1	2	–	–
Angioblastoma	1	1	–	–	–
Oligodendroglioma	1	1	–	–	–
Epidermoid	1	1	–	–	–
Total	20	12	5	2	1

Table 5. Final outcome respecting the detailed neurologic deficit

Final outcome	No.	Neurologic deficit					
		Without	Slight	Moder-ate	Severe	Needing help	Dead
Medulloblastoma	4	–	3	1	–	–	–
Spongioblastoma	4	–	4	–	–	–	–
Plexuspapilloma	3	–	1	1	–	1	–
Ependymoma	3	1	–	–	–	1	1
Microangioma with hematoma	3	–	3	–	–	–	–
Angioblastoma	1	–	1	–	–	–	–
Oligodendroglioma	1	–	–	1	–	–	–
Epidermoid	1	–	1	–	–	–	–
Total	20	1	13	3	–	2	1

Conclusions

Despite of the variety of histologic diagnosis (8 categories), these 20 patients have corresponding fates in the first period of management, depending on the correlations of the space-occupying lesion to the adjacent tissues and vessels. Preparation has to be done very carefully, stepwise reducing the size of the tumor in order to protect all vessels and functioning tissue of the brain stem and its junctions to the cerebellum. Especially in ventral or ventrolateral localization one has to act very cautiously. The patient who died from aspiration and the two patients needing help in my opinion are witnesses of this doctrine. Beyond the advantages of microneurosurgery and bipolar coagulation technique, ultrasonic surgical instruments and laser surgery will further improve the results.

Summary

Out of a total of 282 operations of processes in the posterior fossa within 5 years, in 20 patients space-occupying lesions of the fourth ventricle and the aquaeductus were found. They belong to 8 different histologic groups but are regarded as a corresponding group because of localization and their correlation to the adjacent tissue. The operative approach was via Foramen Magendi for the processes in the lower part or via Pyramis-Uvula-point for the upper region of the fourth ventricle and the aquaeductus. Prerequisition to operation is the very cautious (microsurgical) preparation of the tissues under strict protection of all vessels in order to avoid failures of treatment and impairment.

References

1. Gökalp HZ et al. (1981) A giant meningioma of the fourth ventricle associated with Sturge-Weber disease. Acta Neurochir (Wien) 57: 115–120
2. Kobayashi H, Kawano H, Ito H, Hayashi M, Yamamoto S (1984) Hemangioma calcificans in the fourth ventricle. Neurosurgery 14: 737–739
3. Korosue K, Tamaki N, Fujiwara K, Matsumoto S (1983) Arachnoid cyst of the fourth ventricle manifesting normal pressure hydrocephalus. Neurosurgery 12: 108–110
4. Luyendijk W (1976) The operative approach to the posterior fossa. In: Krayenbühl H (ed) Advances and technical standards in neurosurgery, vol 3. Springer, Wien New York, p 81–101
5. Occhiogrosso M, Carella A, D'Aprile P, Vailati G (1983) Brain-stem hemangioma calcificans. Case report. J Neurosurg 59: 150–152
6. Pascual-Castroviejo I et al. (1982) Choroid plexus papillomas of the fourth ventricle. Report of 3 cases. Child's Brain 9: 373–380
7. Rosario M et al. (1981) Epidermoid tumors involving the fourth ventricle. Neurosurgery 9: 9–13
8. Seeger W (1980) Microsurgery of the Brain. Anatomical and technical principles. Springer, Wien New York
9. Tsuboi K, Nose T, Maki Y (1983) Meningioma of the fourth ventricle: a case report. Neurosurgery 13: 163–166
10. Wilcke O (1984) Infratentorielle Tumoren. In: Dietz H, Umbach W, Wüllenweger R (eds) Klinische Neurochirurgie, Bd. II: Klinik und Therapie. Thieme, Stuttgart New York, p 130–165

Some Considerations on the Successful Total Extirpation of Hemangioblastoma Originating in the Medulla Oblongata – A Report of Two Cases

N. NAKAMURA, H. SEKINO, Y. TAGUCHI, and T. FUSE, Tokyo/Japan

Introduction

The vicinity of the calamus scriptorius and obex of the medulla oblongata is one of the commonest sites of hemangioblastoma. Complete excision of these tumors was, however, once considered extremely risky, unlike the removal of hemangioblastomas arising in the cerebellum.

The introduction of the surgical microscope has changed the surgical prospects for patients with brain stem hemangioblastomas, and several neurosurgeons have reported the successful total removal of these tumors. We recently operated on two patients with this tumor, and succeeded in total excision in both of them.

The purpose of our paper is to present these two cases and discuss briefly the problems we encountered during as well as immediately after the operation.

Report of Two Cases

The first case is a 42-year-old male who presented with numbness of all four extremities, predominantly on the right side. He also complained of dysphagia and dysarthria. All these symptoms had developed in sixteen months prior to admission.

On admission in April 1982, there was no choked disc, but a variety of neurologic deficits were observed which are summarized in Table 1.

A CT scan revealed low density mass, 2 cm in diameter, extending from the caudal vermis to the medulla oblongata. Enhancement was marked, and a small low

Table 1. Case history and neurological findings on admission

42-year-old male	
January 1981	Numbness in fingers of the right hand which gradually extended to the entire right side of the body.
January 1982	Dysphagia, dysarthria, hoarseness.
April 1982	Admitted Rt-V, IX, XI involvement Lt-VII, IX, X involvement Bilateral limb ataxia Bilateral sensory disorders below the 8th thorax level Bilateral exaggerated deep tendon reflexes No choked disc

density area was evident in front of the tumor mass. Vertebral angiography demonstrated a vascular tumor that was fed by both posterior inferior cerebellar arteries (Figs. 1, 2).

On May 18, 1982, a suboccipital craniotomy combined with laminectomy of the atlas was performed with the patient in a sitting position.

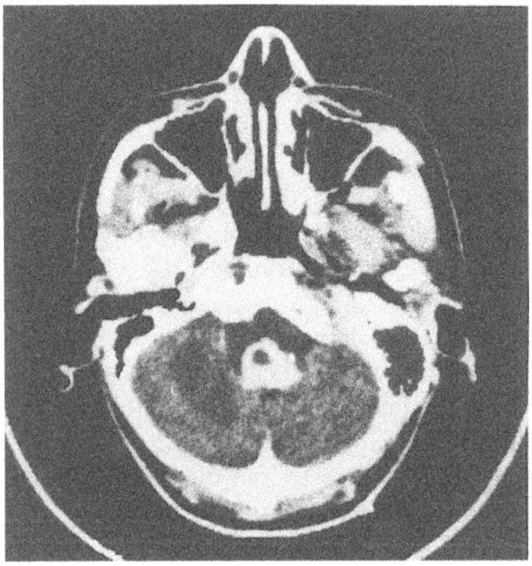

Fig. 1. Case 1. Computed tomogram showing a highly enhanced mass

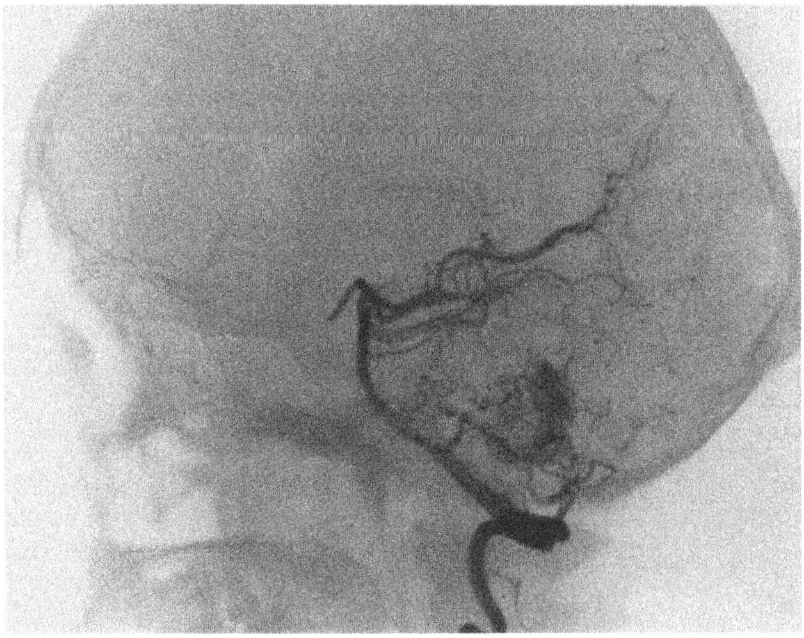

Fig. 2. Case 1. Vertebral angiogram showing a vascular tumor, fed by both posterior inferior cerebellar arteries

We incised the swollen vermis longitudinally and uncovered a chestnut-sized tumor, filling the fourth ventricle. One quarter of the tumor was buried in the caudal medulla.

With the aid of bipolar electrocoagulation instrument and a surgical microscope, we separated the tumor deliberately from the surrounding brain parenchyma without incident.

However, when we approached the obex, the patient experienced transient episodes of tachycardia and elevated blood pressure. Following enblock removal of the tumor the systolic pressure suddenly dropped to 60 mm Hg and dopamine and epinephrine were ineffective. We immediately closed the skull. Postoperative respiration rate was only five per minute, and blood pressure hypotension did not recover to normal until the fifth day.

A second case was a 41-year-old female who complained of numbness of the right arm, unsteady gait and repeated vomitings. The symptoms had progressed in six months prior to admission.

Neurologic findings on admission in June 1982 are shown on Table 2.

Table 2. Case history and neurologic findings on admission

41-year-old female	
January 1982	Difficulty in hand-writing and numbness of the right hand Unsteady gait and vomiting appeared and got worse gradually
June 1982	Admitted Lt-V involvement Bilateral limb ataxia Bilateral sensory disorders on both arms and legs. Lt-pyramidal sign No choked disc

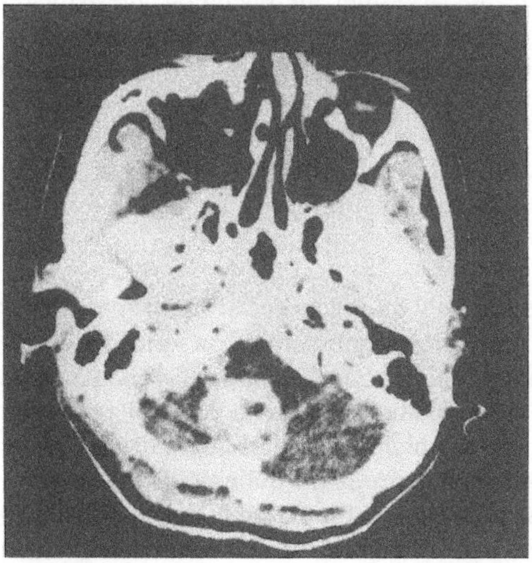

Fig. 3. Case 2. Computed tomogram showing a highly enhanced mass

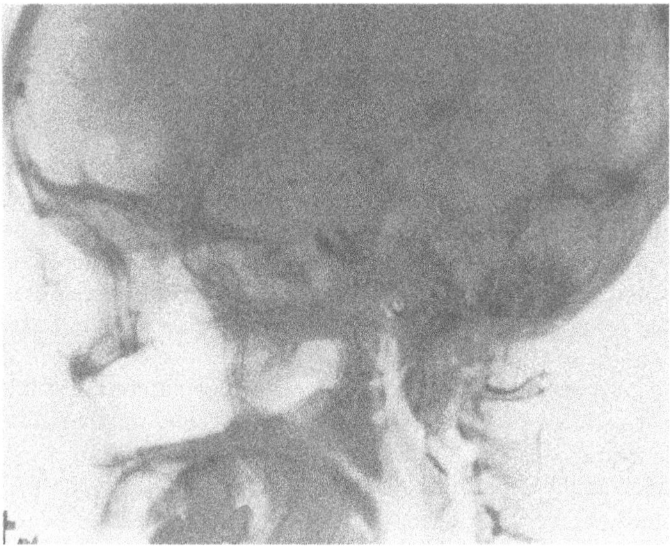

Fig. 4. Case 2. Vertebral angiogram showing heterogenous tumor staining

A CT scan revealed an isodensity tumor, 2.5 cm in diameter, which was located in the medial portion of the posterior margin of the foramen magnum. Vertebral angiography confirmed the presence of a vascular tumor fed bilaterally by the posterior inferior cerebellar arteries (Figs. 3, 4).

The patient underwent an operation on June 21. A chestnut-sized tumor originated in the caudal medulla, was compressing the tonsils bilaterally, and one fifth of the mass was buried in the medulla. The tumor margin was undefined on the caudal side and bradycardia occurred immediately when we attempted to excise this portion. Therefore, we left a small area of the tumor in place in the obex which was electrically cauterized. Not only during but also after the operation, the patient's blood pressure fluctuated significantly, with systolic pressure ranging from 80 to 100 mm Hg. The postoperative respiration was weak. These stormy responses stabilized within four days.

Discussion

Now we would like to focus the discussion only on the technical problem of tumor removal and the postoperative care for the cardiorespiratory storm immediately after surgery. To our knowledge, there have been reported 12 cases of successful total excision of hemangioblastoma arising in the medulla oblongata, including our own cases. Although all the described tumors are highly vascular, and surrounded by tangled arteries and veins, there are features that lessen the difficulty of this surgery. (Small cysts, gelatinous tissue or a clear tumor margin are usually not so difficult to separate from the brain stem parenchyma.) Therefore, if the surrounding blood vessels can be dissected by cauterization it is usually possible to remove the tumor clearly from the brain stem.

Unfortunately, successful excision of the tumor does not always lead to overall surgical success, since complications are frequent and serious. The tachycardia and bradycardia that often occur during the operation may subside if the procedure is suspended. The hypotension, however, is very difficult to control, both immediately and over the long term. Our experience suggests that continuous drip infusion of norepinephrine, phenylephrine or dopamine, plus regulation of respiration is likely to restore normal blood pressure within several days.

The largest postoperative problem is maintenance of respiration, which necessitates mechanical control or assistance for more than several days.

As for our two patients, the breathing was stabilized on the fifth postoperative day in both of them but sleep apnea persisted for about one month in the first case.

In summary it must be stressed that the most important factor in the patient's recovery appears to be avoidance of injury to the brain stem parenchyma.

Summary

Hemangioblastomas of the medulla oblongata were successfully excised in two cases.

The cardiorespiratory complications were the largest problems during as well as immediately after the operation. The most important factor in the patient's recovery appears to be avoidance of injury to the brain stem parenchyma, even though a microsurgical technique has made a great progress in the tumor removal.

Indications for Posterior Fossa Surgery in Syringomyelia

R. VAN DEN BERGH, Leuven/Belgium

In spite of numerous studies dedicated to syringomyelia, and in spite of important results of neurosurgical therapy, there still remain many doubts about the diagnostic and therapeutic management of this disease.

Specifically, the benefit of posterior fossa operations has recently been questioned after many years of claimed success.

On the basis of our own experience of the last twenty years, I would like to summarize the present neurosurgical possibilities, the doubts about posterior fossa surgery and the remaining undisputable indications for posterior fossa surgery.

1. Neurosurgical Possibilities

Originally and for a long time, the neurosurgical therapy was limited to myelotomy with syringostomy, fistulization or marsupialization (Elsberg 1916; Puusepp 1926). After the publication by Gardner of a series of 74 cases in 1965, posterior fossa operations, which previously were applied mostly in cases of arachnoiditis and of Arnold-Chiari malformation, were generalized. In the late sixties this technique expanded quickly (Newton 1969; Conway 1967; Hankinson 1970).

Because of a certain mortality and morbidity and because of a number of recurrences after posterior fossa surgery other types of operation were soon proposed. Gardner himself switched to terminal ventriculostomy, which in fact is a form of myelotomy and consists of an excision of the filum terminale and the tip of the conus terminalis (Gardner et al. 1977). Many neurosurgeons including Krayenbühl and Benini (1969, 1971) proceeded to ventriculocardial or ventriculoperitoneal shunting. Others, however, taking advantage of new and more inert materials, returned to the use of one or other variation of syringostomy, for example the syringosubarachnoidal shunt (Tator et al. 1982). More recently the syringoperitoneal shunt was added to the range of possibilities (Phillips and Kindt 1981; Pecker et al. 1983).

2. Doubts About Posterior Fossa Operations

Why are posterior fossa operations less often applied during the last years? The hydrodynamic theory of Gardner (1965), which originally was well accepted, postulates a failure of normal perforation of the rombic roof leading to a persistence of the central canal of the spinal cord in communication with the ventricular system.

The block of the fourth ventricle is believed to be responsible for a variable degree of hydrocephalus and Arnold-Chiari malformation with low position of the tonsillae cerebelli. The arterial pulsations of the choroid plexus should give rise to a dilatation of the central canal, eventually leading to hydromyelia and syringomyelia.

Williams (1969, 1970) believes that the force, which leads to the dilatation of the central canal, originates from the liquor movements, due to the sudden expansions of the spinal epidural venous plexus caused by coughing, straining, etc. He and also other authors (Williams 1977; Newman et al. 1981) think that a traumatic birth plays a determining role in the provocation of syringomyelia in individuals with the malformations mentioned.

After years, it became clear that Gardner's ideas did not fit reality in many cases. Often there is no block at all of the IVth ventricle and furthermore collapsing cysts are not always connected with the ventricular system. Aboulker (1979) argued in an ample report for an alternative explanation of the pathogenesis of syringomyelia. Together with other authors such as Ball and Dayan (1972), he believes that syringomyelic cavities can be filled from the perimedullar subarachnoidal space either by small clefts and breaches along the dorsal roots or via the perivascular Virchow-Robin spaces. Doubts about the theoretical basis of Gardner's operation as well as rather poor results and some disadvantages brought about a growing defection from posterior fossa operations. In a remarkable "critical appraisal of posterior fossa surgery for communicating syringomyelia", Williams (1978) incriminated the following possible complications: worsening of neurologic deficit, exacerbation or even beginning of hydrocephalus, prolapse of the cerebellar hemispheres through the occipital decompression with, as consequence, a renewed occlusion of the fourth ventricle.

3. Remaining Indications for Posterior Fossa Surgery

In spite of several doubts and objections, we are still convinced that a number of indications for posterior fossa surgery remain indisputable. The decision has to be based upon a complete clinical, neuroradiological and when necessary scintigraphic exploration. In a number of cases posterior fossa surgery is absolutely requested. In other cases it is completely illogical. The applied technique must be the golden mean.

Between 1964 and 1984, 113 patients with syringomyelia were admitted to our department. 19 patients underwent a posterior fossa operation. The result was very good in 9 cases. There was no mortality.

a) Preparatory Investigations

The clinical examination has to show a typical but not necessarily complete syringomyelia syndrome, with lower motor neurone deficit, absent tendon reflexes and thermoanalgesia in one or both upper limbs. A Horner's syndrome, perspiration dysfunction and brain stem signs can be seen. Combination of the suspended cervical cord signs with early pyramidal signs in the lower limbs is an important finding pleading for a communicating syringomyelia, which we consider to be a hydrosyringomyelia.

A complete neuroradiologic work up is strictly necessary and has to be made in a logical sequence.

Plain X-rays examination of the skull and of the craniocervical junction can show typical anomalies.

A CT scan of the skull and of the cervical spine gives an idea of the ventricular system and may show anomalies in the posterior fossa and in the spinal cord. A progressive tomographic pneumoencephalomyelography is one of the most important examinations: it can indicate a collapsing cord and it shows the patency or a block of the IVth ventricle, with or without Arnold-Chiari malformation. Positive contrast myelography, followed by spinal cord CT scan is indicated when the former examination is not conclusive. Transmedullary opacification of a syrinx gives important information as well.

Positive contrast ventriculography is indicated if the pneumoencephalography has demonstrated a block of the IVth ventricle and/or tumorlike malformations of the posterior fossa. In this case a vertebralis angiography may be interesting, because of the possibility of the association of syringomyelia and vascular malformations in the posterior fossa.

Nuclear magnetic resonance gives important information about the extent of the spinal cord cyst.

Cisterno-scintigraphy is of great value in exploring the patency of the pericerebral subarachnoid space.

b) Formal Indications

We consider formal indications to be:

1. Complete occlusion of the fourth ventricle as proven by pneumoencephalomyelography and ventriculography; however, if there is an important degree of hydrocephalus, a trial with a ventriculo-atrial or ventriculo-peritoneal shunt may be considered.
2. Cystic or tumoral structure in the posterior fossa.
3. Arnold-Chiari malformation together with clinical signs of paroxysmal tonsillar herniation.

In the three indications the presence of a collapsing spinal cord cyst and the patency of the pericerebral subarachnoid spaces should be proven.

Case Reports

Case 1

A 25-year-old female presented with an acute weakness of the right upper limb and burning sensations in the right hemicorpus under C6. The clinical examination revealed an areflexia in the right upper limb, an anesthesia C3–C6 and a thermoanalgesia D5–D7 at the right side.

A progressive pneumoencephalomyelography showed a collapsing cyst in the cervical cord and passage of the lumbar injected air into the ventricular system. The fourth ventricle was slightly dilated and had an abnormal configuration. Ventriculography with metrizamide showed a cyst above the foramen magnum. A posterior fossa operation revealed an incomplete occlusion of the foramen Magendie, a low position of the tonsils and a cyst imprisoned in tight membranes. After the operation the complaints disappeared completely.

Case 2

A 28-year-old male complained of an uncertain feeling in the lower limbs, and of severe occipitonuchal pain attacks after coughing, straining and laughing, as typically seen in paroxysmal tonsillar herniation with craniospinal pressure dissociation. Clinically we noticed a complete areflexia and a hypo-esthesia C2–C3. The plain radiographs showed a malformation with occipitalization of an asymmetrical atlas.

Air myelography showed a collapsing cord with Arnold-Chiari malformation and occlusion of the fourth ventricle. CT scan and NMR confirmed this intramedullary cyst. A metrizamide ventriculography showed a low position of the fourth ventricle and a minimal patency of the foramen Magendie. A posterior fossa operation revealed a spina bifida with unilateral left side occipitalization of C1, an extreme low position of the tonsils and a severe degree of occlusion of the foramen Magendie. After the operation the complaints disappeared completely.

c) Contra-Indications

We consider contra-indications to be:

1. Collapsing cyst, without Arnold-Chiari malformation and with an easy passage of air in a ventricular system with a normal configuration.
2. Syringomyelia after thoraco-lumbar spinal injury.

In the former case we usually did not intervene at all. In the latter case a syringoperitoneal or a spinoperitoneal shunt is most logical, because the cyst is most likely produced by cerebrospinal fluid penetrating from the perimedullar subarachnoid space.

d) Operative Technique

The operative technique has to be a golden mean. Our operative management is as follows:

- Operation in decubitus ventralis position, the neck in moderate flexion and the head slightly above the heart level.
- suboccipital craniotomy and resection of the lamina C1 and if necessary C2.
- Opening of the dura mater in Y.
- Opening of the cisterna magna and removal of cystic or tumoral structures.
- Opening of the IVth ventricle roof at the level of the foramen Magendie or above this level in case of adherent membranes.
- Closure of the dura mater with patch insertion.
- We do not plug the entrance of the central canal and we do not dissect the cerebellar tonsils.

Conclusion

In the neurosurgical treatment of syringomyelia there remains, in spite of doubts and disillusions, a number of formal indications for posterior fossa surgery, especially based upon a complete neuroradiologic investigation. Furthermore certain indications emerge for syringo- and spinoperitoneal shunt.

References

Aboulker J (1979) La syringomyélie et les liquides intrarachidiens. Neurochirurgie [Suppl] 25:1–44
Ball MJ, Dayan AD (1972) Pathogenesis of syringomyelia. Lancet II:799–801
Benini A, Krayenbühl H (1969) Ein neuer chirurgischer Weg zur Behandlung der Hydro- und Syringomyelia. Schweiz Med Wochenschr 99:1137–1142
Conway LW (1967) Hydrodynamic studies in syringomyelia. J Neurosurg 27:501–514
Elsberg GA (1916) Diagnosis and Treatment of Surgical Diseases of the Spinal Cord and its Membranes. Saunders, London
Gardner W (1965) Hydrodynamic mechanism of syringomyelia: its relationship to myelocele. J Neurol Neurosurg Psychiatry 28:247–259
Gardner WJ, Bell H, Poolos P, Dohn D, Steinberg M (1977) Terminal ventriculostomy for syringomyelia. J Neurosurg 46:609–617
Hankinson J (1970) Syringomyelia and the surgeon. Mod Trends Neurol 5:127–148
Krayenbühl H, Benini A (1971) A new surgical approach in the treatment of hydromyelia and syringomyelia. The embryologic basis and the first results. J R Coll Surg Edinb 16:147–161
Newman PK, Terenty TR, Foster JB (1981) Some observations on the pathogenesis of syringomyelia. J Neurol Neurosurg Psychiatry 44:964–969
Newton EJ (1969) Syringomyelia as a manifestation of defective fourth ventricular drainage. Ann R Coll Surg Engl 44:194–213
Pecker J, Javalet A, Boutelis A (1983) La dérivation syringo-péritonéale. Neurochirurgie 29:171–173
Phillips TW, Kindt GW (1981) Syringoperitoneal shunt for syringomyelia: a preliminary report. Surg Neurol 16:462–466
Puusepp M (1926) Traitement opératoire dans deux cas de syringomyélie avec amélioration notable. Rev Neurol (Paris) 1:1171–1179
Tator C, Meguro K, Rowed D (1982) Favorable results with syringosubarachnoid shunts for treatment of syringomyelia. J Neurosurg 56:517–523
Williams B (1969) The distending force in the production of "communicating syringomyelia". Lancet II:189–193
Williams B (1969) The distending force in the production of "communicating syringomyelia". Lancet II:696–697
Williams B (1970) The distending force in the production of "communicating syringomyelia". Lancet II:41–42
Williams B (1977) Difficult labour as a cause of communicating syringomyelia. Lancet II:51–53
Williams B (1978) A critical appraisal of posterior fossa surgery for communicating syringomyelia. Brain 101:223–250

Surgical Technique for Excision of Large Chemodectomas of the Jugular Foramen

G. MEINIG, K. SCHÜRMANN, B. LUDWIG, and J. HELMS, Mainz/FRG

Introduction

On the basis of ten years experience in neurosurgical-otorhinolaryngological team work using combined temporo-suboccipital approach in clival and petroclival tumors [4, 5, 9], we now summarize the results obtained with surgical techniques in glomus jugulare tumors operated in Mainz.

Patients and Methods

From our limited number of glomus jugulare tumors from the last decade, we have selected four cases suffering from large tumors with extra- and intracranial extension. In these patients, we performed a combined suboccipito-temporal approach in cooperation with the ENT surgeon, including removal of mastoid process as well as petrosectomy. Figure 1 shows an example of a patient with a rather large tumor. More than one half of the tumor is located intracranially in the middle and posterior fossa, the other part is located extracranially. The tumor caused destruction of the skull base, especially of the pyramid. A similar defect of the skull base is to be seen in Fig. 4. The angiogram in Fig. 2 shows the extent of the hypervascularized tumor.

Table 1 shows that all four patients we selected suffered from severe cranial nerve palsy, which developed over many years (3, 6, 10, 11 years). The majority of the patients underwent subtotal ENT operation some years ago. Two patients suffered from ataxia or hemiataxia. One case suffered from subarachnoid hemorrhage – probably due to bleeding from the tumor – with consecutive hydrocephalus.

Table 1. Symptoms and case history of four selected patients suffering from a large glomus jugulare tumor

Case no.	Cranial nerve deficit	Duration of deficit	First op.	Additional symptoms
1	VII–X	10 years	–	–
2	V–XII	3 years	Ent 1 year	Ataxia
3	V–XII	6 years	Ent 6 years	–
4	V–XII	11 years	Ent 6 + 11 years	Hemiataxia hydrocephalus after severe SAH

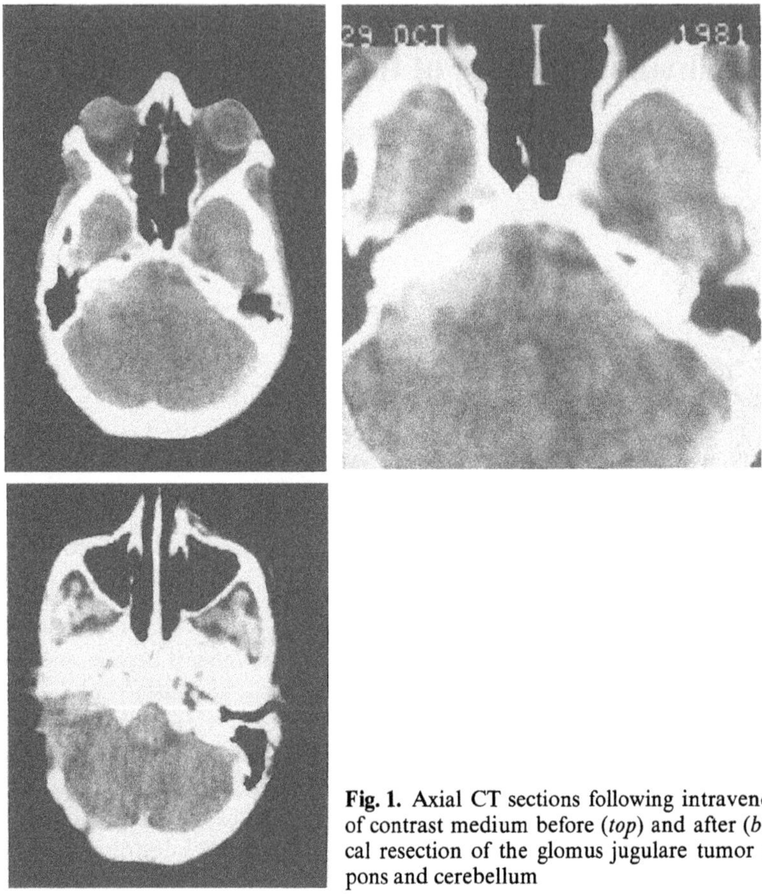

Fig. 1. Axial CT sections following intravenous injection of contrast medium before (*top*) and after (*bottom*) surgical resection of the glomus jugulare tumor extending to pons and cerebellum

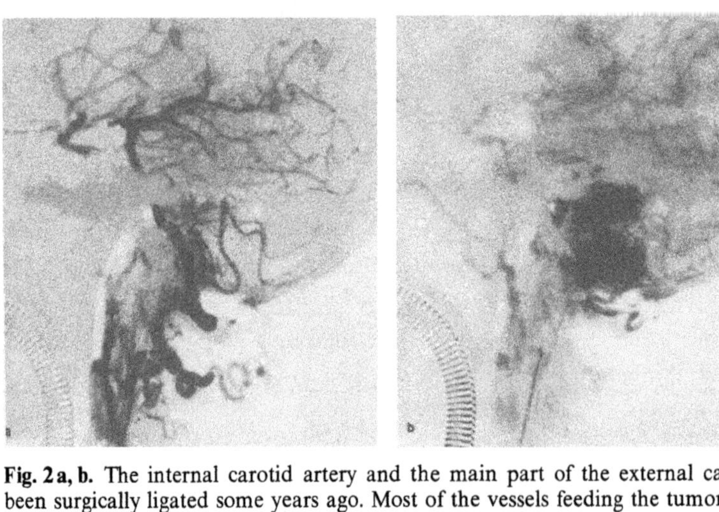

a b

Fig. 2a, b. The internal carotid artery and the main part of the external carotid artery had been surgically ligated some years ago. Most of the vessels feeding the tumor (**b**) can be visualized now by angiography of the vertebral artery which anastomoses with branches of the external carotid artery (**a**)

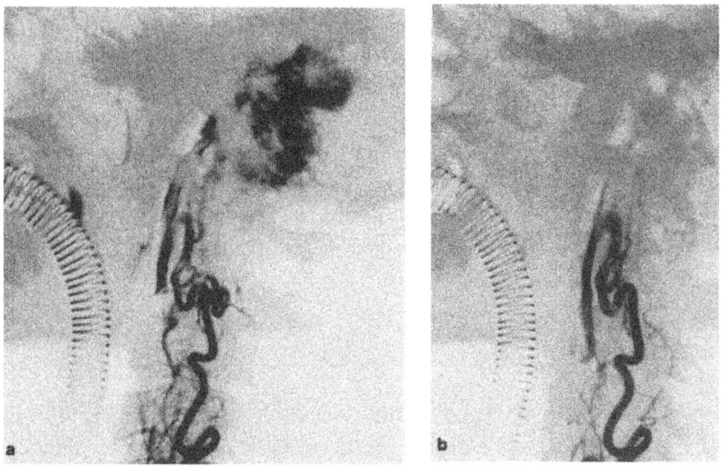

Fig. 3. **a** Opacification of tumors vessels by angiography of the ascending cervical artery. **b** Reduction of tumor staining following embolization via the ascending cervical artery

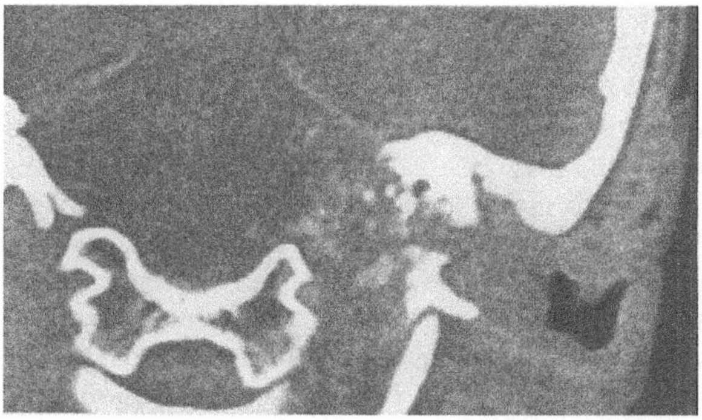

Fig. 4. Coronare CT section of glomus jugulare tumor after intravenous injection of contrast medium: the tumor destroys the skull base and extends into the posterior fossa

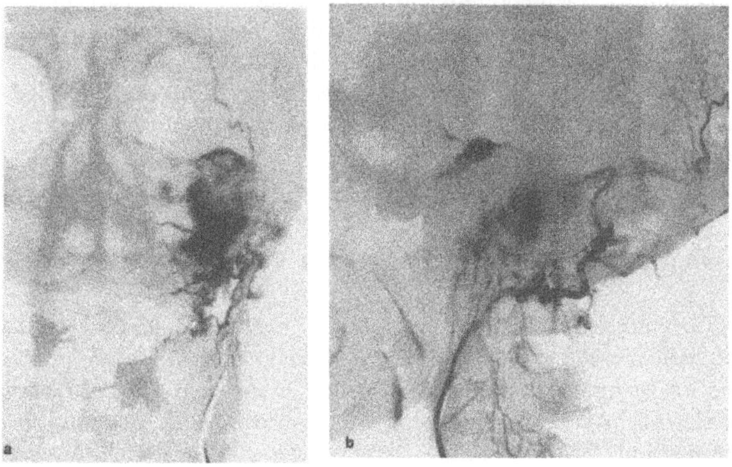

Fig. 5. Angiography of the occipital and ascending pharyngeal arteries (before embolization) demonstrates the marked tumor staining

In our opinion, every patient requires four-vessel angiography with contralateral vessel compression, or temporary intracarotid balloon occlusion test with nrCBF measurement, EEG etc. to assess the collateral circulation. In special cases, an extra-intracranial anastomosis may be of advantage. In all cases, superselective embolization two days preoperatively was performed by our neuroradiologist. Figure 3 gives an other example of preoperative embolization. Here the ascending cervical artery was embolized. Figure 5 shows the situation of an embolized occipital artery as well as ascending pharyngeal artery.

Surgical Procedure

In semi-recumbent position combined with elevation of the lower limbs ("V" shaped) and fixation of the skull in a three-point headholder, a skin incision is performed – slightly arched – from temporal retromastoidal along the sternocleidomastoid muscle. In the supratentorial region an osteoplastic craniotomy and in the infratentorial area a suboccipital craniectomy is performed. The transverse sinus is dissected by the ENT surgeon. A mastoid resection as well as a petrosectomy is performed (Fig. 1). The dura mater is opened along and parallel to the transverse sinus supra- and infratentorially and the transverse sinus can be resected after ligation. The tentorium is incised to the tentorial notch, so that the tentorium as well as the transverse sinus may be rotated upward. Tumor-supplying vessels can now be isolated. The tumor may be reduced in size by bipolar coagulation, laser and CUSA. The dissection is easier along the growth direction of the tumor along the veins and sinuses [1, 2, 3, 6, 7]. However, parts of the veins and the dorsal part of cavernous sinus have to be resected. If necessary, the internal carotid artery is to be dissected up to the entrance into the cavernous sinus, so that the internal carotid artery can be displaced ventrally to 1–2 cm in order to get more space [8]. Because of the wide supra- and infratentorial approach, the isolation of the tumor from the cerebellum and temporal lobe as well as from the rostral parts of medulla, pons, midbrain etc. is normally easier than the dissection of the skull base, so is the isolation of the cranial nerves, and may be possible without additional deficit. The basal dura normally has to be resected and closed by gel foam, or affixed lyodura or a galeaperiosteal gel foam flap. The cavity will be tamponed by flapped muscle and fixed with fibrin adhesive.

Possible Complications – Measures to Prevent Them

Of course there is a number of possible complications – some of them are listed in Table 2 together with measures to prevent them. Due to the team-work of the neurosurgeon and ENT-surgeon, optimal magnification, preoperative embolization, bipolar coagulation and/or laser, we had neither any serious bleeding during the operation nor any postoperative rebleeding. There was no additional cranial nerve deficit in our patient group. However, our intention to demonstrate that additional cranial nerve deficit may be avoided by combined neurosurgical and ENT surgical

Table 2. Possible complications in extirpation of large glomus jugulare tumors as well as measures to prevent them

(Re-)bleeding	Additional cranial nerve defect	Brain stem lesion	Cerebral ischemic events	Aspiration	CSF-fistula infection
	Neurosurgical – ENT approach (petrosectomy)				Careful covering of dura defect
	Optical magnification				
Pre-op-embolization Attention to the growth direction along the veins Bipolar coagulation/laser	Mandibular resection		Careful dissection of ICA to cavernous sinus EC/IC anastomosis Arterial reconstruction	Tracheotomy Deglutition operation	Careful closure of eustachian tube and acoustic meatus etc. Rotation of a muscle into the cavity Fibrin glue

approach could not materialize since this patient group had already severe cranial nerve deficit preoperatively (Table 1) because of the extension of the tumor. No patient showed additional neurologic deficits, there was no cerebral ischemic event, no patient needed extra-intracranial anastomosis or arterial reconstruction. Only one patient underwent tracheotomy and another deglutition reconstructive operation. We had no infection, however CSF-fistula appeared in two patients since we failed to rotate a muscle flap primarily into the tumor cavity, so we had to do this in a second operation. At all events, CSF fistula can be avoided at the first attempt.

Summary

The combined neurosurgical and ENT surgical temporo-suboccipital approach including removal of mastoid and pyramid with optical magnification and preoperative superselective embolization allows complete removal of large glomus jugulare tumors without additional cranial nerve or neurological deficit. Since size and extension of the tumors vary, choice and modification of the different approaches have to be adapted to the individual situation.

References

1. Denecke HJ (1978) Die Chirurgie ausgedehnter Tumoren des Felsenbeins und der Otobasis. Laryngol Rhinol Otol (Stuttg) 57:287–290
2. Draf W, Samii M (1977) Otorhinolaryngologisch-neurochirurgische Probleme an der Schädelbasis. Laryngol Rhinol Otol (Stuttg) 56:1007–1020
3. Draf W, Samii M (1982) Diagnostik und operative Strategie bei großen Glomustumoren der lateralen Schädelbasis. Aktuelles in der Otorhinolaryngologie. Thieme, Stuttgart New York, S 61–70

4. Helms J, Schürmann K (1986) The removal of the petrous pyramid to improve neurosurgical access to the brain stem. In: Samii M (ed) Surgery in and around the Brain Stem and the Third Ventricle. Springer, Berlin Heidelberg New York, S 457–459
5. Helms J, Schürmann K (1984) Interdisciplinary approach to benign tumors of the lateral skull base. Int. Congr. Skull Base, Mainz
6. Menzel J, Denecke HJ, Penzholz H (1978) Surgery of extensive glomus jugulare tumors. In: Frowein RA, Wilcke O, Karimi-Nejad A, Brock M, Klinger M (eds) Advances in Neurosurgery, vol 5. Springer, Berlin Heidelberg New York, S 259–265
7. Menzel J (1978) Neurochirurgische Therapie extensiver Glomus-jugulare-Tumoren. Laryngol Rhinol Otol (Stuttg) 57:281–286
8. Samii M, von Wild K (1981) Operative treatment of lesions in the region of the tentorial notch. Neurosurg Rev 4:3–10
9. Schürmann K, Meinig G, Helms J (in press) The strategy for approaching Petroclival and Clival Tumors

Stereotactic Intervention, Radiotherapy, Chemotherapy

CT-Guided Stereotactic Biopsy and Interstitial Curie-Therapy with ^{192}Ir and ^{125}I of Non-Resectable Midline and Brain Stem Gliomas

F. MUNDINGER, Freiburg/FRG

Summary

From a total number of 1587 (until Dec. 31. 1984) stereotactically irradiated cases (Table 1) treated either by permanent implantation with radioisotopes of a low dose rate (Curie-therapy) or by temporary implantation with high dose rate nuclides (after-loading brachy-Curie-therapy), a series of 664 gliomas of the midline is reported on. Life expectancy figures are given for patients after 1, 3, 5 and 10 years (the 10 year statistics are not yet complete) since treatment with Curie-therapy; 197 of these cases were irradiated with ^{192}Ir wires (1965–1984) and 202 with ^{125}I seeds[1] (February 1979–1984).

All stereotactic irradiation procedures were, within the same session, directly preceded by bioptic confirmation. The biopsies were evaluated according to classification, dignity as well as localization (hypothalamic, thalamic, mesencephalic, brain stem/pons). The CT stereotaxy today is the method of choice. For our polar-coordinated stereotactic device (Riechert and Mundinger [35], in the computer compatible modification of Birg and Mundinger [2]) the intracranial targets and trephination points as well as the corresponding coordinates are, in an uncomplicated way, taken directly from the CT scans.

Table 1. Radionuclides and number of stereotactic interstitial irradiation procedures 1952–Dec. 31. 1984

^{32}P	6
^{60}Co	179
^{90}Y	44
^{182}Ta	21
^{198}Au	129
^{125}I	331
^{125}I Brachy Curie	35
^{192}Ir GammaMed	284
^{192}Ir	558
Total	1,587

[1] (In the preparation according to Hilaris [8])

Introduction

With the modern image-producing techniques such as X-Ray Transmission Computer Tomography (CT) and Magnetic Resonance Imaging (MRI), it is possible to locate accurately and reliably intracranial processes. With regard to a morphologic diagnosis, however, we have been able to show in fact that, for example, 164 out of 904 intracranial lesions, which we stereotactically biopsied and which had been previously diagnosed as tumors because of their ring-shaped structures, were bioptically found not to be tumors at all. The foci were bioptically diagnosed as hemorrhages, necroses, abscesses or even multiple sclerosis foci. Infiltrating processes which are surgically non-resectable, located around the 3rd ventricle and in the brain stem and which are presumed to be tumors, are still today treated conservatively or by external radiation without a histologic diagnosis having been established. Due to the lack of an optimum therapy, one finds many examples of unsuccessful treatment [31].

The CT stereotactic biopsy, however, succeeds in establishing an accurate and reliable histologic diagnosis. By including the intraoperative diagnosis with the smear preparation, optimum therapeutic measures can immediately be taken [1, 4, 5, 12, 20, 32, 33, 42].

Method

For carrying out the stereotactic biopsy and interstitial implantation of radioactive material, we use our own stereotactic device (Riechert and Mundinger [35] in the computer-compatible version (Mundinger and Birg [2]). Its principles and technique have been described in other publications [25, 27]. Through the same burrhole of 7 mm in diameter, several puncture tracks for biopsies and radionuclide implantation have to be performed in different directions, using the transcerebral or transcerebellar approach. The accuracy of location is 0.6 mm [26]. Our biopsies are carried out with biopsy forceps of 0.8 mm diameter which are directed in a 1.0 mm diameter cannula. Step by step, in intervals of millimeters, tissue of about ⅓ mm^3 volume is taken. This amount of tissue is sufficient for histologic purposes [12, 22]. Material is taken from the same site for both the intraoperative histology in the smear preparation and the conventional examination. By using this method, a morphologic profile of the focus is established. This is most important with regard to the decision as to the tumor pathology [9, 36]. The decision on which further therapeutic measures should be taken during the same operation is made immediately after the intraoperative histologic examination (Table 2).

Results

To date, we have performed stereotactic biopsies in more than 2200 cases, including the CT-stereotactic biopsy (since January 1981).

Table 2 indicates the kinds of therapy which, in a series of 1293 cases, followed the stereotactic biopsies.

Table 2. Type of subsequent treatment after stereotactical diagnostic biopsy (1965 – June 30, 1984) in a series of 1,293 cases

Type of procedure	No. of cases	(%)
Permanent interstitial Curie-therapy ^{192}Ir	254	20
^{125}I	298	23
+ external irradiation	78	7
Temporary interstitial (Brachy-) Curie-therapy	75	7
External irradiation	215	17
Cyst drainage (catheter implantation)	88	7
Tumor resection	79	6
No subsequent therapy	389	30

Table 3. Complications after stereotactic biopsy (1,293 cases) (1965–June 30, 1984)

	No. of cases	(%)
Operative mortality	8	0,6
Operative morbidity		
– Transient complication	52	4
– Persistent complication	33	3
Type of complications		
– Hemorrhage	26	2
– Paresis	25	2
– Aphasia	16	1
– Seizure	38	3

Table 4. Localization of stereotactically biopsied lesions (1965–June 30, 1984)

Site	No. of cases
Midbrain-pons-region	221
Basal-ganglia	270
Diencephalic region	173
Total	664

Table 3 indicates the rates of mortality and the morbidity of the last series which is usually characterized by an aggravation of the neurologic symptoms.

Table 4 shows the topographic distribution of our stereotactic biopsies in cases of midline tumors. Table 5 indicates the localization and therapy of non glial-midline tumors. The following Table 6 indicates the life expectancy of midline tumor patients treated with Curie-therapy as compared to those cases which were only biopsied. These patients are nevertheless comparable. They had been either selected prospectively or the implantation had not been carried out for technical reasons because, for example, the necessary radioactivity had not been available. Other cases had been referred to us from outside hospitals in order to perform the biopsy only. Table 6 depicts the life expectancy in cases of low-grade gliomas in the chiasma area, optic tract and hypothalamic area. What is not expressed in these tables is the remarkable symptomatic improvement of those tumors which had implantations, combined with a considerable regression and in some cases even a complete disappearance of the tumor. In cases of low-grade gliomas of the quadrigeminal region (Table 6), irradiation with ^{192}Ir has clearly shown the better life expectancy figures. In cases of anaplastic thalamic gliomas, the medium survival time of the implanted cases has also proved to be longer (Table 6). Especially for thalamic low-grade glio-

Table 5. Stereotactic treatment (December 31, 1984)

	Biopsy only	Since 1979 ^{125}I	Since 1965 ^{192}Ir	Total
	Hypothalamic region			
Non glial tumors				
Ependymoma	–	3	1	4
Papilloma	2	–	1	3
Meningioma	1	1	–	1
Germinoma	1	–	–	1
PNET	2	1	1	4
Medulloblastoma	4	–	–	4
Craniopharyngioma	39	8	6	53
Teratoma	3	1	1	5
Epidermoid	1	–	1	2
Metastasis	5	1	–	6
Unclassified tumor	1	1	–	2
	59	16	11	85
Non tumoral lesions				
Colloid cyst	15	–	1	16
Hemorrhage	–	–	–	–
Gliosis	5	–	–	5
Abscess	2	–	–	2
	22	–	1	23
	Thalamic region			
Non glial tumors				
Ependymoma	2	3	1	6
Germinoma	2	–	–	2
PNET	1	–	–	1
Teratoma	1	–	1	2
Metastasis	20	4	1	25
Unclassified tumor	2	–	1	3
	28	7	4	39
Non tumoral lesions				
Hemorrhage	18	–	–	18
Gliosis	9	–	1	10
Abscess	1	–	–	1
	28	–	1	29
	Midbrain-pons region			
Non glial tumors				
Ependymoma	2	1	4	7
Papilloma	–	1	3	4
Meningioma	1	1	–	2
Germinoma	15	10	7	32
PNET	8	8	3	19
Medulloblastoma	1	1	–	2
Craniopharyngioma	1	–	1	2
Teratoma	5	–	1	6
Epidermoid	1	–	1	2
Metastasis	2	2	–	4
Unclassified tumor	–	–	2	2
	36	24	22	82

Table 5. (continued)

	Biopsy only	Since 1979 ^{125}I	Since 1965 ^{192}Ir	Total
Non tumoral lesions				
Hemorrhage	4	–	–	4
Gliosis	5	–	–	5
Abscess	1	–	–	1
	10	–	–	10

Table 6. Life expectancy of stereotactic interstitial irradiation with ^{125}I or ^{192}Ir of patients with low grade gliomas in comparison with biopsy only – June 30, 1984

	Tumor type		No. of	1 yr (%)	3 yrs	5 yrs	10 yrs
Chiasm and optic tract	Astro I	^{125}I	7	86	69	51	–
		^{192}I	4	75	75	33	–
		Biopsy only	13	92	76	51	–
Hypothalamic region	Astro I	^{125}I	8	87	58	41	–
		^{192}Ir	5	82	51	38	–
		Biopsy only	6	82	75	75	–
Quadrigeminal region	Astro I	^{125}I	14	93	73	73	–
		^{192}Ir	12	100	56	37	–
		Biopsy only	10	100	82	68	–
	Astro II	^{125}I	6	100	45	45	–
		^{192}Ir	5	78	78	39	–
		Biopsy only	17	56	46	–	–
Thalamic region	Astro I	^{125}I	24	100	68	55	–
		^{192}Ir	20	94	88	82	63
		Biopsy only	7	69	50	50	21
	Astro II	^{125}I	23	86	28	28	–
		^{192}Ir	25	86	43	31	28
		Biopsy only	21	86	9	5	–

Median survival time in months of patients with anaplastic thalamic gliomas (n = 84) – June 1984

Tumor type	^{125}I	^{192}Ir	Biopsy only
Astro III	5	16	3
Astro IV	8	6	3

mas (WHO I and II), life expectancy rates have clearly improved after ^{192}Ir Curie-therapy, although the results after 10 years of the ^{125}I series are not yet available (Table 6).

Discussion and Indications

Our experience with CT-stereotactic biopsies has shown that 17% of the processes which, using the image-producing diagnostic method, were previously diagnosed as tumors, are in fact non-tumoral lesions [22, 26]. Our results show that, considering the minimal risk and high reliability of the bioptic procedure, no conservative or percutaneous radiation therapy should be carried out today on patients with space-occupying processes without a previous histologic diagnosis. Diagnostic errors, especially false or omitted therapy, can in this way be avoided. In cases of non-resectable infiltrating tumors or recurrencies after operations and/or external radiation of midline tumors, the biopsy can be immediately followed by the interstitial Curie-therapy within the same procedure.

Application technique and dosimetry of ^{192}Ir and ^{125}I for carrying out the Curie-therapy have been described extensively in other publications [21, 23, 24]. In cases of anaplastic midline tumors or tumors between Grade II and III, the interstitial Curie-therapy is carried out and possibly followed by supporting measures such as tumor cyst catheter drainage, as well as a saturation of the focal dose by means of external beam irradiation and chemotherapy (Fig. 1a, b). In cases of Grade I and Grade II tumors which are not clearly demarcated, we perform the continuous low-dose-rate radiation by permanent implantation of ^{192}Ir seeds. The peripheric tumor dose (= tumor surface) should be 120 Gy.

In cases of sharply demarcated tumors we permanently implant ^{125}I seeds, using a peripheric tumor dose of 100 Gy.

The life expectancy after the application of the Curie-therapy has proved to be clearly higher compared with the cases which were only biopsied.

The optimum therapy of the optic glioma (Grade I) is still under debate [6, 11, 39]. Our experience has shown that Curie-therapy is indicated in cases of continuing tumor growth or recurrences, if no resection is performed. In cases of infiltrating low-grade gliomas or recurrences of tumors of the diencephalon, mesencephalon and brain stem/pons region, Curie-therapy is the method of choice [28–30]. It is indicated for gliomas which are clearly defined, so that an exact dosimetry can be done, sparing to surrounding neurologic structures and pathways.

Moreover, the Curie-therapy does not eliminate the possibility of a nuclide-reimplantation or external beam irradiation later on if the tumor starts to grow again.

In contrast to surgery of hemispheric low grade tumors [13, 15, 40], a comparison of our results of non-resectable tumors with those of other therapeutic methods, especially the external beam irradiation, is handicapped by the fact that an overwhelming majority of the reported midline tumors were not biopsied. Moreover, the actual number of such cases is quite small [3, 14, 16–19, 34, 37, 40, 41, 43].

Our extensive experience has shown that in cases of such tumors of the midline the application of interstitial brachy-Curie-therapy, using a single high-dose-rate afterloading technique such as the ^{192}Ir contact radiation device "GammaMed" [21] a 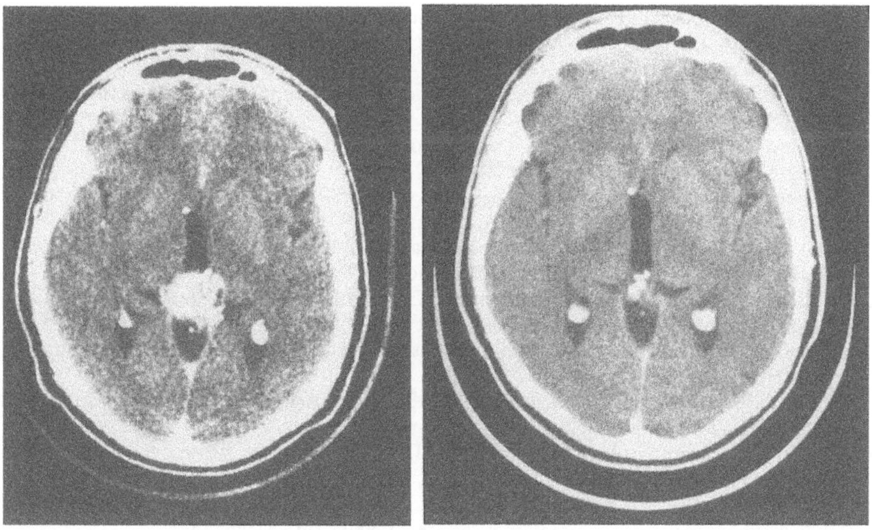 b

Fig. 1. **a** Primitive neuroectodermal tumor (PNET) in the pineal region. Recurrence after open surgery and external beam irradiation before Curie-therapy. **b** 6 months after Curie-therapy with ^{125}I. Peripheral tumor dose: 100 Gy. Except the artefacts of ^{125}I seeds tumor not detectable any more

or the highly-active ^{125}I catheters [7, 10, 38], is not well tolerated by the patients. After applying this therapy, the palliative effect usually diminishes. The combination of several interstitially applied fractions of high dose rates and an additional saturation of the focal dose with external beam radiation – as we already did in the fifties [21] – offers an alternative for the treatment of malignant tumors.

Acknowledgment: I want to thank Dr. K. Weigel for helping me in the statistic evaluation of the series.

References

1. Apuzzo MLJ, Zelman V, Jepson J, Chandrasoma P (1984) Observations with the Utilization of the Brown-Roberts-Wells stereotactic system in the management of intracranial mass lesions. Acta Neurochir (Wien) [Suppl] 33:261–263
2. Birg W, Mundinger F (1973) Computer calculations of target parameters for a stereotactic apparatus. Acta Neurochir (Wien) 29:123–129
3. Bouchart J (1973) Central nervous system. In: Fletcher GH (ed) Textbook of radiotherapy, ed 2. Philadelphia, Lea & Febiger, p 336–348
4. Daumas-Duport C, Monsaingeon V, N'Guyen JP, Missir O, Szikla G (1984) Some correlations between histological and CT aspects of cerebral gliomas contributing to the choice of significant trajectories for stereotactic biopsies. Acta Neurochir [Suppl] (Wien) 33:185–194
5. Galanda M, Nádvornik P, Sramka M, Basandova M (1984) Stereotactic biopsy of brainstem tumors. Acta Neurochir [Suppl] (Wien) 33:213–217
6. Glaser J, Hoyt W, Corbeit J (1971) Visual morbidity with chiasmal glioma. Long term studies of visual fields in untreated and irradiated cases. Arch Ophthalmol 85:3–12

7. Gutin PH, Phillips TL, Hosobuchy Y, Wara WM, Mackay AR, Weaver KA, Lamb S, Hurst S (1981) Permanent and removable implants for the brachytherapy of brain tumors. Int J Radiat Oncol Biol Phys 7: 1371–1381
8. Hilaris BS (ed) (1975) Handbook of interstitial brachytherapy. Acton, Massachusetts·Publishing Sciences Group, Inc
9. Hoshino T (1984) A commentary on the biology and growth kinetics of low-grade and high-grade gliomas. J Neurosurg 61:895–900
10. Hosobuchi Y, Phillips TL, Stupar TA, Gutin PH (1980) Interstitial brachytherapy of primary brain tumors: Preliminary report. J Neurosurg 53:613–617
11. Hoyt W, Baghdassarian S (1969) Optic glioma of childhood: Natural history and rationale for conservative management. Br J Ophthalmol 53:793–798
12. Kiessling M, Anagnostopoulos J, Lombeck G, Kleihues P (1982) Diagnostic potential of stereotactic biopsy of brain tumors. A report of 400 cases. In: Voth D, Gutjahr P, Langmaid C (eds) Tumours of the central nervous system in infancy and childhood. Springer, Berlin Heidelberg New York, p 247–256
13. Kuhlendahl H, Miltz H, Wüllenweber R (1973) Die Astrocytome des Großhirns. Acta Neurochir (Wien) 29: 151–162
14. Lassiter K, Alexander E, Davis C, Kelly D (1971) Surgical treatment of brain stem gliomas. J Neurosurg 34:719–725
15. Laws ER Jr, Taylor WF, Marvin BC, Okazaki H (1984) Neurosurgical management of low-grade astrocytoma of the cerebral hemispheres. J Neurosurg 61:665–673
16. Leibel SA, Sheline GE, Wara WM et al. (1975) The role of radiation therapy in the treatment of astrocytomas. Cancer 35: 1551–1557
17. Liebner E, Pretto J, Hochhauser M, Kassaraba W (1964) Tumors of the posterior fossa in childhood and adolescence. Their diagnostic and radiotherapeutic patterns. Radiology 82: 193–201
18. Lütolf UM, Glanzmann CH, Aberle HG, Horst W (1978) Ergebnisse der Radiotherapie bei 68 inoperablen Hirntumoren (1950–1975). Strahlentherapie 154:8–10
19. Marsa GW, Probert JC, Rubinstein LJ, Bagshaw MA (1973) Radiation therapy in the treatment of childhood astrocytic gliomas. Cancer 32:646–655
20. Monsaingeon V, Daumas-Duport C, Mann M, Miyahara S, Szikla G (1984) Stereotactic Sampling Biopsies in a Series of 268 Consecutive Cases – Validity and Technical Aspects. Acta Neurochir. [Suppl] (Wien) 33: 195–200
21. Mundinger F (1970) The treatment of brain tumors with interstitially applied radioactive isotopes. In: Wang Y, Paoletti P (eds) Radionuclide applications in neurology and neurosurgery. Thomas, Springfield Ill, USA, p 199–265
22. Mundinger F (1982) CT-stereotactic biopsy of brain tumors. In: Voth D, Gutjahr P, Langmaid C (eds) Tumours of the central nervous system in infancy and childhood. Springer, Berlin Heidelberg New York, p 234–246
23. Mundinger F (1982) Implantation of radioisotopes (curie-therapy). In: Schaltenbrand G, Walker AE (Hrsg) Stereotaxy of the human brain, 2. Aufl. Thieme, Stuttgart, S 410–435
24. Mundinger F (1985) Technik und Ergebnisse der interstitiellen Hirntumorbestrahlung. In: Heilmann HP (Hrsg) Handbuch der medizinischen Radiologie. Band XIX/4: Spezielle Strahlentherapie maligner Tumoren. Springer, Berlin Heidelberg New York Tokyo, S 179–214
25. Mundinger F, Birg W (1984) Stereotactic biopsy of intracranial processes. Acta Neurochir [Suppl] (Wien) 33:219–224
26. Mundinger F, Birg W (1984) CT-Stereotaxy in the clinical routine. Neurosurg Rev 7:219–224
27. Mundinger F, Birg W (1984) CT-guided stereotaxy for Diagnoses and Treatment of Intracranial Processes (Biopsy, Catheter/Electrode-Implantation, Interstitial Irradiation with Radioisotopes). 7th CARVAT (New Imaging In Radiology), Rom, February 6–10, 1984
28. Mundinger F, Weigel K (1983) CT-stereotactic biopsy and interstitial radiotherapy of pineal region tumors. VIII. Mexican Congress of Neurological Surgery. 26.–30. 7. 1983, Acapulco/Mexico
29. Mundinger F, Weigel K (1984) Indication and results of stereotactic curie-therapy with iridium-192 and iodine-125 for non-resectable tumors of the hypothalamic region. Acta Neurochir [Suppl] (Wien) 33:323–350

30. Mundinger F, Weigel K (1984) Stereotactic curie-therapy of thalamic tumors. J Neurol Oncol 2:278/64
31. Mundinger F, Weigel K, Mohadjer M (1984) CT-stereotaktische Biopsie und/oder interstitiell-extern kombinierte Strahlenbehandlung von Hirnmetastasen. In: von Heyden HW, Krauseneck P (Hrsg) Hirnmetastasen. Pathophysiologie, Diagnostik und Therapie. Aktuelle Onkologie 13, Zuckschwerdt, München, S 128–143
32. Ohye C, Nakajima H, Matsushima T, Komatsu T, Hirato M, Kawashima Y (1984) CT Assisted Stereotactic Biopsy of Deep Cerebral Lesions and the Results. Acta Neurochir [Suppl] (Wien) 33:257–259
33. Pecker J, Scarabin JM, Brucher JM, Vallee B (1979) Démarche stéréotaxique en neurochirurgie tumorale. Pierre Fabre, Paris, p 1–301
34. Redmond J (1961) The roentgen therapy of pontine gliomas. Am J Roentgenol 86:644–648
35. Riechert T, Mundinger F (1956) Beschreibung und Anwendung eines Zielgerätes für stereotaktische Hirnoperationen (2. Modell). Acta Neurochir (Wien) 3:308–337
36. Rubinstein LJ (1972) Atlas of tumor pathology, second series, fasc 6, Tumors of the central nervous system. Washington, DC Armed Forced Institute of Pathology, p 19–85
37. Sheline G, Phillips T, Boldrey E (1965) The therapy of unbiopsied brain tumors. Am J Roentgenol 93:664–670
38. Szikla G, Peragut JC (1975) Irradiation interstitielle des gliomes. Neurochirurgie [Suppl 2] 21:187–228
39. Taveras J, Mount L, Wood E (1956) The value of radiation therapy in the management of glioma of the optic nerves and chiasm. Radiology 66:518–528
40. Uihlein A, Colby MY Jr, Layton DD et al. (1966) Comparison of surgery and surgery plus irradiation in the treatment of supratentorial gliomas. Acta Radiol (Ther) 5:67–78
41. Urtasun R (1972) ^{60}Co radiation treatment of pontine gliomas. Radiology 104:385–387
42. Weigel K, Mohadjer M, Mundinger F (1983) CT-Stereotaxy for differential diagnosis and radiotherapy of intracranial metastases. In: Piotrowski W, Brock M, Klinger M (eds) CNS Metastases Neurosurgery in the Aged. Advances in Neurosurgery 12. Springer, Berlin Heidelberg New York, p 87–89
43. Whyte T, Colby M, Layton D (1969) Radiation therapy of brainstem tumors. Radiology 93:413–416

Computed Tomographic Guidance Stereotaxis in the Management of Ninety-Four Lesions of the Third Ventricular Region

M. L. J. APUZZO, Los Angeles, CA/USA

Introduction

The advent of computed tomographic radiologic imaging has changed and enhanced the neurosurgeons perspective regarding definitions and strategies of mass lesion management within the intracranial space. The structural definition of the nature and extent of intra- and extraaxial mass processes has been developed to levels that have been previously unappreciated. Wedding of stereotactic instrumentation with such imaging techniques offers the surgeon important management options when faced with intracranial mass pathology (Apuzzo et al. 1984a; Apuzzo et al. 1984b; Apuzzo and Sabshin 1983; Heilbrun et al. 1983). Nowhere is this more appreciated than in the third ventricular region where direct surgical approaches are undertaken with appreciable risk, and outcome is often only biopsy or surgical reduction of an inoperable lesion. This paper presents the utilization of computed tomographic guidance stereotactic techniques in the evaluation and management of 94 lesions of the third ventricular region.

Case Material

Review of 300 consecutive cases who underwent CT guidance stereotaxy at the University of Southern California Medical Center disclosed 94 cases of third ventricular region lesions. The majority of patients presented with masses without previous operation or absolute definition of a specific pathologic process.

Target Masses

8 lesions were limited to the third ventricular cavity, 13 occurred in the anterior, and 19 in the posterior third ventricular region; 54 masses were located primarily lateral to the ventricle, but all deformed the adjacent lateral ependymal surface (Fig. 1).

Procedural Objectives

Surgical objectives related to the stereotactic procedures were variable and related to clinical and radiographic issues attendant on a given lesion. These included biopsy, culture, aspiration, drainage, conduit placement, endoscopic visualization with biopsy, excision or aspiration (Table 1).

Instrumentation and Technique

A Brown-Roberts-Wells stereotactic system was used with both a General Electric 8800 or Phillips Tomoscan 310 scanning systems for data collections; data processing was accomplished employing a Hewlett Packard programmable calculator (HP41CV) and more recently an Epson HP-20 programmable computer.

All surgical aspects of each procedure were performed in a neurosurgical operating room. All adult procedures were performed with local anesthesia and mild sedation with anesthesia standing by.

Details of techniques for calvarial entry and instrumentation at the target point were similar to those of our previous reports.

Table 1. Initial stereotactic procedure objectives (94 cases), 3rd ventricular region

Biopsy (60)	Temporary drainage (4)
Biopsy, culture (10)	Biopsy, texture assessment (3)
Biopsy, aspiration (6)	Endoscopic visualization, biopsy (4)
Biopsy, Rickham drainage (5)	Endoscopic visualization, aspiration (2)
97 – Point placements	
300 – Point specimens	

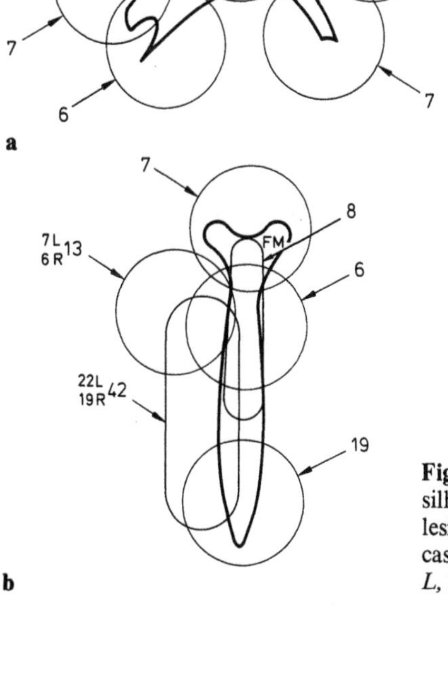

Fig. 1. Lateral (**a**) and superior (**b**) 3rd ventricular silhouettes with *circles* representing the areas of lesion location. The *numbers* indicate the number cases. *FM,* foramen of Monro; *R,* right-sided; *L,* left-sided

Results and Complications

In 94 procedures there were 97 point placements with more than 300 tissue specimens retrieved. Procedural objectives were accomplished in 93 of 94 cases. In one individual with a 2 cm cystic lesion of the suprasellar region, cyst penetration and drainage could not be accomplished; manipulation for entry and biopsy were attended by complaints of headache and transient scotomata.

In the remaining cases either histologic or microbiologic verification of a disease process was obtained.

Three of the cases proved to be developmental, 66 neoplastic, 22 infectious, and 2 cavernous angiomas (Table 2).

One death occurred in a patient with a contrast enhancing diffuse lesion of the right posterior thalamus, that was avascular on angiography. Two previous biopsies at another institution had been nondiagnostic. Our specimen was consistent with a cavernous angioma. During biopsy the patient experienced mild transient headache, but was completely asymptomatic until five hours post biopsy when he suddenly became comatose. CT scanning revealed a massive thalamic and intraventricular hemorrhage. Case review indicated that the patient probably experienced acute third ventricular outlet obstruction secondary to the biopsy manipulation with subsequent alteration of systemic arterial pressure and the acute hemorrhagic event. Based on this occurrence all patients with evidence of minimal ventriculomegaly who were candidates for manipulation at the ventricular outlet had placement of a ventriculostomy prior to point placement of instrumentation. No further hemorrhagic events have been noted in over 40 subsequent cases.

There were no other complications attendant on the procedures that were generally completed in 60 to 90 minutes. All patients recovered satisfactorily within six hours and were ready to proceed with further levels of therapy as indicated.

Table 2. Pathologic lesions substantiated (93 cases), 3rd ventricular region

Developmental (3)	*Infections (22)*
Colloid cyst (3)	Herpetic encephalitis (1)
Neoplastic (66)	Bacterial abscess (6)
Metastatic carcinoma (14)	Tuberculous abscess (3)
Astrocytoma (10)	Tuberculous granuloma (1)
Ependymoma (2)	Toxoplasmosis granuloma (6)
Anaplastic glioma (8)	Coccidiomycosis abscess (1)
Glioblastoma multiforme (9)	Cysticercosis (4)
Ganglioglioma (1)	*Vascular (2)*
Primitive neuroectodermal (1)	Cavernous angioma (2)
Pituitary adenoma (2)	
Meningioma (2)	
Ectopic pinealoma (1)	
Craniopharyngioma (8)	
Pineocytoma (1)	
Pineoblastoma (2)	
Medulloblastoma (2)	
Atypical teratoma (4)	

Table 3. Treatment initiatives following stereotactic procedure (94 cases), 3rd ventricular region

A. Craniotomy (15)
B. Radiotherapy, craniotomy (1)
C. Radiotherapy (26)
  1. Teletherapy (20)
  2. Brachytherapy (8)
    a. Point source (5)
    b. Colloid (3)
D. Radiotherapy, chemotherapy (28)
  1. Teletherapy, brachytherapy (13)
  2. Teletherapy (15)
E. Antibiotic, antiviral (21)
F. Ventriculoperitoneal shunting (52)

Information obtained during the stereotactic procedures allowed for therapeutic action based on the logic of precise histologic and microbiologic data (Table 3). Treatment initiatives included craniotomy in 15 cases or approximately $1/6$ of the patient group. The majority of these procedures were undertaken for excision of histologically benign potentially excisable lesions. 55 cases were subsequently managed by radiotherapy with brachytherapy employed in 21 and teletherapy in 48. Antibiotic medications were administered in 21 cases with ventriculoperitoneal shunting performed in 52. In all cases, subsequent courses and lesion responses testified to the appropriate selection of management modes.

Discussion

A number of authors have stressed the prudence of stereotactic exploration of deep brain regions as an alternative to immediate craniotomy which often, at best, may have at its endpoint only biopsy and establishment of an appropriate "tissue diagnosis" (Apuzzo et al. 1984a; Bosch 1980; Pecker et al. 1979). The advent of CT guidance stereotaxy and the development of standardized related instrumentation would logically enhance the precision, diagnostic yield and safety of such a procedure, particularly in the third ventricular region. Our observations speak for the credibility of the approach which had a precise diagnostic yield in 93 of 94 cases and only one death which we feel could have been avoided if a ventriculostomy had been placed prior to biopsy. 92 of the procedures were performed with local anesthesia with full post procedural recovery evident within six hours, with only 16 subsequent craniotomies required for benign and potentially circumscribed lesion management.

Cystic lesions may be satisfactorily managed by these techniques (Apuzzo et al. 1984a). Cysticercosis cysts may be totally excised and colloid cysts aspirated under direct vision with concurrent use of the stereotactic instrument and appropriate miniature cerebroscopic devices. Fiberoptically conducted laser energy may be employed via ventriculoscopic conduits to control hemorrhage and reduce tissue mass.

Based on these data, it would seem advisable to consider imaging guidance stereotactic techniques as an alternative to initial craniotomy in all third ventricular region lesions (Apuzzo et al. 1984a; Bosch 1980; Pecker et al. 1979) that: (1) seem to be intrinsic or of invasive neoplastic origin, (2) are possibly of infectious etiology, (3) are potentially radiosensitive or, (4) are not diagnosed with assurance.

References

Apuzzo MLJ, Sabshin JK (1983) Computed tomographic guidance stereotaxis in the management of intracranial mass lesions. Neurosurgery 12:277–285

Apuzzo MLJ, Chandrasoma PT, Zelman V, Giannotta SL, Weiss MH (1984a) Computerized tomographic guidance stereotaxis in the management of lesions of the third ventricular region. Neurosurgery 15:502–508

Apuzzo MLJ, Jepson JH, Luxton G, Little FM (1984b) Ionizing and non-ionizing radiation treatment of malignant cerebral gliomas: Specialized approaches. Clin Neurosurg 31:470–496

Bosch DA (1980) Indications for stereotactic biopsy in brain tumors. Acta Neurochir (Wien) 54:167–179

Heilbrun MP, Roberts TS, Apuzzo MLJ, Wells TH, Sabshin JK (1983) Preliminary experience with Brown-Roberts-Wells computerized tomographic stereotaxic guidance system. J Neurosurg 59:217–222

Pecker J, Scarabin JM, Vallee B, Brucher JM (1979) Treatment in Tumours of the Pineal Region: Value of Stereotaxic Biopsy. Surg Neurol 12:341–348

Computed Tomography-Guided Thalamotomy

L.V. Laitinen, Umeå/Sweden

Recent development of computed tomography (CT)-guided stereotaxis has opened a new era in functional stereotactic surgery. Until recently, contrast-medium enhanced ventriculography only gave information of the internal boundaries of the third ventricle, but nothing could be seen of the posterior and lateral extensions of the thalamus. Additionally, ventriculography could cause a dilatation and displacement of the third ventricle. The headaches and nausea increased the surgical risks of thalamotomy. With CT it is possible to define the posterior (cisterna ambiens) and lateral (internal capsule) margins of the thalamus and thus increase the chances of proper positioning of the therapeutic lesions.

In Umeå air ventriculography was abandoned in March 1984 when a new CT adapter had been developed (Laitinen et al. 1985). Since then all functional stereotaxis has been done with CT-guidance only. The CT adapter consists of a duraluminium framework which is non-invasive and easy and fast to mount on the patient's head (Fig. 1). Repeated mountings are highly reproducible. The surgical target from the CT study can be determined with the x, y and z coordinates in relation to the adapter which can then be removed (Fig. 2). Surgery can be performed any time, even months after the CT study. The adapter is remounted and the stereotactic frame is fixed rigidly to the skull without contact with, or given relation to, the adapter. The stereotactic intervention can be carried out with conventional radio-

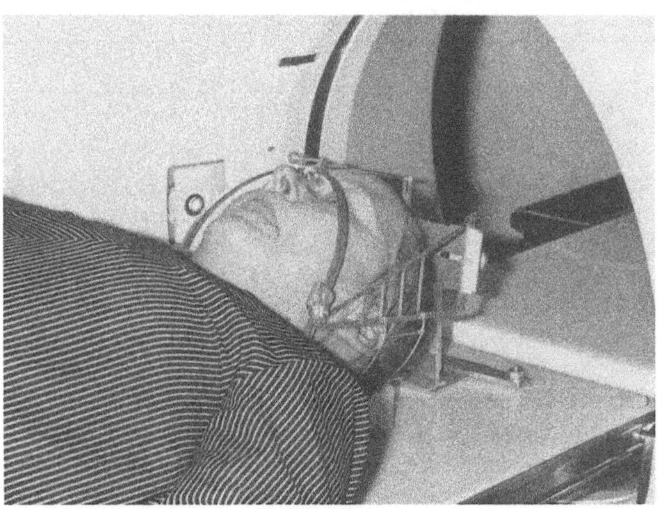

Fig. 1. The CT adapter

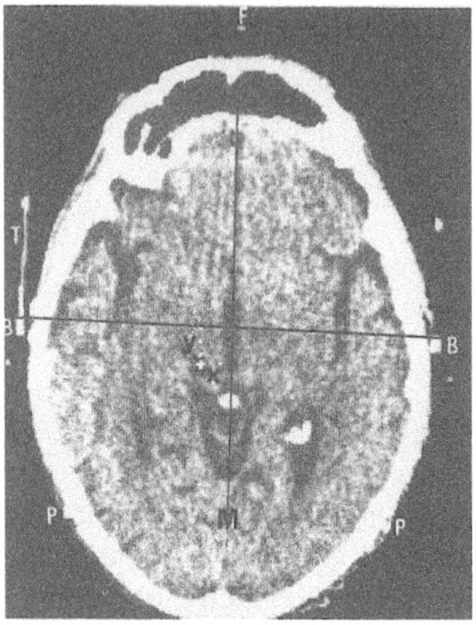

Fig. 2. A surgical lesion one month postoperatively in the right ventralis posterolateralis nucleus of the thalamus (*dotted circle*). The *white cross* in the anterior part of the low-attenuating area shows the original surgical target. The target is determined with an x coordinate in relation to the adapter's mid-plane (*F-M*) and with an y coordinate in relation to the interaural plane (*B-B*). The z coordinate is obtainable from the height difference between the target level and the level of the transverse bars (*T*) of the adapter

Table 1. CT-guided ablative stereotaxis. (*Vim* = ventralis intermedius nucleus of the thalamus; *Pall* = medial pallidum; *Pulv* = medial pulvinar; *CM* = centrum medianum; *VPL* = ventralis posterolateralis nucleus; *Parafasc* = parafascicularis nucleus; *Dentate* = dentate nucleus; *Ant Capsule* = capsula interna anterior; *Post-Med-Hypothal* = nucleus postero-medialis hypothalami; *bilat* = bilateral lesions at one session)

Diagnosis	No of cases	Target	Complications	
Parkinson's disease	10	Vim 9, Pall 1	–	
Intention tremor	3	Vim	–	
Deafferentation pain	7	Pulv 5, CM 2	2	Pulv 2: no effect
Cancer pain	3	VPL 1, Parafasc 2,		Parafasc 1: no effect
		bilat 1	1	3rd n palsy
Cerebral palsy	2	Dentate bilat	–	
Anxiety neurosis	1	Ant Capsule bilat	–	
Obsessive neurosis	1	Ant Capsule bilat	–	
Schizophrenic aggressions	1	Post-Med-Hypothal bilat	–	
Total	28		3	

graphy, where the shadows of the adapter permit the transfer of the CT target to the stereotactic frame. But the stereotactic intervention can also be performed without X-ray, if the stereotactic instrument is placed around the adapter in such a way that the brain target conincides with the mid-point of the spherical stereotactic system.

A repeated CT study after surgery not only shows the high reproducibility of the adapter's mounting, but also corroborates the actual site and size of the surgical lesion (Fig. 2).

Table 1 shows the present clinical material of ablative stereotaxis performed with CT-guidance only. The clinical results have so far been clearly better than after the previous ventriculography-guided surgery. The difference is possibly due to a more exact positioning of the lesions than before, but the lack of nausea and headaches may also have contributed to the positive outcome. The patients can be mobilized a few hours after surgery and are discharged home 1–5 days postoperatively.

The new technique seems to improve the chances to operate on old people who previously were considered to be inoperable. Also cancer patients in poor general condition seem to tolerate ablative thalamotomy far better than percutaneous cordotomy.

Reference

Laitinen LV, Liliequist B, Fagerlund M, Eriksson AT (1985) An adapter for computed tomography (CT) guided stereotaxis. Surg Neurol 23:559–566

Interstitial Irradiation of Inoperable Brain Stem Tumors

F. Oppel, H. W. Pannek, J. Voges, and M. Brock, Berlin/FRG

Introduction

The long-term prognosis of patients with malignant brain stem and midbrain tumors must be regarded as unfavorable. Mean survival rates of 5–15 months have been reported [1]. Several studies show a correlation between prognosis and localization or histology. Most tumors in the cranial pons and in the midbrain are well differentiated astrocytomas, whereas tumors caudal to the pons and in the medulla are usually more malignant [1]. Treatment of these tumors must not be considered curative, its purpose being to increase survival time and improve life quality.

These goals may be attained by:

1. percutaneous irradiation combined with chemotherapy
2. interstitial irradiation in the form of permanent and temporary implantation of isotopes and so-called afterloading. We have lately applied the technique fractionated afterloading to the treatment of inoperable brain gliomas (Oppel et al. 1985 [4]).
   Interstitial irradiation makes it possible to attain a much higher radiation dose than percutaneous irradiation thus improving therapeutic efficiency.

During the past 5 years, 17 patients (6–73 years of age) – 6 with tumors of the brain stem and 11 with tumors of the midbrain – were submitted to interstitial irradiation by permanent implantation of ^{192}Ir seeds. The procedure of fractionated afterloading was applied in two patients.

Method

The dose required for interstitial irradiation was calculated according to the tumor volume and the configuration as determined by angiography, computerized tomography (CT) and magnetic resonance tomography (MR). The marginal tumor dose was limited to 6000–8000 rad in the brain stem and to 8000–10000 rad in the midbrain. Tumor biopsy and isotope implantation were performed by conventional stereotactic technique using an adapted biopsy forceps and an implantation catheter. In order to ensure the diagnosis and verify the exact target determination, 4–6 tumor biopsies were taken and evaluated immediately. The material thus obtained was sufficient to establish diagnosis in all cases.

Depending on the location, extent and shape of the tumor, the needle-path must be chosen so as to permit alignment within the tumor (Fig. 1). While, as a rule, ac-

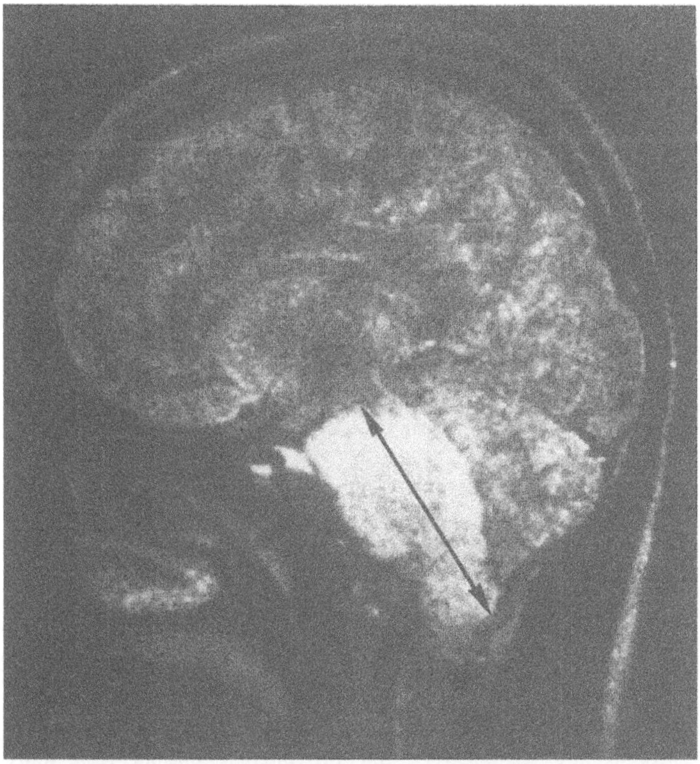

Fig. 1. Magnetic resonance picture of a brain stem tumor (astrocytoma II). Tumor localization and spreading is largely cranio-caudal. Accordingly, ^{192}Ir must be implanted in the longitudinal axis of the tumor. A transcerebellar access would not allow such an alignment of the seeds

cess to the midbrain does not present any problem, access to the brain stem may be hampered by the tentorium, the vessels in the pineal region, or the petrous bone. Since brain stem tumors are partly supra- and infratentorial in location, direct (easier) infratentorial access does not permit optimal seed positioning. For this reason, we have chosen the frontal access through the tentorial notch. As shown in Figs. 2 and 3, the implantation catheter passes between the corpus callosum and the internal capsule and through the thalamus and tentorial notch without affecting the pineal vessels. In order to eliminate the radiation problems caused by temporary interstitial irradiation, we have recently devised a technique for fractionated afterloading by modification of a technique used in the field of gynecology [5].

Our method consists of inserting a catheter (outer diameter: 3 mm) through the longitudinal access of the tumor, the target for the catheter tip being the midpoint of the distal tumor margin. The first step consists of making a burrhole into the calvarium (diameter: 8 mm) and in cutting a winding into the walls of this burrhole. This winding serves for the firm fixation of a screw bolt through which the catheter is inserted, and to which it is fixed. The skin is closed over the bolt, the catheter opening surpassing the skin surface by 2 mm (Figs. 4, 5). The patient can move unrestricted with this implanted catheter, the distal tip of which is closed. The radia-

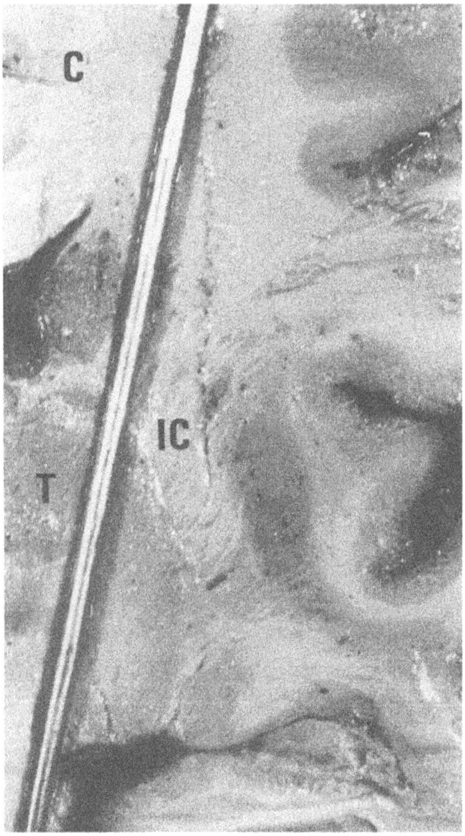

Fig. 2. Anatomic specimen. The stereotactically inserted implantation catheter passes between the corpus callosum (*C*) and the internal capsule (*IC*) transthalamically (*T*) down to the tentorial notch. (Material kindly provided by Prof. J. Lang, Würzburg)

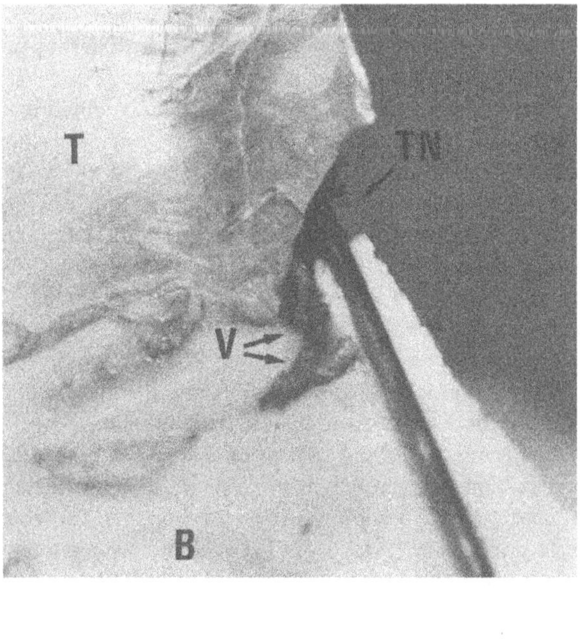

Fig. 3. Anatomic specimen. The implantation catheter passes through the tentorial notch (*TN*) without affecting the vessels of the pineal region (*V*). *T* = tentorium, *B* = brain. (Material kindly provided by Prof. J. Lang, Würzburg)

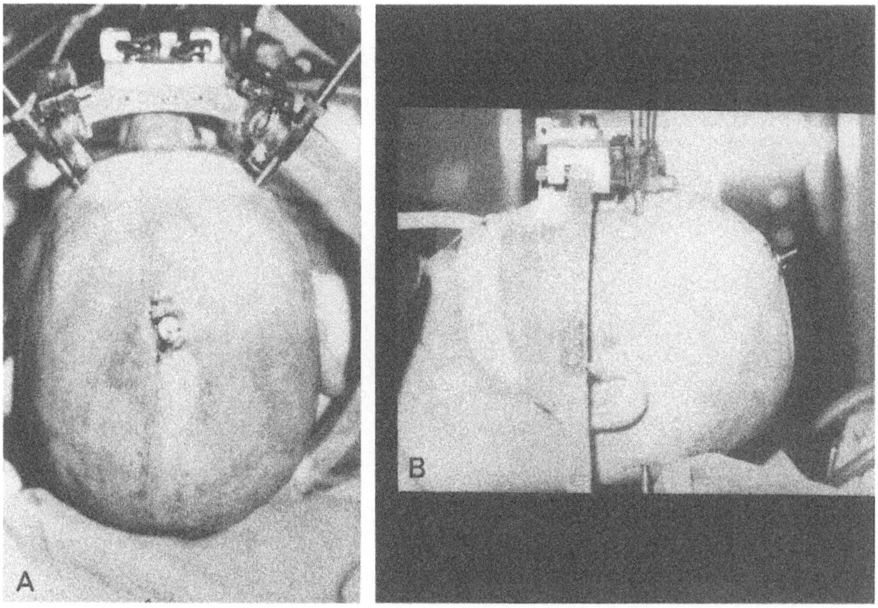

Fig. 4. A Patient fixed in the stereotactic ring. Skin closure is performed after insertion and fixation of the catheter in the screw bolt. **B** Lateral view showing the protruding catheter for later introduction of the radiation source

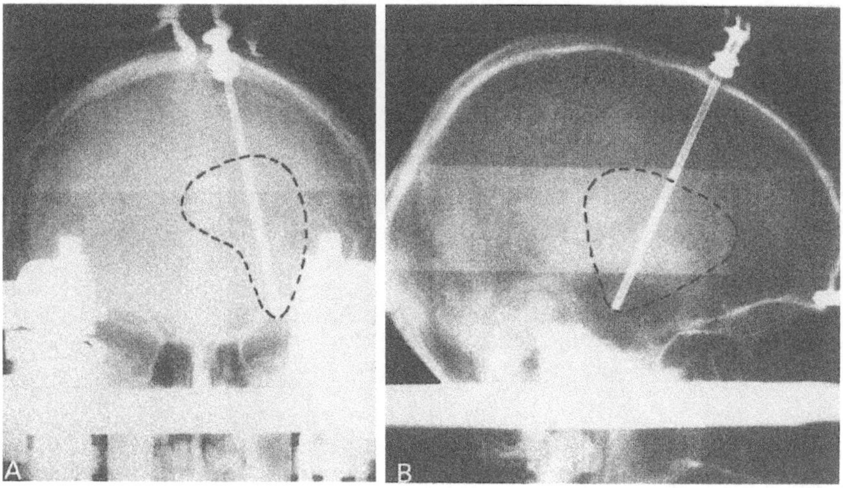

Fig. 5A, B. X-rays showing the indwelling catheter for intermittent afterloading (with tumor contour). **A** a.p., **B** lateral view

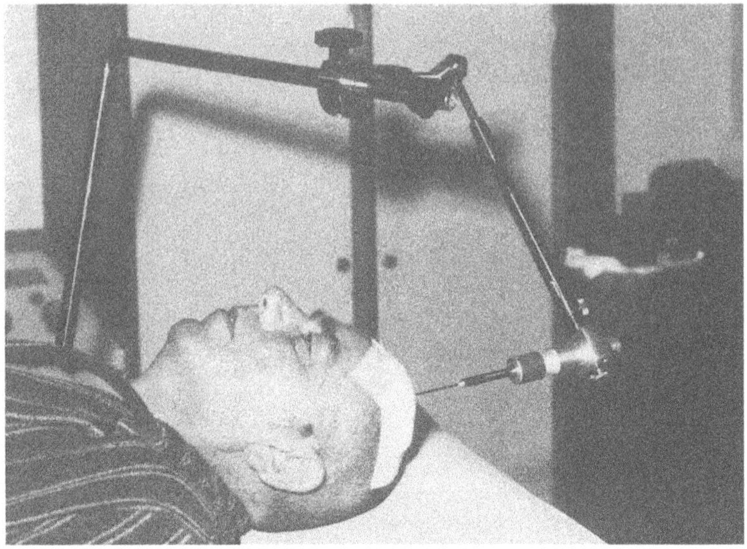

Fig. 6. Patient in the radiation chamber after introduction of the radiation source

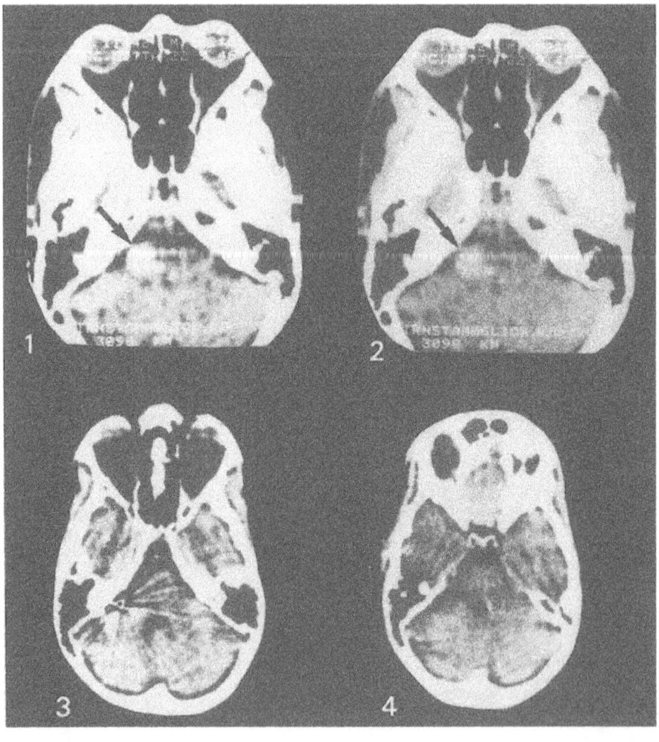

Fig. 7. CT of a pons glioma before (*1, 2, arrows*) and six months after (*3, 4*) interstitial ^{192}Ir irradiation. In the late follow-up, the tumor is no longer visible and the basal cisterns are fully open

tion source has the form of a trocar and is driven into the catheter by remote control once a day for 3–4 minutes (Fig. 6). The required radiation dose, adjusted to the tumor volume, is achieved in up to 10 sessions. After conclusion of radiotherapy, the catheter and thread bolt can be easily removed under local anesthesia. In addition, percutaneous irradiation may be performed after an interval of 3 weeks. In this way, the total radiation dose applied can be significantly increased.

Tables 1–3. Histologic diagnosis, maximal tumor spread, radiation activity and survival time of the dead (*N*) and the still living patients (*S*)

Table 1. Basal ganglia

Pat. no.	Age (years)	Sex	Pathology	Diameter max (mm)	Activity (mCi)	Survivors (S) Non-survivors (N)	Survival time
1. H. D.	57	M	Oligodendro-astrocytoma II	50	4.6	S	2 months
2. D. Z.	46	M	Oligodendroglioma II	40	4.0	N	7 months
3. G. H.	33	M	Astrocytoma II–III	40	1.6	S	8 months
4. G. L.	26	M	Astrocytoma	40	2.0	S	8 months
5. B. B.	45	F	Astrocytoma II–III	40	1.6	N	4 months

Table 2. Thalamus

Pat. no.	Age (years)	Sex	Pathology	Diameter max (mm)	Activity (mCi)	Survivors (S) Non-survivors (N)	Survival time
1. H. Sch.	54	F	Astrocytoma	35	3.4	N	4 days
2. G. L.	67	F	Astrocytoma I	40	1.5	S	3 months
3. A. K.	30	F	Astrocytoma II	30	1.6	S	16 months
4. H. G.	22	M	Astrocytoma I	40	3.0	S	8 months
5. B. H.	26	F	Oligodendro-Astrocytoma III	50	3.2	S	6 months
6. H. D.	35	F	Astrocytoma	40	3.1	S	16 months

Table 2. Brain stem

Pat. no.	Age (years)	Sex	Pathology	Diameter max (mm)	Activity (mCi)	Survivors (S) Non-survivors (N)	Survival time
1. J. Z.	32	M	Astrocytoma I	45	4.2	S	8 months
2. G. S.	70	M	Metastatic Ca.	30	1.3	S	10 days
3. F. B.	59	M	Astrocytoma II	50	5.5	N	5 days
4. H. G.	40	M	Astrocytoma III	40	2.1	N	8 months
5. N. H.	5	M	Oligodendroglioma II	60	3.3	S	4 months
6. R. Y.	37	F	Astrocytoma II	40	2.1	S	23 months

Results

Various degrees of neurologic improvement were achieved in all patients with permanent implantation of ^{192}Ir, in few cases (Fig. 7, Tables 1–3), computerized tomography gave the impression of complete tumor remission for periods up to 2 years. In other cases, tumor growth could not be checked (Tables 1–3). Age, sex, tumor size, marginal tumor dose and survival rates are shown in Tables 1–3. The results must be considered individually and are probably to a large extent dependent on the histology. No complications occurred.

Discussion

At present, interstitial irradiation through permanent ^{192}Ir implantation must be regarded as the most effective therapeutic possibility for treating inoperable tumors of the brain stem, the thalamus and the basal ganglia [2, 3]. Stereotactic technique permits optimal positioning of the seeds and allows bioptic diagnosis. Only tumors of low malignancy can be considered for this therapy, since the radiation effect must correspond to the tumor proliferation. In contrast, rapidly growing tumors can only

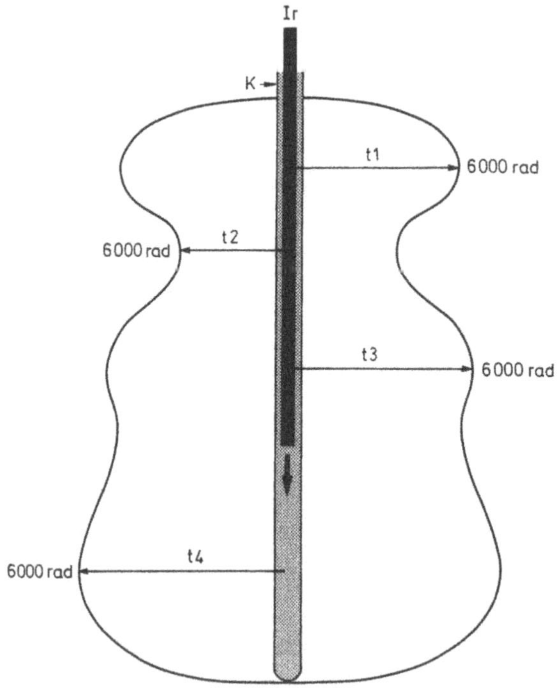

Fig. 8. Schematic representation of a tumor with irregular contours. A catheter (*K*) has been introduced through the longitudinal axis of the tumor for interstitial irradiation by fractionated afterloading. The radiation source (*Ir*) remains (*arrow*) at each point of the tumor for the individual length of time (*t 1–4*) required, the purpose being to attain a marginal tumor dose of 6000 rad through different durations of exposure

be treated and checked in their growth by a short-term high radiation dose. The technique of afterloading seems particularly suitable for this purpose, since high radiation dose can be applied without exposure of family members and nursing personnel. A further advantage is the adjustment of the radiation dose to the tumor contours (Fig. 8), the CT technique now permitting 3-dimensional tumor depiction and thus volumetry. Whenever adequate irradiation of peripheral tumor regions poses difficulties, association of interstitial and percutaneous irradiation may be useful.

Our results (Tables 1–3) show a better response to permanent interstitial ^{192}Ir irradiation in gliomas of low malignancy. This is in agreement with the findings of others [2, 3]. It must be emphasized that initially all patients experience a neurologic improvement. In patients surviving for a long time, the quality of life is markedly improved to completely normal. Patients in whom interstitial irradiation fails to stop tumor growth usually only survive for a short period of time. These patients, as a rule, die of cardiovascular complications. So far, we have not seen complications such as hemorrhages or radiolesions in the surrounding tissue. Local brain edema, the extent of which may vary, can be treated by dexamethasone. Interstitial irradiation of inoperable brain tumors in the brain stem and around the 3rd ventricle can be carried out effectively and without danger in cases of glioma of low malignancy. The new technique of fractionated afterloading seems promising for tumors of higher malignancy. However, conclusive results are not available yet.

References

1. Gutin PhH, Levin VA (1983) Surgery, radiation, and chemotherapy in the treatment of malignant brain tumors. In: Thompson RA, Green JR (eds) Controversies in Neurology. Raven Press, New York, pp 67–86
2. Mundinger F (1983) Stereotaktische intrakranielle Bestrahlung von Tumoren mit Radioisotopen (Curie-Therapie). In: Dietz H, Umbach W, Wüllenweber R (Hrsg) Klinische Neurochirurgie. Thieme, Stuttgart New York, S 519–565
3. Mundinger F (1981) Stereotaktische Therapie nicht resezierbarer intrakranieller Tumoren mit ^{192}Ir und ^{125}J. In: Wannemacher, Schreiber (Hrsg) Kombinierte chirurgische und radiologische Behandlung maligner Tumoren. Urban und Schwarzenberg, München, S 90–112
4. Oppel F, Pannek HW, Brock M (1985) Die interstitielle Bestrahlung maligner inoperabler Hirntumoren nach dem Prinzip des „after loading“. Psycho 11:422–424
5. Rotte K (1983) Das ferngesteuerte Nachladeverfahren (Remote controlled after loading) für intrakavitäre Kontakttherapie (brachy therapy) gynäkologischer Karzinome. Radiologie 23:20–23

Aspiration of Intracerebral Hematomas and Biopsy of Deep Brain Tumors Using CT-Guided Stereotaxic Technique

H. NIIZUMA, T. OTSUKI, R. KATAKURA, and J. SUZUKI, Sendai/Japan

Introduction

Accurate diagnosis of the site and configuration of brain tumors and intracerebral hematomas etc. became possible with the advent of CT-scanning and, through the development of a CT-stereotaxic system (Leksell and Jernberg 1980; Perry et al. 1980; Birg and Mundinger 1982), stereotaxical techniques have developed beyond the traditional boundaries of functional neurosurgery. In the present paper, we report on the aspiration of intracerebral hematomas and biopsy of suspected deep brain tumors.

Aspiration of Intracerebral Hematomas

Thus far, we have performed CT-guided stereotaxic aspiration in a total of 68 cases (Table 1). Ages of the patients were between 28 and 76 years and the level of consciousness on admission was: alert in 14, confused in 28, somnolent in 9, stuporous in 12 and semicomatose in 5. The estimated hematoma volume was 6–20 ml in 23 cases, 21–40 ml in 25 cases and 41–100 ml in 20 cases. Among the operated cases with estimated volumes of less than 20 ml, there were 13 thalamic and 8 putaminal hemorrhage cases – all of these patients were incapable of raising and lowering the limbs on the affected side, and 2 cases of cerebellar hemorrhage.

Six of the cases were operated between 4 and 11 hours after onset, 29 between 12 and 48 hours, 22 between 3 and 7 days, 9 between 8 and 14 days and 2 after 15 days.

Methods

The entire surgical operation was performed in the CT room (Fig. 1). Under local anesthesia, the patient's head was placed in a Leksell's CT-stereotaxic frame (Lek-

Table 1. Location of the hematomas

Site	No. of cases
Putamen	38
Thalamus	17
Cerebellum	7
Cerebral subcortex	6
Total	68

sell and Jernberg 1980). After taking CT-scans, the three-dimensional coordinates of the center of the hematoma were determined and, after moving the CT bed to the rostral side, a burr hole was made. In the case of cerebellar hemorrhage, the head was tilted 30–40° toward the healthy side and a lateral approach was used. Aspiration of the hematoma was done manually using a syringe and lengthened Dandy's ventricular cannula (220 mm long, 3 mm external diameter) (Fig. 2). After aspiration, a silastic drainage tube was inserted to the hematoma cavity and 6000 units of Urokinase dissolved in 2–3 ml of saline solution was injected. Twenty-four hours later, the dissolved hematoma was aspirated through the drainage tube. If required, injection of Urokinase can be repeated several times until the bulk of the hematoma has been removed (Figs. 3, 4, 5).

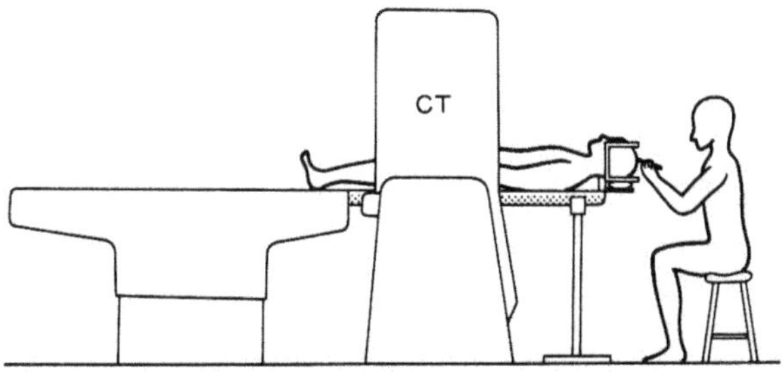

Fig. 1. The stereotaxic operation is performed in the CT room

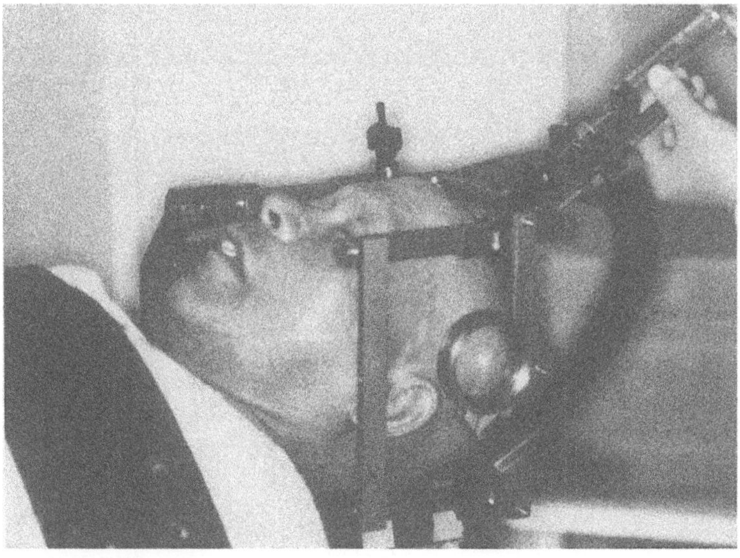

Fig. 2. Aspiration of the hematoma

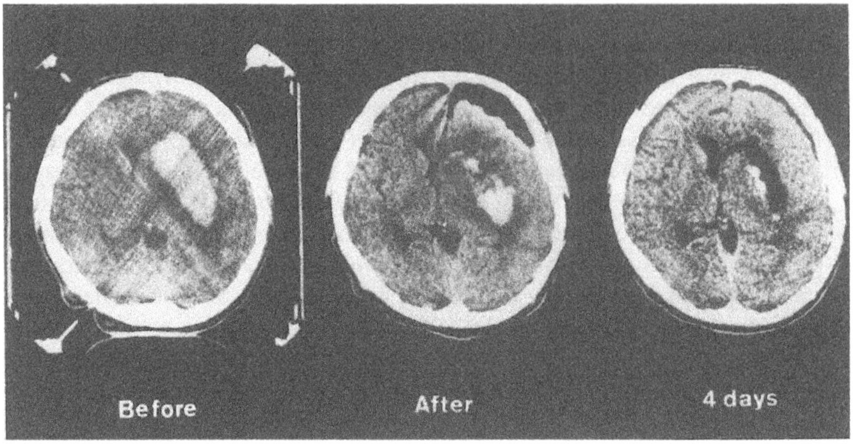

Fig. 3. Putaminal hemorrhage

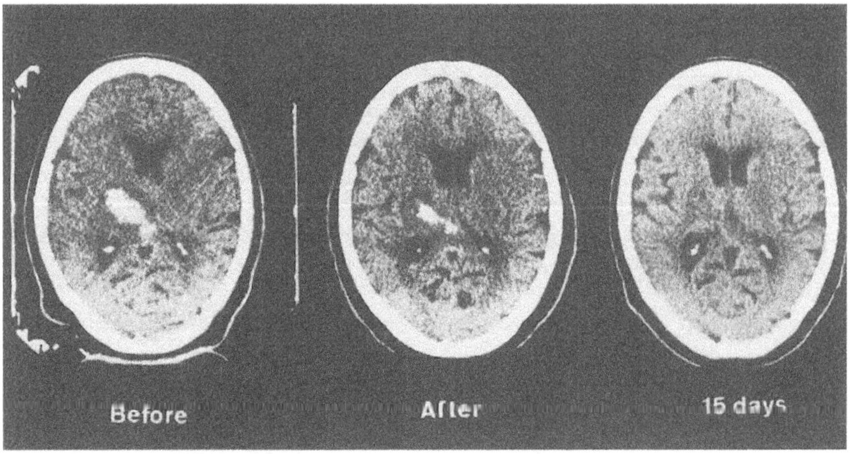

Fig. 4. Thalamic hemorrhage

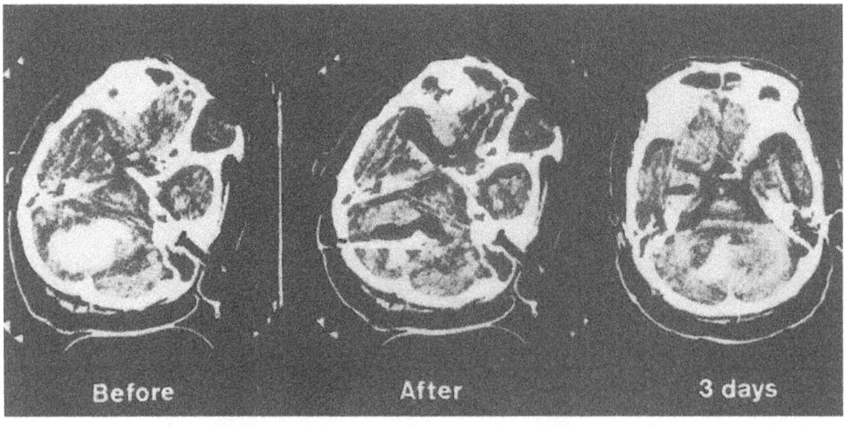

Fig. 5. Cerebellar hemorrhage

Results

It was possible to remove more than 80% of the hematoma in 48 cases; between 50 and 70% was removed in 14 cases and between 30 and 40% was removed in 4 cases. Among the cases in which aspiration of only 30–70% was possible, there were 3 cases in which reaccumulation occurred during the postoperative aspiration of the hematoma. In 2 other cases, postoperative hematoma increased slightly. One was a patient with thalamic hemorrhage in which rebleeding occurred after removal of the drainage tube, but symptoms remained unchanged and she was treated conservatively. The other patient had putaminal hemorrhage which showed slight increases in the hematoma volume at CT-scans taken one hour postoperatively. Symptoms also worsened somewhat, so that the hematoma was immediately removed by conventional craniotomy, and he was able to walk unassisted within one week.

In comparison with conservative treatment or conventional craniotomy, the postoperative recovery following stereotaxic aspiration is extremely rapid in many cases and 48 of our patients (71%) showed improvements in neurologic symptoms on the day following surgery. The drainage tubes were left in place for 1–6 days (most for less than 4 days), but no cases of meningitis were experienced. Our one fatality was a patient in a stuporous state, who had a 98 ml of combined-type hematoma. Fifty percent of hematoma was aspirated, but the patient died of pneumonia 39 days postoperatively.

Among the 31 patients who have been followed for 6 months postoperatively, 25 have returned to normal social lives or are in good condition and capable of unassisted domestic life. Four patients are partially disabled and living at home, and two are in poor condition – totally disabled or bedridden.

Biopsy of Deep Brain Tumors

The biopsy method was nearly identical to the method used for hematoma aspiration. The tissue sample was collected using a Backlund spiral biopsy needle. Prior to biopsy, angiography was performed in all cases and biopsy was performed in 57 cases of suspected brain tumor – excluding only two cases of hypervascular tumor. The site of the lesion was in the temporal lobe in 14 cases, the frontal lobe in 12 cases, the parieto-occipital lobe in 7 cases, the thalamus in 7 cases, the basal ganglia in 7 cases, the corpus callosum in 4 cases, the pineal region in 3 cases, the third ventricle or suprachiasmal region in 2 cases and the pons in one case.

Results

In 2 cases of cystic tumor following irradiation therapy, the wall of the tumor was too hard to allow biopsy and in 7 cases of inadequate sampling diagnosis was impossible. These 7 cases included 2 cases of cystic tumor with thin walls, 2 cases showing low density regions without contrast enhancement in CT scans, and one case of central low density with faint ring enhancement. In the remaining 48 cases (84%), diagnosis from the biopsied tissue was possible (Table 2). Minimal bleeding was found in 3 patients in postoperative CT scans, but symptoms did not become aggra-

Table 2. Pathologic diagnosis

Glioblastoma	11
High grade astrocytoma	12
Low grade astrocytoma	12
Oligodendroglioma	3
Malignant lymphoma	2
Metastasis	2
Germinoma	2
Others	4
Inadequate sampling	7
Total	55

vated. In one case, postoperative intracranial hypertension worsened, but no changes in the CT scans were noted and the symptoms were transient.

Discussion

By means of CT guidance, the CT-guided stereotaxic technique makes the stereotaxic operation a safer, minimally invasive method. Since the operation can be performed under the administration of a local anesthetic, it is relatively easy to perform in elderly patients. Sixteen of the 125 patients in the present series were over 70 years of age, but the operative invasion itself did not become a problem in any case. The greatest disadvantage of this technique is that, when bleeding has been brought about, it is then difficult to begin surgery in counteract to the hemorrhage. Nonetheless, by means of careful handling of the site and control of blood pressure, a fatal outcome from the hemorrhage is thought to be unlikely.

In hypertensive intracerebral hemorrhage cases where there is rebleeding, the cause seemed to be excessive aspiration during the operation and changes in the position of the drainage tube while using Urokinase postoperatively. While aiming for total removal of the hematoma in most cases, it is thought safe and appropriate to achieve subtotal evacuation in some cases, as Backlund and Holst (1978) have previously indicated in his first report on stereotaxic aspiration. Recently, we have considered evacuation of 80–90% of the hematoma volume to be sufficient. In order to aspirate the hematoma, various methods, including the use of a rotating helical mandrel, have been reported (Backlund and Holst 1978; Higgins and Nashold 1980; Doi et al. 1982), but if the hematoma is approached along its long axis, some 50–80% of the hematoma can be aspirated during the surgery using a lengthened ventricular cannula. By injection of Urokinase to dissolve the remaining hematoma, the majority of the hematoma can be removed in most cases.

Sufficient follow-up study to allow for meaningful comparisons between this stereotaxic technique, conservative therapy and conventional surgical techniques has not yet been undertaken, but the stereotaxic technique shows promise both in terms of the rapid postoperative recovery and the safety even when used in elderly patients. Moreover, it is thought that, because of the minimal operative invasion required in the stereotaxic method, its applicability may eventually be much wider than currently believed – particularly in cases of small hematomas or deep-seated hematomas in the thalamus, etc., for which surgical invasion has not previously been indicated.

With regard to CT-guided stereotaxic biopsy, we have found that such biopsies are easy to perform and can be done with great accuracy (Niizuma et al. 1984). The rate of diagnosis, however, has not yet approached 100% – primarily due to insufficient sampling of active tumor cells. Insufficient sampling was generally a consequence of the fact that the tumor had previously undergone irradiation, the tumor itself was cystic with thin walls or bulk of the tumor was necrotic. Nonetheless, an accurate diagnosis is normally possible in contrast enhanced tumors from which a sufficient sample has been obtained. Provided that the tumor is checked angiographically prior to surgery and that an unnecessarily large sample is not obtained, the CT-guided stereotaxic biopsy technique is thought to be very safe and effective.

References

1. Backlund EO, Holst H (1978) Controlled subtotal evacuation of intracerebral hematomas by stereotaxic technique. Surg Neurol 9:99–101
2. Birg W, Mundinger F (1982) Direct target point determination for stereotactic brain operations from CT data and the calculation of setting parameters for polar-coordinate stereotactic devices. Appl Neurophysiol 45:387–395
3. Doi E et al. (1982) Stereotactic evacuation of intracerebral hematomas. Neurol Med Chir (Tokyo) 22:461–467
4. Higgins AC, Nashold BS (1980) Modification of instrument for stereotactic evacuation of intracerebral hematoma: Technical note. Neurosurg 7:604–605
5. Leksell L, Jernberg B (1980) Stereotaxis and tomography – A technical note. Acta Neurochir (Wien) 52:1–7
6. Niizuma H et al. (1984) CT-guided stereotaxic brain tumor biopsy. Neurol Surg 12:55–61 (in Japanese)
7. Perry JH et al. (1980) Computed tomography-guided stereotactic surgery: Conception and development of a new stereotactic methodology. Neurosurg 7 (4):376–381

Thalamic Stimulation: Effects on Deafferentation Pain and Movement Disorders

J. SIEGFRIED and H. VAN LOVEREN, Zürich/Switzerland

Introduction

Pain is a dynamic process which may eventually by-pass any iatrogenic block in the nervous system whether induced by drugs or by the destruction of specific pathways. Therefore the attention of those who would treat chronic pain remains focused upon stimulation techniques which can modify pain in a reversible and adjustable fashion. The two preferred targets for deep brain stimulation are the periaqueductal gray substance (PAG) and the thalamic sensory relay nuclei: ventroposteromedialis (VPM) and ventroposterolateralis (VPL). PAG stimulation has demonstrated effectiveness in the treatment of somatogenic (nociceptive) pain – pain due to involvement of non-nervous tissues, typically due to cancer. It has little effect, however, on neurogenic pain which is due to direct involvement of nervous tissues and has deafferentation as a prominent feature (Meyerson 1983). This is corroborated by our own experience with nine cases of deafferentation facial pain treated in 1977 by PAG stimulation without success. In contrast, our results in 80 patients followed for 1 to 62 months indicate that stimulation of the thalamic sensory nuclei is very effective in the treatment of deafferentation pain. During this study we were also able to observe the beneficial effect of thalamic stimulation on the involuntary movement disorders of 6 patients with associated chronic pain disorders.

Materials and Methods

During the six year period from October 1978 to December 1984, 103 patients with chronic, intractable pain were judged appropriate candidates for thalamic sensory stimulation. Each patient underwent trial stimulation for 2 to 7 days via a stimulating electrode stereotactically implanted into the somatotopic region of the thalamic sensory nucleus which corresponded to the distribution of pain. Eighty of these 103 patients (78%) reported significant pain reduction and subsequently underwent implantation of a permanent subcutaneous receiver (Model Pens; Avery, Farmingdale, New York) or total programmable implant (Model Itrel; Medtronic, Minneapolis, Minnesota). Results obtained from these eighty patients form the basis of this report.

This series consisted of 46 males and 34 females ranging in age from 19 to 83 years; average age 54.5 years. Pain was neurogenic in 76 patients, somatogenic in 4 patients and mixed in 4 patients. The duration of pain prior to stimulation was from

1 to 10 years and averaged 4 years. The most common diagnosis was anesthesia/hypesthesia dolorosa (20 cases) followed by post-herpetic neuralgia (19 cases) (Table 1). The majority of patients had pain localized to the face.

Follow-up ranged from 1 to 62 months; average 32 months. Pain was assessed prior to stimulation and at regular follow-up intervals using standardized protocols. The most subjective of these was the visual analog-scale which consisted of a line divided into four quarters (0–25, 25–50, 50–75, 75–100) along which a patient could rate his/her pain level (Fig. 1). The most objective assessments were occu-

Table 1. Etiology of pain

Diagnosis	Male	Female
Somatogenic	4	4
Arachnoiditis	1	2
Carcinoma	1	2
Other	2	0
Neurogenic	45	31
Anes./hyp. dol.	12	8
Causalgia	1	0
Phantom pain	5	3
Stump pain	3	1
Nerve lesion	2	3
Herpes zoster	7	12
Brachial plexus	9	1
Thalamic	8	4
Carcinoma	6	2
Other	4	1

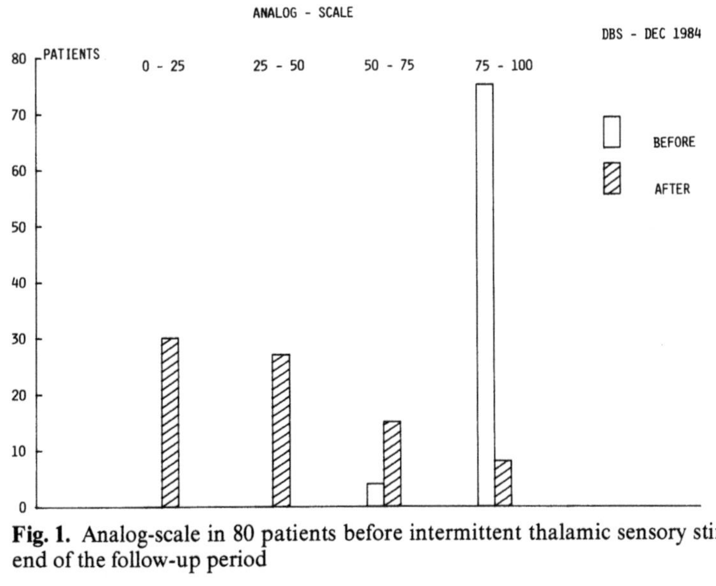

Fig. 1. Analog-scale in 80 patients before intermittent thalamic sensory stimulation and at the end of the follow-up period

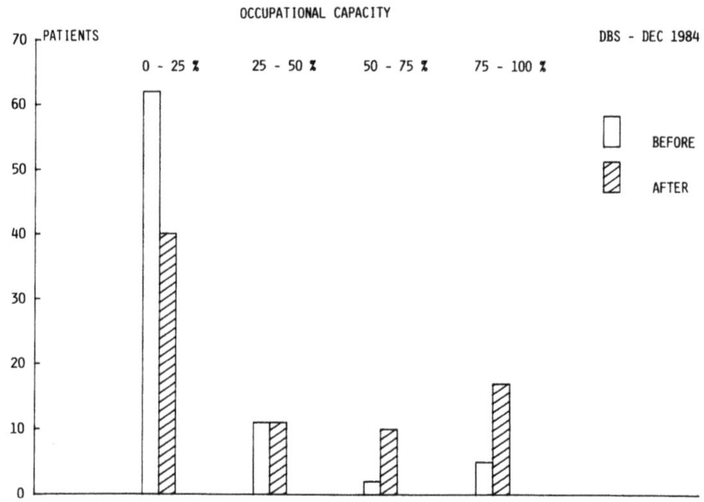

Fig. 2. Occupational capacity in 80 patients before intermittent thalamic sensory stimulation and at the end of the follow-up period

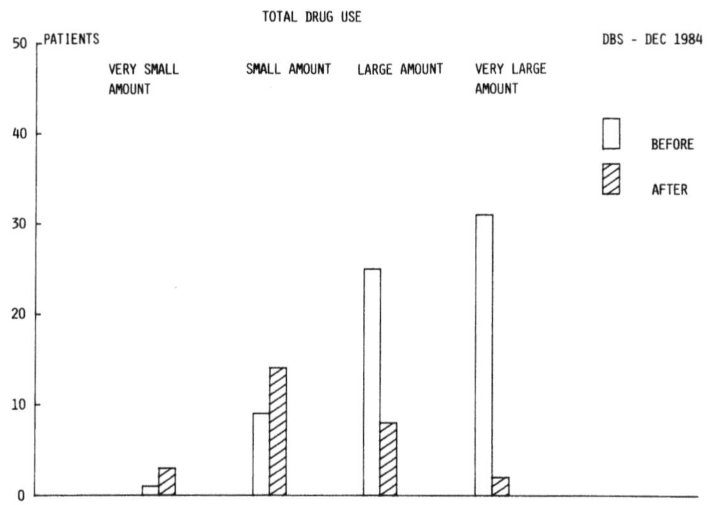

Fig. 3. Total drug use (including anxiolytics, anti-depressants, analgesics and narcotics) in 80 patients before intermittent thalamic stimulation and at the end of the follow-up period. Patients without any drug use are not depicted but account for 53 patients at the end of the follow-up period

pational capacity and drug use (Figs. 2, 3). Pain was also assessed using a five grade rating score, the pain profile, which took into consideration:

1. the duration of pain,
2. intensity of pain,
3. level of activity,
4. influence on mood and behavior and
5. use of drugs (Fig. 4).

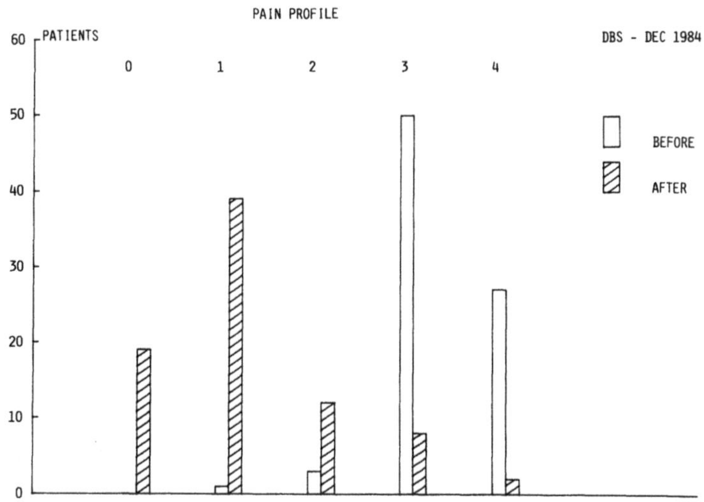

Fig. 4. Pain profile in 80 patients before intermittent thalamic stimulation and at the end of the follow-up period. See text for details of rating scale

The coordinates for the thalamic sensory nuclei were as follows: VPM for pain in the facial region – 3 mm anterior to the posterior commissure on the AC-PC line, 1 to 2 mm below this line and 9 mm lateral to the midline; VPL_1 for the upper extremity – 3 mm anterior to the posterior commissure on the AC-PC line, 1 to 2 mm below this line and 13 mm lateral to the midline; VPL_2 for the lower extremity – 16 mm lateral to the midline.

The 80 patients in this series underwent a total of 101 operations with 89 electrode implantations (three patients were operated on bilaterally). The electrode targets were as follows: 44 VPM, 27 VPL_1, 16 VPL_2 and 2 PAG. Earlier patients in this series received a subcutaneous receiver while a total programmable implant was used in the final procedures.

Results

1. Stimulation Parameters

The initial stimulus intensity required to produce paresthesia in the distribution of pain ranged from 0.3 to 3.0 volts. At the time of last follow-up in patients with pain controlled, the mean intensity for effective stimulation was 1.69V ± 0,86 in cases of total implant and 1.87V ± 1.98 in cases with a subcutaneous receiver. The initial mean frequency of stimulation was 42 Hz which was gradually increased to 45.19 Hz by patients with a total implant and 53.39 Hz by patients with a subcutaneous receiver. Other parameters for the total implant included an impulse duration of 191.25 msec ± 37.7 with programmed stimulation alternating ON 22.43 seconds and OFF 11.81 minutes for an average stimulation time of 44.18 minutes per day. Parameters for the subcutaneous receiver were impulse duration 205.16 msec ± 63.6 with stimulation ON for an average of 56.24 minutes per day.

2. Pain Control

Eighty patients undergoing thalamic stimulation were followed for 1 to 62 months; average follow-up 32 months. According to the parameters applied, pain decreased remarkably during the initial four months of stimulation and then slowly increased to a new steady state below the pre-stimulation level at about 6 months. Parameters were compared prior to stimulation and at the end of the follow-up period, December 1984. The visual analog-scale indicates that 71% of the patients who rated their pain level in the upper half of the scale prior to stimulation, rated their pain level in the lower half at the last evaluation (Fig. 1). Total drug use was "large" or "very large" in 70% of patients before stimulation and in only 12.5% at last follow-up (Fig. 3). Occupational capacity, perhaps the most critical parameter socioeconomically, showed the least improvement. However, prior to stimulation only 9% of patients had greater than 50% working capacity compared to 35% at last follow-up (Fig. 2). The pain profile which attempts to summarize the psychologic, social, medical and economic parameters visually demonstrates the overall benefit of stimulation (Fig. 4).

Analysis of these parameters for each diagnosis revealed comparable results for each category including somatogenic pain. Best results were obtained with anesthesia or hypesthesia dolorosa and postherpetic neuralgia. Phantom pain unresponsive to dorsal cord stimulation did respond to thalamic stimulation. As might be expected, the success in treatment of thalamic pain syndrome appeared to be inversely proportional to the size of the lesion on computerized tomography.

3. Movement Disorders

Four patients with thalamic pain syndrome had an associated dyskinesia of the hand. Stimulation of the VPL_1 thalamic nucleus according to standard parameters relieved pain but was also observed to arrest the dyskinesia of the hand during and for several minutes after stimulation. Two paraplegic patients with deafferentation pain had associated bilateral spontaneous clonus and spasticity. During and for several minutes after bilateral VPL_2 thalamic nucleus stimulation, spontaneous clonus was arrested and spasticity was markedly reduced.

4. Complications

One patient suffered a slight hemiparesis after placement of a non-hollow-core electrode. Three systems had to be removed due to a foreign-body rejection reaction and 4 others due to local infection. Four patients underwent re-operation to replace a defective component and 6 for electrode dislocation. Four cancer patients died due to complications of their primary diagnosis at 1, 2, 6 and 15 months post-stimulation. One patient suffered a cerebral infarction contralateral to the side of stimulation with sufficient mass effect to dislocate the electrode.

Discussion

The original observation of stimulation-produced analgesia (Reynolds 1969) and subsequent discovery of an endogenous pain controlling system in the upper brain stem (Mayer 1979) opened a new era in pain therapy. The region of effective stimulation in experimental animals, the raphe nucleus, was not safely accessible in humans. Therefore attention has been directed to regions surrounding the third ventricle made accessible by recent advances in stereotactic technique and instrumentation.

The analgesic effect of electrical activation of the thalamic sensory relay nucleus was first observed by Mazars (Mazars et al. 1973) and subsequently described by Richardson and Akil who performed thalamic stimulation prior to stereotactic thalamotomy (Richardson and Akil 1977). The neuronal pathway for this pain inhibition is not known. A supraspinal gating mechanism based on the gate-control theory of pain has been suspected due to similarities to dorsal cord stimulation (DCS) such as the prerequisite paresthesia, time course to relief and post-stimulatory duration of relief (Meyerson 1983). Neither modality is naloxone-reversible (Hosobuchi et al. 1980) and therefore would not be expected to be of benefit for opioid-sensitive somatogenic pain. Reports to the contrary are noted (Tsubokawa et al. 1984), especially experimental reports that thalamic stimulation facilitates neurons of the raphe nucleus (Tsubokawa et al. 1981) implying a common pathway for thalamic and PAG stimulation. Spinal cord dorsal horn interneurons which normally respond to noxious stimulation can be inhibited by stimulation of the PAG (Carstens et al. 1979) and raphe nucleus (Guilbaud et al. 1977). Subsequent demonstration of inhibition of spinothalamic tract cells during and after stimulation of the VPL thalamic nucleus (Gerhart et al. 1981) offers an experimental correlate to the clinical effect of thalamic stimulation.

PAG stimulation, which is naloxone-reversible, increases CSF β-endorphin concentration (Tsubokawa et al. 1984). Such an effect had not been demonstrated for thalamic stimulation (Hosobuchi et al. 1980). Recent studies indicate that CSF β-endorphin concentration may be lower in patients with chronic pain than in normal controls. This concentration increases with thalamic stimulation but neither exceeds control levels nor correlates with clinical relief of pain (Tsubokawa et al. 1984).

Mazars has advocated thalamic stimulation since 1973 and subsequently reported almost total relief of pain in 90% of some 100 patients with deafferentation pain (Mazars et al. 1979). Pain relief has also been reported with stimulation of other targets along the somatic afferent system including the sensory limb of the internal capsule (Hosobuchi et al. 1973) and the medial lemniscus (Mundinger and Salomao 1980). Mazars' results have been difficult to reproduce (Lazorthes 1979). The results of this study, however, corroborate other studies which justify the continued application and investigation of thalamic sensory stimulation in the treatment of chronic pain.

Deep brain stimulation for involuntary movement disorders was introduced by Cooper (Cooper et al. 1982) and Mundinger (Mundinger 1977). There is neither sufficient clinical data nor experimental rationale to justify widespread application of thalamic stimulation using movement disorders as a primary indication. The temporary resolution of dyskinesia and clonus in our 6 patients is encouraging and warrants further observation and investigation.

References

Carstens E, Yokota T, Zimmermann M (1979) Inhibition of spinal neuronal responses to noxious skin heating by stimulation of mesencephalic periaqueductal gray in the cat. J Neurophysiol 42:558–568

Cooper IS, Upton ARM, Amin I (1982) Chronic cerebellar stimulation and deep brain stimulation in involuntary movement disorders. Appl Neurophysiol 54:209–217

Gerhart KD, Yezierski RP, Wilcox TK, Grossman AE, Willis WD (1981) Inhibition of primate spinothalamic tract neurons by stimulation in ipsilateral or contralateral ventral posterior lateral (VPL_c) thalamic nucleus. Brain Res 229:514–519

Guilbaud G, Oliveras JL, Gisler G Jr, Besson JM (1977) Effects induced by stimulation of the centralis inferior nucleus of the raphe on dorsal horn interneurons in cat's spinal cord. Brain Res 126:355–360

Hosobuchi Y, Adams JE, Rutkin B (1973) Chronic thalamic stimulation for the control of facial anesthesia dolorosa. Arch Neurol 29:158–161

Hosobuchi Y, Rossier J, Bloom FE (1980) Oral loading with L-tryptophan may augment the simultaneous release of ACTH and beta-endorphin that accompanies periaqueductal stimulation in humans. In: Costa E, Trabucchi M (eds) Neural Peptides and Neuronal Communication. Raven Press, New York, p 563–570

Lazorthes Y (1979) European Study on Deep Brain Stimulation. Résumé of the 3rd European Workshop on Electrical Neurostimulation. Medtronic, Paris

Mayer DJ (1979) Endogenous analgesia systems: Neural and behavioral mechanisms. In: Bonica JJ, Liebeskind JC, Albe-Fessard DG (eds) Advances in Pain Research and Therapy, vol 3. Raven Press, New York, p 385–410

Mazars GJ, Mérienne L, Cioloca C (1973) Stimulations thalamiques intermittentes antalgiques. Rev Neurol 128:273–279

Mazars GJ, Mérienne L, Cioloca C (1979) Comparative study of electrical stimulation of posterior thalamic nuclei, periaqueductal gray, and other midline mesencephalic structures in man. In: Bonica JJ, Liebeskind JC, Albe-Fessard DG (eds) Advances in Pain Research and Therapy, vol 3. Raven Press, New York, p 541–546

Meyerson BA (1983) Electrostimulation procedures: Effects, presumed rationale, and possible mechanisms. In: Bonica JJ, Liebeskind JC, Albe-Fessard DG (eds) Advances in Pain Research and Therapy, vol 5. Raven Press, New York, p 495–534

Mundinger F (1977) Neue stereotaktisch-funktionelle Behandlungsmethode des Torticollis spasmodicus mit Hirnstimulatoren. Med Kin 72:1982–1986

Mundinger F, Salomao JF (1980) Deep brain stimulation in mesencephalic lemniscus medialis for chronic pain. Acta Neurochir [Suppl] (Wien) 30:245–258

Reynolds DV (1969) Surgery in the rat during electrical analgesia induced by focal brain stimulation. Science 164:444–445

Richardson DE, Akil H (1977) Pain reduction by electrical brain stimulation in man. J Neurosurg 47:178–183

Tsubokawa T, Yamamoto T, Katayama Y, Moriyasu N (1981) Diencephalic modulation of activities of raphe-spinal neurons in the cat. Exp Neurol 74:561–572

Tsubokawa T, Yamamoto T, Katayama Y, Hirayama T, Sibuya H (1984) Thalamic relay nucleus stimulation of relief of intractable pain. Clinical results and B-endorphin immunoreactivity in the cerebrospinal fluid. Pain 18:115–126

Stereotaxic Hypothalamotomy in Aggressive Behavior

B. RAMAMURTHI and V. BALASUBRAMANIAM, Madras/India

Stereotactic surgery provides a safe and effective method of making lesions in the deep structures in the brain to control specific functional neurologic problems. In spite of various advances that have taken place in neuro- and psychopharmacology stereotactic surgery still continues to have a useful place in the treatment of some types of movement disorders, psychiatric illnesses and behavior problems. Placing a lesion in the VL thalamus is even now the ideal way of treating unilateral parkinsonism tremors in younger people especially when there is no response to the latest drugs. In psychiatric disorders, discrete lesions placed in the cingulum bundle and the baso-frontal region provide an effective way of helping patients suffering from severe depression and from obsessive disorders (Ramamurthi et al. 1982).

For behavior disorders in children, stereotactic surgery of the limbic system and the hypothalamus provides a useful method of therapy (Narabayashi et al. 1963; Sano et al. 1966). In children, who have behavior disorders where the chief symptoms are aggression and violence, lesions in the amygdala and/or in the hypothalamus have proved effective (Balasubramaniam and Ramamurthi 1970; Balasubramaniam et al. and Ramamurthi 1973; Ramamurthi 1977).

Stereotactic hypothalamotomy was performed by Spiegel and Wycis as early as 1951 to control aggression in schizophrenics. In 1962 Sano introduced the term Sedative Neurosurgery and showed that hypothalamic lesions control aggression. Following the lead given by Sano, we in Madras have practised stereotactic hypothalamotomy in children with aggressive behavior disorders.

Of the 1775 stereotactic procedures performed in Madras over a period of 25 years, 603 operations were done in children who had behavior disorders with or without epilepsy. Of these 480 were amygdalotomies and 123 were hypothalamotomies. All the patients included in this series have been children below 15 years and have been on medical therapy for a minimum period of two years. When such therapy has not given the desired benefit and when the problem becomes uncontrollable stereotactic surgery has been offered as an effective therapy. The common cause of such aggressive behavior is an encephalitis, the behavior disorder arising as a postencephalitic sequel. In some children frequent epileptic attacks have led to a change in the personality and when the fits got controlled, aggression became the dominant problem. The types of behavior disorder include violence, restlessness, wandering tendency, pyromania, self destruction etc. In our experience bilateral stereotactic amygdalatomy is the ideal first choice for treating such children (Balasubramaniam and Ramamurthi 1970). In cases where bilateral stereotactic amygdalatomy has not succeeded and also primarily as a first procedure, stereotactic hypothalamotomy has been performed in 123 cases over a period of 20 years. 50 were primary and 73 were secondary hypothalamotomies. The armamentaria has been kept quite simple. Leksell's stereotactic apparatus is used and pneumoencephalography helps to locate the midline structures in the brain for the necessary calculations.

Depth electrode recordings have not been helpful in locating the target. The target is identified by sympathomimetic responses to stimulation and include respiratory changes like tachypnoea or apnoea, pupillary dilatation, ocular movements including convergence and increase in the blood pressure. This apnoea has not been reported by earlier workers. We consider apnoea as a characteristic of limbic system stimulation. The apnoea was seen both in primary hypothalamotomy cases and in children where bilateral amygdalatomy has been done earlier, thus confirming the effector and 'distal' nature of the role of the hypothalamus in the limbic complex.

Balasubramaniam and myself have found from our experience that the best area to make the lesion is slightly different from that proposed by Sano 1962 (Balasubramaniam et al. 1972). This target is a little forward and below the Sano's target, though lying within the ergotropic triangle. We found that the maximum responses were elicited from this area, and lesions in this field caused the best improvement in the aggressive behavior disorder. There have been few postoperative complications, transient diabetes insipidus being one of them. We have performed the hypothalamotomy on the two sides in two stages with an interval of a week or ten days.

An interesting finding during the course of our studies in some of these patients has been the correlation of function between the amygdala and the hypothalamus in humans. Recordings were made of the electrical activity of the amygdala during hypothalamotomy. There was a change in the pattern of discharges from the amygdala immediately after the hypothalamic lesion was made, thus effectively proving the close functional relationship between these two structures.

Another observation made during the operations related to gastric acid secretion. It has been shown by us that stimulation of the amygdala as well as the hypothalamus results in an increase in gastric acid secretion. Following lesions in these structures, there was a significant fall in gastric acid secretion (Ramamurthi et al. 1977).

The immediate results of primary hypothalamotomy are similar to those of amygdalatomy; one third of the patients improving remarkably and one third moderately. When hypothalamotomy is performed in a child where bilateral amygdalatomy has failed, good results are obtained in 50% of these patients. Long term assessment with a follow-up of 3 to 20 years show that 55% of children who had hypothalamotomy showed good results, 30% showed some improvement while 15% showed failure (Ramamurthi 1977). It is possible to correlate the positive responses with two features namely the presence of associated epilepsy and the presence of violence. Where the results have been good, the children have become free from fits and aggression and have progressed mentally within the limits of their damaged brain function.

Conclusions

Stereotactic hypothalamotomy has a useful place in the treatment of aggressive behavior disorder in children and can be performed in a simple set up. Stimulation response are the best guide to identifying the target. Long term follow-up reveals good improvement in one third of the patients and moderate improvement in another third.

References

Balasubramaniam V, Ramamurthi B (1970) Stereotaxic amygdalotomy in behavior disorders. Confin Neurol 32:367–373

Balasubramaniam V, Kanaka TS, Ramanujam PB, Velmurugendran CU, Ramamurthi B (1972) Electrophysiological studies during sedative neurosurgery. Neurol India [Suppl 2] 20:175–178

Balasubramaniam V, Kanaka TS, Ramanujam PB, Ramamurthi B (1973) Stereotaxic hypothalamotomy. Confin Neurol 35:138–143

Narabayashi H, Nagao T, Saito Y, Yoshida M, Nagahata M (1963) Stereotaxic amygdalotomy for behavior disorders. Arch Neurol 9:1–16

Ramamurthi B (1977) Surgery for aggressive behaviour disorders. Excerpta medica international congress series No. 433. Proceedings of the Sixth international congress of neurological surgery. Brazil, p 19–25

Ramamurthi B, Mascreen M, Valmikinathan K (1977) Role of amygdala and hypothalamus in the control of gastric secretion in human beings. Acta Neurochir [Suppl] (Wien) 24:187–190

Ramamurthi B, Ravi R, Narayanan R (1982) Long term follow-up of functional neurosurgery in psychiatric disorders. Appl Neurophysiol 45:538

Sano K (1962) Sedative neurosurgery with special reference to posteromedial hypothalamotomy. Neurol Med Chir (Tokyo) 4:112–142

Sano K, Yoshioka M, Ogashiwa M, Ishijima B, Ohye C (1966) Postero-medical hypothalamotomy in the treatment of aggressive behaviors. Confin Neurol 27:164–167

Spiegel EA, Wycis HT (1951) The central mechanism of emotion. Am J Psychiatry 108:426–431

Stereotactic Radiosurgery in Rabbit Eye Melanoma

R. W. Rand, A. Khonsary, W. J. Brown, J. Winter, E. Holly, H. D. Snow, and T. Geiger, Los Angeles, CA/USA

Melanoma of the eye is one of the most common eye malignancies in humans. One of the more effective ways of treating such neoplasms is by the use of focused radiation energy using the heavy particles delivered by a cyclotron. These Bragg peak radiation programs are being carried out successfully in Boston, Mass. and Berkeley, Ca.

The Leksell Stereotactic Gamma Unit developed in 1970 for the treatment of selected small brain tumors and arteriovenous malformations has been used in Stockholm, Sweden, in a few human cases of melanoma of the eye.

The UCLA stereotactic radiosurgical system focuses 178 ^{60}Cobalt needle sources to a small area within the radiation chamber. This system is rated currently at 110 rads per minute. Therefore, a 7000 rad treatment to an eye neoplasm can be delivered in slightly over one hour.

Appropriate anesthesia is used for the rabbits in whom the melanoma has been implanted into the anterior chamber. Within one week after treatment, these tumors are significantly reduced in size and have disappeared four weeks thereafter. Follow-up histologic studies in nine months have indicated no recurrence of tumor growth. The control rabbits continue to show rapid growth of the melanoma.

The experimental melanoma model was provided by Linn Murphree, M. D. and Charles Gomer, Ph. D., Division of Ophthalmology, Los Angeles Childrens Hospital.

Stereotactic radiosurgery was introduced by Leksell in 1971 as a ^{60}Cobalt single dose treatment for selected small brain tumors, arteriovenous malformations, and to control severe cancer pain. The original radiosurgical instrument was fabricated to accomplish this new concept of bloodless stereotactic surgery using focused gamma beams from 179 ^{60}Cobalt needles arranged in a partial hemisphere design within a radiation chamber (Fig. 1). The size of the focal area in the radiosurgical instrument used in the current rabbit eye melanoma experiments was 4 mm at the 90% dosimetry zone (Fig. 2). This radiation focus area can be increased by substituting other gamma beam collimators. The current UCLA Radiosurgical Instrument can deliver a radiation dose of 110 rads per minute, and, therefore, can deliver up to 10000 rads in a relatively short period of time to a surgical target (Fig. 3).

The radiosurgical target is located either by CT scans or plain films and is then applied to the Leksell coordinate localizer. The stereotactic coordinates of the surgical target are determined as the X axis (side to side), the Y axis (front to back), and

---

Key Words: Stereotactic ^{60}Cobalt Radiosurgery – Experimental Melanoma – Rabbit Eye.

the Z axis (depth from vertex). Once the XYZ coordinates of the center of the surgical target are determined, the volume of the tumor is calculated by the medical physicist in order to ascertain the radiosurgical gamma dose to be delivered.

Considerable research has been done using a variety of dosimetry techniques to measure accurately the gamma radiation at the 90 percentile, 50 percentile, and 10 percentile zones from the center of the radiosurgical lesion [14]. These dosimetry zones are very narrow, so within a predetermined area a central radiosurgical dose of 6000 rads would be only 3000 rads delivered at the 50% zone a few millimeters away and 600 rads at the 10% zone (Fig. 2). Consequently, when the tissue target is radiated at the radiosurgical focus within the radiation chamber, the edge between

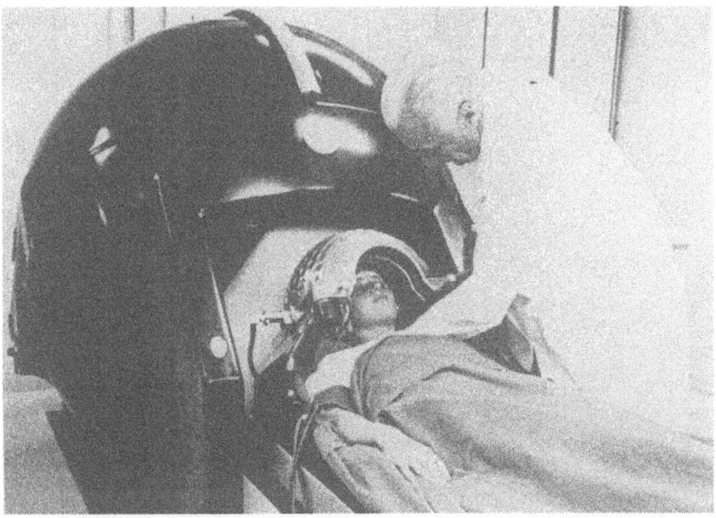

Fig. 1. The Leksell Stereotactic Radiosurgical Unit or "Gamma Knife" containing 179 ^{60}Cobalt needles directed to a focal point within the radiation chamber. Professor Lars Leksell is shown treating a patient with a small pituitary tumor having determined the stereotactic XYZ coordinates and the proper collimator helmet to further focus the gamma radiation from the Cobalt^{60} needles

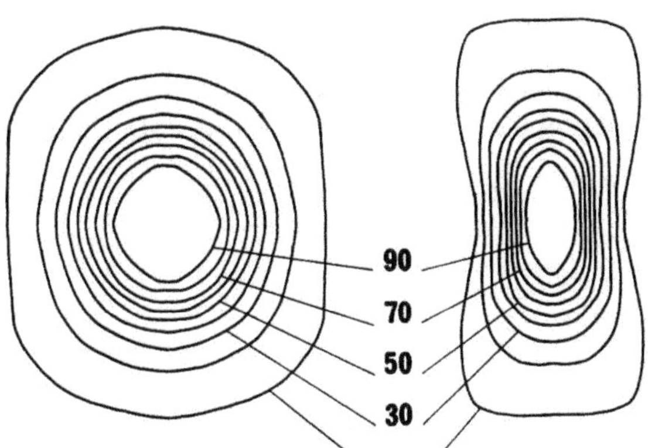

Fig. 2. Diagram of dosimetry configuration in anterior, posterior and lateral views demonstrating the narrow radiation field from the 90% to the 10% dosage using a particular set of collimator helmets

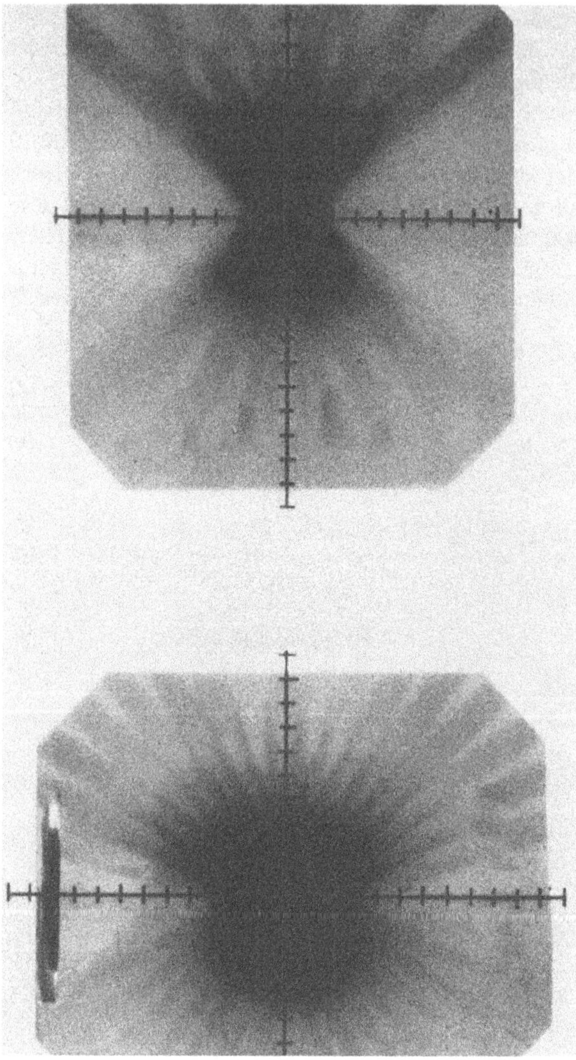

Fig. 3. Film dosimetry with millimeter scale illustrating the concentration of the ^{60}Cobalt radiation field within the radiation chamber of the "Gamma Knife". It is possible to deliver 6000 to 10000 rads in a relatively short time as a single radiosurgical treatment. The current radiation rate of the UCLA unit is 110 rads per minute

normal cells and necrosed cells is a matter of one millimeter. As a result of these observations, the Leksell Stereotactic Radiosurgical Instrument has also become known as the "Gamma Knife".

Materials and Methods

Albino and pigmented rabbits were used in nine consecutive experiments. Under general anesthesia of acepromazine, ketamine and atropine, a suspension of amelanomic epithelioid melanoma cells was injected into upper quadrant of the anterior chamber of the right eye using approximately 7 million cancer cells to create the tu-

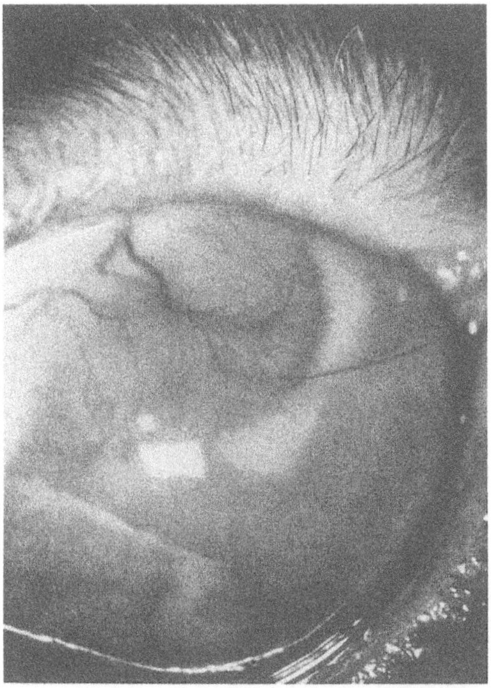

Fig. 4. Amelanomic epithelioid melanoma growing in the anterior chamber of a pigmented rabbit. This neoplasm was created by a single injection of approximately 7 million cancer cells as a suspension into that chamber of the eye. The melanoma grew to the present size in 10 days

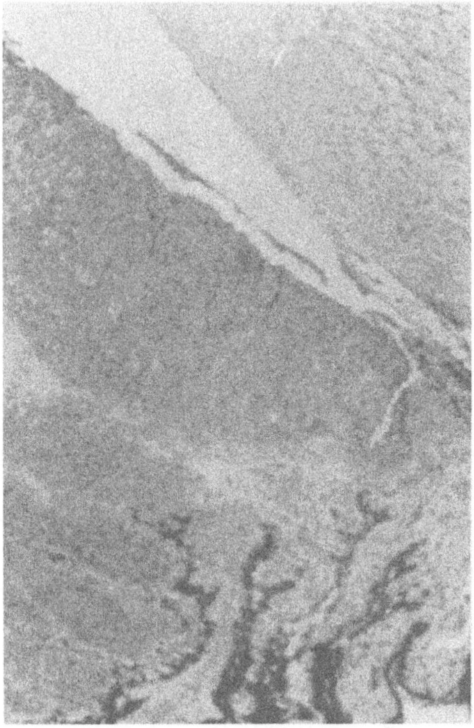

Fig. 5. Photomicrograph of paraffin section stained by H and E technique showing the untreated melanoma at 10X magnification growing and invading the iris and ciliary body in the anterior chamber of the pigmented rabbit of the type in Figure 4

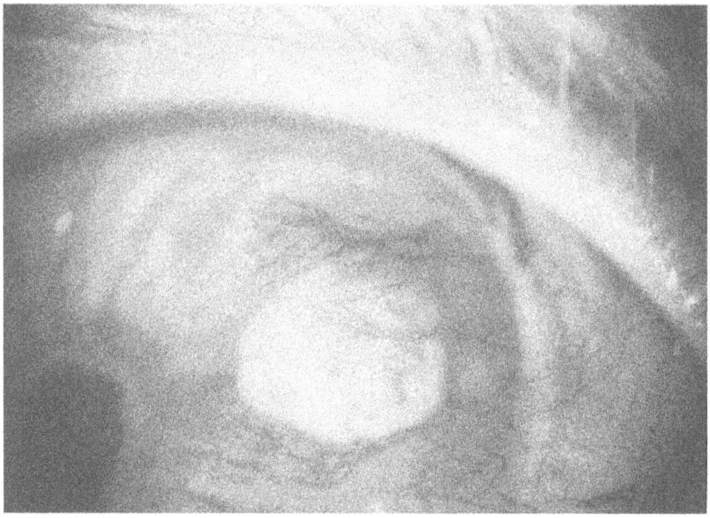

a

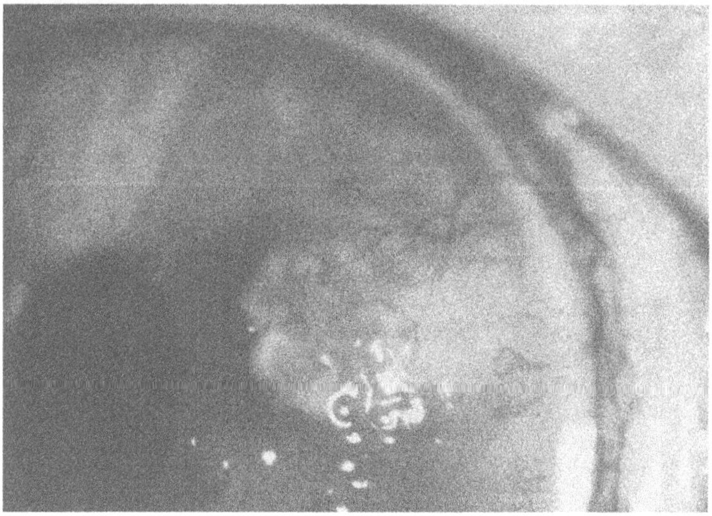

b

Fig. 6. **a** Small melanoma in the anterior chamber of albino rabbit prior to stereotactic radiosurgery treatment. **b** Appearance of rabbit eye melanoma 9 days following focused Gamma Knife ^{60}Cobalt radiation of 6450 rads directed at the 90% dosimetry zone. **c** Forty days after stereotactic radiosurgery, the melanoma appears as a quite small necrotic scar in the iris. No active cancer growth can be identified. **d** Photomicrograph of anterior chamber of albino rabbit at site of prior melanoma demonstrating complete absence of neoplasm. There is an increase in collagen and some edema present in the iris and ciliary body

mor model. The neoplasms formed consistently in the anterior chamber. The growth of the tumor model was rapid, becoming as large as 3 to 4 mm within a 7-day period with no spontaneous regression of tumor growth (Figs. 4, 5). Photographs were taken of the eyes during the development of the tumor, at the time of treatment, and periodically following the stereotactic radiosurgery (Fig. 4).

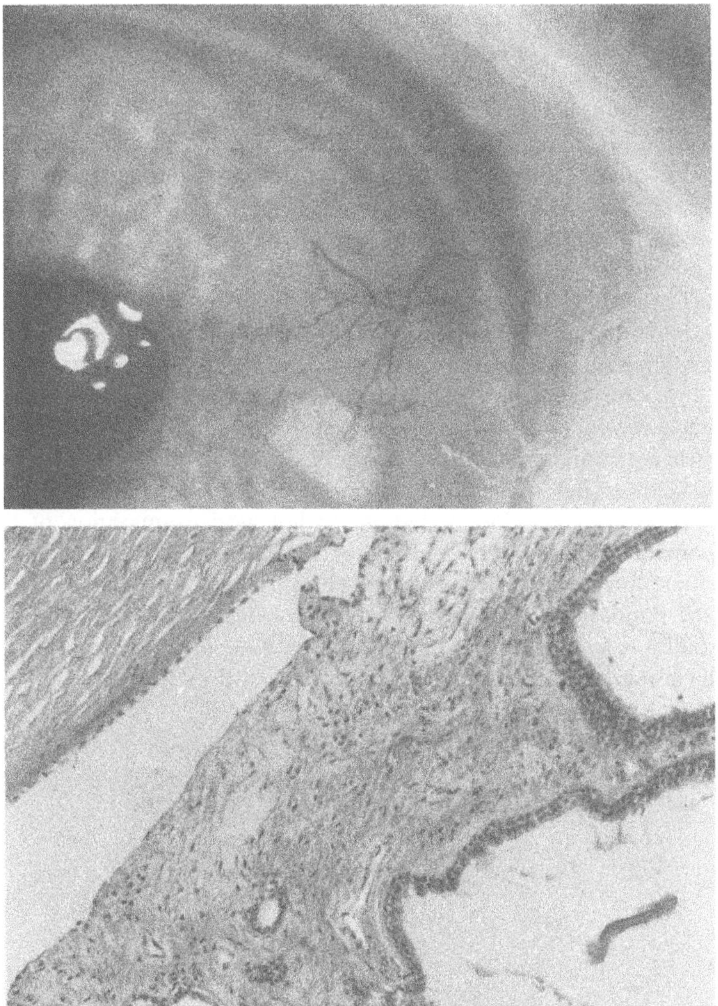

c

d

Fig. 6 c, d

The first pigmented rabbit eye tumor treated in April of 1983 was given 7000 rads in one dosage. This rabbit's tumor regressed and disappeared within 30 days as demonstrated by periodic ocular examination and photographs. Twenty-three months following the radiosurgery, there is no evidence of tumor recurrence, and the rabbit remains in excellent health with preserved vision.

The second pigmented rabbit had a similar size tumor treated in August, 1983 under the same general anesthesia protocol with a single dose of 7000 rads using the stereotactic radiosurgical principles and obtaining accurate location of the XYZ coordinates with the standard Leksell stereotactic frame and a specifically designed inner frame technique. This neoplasm also regressed and disappeared completely to ocular examination and photographs within 30 days. The animal was sacrificed five months later in January, 1984. Serial Hematoxylin and Eosin paraffin sections revealed no evidence of the melanoma. Some increase in collagen and decrease in microvascularity consistent with radiation was observed at the site where neoplasm had been located.

The third albino rabbit also developed a similar tumor model and was treated with 6450 rads of radiation (Figs. 6a, b). The tumor regressed and disappeared leaving a small scar that could be identified in the anterior chamber measuring less than one millimeter in size (Fig. 6c). Serial paraffin Hematoxylin and Eosin sections of the affected eye done 40 days after treatment demonstrated some scar tissue but no viable neoplasm (Fig. 6d).

The fourth rabbit's tumor was approximately 4 mm in size when treated with 7000 rads. The neoplasm continued to grow because the focused radiation did not cover the entire tumor due to a 2 mm incorrect stereotactic localization. This animal was sacrificed four weeks after a treatment at which time the neoplasm had grown to involve the entire anterior chamber of the right eye.

The fifth and sixth albino rabbits had tumors of similar sizes, and both were treated with 7000 rads of single-dose radiation. Pathological examination of the sixth rabbit demonstrated plasma cells and necrotic tumor tissue 27 days after the stereotactic radiation, however, no viable cancer cells could be identified (Fig. 7). In the fifth rabbit, the tumor has continued to regress in a manner observed in rabbits 1, 2 and 3. This rabbit is living and without evidence of recurrence eight months after treatment. The vision remains normal by electroretinography (ERG).

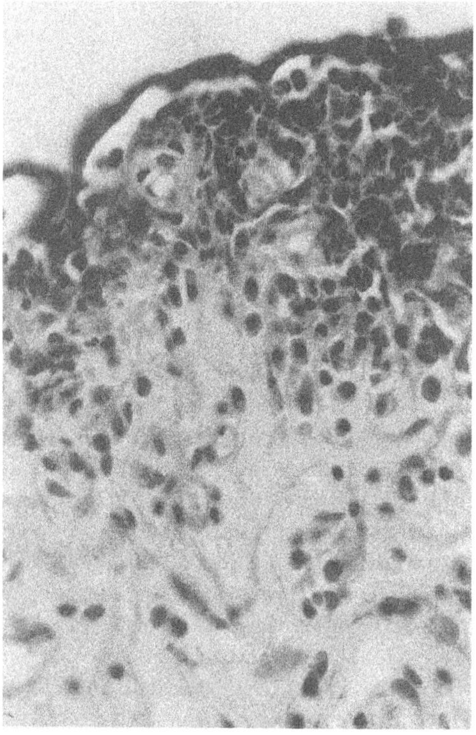

Fig. 7. Photomicrograph of pigmented rabbit 6, 27 days after 7000 rads of gamma radiation to the 90% dosimetry zone using the Leksell "Gamma Knife" Unit. No viable melanoma cells are identified; necrotic cancer cells and plasma cells, however, are present

Rabbit No. 7 had a 4 mm tumor that was not covered completely by the focal point of the collimator of the stereotactic radiosurgical unit, again, because of a millimeter error in calibration of the XYZ coordinates. Therefore, the tumor continued to grow. This animal was sacrificed 5 weeks after treatment and pathologic examination showed active cancer cells.

The 8th and 9th rabbit models were treated with a single dose of 9000 rads of radiation respectively. The tumor is necrosed and regressed in rabbit No. 8. In rabbit No. 9, however, the tumor continued to grow. It is believed by the investigators that in this rabbit the tumor was too large to be treated by this particular collimator and inadequate radiation was delivered at the 50% dosimetry zone.

Investigations utilizing the rabbits adhered to the ARVO resolution. Control rabbits with eye melanoma have not shown regression of the neoplasm which eventually involved the entire eye and was spreading into the orbit at the time of sacrifice.

Results and Discussion

The current experiments indicate that a focused single radiation treatment with a dose of 6000 to 9000 rads delivered to the 90% zone through a collimator of the Leksell Stereotactic Radiosurgical Unit or "Gamma Knife" to the rabbit eye melanoma model is capable of destroying the cancer totally and thus effecting a cure.

The beneficial effect in these rabbit eye melanoma experiments appears to be similar to the results obtained by physicians using the Harvard and Berkeley cyclotrons in treating malignant melanomas in the human eye [1–13].

Therefore, it is proposed by the authors that the Stereotactic Radiosurgical Unit can be used in patients similar to those selected for the cyclotron systems if the tumor size is sufficiently small to be covered by the current collimator within the 90% dosimetry. Furthermore, the human neoplasms can be identified on an enhanced high resolution CT scan so that the XYZ stereotactic coordinates can be determined accurately by the latest design of the Leksell Stereotactic system. Under these circumstances, such radiation, if successful, would be preferable to surgical enucleation of the diseased eye.

Conclusion

In summary, 6 of 9 rabbits showed melanoma regression after stereotactic radiosurgery of the eye. In rabbits 2, 3 and 6, no viable cancer cells in the eye could be identified at autopsy. Rabbits 1, 5 and 8 are continuing to be observed and melanoma is not present in the first rabbit and has regressed completely in rabbits 5 and 8. The tumor continued to grow in rabbits 4, 7 and 9 because of either very slightly incorrect calculation of the XYZ stereotactic coordinates, or because the cancer was too large to be treated with this particular collimator. This inaccuracy of localization has been identified and corrected. The results prove that this rabbit eye melanoma model can be destroyed totally by stereotactic radiosurgery.

References

1. Gragoudas ES, Goitein M, Koehler AM, Verhey L, Tepper J, Suit HD, Brockhurst R, Constable IJ (1977) Proton irradiation of small choroidal malignant melanomas. Am J Ophthalmol 83:665–673
2. Gragoudas ES, Goitein H, Koehler A, Constable IJ, Wagner MS, Verhey L, Tepper J, Suite HD, Brockhurst RJ, Schneider RJ, Johnson KN (1978) Proton irradiation of choroidal melanomas. Preliminary results. Arch Ophthalmol 96:1583–1591
3. Gragoudas ES, Goitein M, Koehler A, Wagner MS, Verhey L, Tepper J, Suite HD, Schneider RJ, Johnson KN (1979) Proton irradiation of malignant melanoma of the ciliary body. Br J Ophthalmol 63:135–139
4. Char DA, Castro JR, Quivey JM, Chen GT, Lyman JT, Stone RD, Irvine AR, Barricks M, Crawford JB, Hilton GF, Lonn LI, Schwartz A (1980) Helium ion charged particle therapy for choroidal melanoma. Ophthalmology 87:565–570
5. Gragoudas ES, Goitein M, Verhey L, Munzenreider J, Suit HD, Koehler A (1980) Proton beam irradiation. An alternative to enucleation for intraocular melanomas. Ophthalmology 87:571–581
6. Suit HD, Goitein M, Munzenreider JE, Verhey L, Gragoudas E, Koehler AM, Urano M, Shipley WU, Linggood RM, Friedberg C, Wagner M (1980) Clinical experience with proton beam radiation therapy. J Can Assoc Radiol 31:35–39
7. Zinn KM, Stein-Pokorny K, Jakobiec FA, Friedman AH, Gragoudas ES, Tich R (1981) Proton beam irradiated epithelioid cell melanoma of the ciliary body. Ophthalmology 88:1315–1321
8. Char DH, Castro JR (1982) Helium ion therapy for choroidal melanoma. Arch Ophthalmol 100:935–938
9. Gragoudas EE, Goitein M, Verhey L, Munzenreider J, Urie M, Suit H, Koehler A (1982) Proton beam irradiation of uveal melanoma. Results of 5½-year study. Arch Ophthalmol 100:928–934
10. Suit H, Goitein M, Munzenreider J, Verhey L, Blitzer P, Gragoudas E, Koehler AM, Irie M, Gentry R, Shipley W, Urano M, Duttenhaver J, Wagner M (1982) Evaluation of the clinical applicability of proton beam in definitive fractionated radiation therapy. Int J Radiat Oncol Biol Phys 8:2199–2205
11. Char DH, Crawford JB, Castro JR, Woodruff KH (1983) Failure of choroidal melanoma to respond to helium ion therapy. Arch Ophthalmol 101:236–241
12. Char DH, Saunders W, Castro JR, Quivey JM, Irvine AR, Stone RD, Crawford JB, Barricks M, Lonn LI, Hilton GF (1983) Helium ion therapy for choroidal melanoma. Ophthalmology 90:1219–1225
13. Seddon JM, Gragoudas ES, Albert DM (1983) Ciliary body and choroidal melanomas treated by proton beam. Arch Ophthalmol 101:1402–1408
14. Leksell L (1971) Stereotaxis and radiosurgery, an operative system. Charles C. Thomas, Publisher, Springfield, Ill.

Stereotactic Radiosurgery of Acoustic Neuromas

A. KHONSARY, R. W. RAND, and G. H. WILSON, Los Angeles, CA/USA

Introduction

Acoustic neuromas have been treated primarily in the past twenty-two years by microsurgery using the Rand-Kurze suboccipital transmeatal operation, the Panse-House translabyrinthine operation or the House-Kurze subtemporal operation. The results have been published in numerous articles over the years, but they are well summarized in several chapters of the most recent third edition of Microneurosurgery by Rand, published in 1985 by C. V. Mosby [3].

In 1971, Leksell introduced his concept of Stereotactic Radiosurgery. Initially, the radiosurgical unit was employed to treat intractable cancer pain and Parkinson's Disease [1, 5]. However, Leksell applied the "Gamma Knife" to small acoustic neuromas, modifying the collimators to accommodate the necessary lateral shift of the patient's head to bring the center of the acoustic neuroma to the focal point of the 179 $Cobalt^{60}$ needle beams of the gamma radiation [4, 2]. These results were successful in either shrinking the neoplasm or arresting its growth.

Consequently, when the Mark II Stereotactic Radiosurgical Unit (Gamma Knife) was constructed, the internal diameter of the collimators was enlarged to more easily accommodate the treatment of acoustic tumors up to 20 mm in diameter.

The current report deals with seven patients referred by Rand and treated in the Mark II Model by Leksell and associates between 1979 and 1985.

Case Reports

Case 1

A 44-year-old woman was referred because of left-sided hearing loss. She had an audiogram in October 1979 which showed 9% loss of speech discrimination on the left side. The CT scan demonstrated a 21.5 × 15 mm mass in the left cerebellopontine angle (Fig. 1). She underwent a stereotactic radiosurgery in December 1979.

In June 1980, the patient developed a transient trigeminal neuralgia which disappeared spontaneously. The CT scan, at the time, showed no significant change in tumor size, which measured 22 mm. The tumor measured the same in December 1980 and June 1981 by CT scans, but showed most of the tumor to be hyperdense with only a small component of its volume in the central part remaining as hypodense. The CT scan of December 1981 and June 1982 showed no change in the

1 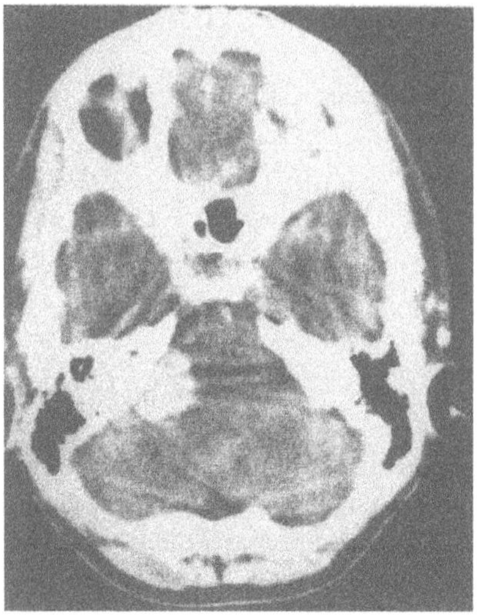 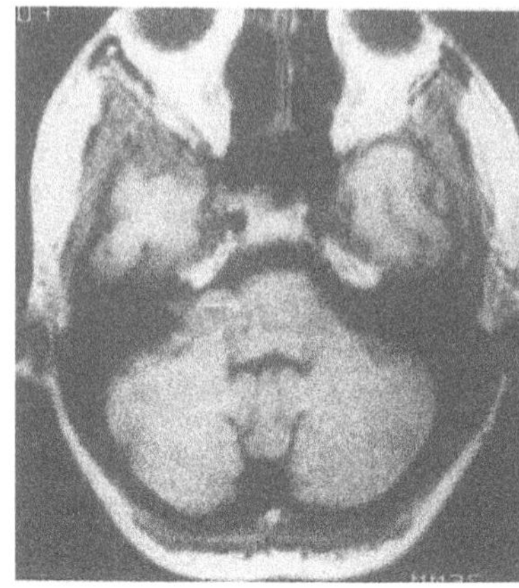 2

Fig. 1. Case 1, Ct scan preoperatively showing the 21.5 × 15 mm mass in the left C.P. angle

Fig. 2. Case 1, NMR postoperatively showing the 11.6 × 19.5 mm mass in the left C.P. angle

size of the tumor. Another CT scan was done in September 1984 which demonstrated the tumor to be 18 mm in size. The NMR performed in February 1985 measured the tumor as 11.6 by 19.5 mm, including the intracanalicular part. Excluding this part, the size of the tumor was 10.1 by 11.6 (Fig. 2).

Case 2

A 25-year-old woman was referred because of headaches and dizziness without a history of hearing loss or tinnitus. The CT scan demonstrated a 22 mm mass on the left cerebellopontine angle in December 1979.

Since the tumor was larger than the size which could be treated by the stereotactic Gamma Unit, it was decided to do a subtotal resection and then treat the residual tumor by the Gamma Unit.

In April, 1980, the patient underwent a subtotal resection of the left-sided tumor, decreasing the size to 17 mm. The tumor macroscopically looked very vascular in comparison to the other acoustic tumors. The pathologic examination was consistent with a benign acoustic schwannoma. Postoperatively, the patient had normal facial movements, but she developed fluctuating hearing on the left side. Four months later, in August 1980, a CT scan showed that the tumor size had increased to 27 × 29 mm (Fig. 3), which was beyond the protocol of treatment. Finally, however, it was decided to try to treat this large sized tumor. Two 14 mm and one 8 mm radiation fields were used and 5000 rads were given to the center on all three targets. The dose for the periphery was inhomogeneous, with a minimum dose of 20% of the central dose in some small areas. In October 1980, the patient developed fifth, sixth, seventh, eighth and ninth cranial nerves palsy associated with dizziness and dysequilibrium due to vestibular nerve involvement. Repetitive CT scans in September,

3 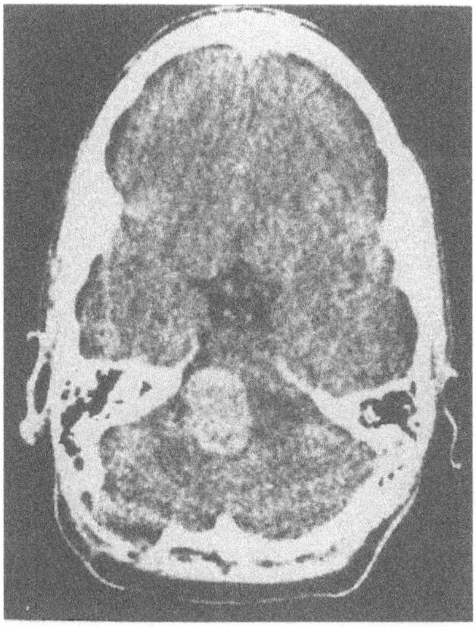

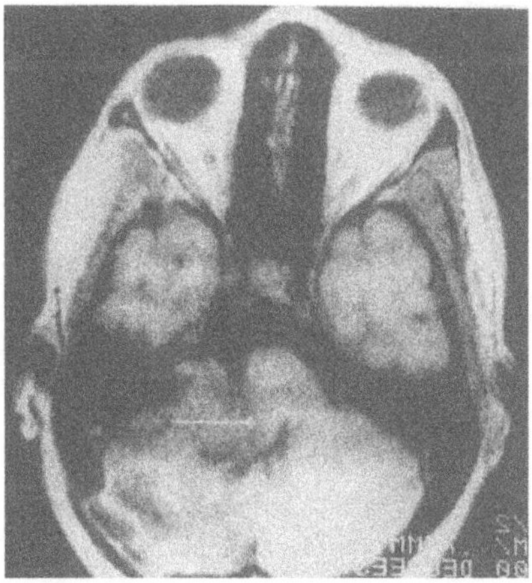 4

Fig. 3. Case 2, preoperative C.T. scan demonstrating 27×29 mm left acoustic tumor

Fig. 4. Case 2, postoperative NMR showing 22.9×28.6 mm mass

October, and December 1980, demonstrated no change in the size of the tumor, but there was evidence of massive central necrosis (29 mm). In January 1981, a tarsorrhaphy was done to protect the cornea. The CT scan of October 1981 showed a striking shrinkage of the tumor. In March 1982, the tarsorrhaphy was removed; the facial movements were much improved as was the balance and walking. The NMR in October 1983 showed a 30 mm left-sided mass including the extension into the left internal acoustic canal. In November 1983, she had a satisfactory facial expression, and the left eye appeared to be normal. The facial nerve function was much improved by February 1984, but she had a burning sensation over her left cheek. The NMR in January 1985 revealed that the tumor size was 22.9×28.6 mm without the intracanalicular part (Fig. 4). There was an additional 14.3 mm intracanalicular part. The facial weakness is very minimal. She can close her left eye. Her gait is much improved. No hearing is on the left side.

Case 3

A 35-year-old woman was referred in June 1980 because of right cerebellopontine angle mass measuring 19 mm in diameter. A few weeks before coming, she had a car accident following which a CT scan was performed and the cerebellopontine angle mass identified. It was learned that the patient had noticed a hearing loss three months before the car accident. The audiogram showed speech discrimination (SDS) of 76% on the right.

The patient underwent stereotactic radiosurgery in August 1980 (Fig. 5). The radiation dosage used was 4000 rads to the center and 2000 rads to the periphery of the neoplasm. The CT scan done in February 1981 showed no significant change in tumor size. The audiogram of the same day revealed increased hearing loss, SDS of 52%.

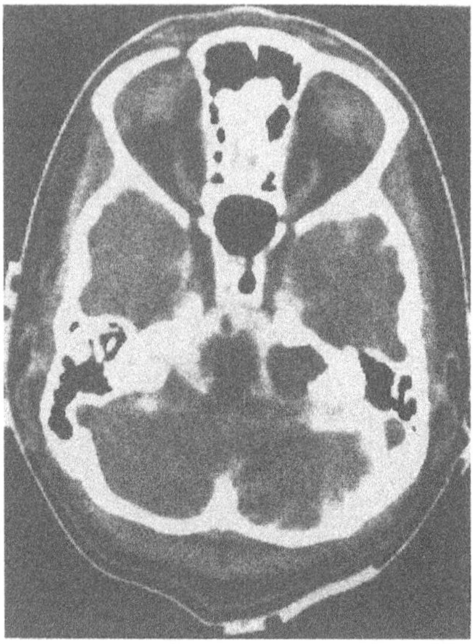

5

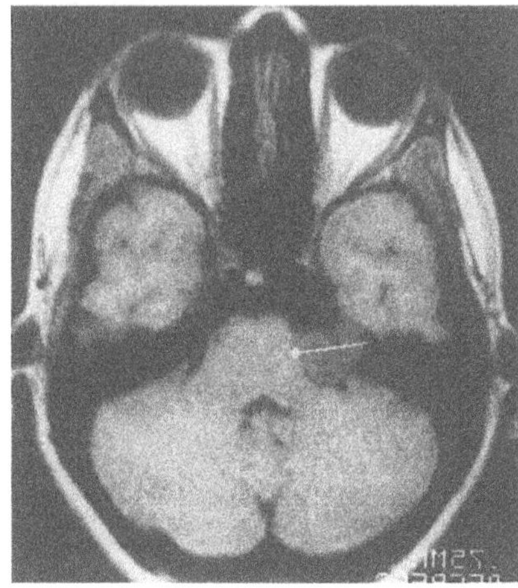

6

Fig. 5. Case 3, preoperative C.T. scan indicative of 19 mm mass in the right C.P. angle

Fig. 6. Case 3, postoperative NMR revealing 17.7 × 19.9 mm mass

A repeated CT scan in February 1982 showed an 18 mm right-sided mass while audiometry in November 1982 revealed severe right-sided hearing loss with very poor discrimination. The CT scan in February 1983 demonstrated a slight increase in size and in August 1983 a CT scan demonstrated the size to be 20 mm. The CT scan of February 1984 revealed a decrease in the tumor size to 15 mm. The patient also developed a very slight right-sided hemifacial spasm of unknown cause. She had her last NMR in February 1985, which showed the tumor size to be 17.7 × 19.9 including the intracanalicular part (Fig. 6).

Case 4

A 34-year-old man was referred in April, 1980 because of right cerebellopontine angle mass. The CT scan showed a 6 mm mass on the right CPA (Fig. 7). The audiometry manifested a decrease in speech discrimination score on the right (88%) in comparison to the left (100%). Five months later, it was 92% on the right and 100% on the left. The patient had a stereotactic radiosurgery in November 1980. The size of the tumor at this time was 10 mm in diameter, and during the treatment only the extracanalicular portion was irradiated with 7000 rads to the center and 3500 rads to the periphery. One month later, the hearing decreased on the right, and decadron was started. An improvement of hearing was noted four days later. In February 1981, the hearing on the right decreased by 20% when tested by SDS. Another course of treatment of decadron was started and the hearing again improved both subjectively and by SDS. In October 1981, SDS was decreased from 76% to 20% in a six-month period. Again, another course of decadron treatment was begun and SDS improved to 60% in the right ear. In November 1981, another course of decadron

7 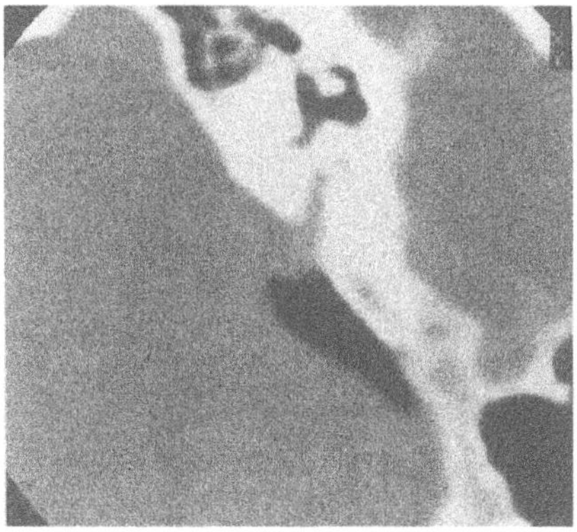 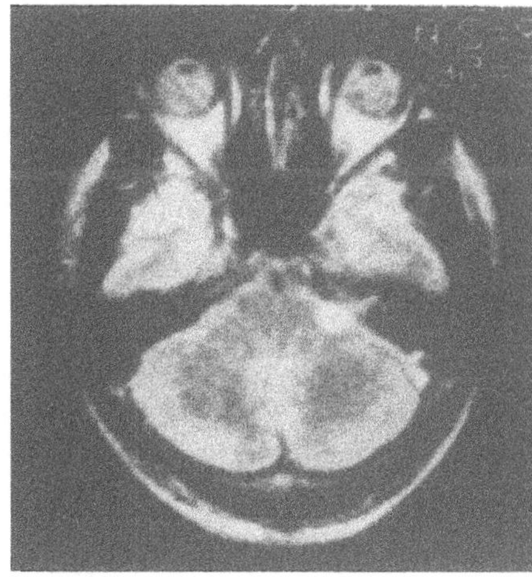 8

Fig. 7. Case 4, preoperative C.T. scan showing 6 mm mass in the right C.P. angle

Fig. 8. Case 4, postoperative NMR showing 14 mm mass

was introduced and the hearing improved by SDS to 72%. By October 1982, the patient had completely normal facial movements, but distinct hearing loss on the right. The patient showed further diminution of hearing in the right side in January 1983 and slight weakness in closing the right eyelid, and some spasm of face occasionally was observed by the patient. Decadron was again started, and improvement of the above mentioned symptoms was observed as less twitching of the face.

In June 1983, the patient had his second course of treatment by stereotactic Gamma Unit in which 4000 rads were used for the target zone, covering the intrameatal part. The CT scan in October 1983 demonstrated an 18 mm tumor and, at that time, the patient had no facial weakness at all. The numbness of the face also disappeared.

The NMR performed in November 1983 showed an 18 mm tumor. In December 1984, the patient had right facial twitching. The comparative NMR showed a definite decrease of the size of the tumor to 14 mm (Fig. 8).

Case 5

A 58-year-old man was referred in November 1977 because of an increase in right-sided hearing loss. He gives a history of right-sided hearing loss after exposure to an explosive in 1968 and a further history of hearing difficulties on the right since 1972 but no history of tinnitus or vertigo.

The audiometry revealed definite loss of hearing, both by pure tone and speech discrimination testing on the right side. Plain films showed definite signs of asymmetry of right internal auditory meatus. The tomograms manifested some widening and erosion of right internal auditory meatus and canal. The electronystagmography showed normal labyrinthine function. The CT scan done in January 1978 was negative. However, cisternography showed no filling in the right internal auditory canal. The patient was referred to Sweden for treatment, but, since the tumor was small in

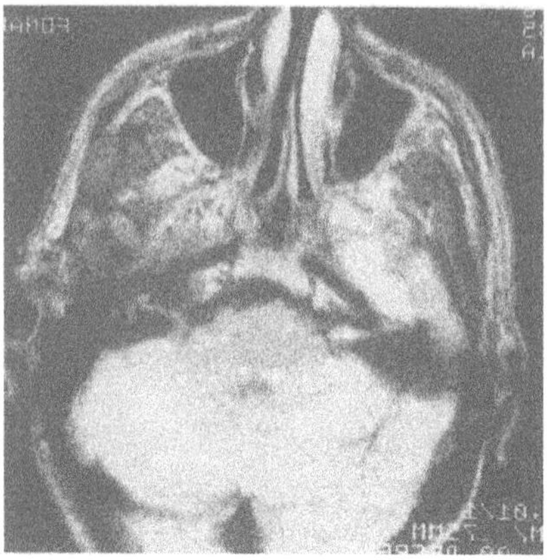

Fig. 9. Case 5, postoperative NMR manifesting a 7.1×7.9 mm mass on the right

size, they refused to treat him at that time. In July and September 1980, the patient noticed further hearing loss on the right side. Therefore, in December 1980, he underwent a CT scan associated with cisternography which showed a right-sided intracanalicular mass with a 2 mm extension outside the meatus. The audiometry in February 1981 demonstrated a little progression of hearing loss on the right. Finally, the patient underwent a stereotactic Gamma Knife treatment in June 1982 with 3000 rads to the center. The exact tumor size at the time of treatment was not known to us.

The patient developed a right-sided facial palsy in July 1983, for which decadron was started and almost one month later, 90% improvement of the palsy was achieved. In the meantime, he noticed a marked decrease in hearing on the right side.

The NMR done in July 1984 showed an 8 mm intracanalicular acoustic tumor. The repeated NMR in February 1985 showed the tumor to be 7.1×7.9, including the intracanalicular part (Fig. 9). We believe the tumor will decrease further in size.

Case 6

A 50-year-old man was referred because of long duration of a slowly progressive hearing loss in the left ear. He was exposed to a major explosion when he was young. The preoperative audiogram showed bilateral symmetrical high frequency hearing loss with a major loss of speech discrimination on the left side. The transorbital and stenvers X-rays showed a wider left internal auditory meatus. The warm and cold caloric testing demonstrated no response on the left. The electronystagmography (ENG) showed no nystagmus on Hennebett test. The CT scan done in August 1983 revealed a 20 mm mass in the left cerebellopontine angle consistent with an acoustic neuroma (Fig. 10).

In December 1983, the patient had the stereotactic radiosurgery in Stockholm, Sweden. The maximum dose in the center of the tumor was 3600 rads with a minimum radiation dose of 1800 rads at its border. In June 1984, the patient noticed a rather precipitous decline in hearing which was documented. One month later, the patient was unable to hear any sounds with the left ear. Prednisone was started and given for 10 days, but no improvement was noted. Facial palsy never occurred.

10 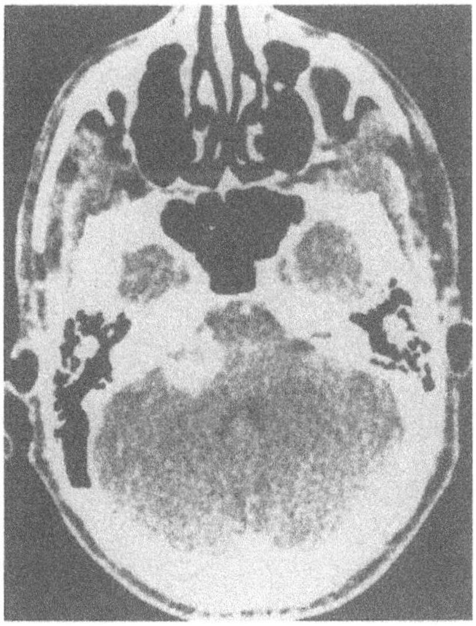

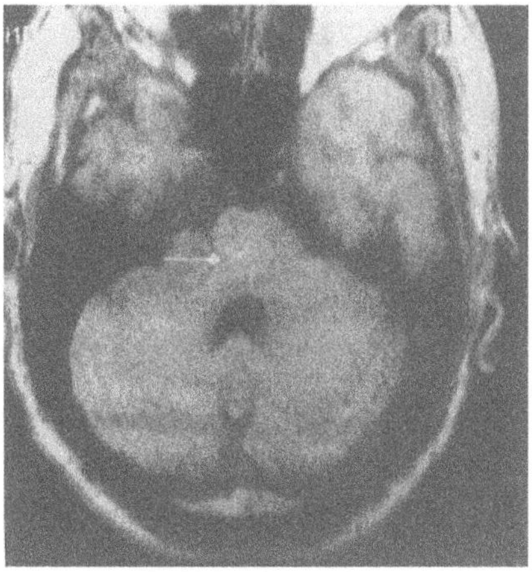 11

Fig. 10. Case 6, preoperative C.T. scan signifying a 20 mm mass on the left

Fig. 11. Case 6, postoperative NMR demonstrating a 16×13.5 mm mass

The NMR in January 1985 showed a significant shrinkage of the tumor to the size of 16×13.5 mm (Fig. 11).

Case 7

A 57-year-old woman was referred because of decreased hearing in the right side, associated with headaches, right ptosis and frozen burning feeling on the right side of the tongue in March 1977. The audiogram showed a conductive hearing loss in the right side. The CT scan at the time was consistent of 20 mm right cerebellopontine angle mass. The vertebral angiogram showed a quarter size tumor in the right CPA. In May 1977, the patient underwent a right temporal craniotomy with transtentorial total resection of the acoustic tumor. The anatomic preservation of the fifth and seventh cranial nerves, cochlear and the remaining vestibular nerves was accomplished. The pathologic examination was consistent with an acoustic schwannoma. Postoperatively, she developed a right facial palsy for two months which was resolved gradually. In January 1979, she had regained almost 90% of her facial function. Her trigeminal nerve function was within normal limits. She had no hearing on the right ear, and had headaches and constant horrible bad taste of her tongue. The CT scan showed no tumor.

The NMR performed in February 1984 showed a 20 mm mass on the right CPA. The repeated NMR in April 1984 showed a slight increase in the size of the mass. The patient underwent a stereotactic Gamma Knife treatment in June 1984 (Fig. 12), with 4000 rads to the center and 1800 rads to the periphery. The repeated NMR in December 1984 showed a decrease in the tumor size to 16.5×15.8 mm, excluding the intracanalicular part (Fig. 13). There was a 3 mm intracanalicular part (Fig. 14).

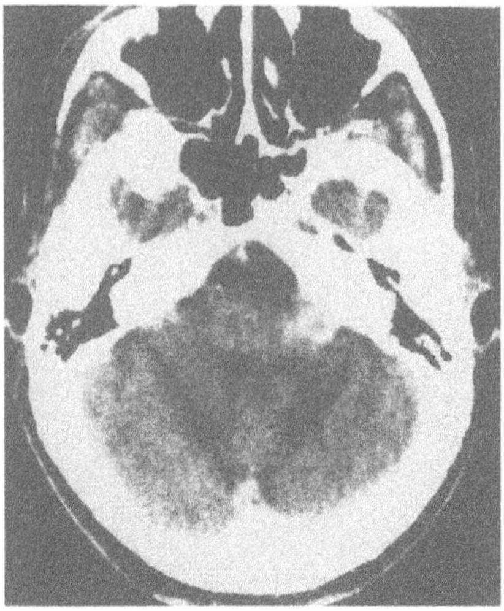

12

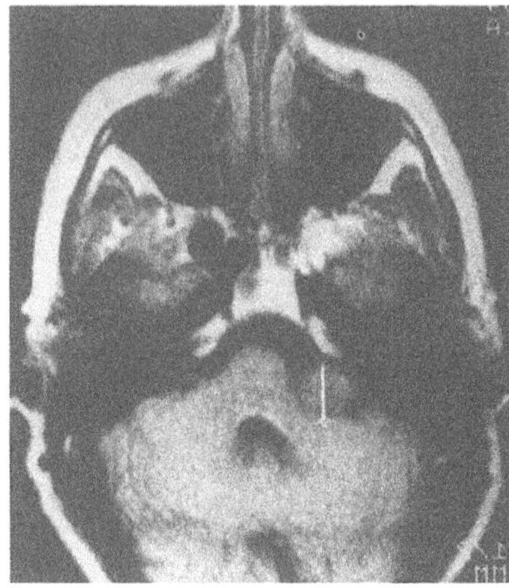

13

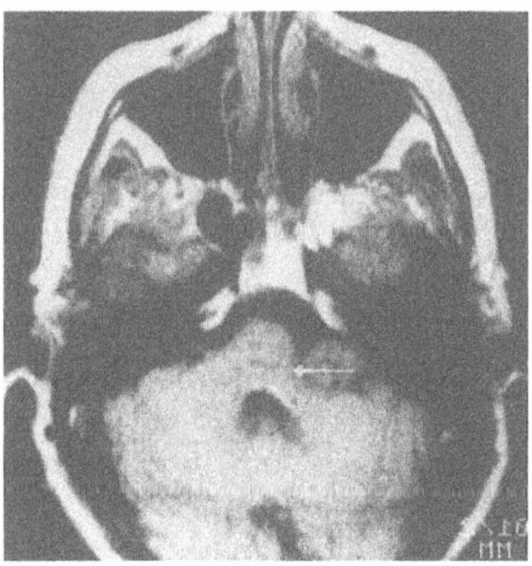

14

Fig. 12. Case 7, preoperative C.T. scan showing a 20 mm mass on the right

Fig. 13. Case 7, postoperative NMR manifesting the 16.5×15.8 mm mass, excluding the intracanalicular part

Fig. 14. Case 7, postoperative NMR showing the 3 mm intracanalicular part

Discussion

The anatomy of the internal acoustic meatus and canal and the related nerves and vessels are well described by Rand and Rhoton [6, 3]. Five nerves reside in the internal auditory canals. The facial nerve being anterior superior, the cochlear nerve anterior inferior, the superior vestibular nerve posterior superior, the inferior vestibular nerve posterior inferior and the intermediate nerve which is a component of the facial nerve running between the facial and the acoustic nerves. This relationship is rather constant and is necessary to understand using any of these surgical approaches.

The origin of an acoustic neuroma is almost universally from the posteriorly located vestibular nerves. The cochlear nerve is softer and more friable than the facial nerve and is affected by the neoplasm sooner than the facial nerve. Furthermore, the cochlear nerve is sensory as compared to the facial nerve which is motor and more subject to dysfunction by compression.

After reviewing these cases, especially the recurrence in case 7, the authors would recommend that excision of the non-involved vestibular nerves should be considered during the operation. Case 7 is an excellent example of the fact that total removal of the tumor was performed, but after seven years the neoplasm regrew presumably from the remainder vestibular nerve. The authors would like to suggest that the use of the Gamma Knife treatment should be considered in such cases of tumor recurrence. In order to follow patients after surgery more closely and avoid further radiation from CT scans, the NMR imaging technique also known as the MRI technique is now available. The NMR follow-up studies which were performed in our patients have the following criteria, except for case 4 which was done at another facility. Magnetic resonance was performed on a 0.3 T permanent magnetic imaging system. All patients were scanned in the axial projection: in some, the coronal projection was added. Two spin-echo sequences were used: 500/28 and 2000/112. Measurements were made using a cursor.

The T_1 and T_2 of acoustic neuroma is greater than brain, so that on the short echo (28 msec) the tumor is of lower intensity, and on the long echo (112 msec) the tumor has a higher signal intensity. Therefore, a line of demarcation can be seen between the tumor and the brain. The intracanalicular portion of the tumor is also well demonstrated because of the lack of signal from the bone.

The current authors recommend the use of NMR imaging as compared to CT techniques because of a higher resolution of the pathology, reduced artifact in the image and lack of radiation on the scanning.

As our results show (Table 1), five of the patients have shown shrinkage of their tumor. However, cases 2 and 4 have shown some different growth behavior. For example, in case 2 there was an unusual increase of tumor growth which was very rapid following her initial suboccipital surgery. Within four months, it had grown from 17 mm to 27 mm in diameter in spite of the fact that the tumor appeared on pathologic examination to be quite benign. The explanation for this rapid period of growth is unknown. During the 4½ years since the stereotactic radiosurgery, the tumor growth in the cerebellopontine angle has been controlled and actually has shown shrinkage. However, there appears to be tumor growth activity within the internal auditory canal. If this proves to be the case in future NMR examinations, that portion of the tumor will need to be removed by the translabyrinthian operation.

In case 4, we believe that the tumor over-reacted to the stereotactic radiosurgical radiation and actually doubled in size initially. Fortunately, however, it is now in a shrinking stage and it is anticipated to shrink further. It certainly is not causing the patient any problems and he is completely well.

Conclusion

Leksell Stereotactic Radiosurgery should be considered by otological surgeons and neurosurgeons as a primary treatment of selected cases of acoustic neuroma of 20 mm or less in diameter. Our patients had been uniformly pleased by these operations of radiosurgery because it can be done as an outpatient in one treatment with

Table 1

Case	Age, sex	Side R	Side L	History of surgery	Date of treatment	Dosage of radiation: Center	Dosage of radiation: Periphery	Preoperative size	Follow-up period	Postop size	Facial palsy
1	44 F		+	No	12/79	Unk	Unk	21.5 × 15	62 m (5 yrs, 2 m)	11.6 × 19.5 (including intracanalicular part)	No
2	25 F		+	Yes (partial resection, 4/80)	8/80	5000	Unk	27 × 29	53 m (4 yrs, 5 m)	22.9 × 28.6 (additional 14.3 mm intra-canalicular part)	Yes (recovered finally)
3	35 F	+		No	8/80	4000	2000	19	54 m (4.5 yrs)	17.7 × 19.9	No
4	34 M	+		No	11/80 6/83	7000 4000	3500	10 Unk		14	Yes (some weakness which dis-appeared)
5	58 M	+		No	6/82	3000	Unk	Intracanal-icular tumor with 1–2 mm extending to CPA	32 m (2 yrs, 8 m)	7.1 × 7.9	Yes temporary
6	50 M		+	No	12/83	3600	1800	20	12 m (1 yr)	16 × 13.5	No
7	57 F	+		Yes (total resec-tion in 1977)	6/84	4000	1800	20	6 m (0.5 yrs)	16.5 × 15.8 (additional 3 mm intra-canalicular part)	No

no risk of death and minimal risk of neurologic deficit. These deficits had been limited to transitory trigeminal neuralgia in one patient and facial palsy in two other patients. Hearing preservation has not been achieved in these cases, and therefore, if patients wish to try for hearing preservation, the Rand-Kurze operation or the House-Kurze operation should be recommended.

Long-term ill effects of focused, single-dose radiation have not been observed in the fifteen years since Leksell introduced stereotactic radiosurgery. Therefore, we recommend this procedure in selected patients with acoustic neuromas.

References

1. Leksell L (1971) Stereotaxis and radiosurgery, an operative system. Charles C. Thomas, Publisher, Springfield, Ill.
2. Rand RW (1982) The stereotactic cobalt 60 gamma unit in the treatment of acoustic neuromas. In: Brackman DE Neurological surgery of the ear and skull base. Raven Press, New York
3. Rand RW, DiTullio MV (1985) The Rand-Kurze suboccipital transmeatal operation for acoustic neuromas. In: Rand RW, Microneurosurgery, Third Ed. C.V. Mosby Co. Missouri
4. Noren G, Arndt J, Hindmarsh T (1983) Stereotactic radiosurgery in cases of acoustic neurinoma: Further Experiences. Neurosurgery 13: 12–22
5. Steiner L, Forster D, Leksell L, Meyerson BA, Boethius J (1980) Gammathalamotomy in intractable pain. Acta Neurochir (Wien) 52: 173–184
6. Rhoton AL (1985) Microsurgical anatomy of the internal acoustic meatus and facial nerve. In: Rand RW, Microneurosurgery, Third Edition C.V. Mosby Co. Missouri

Chemotherapy of Childhood Brain Stem Tumors

M.K. Neidhardt, Augsburg/FRG

The majority of brain stem tumors occur in children (Bloom 1975), and in recent years considerable progress has been obtained with chemotherapy for most pediatric tumors (Mauer et al. 1977; Lampert 1982). It would therefore seem appropriate to have a pediatrician speak on chemotherapy of brain stem tumors.

Unfortunately, brain tumors in general do not represent one of the highlights of multimodal treatment in pediatric oncology. At the present time, radiotherapy has to be considered the mainstay of combined therapy. Median survival periods of brain stem tumors between 5 and 47 months have been reported (Fulton et al. 1981). The five-year survival incidence, however, ranges between 0 and 40% (Gutjahr et al. 1982; Sheline 1975) and thus remains highly unsatisfactory.

Attempts to improve the cure rate of childhood CNS malignancies by the use of cytostatic drugs have been numerous but, on the whole, less successful than those for cancer of other sites, with the exception, possibly, of embryonal tumors with high proliferation rates such as medulloblastoma (Bloom et al. 1982; Evans 1983).

The existing physiologic "barriers" (blood-brain, blood-CSF, CSF-brain) have, in the first place, been held responsible for this disappointing situation. Rall and Zubrod had claimed in 1962 that a cytotoxic drug, in order to be effective on brain tumors, should possess the following properties: high lipid solubility, low degree of ionisation, and small molecular size. However, later studies have shown that these barriers are less impenetrable than originally supposed (Mellet 1977; Vick et al. 1977). A more modern viewpoint is that areas of central necrosis are generally impermeable to lipid-soluble drugs whereas water-soluble drugs do not penetrate into the growing edges of brain tumors (Shapiro et al. 1979).

In trying to appreciate the possible effects of cytostatic drugs in brain stem tumors, we have to be aware of a number of additional pitfalls:

1. These tumors may represent quite variable degrees of histologic "malignancy" as expressed by cellular density, pleomorphism, nuclear hyperchromatism, degree of vascularization and subarachnoid spread (Littman et al. 1980; Albright et al. 1983). Moreover, a well-differentiated astrocytoma is apparently capable of undergoing "anaplastic transformation" (Schmitt and Zeisner 1982). Tumors of the medulla are usually less "mature" than those of the midbrain, with pontine tumors occupying an intermediate position (Reigel et al. 1979; Fulton et al. 1981). It is evident from these observations that, without histologic confirmation, different cohorts of "brain stem tumors" treated at different centers with identical or at least comparable methods may, in fact, be composed quite differently and therefore also possess a different prognosis. It is probably for this reason that therapeutic results at 5 years

reported in the literature are so variable. Thus, there is no well-established "baseline" against which we can measure progress in treatment results.

2. In brain stem tumors, diagnosis of relapse or "progressive disease" is often established on clinical grounds rather than on changes in CT scans (Allen and Helson 1981). Clinical changes, as we all know, are less reliable than the results of objective radiographic measurements, and thus are subject to error. If, however, a patient is started on chemotherapy because of "neurologic deterioration" and later survives for an unexpected number of years, can we be certain in each case that he really had a relapse in the first place and that the "success" obtained is attributable to the treatment employed?

With these limitations in mind, I have tried to collate the accessible literature and compiled Tables 1–4 for an overview of the presently available information. Unfortunately, not all articles contain "hard" data like definition of relapse, criteria and duration of response etc. Large series treated in a uniform manner are practically inexistent. A great number of agents have been tried – water- and lipid-soluble, cycle-specific and non-specific, alkylating and anti-mitotic, administered systemically and intrathecally, single or in combination. Even at the same centers, regimens have changed quite often – a reflection of the dissatisfaction with their efficacy (Bordigoni et al. 1980, Edwards et al. 1980).

The overall results are still inconclusive. Apparently, some tumors (probably those which grow rapidly) respond as well to single-agent as to multiple-agent chemotherapy for a variable (but usually limited) length of time. But the most effective treatment regimen has still to be found, and whether chemotherapy actually improves the cure rate of these tumors remains doubtful (Levin et al. 1984).

Table 1. Single-agent chemotherapy in recurrent pediatric brain stem tumors

Author(s)	Year of publication	Drug employed	Number of patients	Response rate	Survival time (months)	Method of evaluation
Rosen et al.	1977	HD-MTX i.v.	4	2/4	6, 18	Clinical, CT
Djerassi et al.	1977	HD-MTX i.v.	2	2/2	11, 13	Clinical
Fulton et al.	1981	MTX i. th.	2	?	4, 13	Clinical
Fewer et al.	1972	BCNU	3	1/3	?	
Fulton et al.	1981	BCNU	1	?	9	Clinical
Fulton et al.	1981	CCNU	2	2/2	4, 22	Clinical
Edwards et al.	1980	CCNU	5	?	Median, 6	Clinical
Kumar et al.	1974	Procarbazine	1	1/1	?	
Allen and Helson	1981	Cyclophosphamide	4	4/4	3, 9, 9+, 11+	Clinical
Nagai et al.	1980	Interferon	1	1/1	3	Clinical, CT
Khan et al.	1982	Cis-platin	1	1/1	41+	Clinical, CT

Abbreviations used in tables: HD = high dose; MTX = methotrexate; BCNU = 1,3-Bis(2-chloroethyl)-1-nitrosourea; CCNU = 1-(2-chloroethyl)-3-cyclohexyl-1-nitrosourea; 5-Fu = 5-fluorouracil; Proc. = procarbazine, DTIC = dimethyl-triazeno-imidazole carboxamide; Hu = hydroxyurea; 6-MP = 6 mercapto-purine; OPP = vincristine, procarbazine, prednisone; MOPP = OPP + nitrogen mustard

Table 2. Single-agent chemotherapy in primary pediatric brain stem tumors

Author(s)	Year of publication	Drug employed	Number of patients	Response rate	Survival time (months)	Method of evaluation
Newton et al.	1968	MTX i. th.	4	4/4	11, 22, 49+, 55+	Clinical
Fulton et al.	1981	MTX i. th.	1	?	7	Clinical
Rosenblum et al.	1973	CCNU	2	2/2	13+, 15+	Clinical
Fulton et al.	1981	CCNU	3	?	5, 10, 17	Clinical
Bordigoni et al.	1980	Vincristine	7	?	?	Clinical
		Cyclophosphamide	1	?	?	CT
Fulton et al.	1981	BCNU	1	1/1	43+	Clinical
		Hydroxyurea	2	?	3, 3+	Clinical

Table 3. Multiple-agent chemotherapy in recurrent pediatric brain stem tumors

Drugs employed	Author(s)	Year of publication	Number of patients	Response rate	Survival time (months)	Method of evaluation
Vincristine, BCNU	Edwards et al.	1980	4	?	Median, 3	Clinical
	Fulton et al.	1981	2	?	Median, 18	Clinical
Procarbazine, BCNU	Edwards et al.	1980	5	?	Median, 2	Clinical
	Fulton et al.	1981	5	?	Median, 12	Clinical
Procarbazine, CCNU	Fulton et al.	1981	1	1	29	Clinical
5-FU, CCNU	Edwards et al.	1980	1	?	1	Clinical
DTIC, CCNU	Taylor et al.	1975	1	0/1	4	Clinical
Vincristine, BCNU, CCNU	Fulton et al.	1981	1	1/1	22	Clinical
Vincristine, BCNU, MTX i. th.	Fulton et al.	1981	1	1/1	271+	Clinical
Vincristine, CCNU, procarbazine (PCV)	Edwards et al.	1980	10	2/10	4	Clinical
	Fulton et al.	1981	5	?	30	Clinical
CCNU, Proc., 5-FU, HU, 6-MP	Fulton et al.	1981	3	?	18	Clinical
MOPP, OPP	Cangir et al.	1984	1	1/1	22	Clinical
"8 in 1[a]"	Olive et al.	1984	9	4/9	?	?

[a] 8 drugs in 1 day (methylprednisolone, vincristine, CCNU, Proc., HU, DTIC, Ara-C, Cisplatin)

Table 4. Multiple-agent chemotherapy in primary pediatric brain stem tumors

Drugs employed	Author(s)	Year of publication	Number of patients	Response rate	Survival time (months)	Method of evaluation
BCNU, 5-FU	Fulton et al.	1981	1	1/1	12	Clinical
CCNU, 5-FU	Fulton et al.	1981	3	2/3	12	Clinical
Vincristine, cyclophosphamide	Bordigoni et al.	1980	7	?	Median, 24	Clinical
Vincristine, CCNU	Bordigoni et al.	1980	3	?	Median, 24	Clinical
Vincristine, VM 26	Bordigoni et al.	1980	4	?	Median, 24	Clinical
Vincristine, procarbazine, CCNU	Fulton et al.	1981	2	1/1	15	Clinical
CCNU, 5-FU, HU, misonidazole	Levin et al.	1984	28	?	10	Clinical

All progress in pediatric oncology has been obtained with the aid of cooperative, prospective, randomised multi-center studies grouping large numbers of patients. For apparent reasons, such studies are difficult to undertake in such a heterogeneous group of relatively rare tumors as those of the brain stem. One of the prerequisites of a conclusive study, histologic verification of all eligible cases, still remains no more than a theoretical claim.

References

Albright AL, Price RA, Guthkelch AN (1983) Brain stem gliomas of children – a clinicopathological study. Cancer 52:2313–2319

Allen JC, Helson L (1981) High-dose cyclophosphamide chemotherapy for recurrent CNS tumors in children. J Neurosurg 55:749–756

Bloom HJG (1975) Tumours of the central nervous system. In: Bloom HJG, Lemerle J, Neidhardt MK, Voûte PA (eds) Cancer in children – clinical management. Springer, Berlin Heidelberg New York, p 93–119

Bloom HJG, Thornton H, Schweisguth O (1982) SIOP medulloblastoma and high grade ependymoma therapeutic clinical trial: preliminary results (1975–1981). In: Raybaud C, Clement R, Lebreuil G, Bernard JL (eds) Pediatric Oncology. Excerpta Medica, Amsterdam Oxford Princeton, p 309–322

Bordigoni P, Brocard O, Bey P, Montaut J, Picard L, Olive D (1980) Les gliomes du tronc: aspects cliniques, thérapeutiques et évolutifs. Med Hyg 38:589–601

Cangir A, Ragab AH, Steuber P, Land VJ, Berry DH, Krischer JP (1984) Combination chemotherapy with vincristine, procarbazine, prednisone with or without nitrogen mustard (MOPP vs OPP) in children with recurrent brain tumors. Med Pediatr Oncol 12:1–3

Djerassi I, Kim JS, Shulman K (1977) High-dose methotrexate-citrovorum factor rescue in the management of brain tumors. Cancer Treat Rep 61:691–694

Edwards MS, Levin VA, Wilson CB (1980) Chemotherapy of pediatric posterior fossa tumors. Child's Brain 7:252–260

Evans AE (1983) Therapeutic approaches to medulloblastoma and results: the trial of the Children's Cancer Study Group (CCSG) and the Radiation Therapy Oncology Group (RTOG). Proceedings of the 13th International Congress of Chemotherapy, Vienna, Fascicle SY 101–106

Fewer D, Wilson CB, Boldrey EB, Enot, JK (1972) Phase II study of CCNU in the treatment of brain tumors. Cancer Chemother Rep 56:421–427

Fulton DS, Levin VA, Wara WM, Edwards MS, Wilson CB (1981) Chemotherapy of pediatric brain stem tumors. J Neurosurg 54:721–725

Gutjahr P, Voth D, Heidfeld J, Walther B, Kutzner J, Kretzschmar K (1982) Infratentorial tumors – treatment and results in 109 children. In: Voth D, Gutjahr P, Langmaid C (eds) Tumors of the central nervous system in infancy and childhood. Springer, Berlin Heidelberg New York, p 358–364

Khan AB, D'Souza BJ, Wharam MD, Champion LAA, Sinks LF, Woo SY, McCullough DC, Leventhal BG (1982) Cisplatin therapy in recurrent childhood brain tumors. Cancer Treat Rep 66:2013–2020

Kumar ARV, Renaudin J, Wilson CB, Boldrey EB, Enot KJ, Levin VA (1974) Procarbazine hydrochloride in the treatment of brain tumors. J Neurosurg 40:365–371

Lampert F (1982) Childhood cancer studies in West Germany: the first 10 years. Klin Pädiatr 194:195–203

Levin VA, Edwards MS, Wara WM, Allen J, Ortega J, Vestays P (1984) 5-Fluorouracil and CCNU followed by hydroxyurea, misonidazole, and irradiation for brain stem gliomas: a pilot study of the Brain Tumor Research Center and the Children's Cancer Group. Neurosurgery 14:679–681

Littman P, Jarrett P, Bilaniuk LT, Rorke LB, Zimmerman RA, Bruce DA, Carabell SC, Schut L (1980) Pediatric brain stem gliomas. Cancer 45:2787–2792

Mauer AM, Simone JV, Pratt CB (1977) Current progress in the treatment of the child with cancer. J Pediatr 91:523–539

Mellet LB (1977) Physicochemical considerations and pharmacokinetic behavior in delivery of drugs to the central nervous system. Cancer Treat Rep 61:527–531

Nagai M, Arai T, Kohno S, Kohase M (1980) Interferon therapy for malignant brain tumors. In: Kono R, Vilcek J (eds) The clinical potential of interferons. Proc Int Clin Pot Interferons; Jap Med Res Found Publ, No 15, p 257–273

Newton WA jr, Sayers MP, Samuels LD (1968) Intrathecal methotrexate therapy for brain tumors in children. Cancer Chemother Rep 52:257–261

Olive D, Benz E, Philip T, Brunat-Mentigny M, Zucker JM, Vannier JP (1984) Efficacy of "8 drugs in 1 day" regimen in the treatment of childhood brain tumors. 16th meeting of the International Society of Paediatric Oncology, Barcelona (Abstract No. 50)

Rall DP, Zubrod CG (1962) Mechanism of drug absorption and excretion. Passage of drugs in and out of the central nervous system. Ann Rev Pharmacol 2:109–128

Reigel DH, Scarff TB, Woodford JE (1979) Biopsy of pediatric brain stem tumors. Child's Brain 5:329–340

Rosen G, Ghavimi F, Nirenberg A, Mosende C, Mehta BM (1977) High-dose methotrexate with citrovorum factor rescue for the treatment of central nervous system tumors in children. Cancer Treat Rep 61:681–690

Rosenblum ML, Reynolds AF, Smith KA, Rumack BH, Walker MD (1973) Chlorethyl-cyclohexyl-nitrosourea (CCNU) in the treatment of brain tumors. J Neurosurg 39:306–314

Schmitt HP, Zeisner W (1982) The diffuse brain stem astrocytoma in childhood: morphology, course, and prognosis. In: Voth D, Gutjahr P, Langmaid C (eds) Tumors of the central nervous system in infancy and childhood. Springer, Berlin Heidelberg New York, p 149–164

Shapiro WR, Allen JC, Mehta B, Blasberg RG, Kobayshi T, Patlak CS (1979) Pharmacodynamics of entry of methotrexate into brain of humans, monkeys and a rat brain tumor model. In: Paoletti P, Walker MD, Butti G, Knerich R (eds) Multidisciplinary aspects of brain tumor therapy. Elsevier North Holland Biomedical Press, Amsterdam, p 135–142

Sheline GE (1975) Radiation therapy of tumors of the central nervous system in childhood. Cancer 35:957–964

Taylor SG, Nelson L, Baxter D, Rosenbaum C, Sponzo RW, Cunningham TJ, Olson KB, Horton J (1975) Treatment of grade III and IV astrocytoma with Dimethyl Triazeno Imidazole Carboxamide (DTIC) alone and in combination with CCNU or Methyl CCNU. Cancer 36:1269–1276

Vick NA, Khandekar JD, Bigner DD (1977) Chemotherapy of brain tumors. The "blood-brain barrier" is not a factor. Arch Neurol 34:523–526

Chemotherapy of Malignant Brain Stem Tumors in Adults

P. Krauseneck, Würzburg/FRG

In adulthood the chemotherapy of brain tumors is, in contrast to treatment in children, essentially a therapy of supratentorial tumors, especially of malignant gliomas. Only for these gliomas is chemotherapy an established treatment. In brain metastases chemotherapy is becoming more and more accepted as efficient treatment modality, if the primary is breast carcinoma or possibly oat-cell carcinoma of the lung.

Apparently the location of a tumor in the cerebral hemispheres or in the brain stem does not play a major role for the efficacy of chemotherapy, neither in gliomas nor in secondary malignomas.

Before I come back to this point, I would like to give a short review of the possibilities and efficacy of the chemotherapy of brain tumors.

The most important disadvantage of chemotherapy in this field is the blood-brain-barrier, which allows access to the tumor cell only for a few cytostatic agents in very limited concentrations. Although the blood-brain-barrier is going to be impaired by malignant tumor growth, as is demonstrated in the contrast enhancement of malignant tumors in the CT-scan, it does not break down completely. In primary brain tumors the blood-brain-barrier does not exist any more in the inner, often necrotic, parts of the tumor, but in the infiltrative margins and the brain adjacent to the tumor it is well preserved and protects normal and tumor cells against high concentrations of cytostatic drugs. In brain metastases there is some evidence that with the growing of the tumor the blood-brain-barrier is altered qualitatively and, after initially being intact, is damaged to a great extent when the tumor size exceeds a certain volume. (Blasberg et al. 1981; Greig et al. 1983; Hasegawa et al. 1983; Levin et al. 1975; Neuwelt et al. 1982)

Consequently in clinically manifested brain metastases the whole range of cytostatic agents may be applied with some prospect of success, whereas in primary brain tumors up to now only a few lipid soluble cytostatic drugs penetrating the blood-brain-barrier fairly well have proved to be efficacious.

The Brain Tumor Study Group of the USA has worked out the most reliable data referring to the efficacy of chemotherapy in malignant supratentorial gliomas (Walker et al. 1978, 1980; Green et al. 1983, 1984). Similar results were obtained in smaller European (EORTC Brain Tumor Group 1978, Hildebrand 1985; Jellinger et al. 1983, 1985; Krauseneck et al. 1981, 1984) studies.

Summarizing, until now there has been no more effective chemotherapy in malignant gliomas than BCNU monotherapy. A comparison of two successive large studies of the American BTSG shows that the combination of radiotherapy (60 Gy) and BCNU in both studies is superior to radiotherapy alone or radiotherapy plus high-dose methylprednisolone once a week (Green et al. 1983) (Fig. 1). However,

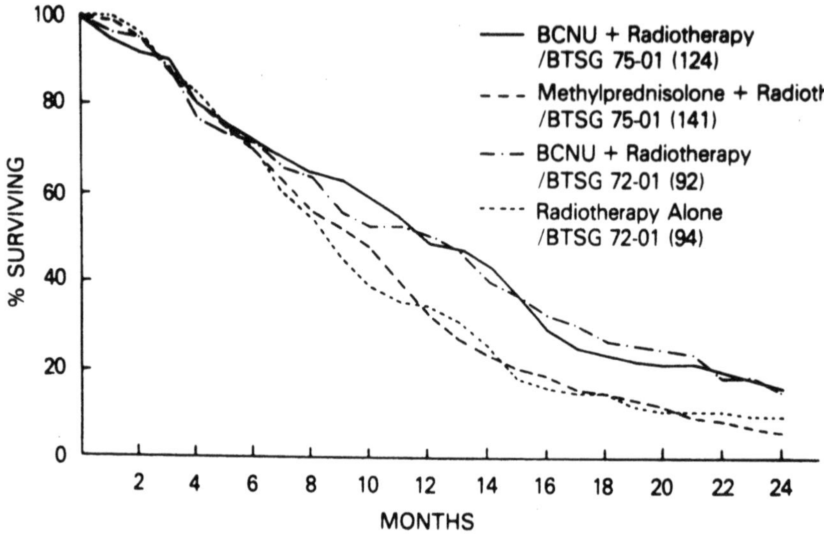

Fig. 1. Survival curves of adult patients with malignant gliomas of the hemispheres with and without chemotherapy in two successive studies of the Brain Tumor Study Group of the U.S. (Green et al. Cancer Treat Rep 1983). All patients received 60 Gray whole brain irradiation. In parentheses the numbers of patients in each treatment arm are given

the survival curves are identical within the first six months after operation. That means that in patients with a very poor prognosis chemotherapy is useless. These data demonstrate also that approximately 30% of the patients harboring a malignant glioma die within six months and these patients have no benefit from the chemotherapy but only have to tolerate the side effects. Unfortunately, we are not able to identify these patients correctly in advance although the most important prognostic factors, age, tumor grade and performance status, are known. About 70% of the patients do benefit from the chemotherapy and this effect is greater as the survival time increases. After two years, three to four times as many patients live in the chemotherapy group as in the only irradiated group which has only about 5% survivors. So, there is no doubt that chemotherapy is effective, though sometimes serious side-effects may impair the therapeutic gain.

Efficacy comparable to BCNU have Methyl-CCNU, Procarbazine and Streptozotocine and probably a few other Nitrosoureas such as ACNU. The widely used, only orally applicable Nitrosourea CCNU was, in randomized studies of the EORTC and the Scandinavian Brain Tumor Group, not effective in malignant gliomas (Hildebrand 1985; Hatlevoll et al. 1985). In one study of the EORTC an effect could be seen, when CCNU was used only after relapse had occurred (EORTC Brain Tumor Group 1978). Other probably efficacious drugs are 5-FU, VM 26, Cisplatin and Dibromodulcitol. Not many data are available for such possibly useful agents as AZQ, Cytosine-Arabinoside, DTIC and Hydroxyurea. As being not effective the following drugs should be considered: antibiotics such as Adriamycine, Vincristine, Cyclophosphamide and their analogues, and the radiosensitizers Metro- and Misonidazole.

Unfortunately, no combination chemotherapy until now has shown clear-cut higher effectiveness in the treatment of malignant primary brain tumors than BCNU alone.

The spectrum of efficacy of the cytostatic drugs is quite different in malignant secondary brain tumors. Here a polychemotherapy is obviously more effective than single agents as in the treatment of most of the possible primaries. In recent years several studies have shown that treatment of brain metastases with agents not penetrating the blood-brain-barrier is also effective (Krauseneck et al. 1977, 1983; Mende et al. 1983; Rosner et al. 1983; Kreuser et al. 1984).

As controlled trials of different chemotherapies in brain metastases are not available, one should use a chemotherapeutic regimen which is known to be effective in the primary and was not used in the particular patient, as it is well known that brain metastases may develop under a chemotherapy being effective in the control of metastases at other sites. Especially in carcinoma of the breast and also in oat-cell carcinoma of the lung high response rates of 60–70% may be expected.

As for other malignant brain tumors in adults, for instance for ependymoma grade III and IV, medulloblastoma, sarcoma and primary cerebral lymphoma no established chemotherapy exists, those tumors can only be treated analogous to the malignant gliomas or to the schedules used in general oncology or pediatry.

After this general review the question remains if brain stem tumors differ in prognosis and chemotherapy from tumors of the hemispheres. As I am not aware of any systematic and controlled therapeutic study of brain stem tumors in adults, I am not able to present conclusive data on these points. In contrast to older statements there are, in recent literature, a few hints that the prognosis of brain stem tumors is not very different from that of hemispheric tumors.

Thus, involvement of the basal ganglia was not an unfavorable prognostic factor in the trials of the American BTSG and the EORTC of supratentorial malignant gliomas. This was the experience made in our studies, too. But this fact needs confirmation as in all of these studies patients were preselected and the number of patients with basal ganglia tumors was small as, in former times, in most of these cases neither operation nor biopsy was done.

Survival times of adolescents and small numbers of adults with malignant brain stem tumors – except medulloblastomas – after radiation therapy are in the range of 8–10 months (Hara and Takeuchi 1977; Levin et al. 1984) and that is exactly the survival time of irradiated patients with malignant gliomas of the hemispheres (Walker et al. 1978). The very few studies of chemotherapy are done almost exclusively on pediatric patients and show, as expected from the small number of patients and the often lacking neuropathologic examination, no clear benefit of the various chemotherapeutic agents used (Fulton et al. 1981; Levin et al. 1984; Reigel et al. 1979). There are preliminary statements that with chemotherapy more long-term survivors are observed and that chemotherapy seems to be more effective after relapse than as adjuvant treatment (Fulton et al. 1981; Levin et al. 1984).

Finally I should mention the intrathecal treatment of leptomeningeal spread. In our limited experience malignant brain stem tumors of adults frequently tend to spread via CSF. In children leptomeningeal spread was described from 4% for an autopsy series of gliomas of various degrees of malignancy (Mantravadi et al. 1982) to 33% in malignant astrocytomas of the brain stem (Kandt et al. 1984; Packer et al.

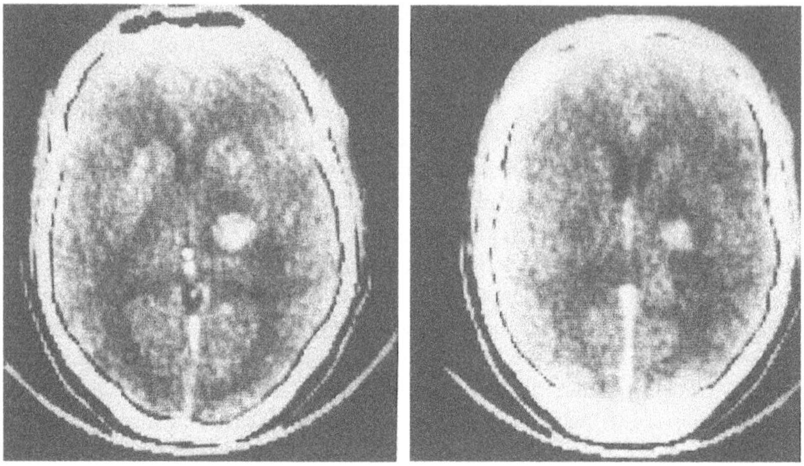

Fig. 2. Right thalamic mass in the CT-scan. Stereotactic biopsy revealed a highly undifferentiated glioma (grade IV WHO)

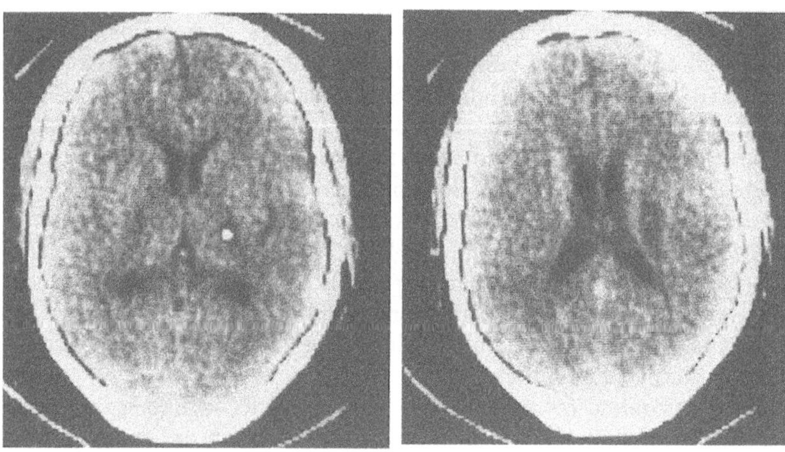

Fig. 3. Six months later after irradiation and chemotherapy the contrast enhanced CT shows only the clip of the biopsy and a small hypodense periventricular area, which resolved completely after further chemotherapy

1983). Therefore, whenever feasible, the CSF should be examined and if malignant cells or clinical signs of spreading are present intrathecal treatment with Cytosine-Arabinoside, Methotrexate or craniospinal irradiation should be performed. We now use diagnostic lumbar punctures in all cases to give a prophylactic injection.

Two short case-records may illustrate the use of chemotherapy in these patients:

In November 1981 stereotactic biopsy of a mass in the right basal ganglia was done and a highly undifferentiated glioma grade IV with giant cells was found (Fig. 2). After irradiation and BCNU chemotherapy the 30-year-old teacher recovered soon and exercised his profession during chemotherapy which was stopped af-

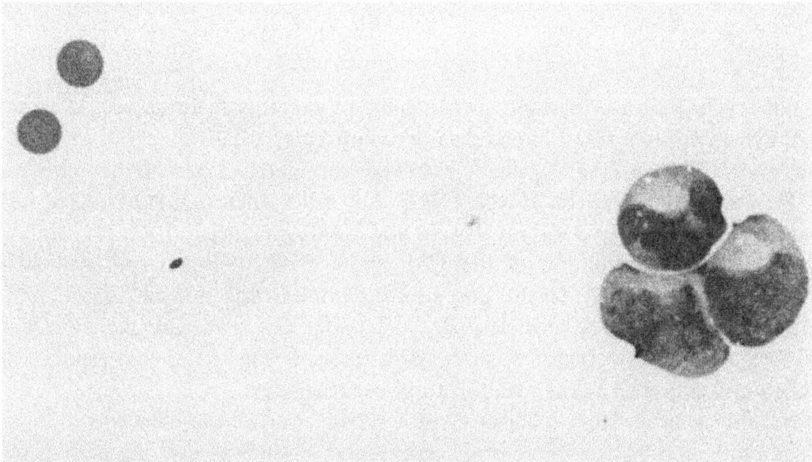

Fig. 4. Malignant astrocytes in the CSF of the patient with the right thalamic mass two and a half years later. At left hand side two erythrocytes

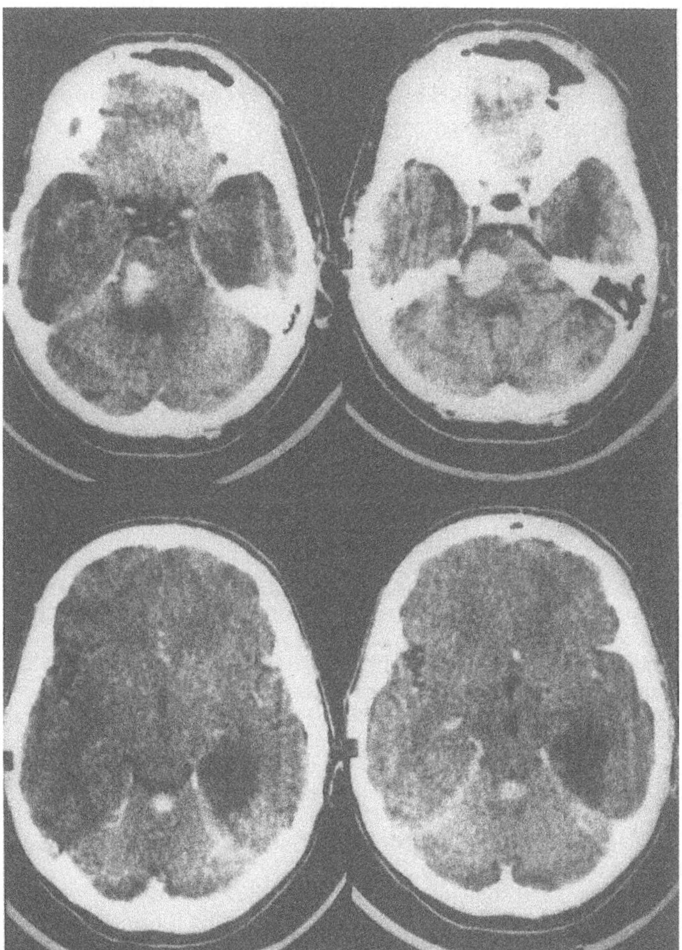

Fig. 5. CT-scan of multiple brain stem metastases of a breast carcinoma before therapy. The metastases showed good, but partial response to irradiation and disappeared completely in the CT only after chemotherapy

ter the sixth cycle because of slight impairment of pulmonary function. After six months of therapy only a small hypodense periventricular area was seen in the contrast enhanced CT-scan (Fig. 3) which resolved completely after further chemotherapy. He was fully active for 2½ years until July 1984 when one generalized seizure led to a deep coma for 3 days. CT-scan and NMR-imaging did not reveal new tumor growth, but examination of the CSF showed slight pleocytosis and 30% malignant astrocytes (Fig. 4). In the past months lumbar injections of Ara-C normalized the cell count but nevertheless 20–30% malignant astrocytes were present and therefore a ventricle catheter was placed to intensify the intrathecal treatment, which eventually achieved again a stabilization of the disease.

Figure 5 shows brain stem metastases of a breast carcinoma.There was a good, but not complete response to whole brain irradiation of 40 Gray and the patient recovered but remained incapable of walking. After chemotherapy according to the FAC-schedule the brain metastases were no longer detectable in the CT-scan and after 3 months the patient was able to walk short distances by herself. She has remained stable for the follow-up period of two years.

Thus, in conclusion we may state: Chemotherapy is effective in malignant brain tumors, but we urgently need better agents and more detailed knowledge in which patients and when in the course of the disease we should apply it.

Acknowledgement: I thank Prof. Dr. Nadjmi, head of the Neuroradiological Department of our university, for the permission to reproduce the CT-scans of these patients.

References

Blasberg R, Groothuis D, Molnar P (1981) Application of quantitative autoradiographic measurements in experimental brain tumor models. Semin Neurol 1:203

EORTC Brain Tumor Group (1978) Effect of CCNU on survival rate, on objective remission and duration of free interval in patients with malignant brain glioma: final evaluation. Eur J Cancer 14:851–856

Fulton DS, Levin VA, Wara WM, Edwards MS, Wilson CB (1981) Chemotherapy of pediatric brain-stem tumors. J Neurosurg 54:721–725

Green SB, Byar DP, Walker MD, Pistenmaa DA, Alexander E Jr, Batzdorf U, Brooks WH, Hunt WE, Mealey J Jr, Odom GL, Paoletti P, Ransohoff J II, Robertson JT, Selker RG, Shapiro WR, Smith KR Jr, Wilson CB, Strike TA (1983) Comparisons of carmustine, procarbazine, and high-dose methylprednisolone as additions to surgery and radiotherapy for the treatment of malignant glioma. Cancer Treat Rep 67:123–132

Green SB, Byar DP, Strike TA, Alexander E Jr, Brooks WH, Burger PC, Hunt WE, Mealey J, Odom GL, Paoletti P, Pistenmaa DA, Ransohoff J, Robertson JT, Selker RG, Shapiro WR, Smith KR (1984) Randomized comparisons of BCNU, streptozotocin, radiosensitizer, and fractionation of radiotherapy in the post-operative treatment of malignant glioma (study 7702). ASCO Proc, vol 3, p 260

Greig NH, Jones HB, Cavanagh JB (1983) Blood-brain barrier integrity and host responses in experimental metastatic brain tumors. Clin Exp Metastasis 1:229

Hara M, Takeuchi K (1977) A temporal study of survival of patients with pontine gliomas. J Neurol 216:189–196

Hasegawa H, Ushio Y, Hayakawa T, Yamada K, Mogami H (1983) Changes in the blood-brain barrier transport in experimental metastatic brain tumors. J Neurosurg 59:304

Hatlevoll R, Lindegaard KF, Hagen S, Nesbakken R et al. (1985) Combined modality treatment of operated astrocytomas grade III and IV. – A prospective and randomized study of

Misonidazole and radiotherapy with two different radiation schedules and subsequent CCNU-chemotherapy (multicenter trial of the Scandinavian Glioblastoma Study Group). In: Voth D, Krauseneck P (eds) Chemotherapy of gliomas. de Gruyter, Berlin New York

Hildebrand J (1985) Chemotherapy of malignant supratentorial gliomas in adults: A ten-year experience of the EORTC brain tumor group. In: Voth D, Krauseneck P (eds) Chemotherapy of gliomas. de Gruyter, Berlin New York, p 317–320

Jellinger K, Volc D, Grisold W, Flament H, Vollmer R, Weiss R (1983) Kombinationsbehandlung maligner Gliome. Wiener Klin Wochenschr 95:407–416

Jellinger K, Volc D, Grisold W, Weiss R, Flament H, Wöber G, Alth G (1985). Combined radiation and polychemotherapy (COMP) in the postoperative treatment of high-grade supratentorial gliomas. In: Voth D, Krauseneck P (eds) Chemotherapy of gliomas. de Gruyter, Berlin New York, p 341–452

Kandt RS, Shinnar S, D'Souza BJ, Singer HS, Wharam MD, Gupta PK (1984) Cerebrospinal metastases in malignant childhood astrocytomas. J Neuro-Oncol 2: 123–128

Krauseneck P, Dommasch D, Lipp F (1977) Cytostatische Beeinflussungsmöglichkeiten von Hirnmetastasen. Verh Dtsch Ges Inn Med 83: 1231–1234

Krauseneck P, Schmidt W, Lorenz R (1981) Treatment of inoperable supratentorial gliomas with radiation, BCNU, and Bleomycin. A multicenter trial. Abstracts 12th World Congress of Neurology, Kyoto, Exc Med Amsterdam, p 301

Krauseneck P, Dommasch D, Ratzka M (1983) CMP-Therapie bei Hirnmetastasen. In: Krauseneck P, Mertens HG (eds) Therapie maligner Neoplasien des Gehirns. Perimed, Erlangen

Krauseneck P, Mertens HG, Richter E, Schmidt M, Halves E, Bogdahn U, Kappos L, Seybold D (1984) Combined chemotherapy of inoperable and operable malignant gliomas. In: Voth D, Krauseneck P (eds) Chemotherapy of gliomas. de Gruyter, Berlin New York, S 353–359

Kreuser ED, Schreml W, Potthoff PC, Keim HM, Neiß A, Schuster Ch (1984) Therapieergebnisse kombinierter und nichtkombinierter Modalitäten bei Hirnmetastasen solider Tumoren. In: von Heyden HW, Krauseneck P (eds) Hirnmetastasen. Zuckschwerdt, München Bern Wien

Levin VA, Freemann-Dove M, Landahl HD (1975) Permeability characteristics of brain adjacent to tumor in rats. Arch Neurol 32:785–791

Levin VA, Edwards MS, Wara WM, Allen J, Ortega J, Vestnys P (1984) 5-Fluorouracil and 1-(2-chloroethyl)-3-cyclohexyl-1-nitrosourea (CCNU) followed by hydroxyurea, misonidazole, and irradiation for brain stem gliomas: a pilot study of the brain tumor research center and the childrens cancer group. Neurosurgery 14:679–681

Mantravadi RVP, Phatak R, Bellur S, Liebner EJ, Haas R (1982) Brain stem gliomas: an autopsy study of 25 cases. Cancer 49: 1294–1296

Mende S, Bleichner F, Stoeter P, Meuret G (1983) Erfolgreiche Behandlung von Hirnmetastasen bei Mammakarzinom mit nicht liquorgängigen Zytostatika und Hormonen. Onkologie 6:58–61

Neuwelt EA, Bigner D, Frenkel EP, Barnett P, Pagel M (1982) The effect of osmotic modification of the blood-brain barrier and adrenal steroid administration on methotrexate delivery to gliomas in rats: The blood-brain barrier is a factor. Proc Natl Acad Sci 79:4420

Packer RJ, Allen J, Nielsen S, Petito C, Deck M, Jereb B (1983) Brain stem glioma: clinical manifestations of meningeal gliomatosis. Ann Neurol 14: 177–182

Reigel DH, Scarff TB, Woodford JE (1979) Biopsy of pediatric brain stem tumors. Child's Brain 5:329–340

Rosner D, Nemoto T, Pickren J, Lane W (1983) Management of brain metastases from breast cancer by combination chemotherapy. J Neuro-Oncol 1: 131–137

Walker MD, Alexander E Jr, Hunt WE, MacCarthy CS, Mahaley MS Jr, Mealey J Jr, Norrell HA, Owens G, Ransohoff J, Wilson CB, Gehan EA, Strike TA (1978) Evaluation of BCNU and/or radiotherapy in the treatment of anaplastic gliomas. Neurosurgery 49:333–343

Walker MD, Green SB, Byar DP, Alexander E Jr, Batzdorf U, Brook WH, Hunt WE, MacCarty CS, Mahaley MS Jr, Mealey J Jr, Owens G, Ransohoff J II, Robertson JT, Shapiro WR, Smith KR Jr, Wilson CB, Strike TA (1980) Randomized comparisons of radiotherapy and nitrosoureas for the treatment of malignant glioma after surgery. N Engl J Med 303: 1323–1329

Chemotherapy of Malignant Brain Stem Tumors in Adults – New Substances, Prospect

G. Haferkamp, Hannover/FRG

The application of the most effective, introduced substances BCNU and CCNU in the chemotherapy of brain tumors is limited by their protracted and cumulative toxicity. Meanwhile, some new CNU derivatives have been developed which, contrary to the first generation, are not only water-soluble, but are also soluble in greasy solutions, and show lesser side effects on the bone marrow whilst having the same cytostatic effect. Up to now, the first clinical results in brain tumors have mainly been with ACNU. Depending on the dosage and interval the patients have to expect leuco- and thrombopenia, nausea appears in a much lesser degree (Saito et al. 1978). So far results of phase I and II studies have not shown any better effects compared to BCNU and CCNU but the side effects were small by a large degree (Shibata 1982; Yumitori et al. 1984). In two trials ACNU was given intra-arterially with the idea of reducing the systemic toxicity while increasing the concentration of ACNU in the tumor itself at the same time (Jaschke 1985; Yamashita et al. 1983). HeCNU is an additional CNU derivative of the third generation. Experimental studies show so far in doses with the same toxicity more antineoplastic effectivity than BCNU. After repeated applications the longterm toxicity and carcinogenity is considerably smaller than with BCNU. A comparison of HeCNU using 100–120 mg/m^2 with ACNU shows significantly smaller nausea and bone marrow toxicity for HeCNU (Eisenbrand 1984). The first clinical phase I-studies confirm the favorable preclinical results, although there have been no clinical studies on brain tumors so far.

AZQ

Azirindinylbenzoquinone (AZQ) represents a group of substances with an interesting potential in the treatment of primary malignancies of the CNS. Their mechanism of antineoplastic action until now remains not completely clear. An interference with DNA metabolism has been discussed, maybe it crosslinks the DNA. Modest toxicity is one of the most attractive features of AZQ: hematologic toxicity is delayed and cumulative (Feun et al. 1984c), but mostly predictable and manageable (Schold jr et al. 1984). It seems encouraging, that patients, failing to respond to nitrosurea, may respond to AZQ, indicating a lack of cross resistance. Further clinical trials with AZQ using different schedules, routes and combinations, seem to be necessary.

Cisplatinum

After the discovery of the growth-limiting effect of platinum-complexes on bacterial cell cultures by Rosenberg 1970 Cisplatinum was introduced to the treatment of malignant neoplasms also of the brain. Further experience with the substance resulted firstly in a direct tumor effect but secondly it was discovered that Cisplatinum also works as a radiosensitizer (Overgaard and Khan 1981). The following mechanisms of X-ray sensibilization are discussed: 1. Sensibilization of hypoxic cells by a factor of 1.7 when given at least 30 minutes before irradiation without important sensibilization of normal tissue except tissue with high rates of proliferation, e.g. intestine. 2. Reaction of Cisplatinum with DNA by which the DNA becomes more sensitive to X-rays and 3. inhibition of repair mechanisms after X-ray induced sublethal or potential lethal DNA damages. The pharmacology of Cisplatinum in the CNS is unknown up to now. The crossing of the blood brain barrier is very limited (Achterrath et al. 1984; Ginsberg et al. 1981; Stewart et al. 1983). Nevertheless, there are high concentrations of Cisplatinum within cerebral tumors and the surrounding brain tissue (Bonnem et al. 1982), also in some cases even after months of the last application (Stewart et al. 1982). The lowest tissue concentration which is necessary for radiosensibilization is 1 μg/ml. Within the intracerebral tumor such levels can be achieved with doses of 20–25 mg/m^2 (Stewart et al. 1982). With the today recommended dosage of 40–60 mg/m^2 every 4 weeks respectively on days 1 and 28 of radiotherapy it seems that the direct antitumor-effect and the radiosensitizing effect of Cisplatinum works together. A problem is the toxicity of the substance especially on kidney and ear functions, which is possibly cumulative. Heavy nausea and vomiting are dose-dependent, also polyneuropathies and myelotoxicity. By intricated hydration-programmes the number of kidney function disturbances was clearly reduced. Nausea and vomiting of 40% of the patients was avoided by combined application of dexamethasone and antiemetics (Aapro and Alberts 1981; Plezia et al. 1983). Especially the nephrotoxicity of Cisplatinum was the reason for the intra-arterial application, because higher local tumor concentrations of Cisplatinum was shown at the same time with lower kidney stress compared to the i.v. application (Stewart et al. 1983). Nevertheless, there is the danger of retinal damage if the catheter is located proximal to the ophthalmic artery origin (Feun et al. 1984b), also, but in a lesser degree, if Cisplatinum is filtered (Lehane et al. 1983). Additionally, lethal incidents by administration of the drug in the vertebral artery were reported (Feun et al. 1984b). Other authors did not see any advantage in the i.a. injection due to the relatively low plasma clearance of Cisplatinum (Campbell et al. 1983). An increased effect using a combination of local hyperthermia with Cisplatinum and radiotherapy has been discussed (Douple and Richmond 1980). Forms of application, dosage and partly amazing results of phase I and II studies with Cisplatinum alone and in combinations in glioblastoma multiforme, astrocytoma grade II and III and ependymomas are presented in Table 1 (Khan et al. 1982; Lehane et al. 1983; Feun et al. 1984a). At this time new derivatives of Cisplatinum with similar antineoplastic activity and lower nephrotoxicity like carboplatin and iproplatin among others are being studied (Achterrath et al. 1984).

Table 1. Cisplatinum in recurrent brain tumor

Tumor type	No. of evol. pts.	CR	PR	SD	PD	Dosage	Author
Glioblastoma	4	–	2	2	2	60 mg/m²/d× 2 i.v./3–4 wks	Khan et al. 1982
	7	–	7	–	–	100 mg/m² i.a./4 wks	Lehane et al. 1983
	15	–	5	4	6	60–120 mg/m² i.v./4 wks	Feun et al. 1984
	8	–	3	1	4	40– 75 mg/m² i.a.+ BCNU/4 wks	Feun et al. 1984
Glioma	2	–	–	1	1	See above	Khan et al. 1982
Grad III	3	–	1	–	2	See above	Feun et al. 1984
Ependymoma	6	2	1	1	2	See above	Khan et al. 1982

CR=complete remission; *PR*=partial remission; *SD*=stable disease; *PD*=progressing disease

Table 2. β-Interferon studies in recurrent brain tumor

Tumor type	No. of evol. pts.	CR	PR	SD	PD	Author	
Glioblastoma	5	1	2	–	2	i.v.	Nagai et al. 1980
	3	–	1	–	2	i.v.	Nakamura et al. 1982
Astrocytoma	26	1	3	13	9	Local	Koyama 1984
	20	–	3	10	7	i.v.	Koyama 1984
Medulloblastoma	3	–	1	2	–	Local	Koyama 1984
	4	2	–	1	1	i.v.	Koyama 1984
	2	2	–	–	–	i.v.	Nagai et al. 1980

CR=complete remission; *PR*=partial remission; *SD*=stable disease; *PD*=progressing disease

Interferon

Human Interferon β (β-IFN) from fibroblasts are shown to be at least partly effective against primary malignant brain tumors. The effects could be explained by a prolongation of the cell-doubling time and also by a distinctive immunostimulation. Up to now it is not known whether Interferon can cross the blood-brain-barrier by i.v. application (Nagai et al. 1980). This can be presumed though, after sole i.v. administration of β-IFN there were pretty good results especially in medulloblastomas. Side-effects were mainly fever and flu-like symptoms like wearyness and limb-pain but also reported are some cases of Interferon encephalopathy with somnolence, confusion, disorientation and gait-abnormalities, appearing 4–14 days after initiation of therapy, slowly resolving after cessation of treatment (Suter et al. 1984). Hematologic toxicity and temporary rise of serum transaminases are more rarely found (Koyama 1984; Nakamura et al. 1982). Table 2 shows the results of the studies known so far (Nagai et al. 1980; Nakamura et al. 1982; Koyama 1984).

Prospect

The present combination of radiotherapy and chemotherapy in primary malignant gliomas of the CNS is better than radiotherapy alone but not at all satisfying. Some new chemotherapeutics were introduced, but also the known data from these substances promise no decisive breakthrough. A main cause for the insufficient effectivity of todays chemotherapy should be found in the fact that human gliomas are very heterogeneous, genotypically and phenotypically as well as in their chemosensitivity (Yung et al. 1982). New aspects for the future also for the neurooncology offers the immunology especially by the possibility to produce different human monoclonal antibodies against gliomas (Phillips et al. 1983; de Tribolet et al. 1984b) and to identify subpopulations in gliomas (de Tribolet et al. 1984c). Furthermore, they could be used as a carrier of toxic agents to the tumor cells (Yashuda et al. 1983). This new technique could also make possible the selection of chemotherapeutics by in vitro-incubation of defined tumor cells with cytostatics (Schlag and Flentje 1984). So far the success of this technique is somewhat limited. Another approach of therapy could result from the observation of cells of glioblastomas setting immun-suppressive factors free (Fontana et al. 1984), the outcome of which is also the proposition to attempt whether these restraining factors could be taken out of the plasma by repeated plasmapheresis (de Tribolet et al. 1984a).

The described techniques allow new successful therapeutical means in the future even if many questions are left to be answered until clinical introduction.

References

Aapro MS, Alberts DS (1981) High-dose dexamethasone for prevention of cis-platin-induced vomiting. Cancer Chemother Pharmacol 7:11–14

Achterrath W, Raettig R, Franks CR, Seeber S (1984) Aktuelle Cisplatin-Derivate. In: Eckhardt S, Holzner JH, Nagel GA (eds) Beitr Onkol, vol 18, Karger, Basel, S 55–82

Bonnem EM, Litterst CL, Smith FP (1982) Platinum concentrations in human glioblastoma multiforme following the use of cisplatin. Cancer Treat Rep 66:1661–1663

Campbell TN, Howell NSB, Pfeifle CE, Wung WE, Bookstein J (1983) Clinical pharmacokinetics of intraarterial cisplatin in humans. J Clin Oncol 1:755–762

Douple EB, Richmond RC (1980) A review of interactions between platinum coordination complexes and ionizing radiation: implications for cancer therapy. In: Prestayko AW, Crooke ST, Carter SK (eds) Cisplatin current status and new developments. Academic Press, New York, p 125–147

Eisenbrand G (1984) Neue Entwicklungen auf dem Gebiet der Nitrosoharnstoffe. In: Eckhardt S, Holzner JH, Nagel GA (eds) Beitr Onkol, vol 18. Karger, Basel, S 18–35

Feun LG, Wallace S, Yung WA, Lee YY, Leavends ME, Moser R, Savaraj N, Burgess MA, Plager C, Benjamin RS, Tang RA, Mavligit GM, Fields WS (1984a) Phase-I trial of intracarotid BCNU and cisplatin in patients with malignant intracerebral tumors. Cancer Drug Delivery 1:239–245

Feun LG, Wallace S, Stewart DJ, Chuang VP, Yung WA, Leavens ME, Burgess MA, Savaraj N, Benjamin RS, Young SE, Tang RA, Handel S, Mavligit G, Fields WS (1984b) Intracarotid infusion of cis-diamminedichloroplatinum in the treatment of recurrent malignant brain tumors. Cancer 54:794–799

Feun LG, Yung WA, Leavens ME, Burgess MA, Obbens EA, Bedikian AY, Savaraj N, Stewart DJ, Benjamin RS, Fields WS (1984c) A phase II trial of 2,5-diaziridinyl 3,6-bis (carboethoxyamino) 1,4-benzoquinone (AZQ, NSC 182986) in recurrent primary brain tumors. J Neuro Oncol 2:13–17

Fontana A, Hengartner H, de Tribolet N, Weber E (1984) Glioblastoma cells release interleukin 1 and factors inhibiting interleukin 2-mediated effects (1984) J Immunol 132:1837–1844

Ginsberg S, Kirshner J, Reich S, Panasci L, Finkelstein T, Fandrich S, Fitzpatrick A, Shechtman L, Comis R (1981) Systemic chemotherapy for a primary germ cell tumor of the brain: a pharmacokinetic study. Cancer Treat Rep 65:477–483

Jaschke H (1985) Intra-arterial therapy of malignant gliomas with ACNU and BCNU in combination with phenobarbital protection (preliminary results). In: Voth D, Krauseneck P (eds) Chemotherapy of gliomas. de Gruyter, Berlin New York, p 383–390

Khan AB, D'Souza JD, Wharam MD, Champion LAA, Sinks LF, Woo SY, McCullough DC, Leventhal BG (1982) Cisplatin therapy in recurrent childhood brain tumors. Cancer Treat Rep 66:2013–2020

Koyama Y (1984) Pharmacokinetics and clinical trials of HuIFN-β in malignant tumors. In: Kishida T (ed) Proceedings of the international symposion on interferons. Organizing committee of the international symposion on interferons Kyoto, p 1–7

Lehane DE, Bryan RN, Horowitz B, DeSantos L, Ehni G, Zubler MA, Moiel R, Rudolph L, Aldama-Leubbert A, Mahoney D, Harper R (1983) Intraarterial Cisplatinum chemotherapy for patients with primary and metastatic brain tumors. Cancer Drug Delivery 1:69–77

Nagai M, Arai T, Kohno S, Kohase M (1980) Interferon therapy for malignant brain tumors. In: Kono R, Vilcek J (eds) The clinical potential of interferons. University of Tokyo Press, p 257–273

Nakamura O, Takakura K, Kobayashi S (1982) Effect of human interferon-β in the treatment of malignant brain tumors. In: Merigan TC, Friedman RM (eds) Interferons. Academic Press New York London, p 465–477

Overgaard J, Khan AR (1981) Selective enhancement of radiation response in a C3H mammary carcinoma by cisplatin. Cancer Treat Rep 65:501–503

Phillips J, Alderson T, Sikora K, Watson J (1983) Localisation of malignant glioma by a radiolabelled human monoclonal antibody. J Neurol Neurosurg Psychiatry 46:388–392

Plezia PM, Aapro MS, Alberts DS, Jones SE, Surwit EA (1983) Double-blind crossover study of the anti-emetic efficacy of high-dose dexamethasone vs high-dose metoclopramide. Clin Pharmacol Ther 33:223–226

Saito Y, Nakaya Y, Muraoka K, Fujiwara T (1978) ACNU, a new nitrosurea in the treatment of malignant brain tumors. Gan To Kagaku Ryoho 5:779–794

Schlag P, Flentje D (1984) Möglichkeiten und Grenzen der Zytostatika-Sensitivitätstestung menschlicher Tumoren mit dem Kolonie-Assai. In: Eckhardt S, Holzner JH, Nagel GA (eds) Beitr Onkol, vol 18. Karger, Basel, S 334–344

Schold SC jr, Friedman HS, Bjornsson TD, Faletta JM (1984) Treatment of patients with recurrent primary brain tumors with AZQ. Neurology (Cleveland) 34:615–619

Shibata S (1982) Postoperative radiotherapy, synchronised radiochemotherapy and radiochemoimmunotherapy in glioma patients, with particular reference to ACNU. Prog Med 2:1237–1246

Stewart DJ, Leavens M, Maor M, Feun L, Luna M, Bonura J, Caprioli R, Loo TL, Benjamin RS (1982) Human central nervous system distribution of cis-diammine-dichloroplatinum and use as a radiosensitizer in malignant brain tumors. Cancer Res 42:2474–2479

Stewart DJ, Benjamin RS, Zimmermann S, Caprioli RM, Wallace S, Chuang V, Calvo III D, Samuels M, Bonura J, Loo TL (1983) Clinical pharmacology of intraarterial cis-diamminedichloroplatinum (II). Cancer Res 43:917–920

Suter CC, Westmoreland BF, Sharbrough FW, Hermann R jr (1984) Electroencephalographic abnormalities in interferon encephalopathy: a preliminary report. Mayo Clin Proc 59:847–850

de Tribolet N, Hamou MF, Mach JP, Carrel S, Schreyer M (1984a) Demonstration of HLA-DR antigens in normal human brain. J Neurol Neurosurg Psychiatry 47:417–418

de Tribolet N, Carrel S, Mach JP (1984b) Brain tumor associated antigens. In: Homburger F (ed) Progr. in experimental tumor research, vol 27. Karger, Basel, p 118–131

de Tribolet N, Piguet V, Diserens AC, Mach JP, Carrel S (1984c) Monoclonal antibodies and gliomas. In: Caciagli F, Giacobini E, Paoletti R (eds) Developmental neuroscience: physiological, pharmacological and clinical aspects. Elsevier Amsterdam, p 273–279

Yamashita J, Handa H, Tokuriki A, Ha YS, Otsuka S-I, Suda K, Taki W (1983) Intra-arterial ACNU therapy for malignant brain tumors. J Neurosurg 59:424–430
Yashuda K, Alderson T, Phillips J, Sikora K (1983) Detection of lymphocytes in malignant gliomas by monoclonal antibodies. J Neurol Neurosurg Psychiatry 46:734–737
Yumitori K, Handa H, Teraura T, Yamashita J (1984) Treatment of malignant brain tumors with ACNU and phenobarbital: Continuous infusion of ACNU into internal carotid artery and systemic administration of phenobarbital. Acta Neurochir (Wien) 70:155–168
Yung WA, Shapiro JR, Shapiro WR (1982) Heterogeneous chemosensitivities of subpopulations of human glioma cells in cultures. Cancer Res 42:992–998

Subject Index

www.ingramcontent.com/pod-product-compliance
Ingram Content Group UK Ltd.
Pitfield, Milton Keynes, MK11 3LW, UK
UKHW051054011026
476163UK00003B/123
* 9 7 8 3 6 4 2 7 1 2 4 2 5 *